MW01056825

PLURAL+PLUS

COMPANION WEBSITE

Foundations of Speech and Hearing: Anatomy and Physiology, Second Edition comes with access to supplementary student and instructor materials on a PluralPlus companion website.

The companion website is located at:
http://www.pluralpublishing.com/publication/fshap2e

STUDENTS:

To access the **student** materials, you must register on the companion website and log in using the access code below.*

Access Code: FSHAP2E-WE9TEP

INSTRUCTORS:

To access the **instructor** materials, you must contact Plural Publishing, Inc. to be verified as an instructor and receive your access code.

Email: information@pluralpublishing.com
Tel: 866-758-7251 (toll free) or 858-492-1555

 Look for this icon throughout the text, directing you to related material available on the companion website.

Note for students: If you have purchased this textbook used or have rented it, your access code will not work if it was already redeemed by the original buyer of the book. Plural Publishing does not offer replacement access codes for used or rented textbooks.

FOUNDATIONS OF SPEECH AND HEARING

Anatomy and Physiology

SECOND EDITION

FOUNDATIONS OF SPEECH AND HEARING

Anatomy and Physiology

SECOND EDITION

Jeannette D. Hoit
Gary Weismer
Brad Story

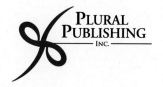

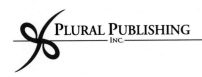

5521 Ruffin Road
San Diego, CA 92123

e-mail: information@pluralpublishing.com
Website: https://www.pluralpublishing.com

Copyright © 2022 by Plural Publishing, Inc.

Typeset in 10/12 Palatino by Flanagan's Publishing Services, Inc.
Printed in China by Regent Publishing Services, Ltd.

All rights, including that of translation, reserved. No part of this publication may be reproduced, stored in a retrieval system, or transmitted in any form or by any means, electronic, mechanical, recording, or otherwise, including photocopying, recording, taping, Web distribution, or information storage and retrieval systems without the prior written consent of the publisher.

For permission to use material from this text, contact us by
Telephone: (866) 758-7251
Fax: (888) 758-7255
e-mail: permissions@pluralpublishing.com

Every attempt has been made to contact the copyright holders for material originally printed in another source. If any have been inadvertently overlooked, the publisher will gladly make the necessary arrangements at the first opportunity.

Library of Congress Cataloging-in-Publication Data

Names: Hoit, Jeannette D. (Jeannette Dee), 1954- author. | Weismer, Gary,
  author. | Story, Brad, author.
Title: Foundations of speech and hearing : anatomy and physiology /
  Jeanette D. Hoit, Gary Weismer, Brad Story.
Description: Second edition. | San Diego : Plural Publishing, Inc., [2022]
  | Includes bibliographical references and index.
Identifiers: LCCN 2020047813 | ISBN 9781635503067 (hardcover) | ISBN
  163550306X (hardcover) | ISBN 9781635503074 (ebook)
Subjects: MESH: Speech—physiology | Speech Perception | Speech Disorders |
  Respiratory System—anatomy & histology
Classification: LCC QP306 | NLM WV 501 | DDC 612.7/8—dc23
LC record available at https://lccn.loc.gov/2020047813

Contents

Preface

The second edition of *Foundations of Speech and Hearing: Anatomy and Physiology* was written for students who are being introduced to the discipline of speech and hearing sciences. This edition includes some reorganization of material, line-by-line revisions of text, and conceptual additions and reductions from the first edition, all done in the service of greater clarity. Many new and revised figures have been included, most created by master illustrator Maury Aaseng. An important addition to this second edition of *Foundations* is a set of highly instructive videos that complement concepts presented in the text and bring these concepts to life. As in the first edition of *Foundations*, only those topics that are ultimately important to understanding, evaluating, and managing clients with speech, hearing, and swallowing disorders are included in this book. In short, it has been written with clinical endpoints and future speech-language pathologists and audiologists in mind.

Although the current text lists three authors, a significant portion of the material was originally conceptualized and written by Tom Hixon (1940–2009) in the writing of our original edition of *Preclinical Speech Science*. Tom's extraordinary vision and effort over a decade ago created the foundation upon which *Foundations* is built.

Sidetracks

Throughout the book you'll find a series of sidetracks. These are short asides that relate to topics being discussed in the main text. Many of the sidetracks in the book are a bit less formal and a bit more lighthearted than the main text they complement. This is intended to enhance your reading enjoyment and to put some fun in your study of the material. We hope you enjoy reading these sidetracks as much as we enjoyed writing them.

Acknowledgments

Many of the people we acknowledge for contributions to this text are the same people we thanked for the first three editions of *Preclinical Speech Science*. Even if their efforts are historical, their influence is reflected in the current textbook. Special thanks to Tim McCulloch and Michelle Ciucci for providing our readers with videos on swallowing, Robin Samlan for laryngeal images, and Adam Baker and Shrikanth Narayanan for magnetic resonance images.

About the Illustrator

Maury Aaseng began illustrating as a freelancer for young-adult nonfiction publications in San Diego, California. While there, his work expanded into the realm of medical and anatomical art. He collaborated with authors and experts to create digitally rendered illustrations for publications that illuminate concepts in the health sciences, the body, and nature. Beyond medical illustration, his range includes cartooning, watercolor, logos, line art, ink, and digital art. Clients include various publishing companies, podcasts, botanical gardens, lawyers, public works utilities, an opera company, and a creative studio in Melbourne, Australia.

His work first won recognition in the juried exhibition Upstream People Gallery in 2008. In 2016, a collection of his watercolor work was displayed at the Great Lakes Aquarium gallery. He has taught classes covering scientific illustration and nature-inspired watercolor and recently has "drawn on" his experience to create books that demonstrate techniques to other budding artists.

Maury resides with his wife, Charlene, a graphic designer, and their two children in Duluth, Minnesota, near the shores of Lake Superior. They enjoy spending time outdoors as much as possible in the surrounding woods and lakes.

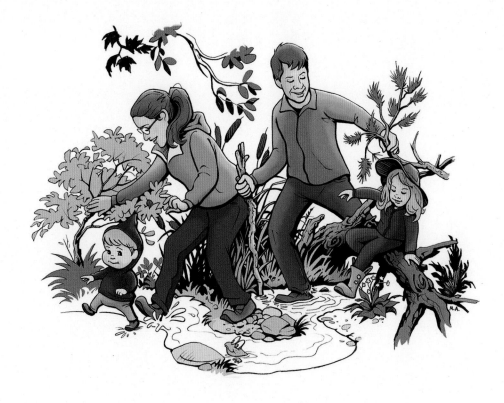

Introduction to Basic Concepts

INTRODUCTION

This book is about the **anatomy** (the study of the structure of organisms and the relations of their parts) and **physiology** (the study of functions of living organisms or their parts) of the speech and hearing mechanisms. In this first chapter, we provide an overview of certain overarching and basic concepts that will make the reading of later chapters much easier. It begins with a general anatomical description of the speech and hearing *subsystems*, anatomic *directions and planes*, and *tissue types*. The next section focuses on *movements and forces*, phenomena that are critical to understanding speech production and certain aspects of hearing. The chapter concludes with a simple description of the *stages of spoken communication*, a general framework meant to guide the reader through the material in the remaining chapters.

SUBSYSTEMS

The human body operates as an elegant, integrated system. Although it cannot actually be divided into parts without sacrificing its functional integrity, it is convenient to discuss separate parts of the system as a way to make the information easier to understand and remember. In this book, we divide the material into *speech* and *hearing* mechanisms, and each of these can be divided into *subsystems*.

Speech Subsystems

Most textbooks divide the speech mechanism into three or four subsystems. The first two, respiratory and laryngeal, are also used in this book. Where this book diverges from the others is in the treatment of the region above the larynx. Some textbooks present this region as a single subdivision of the speech mechanism, often called the *articulatory subsystem* and encompassing the pharyngeal, oral, and nasal cavities and associated structures. Other textbooks present this region as two subdivisions, using terms such as *articulatory* (in this context meaning the oral region) and *resonatory* (usually meaning the velopharyngeal region and sometimes including the nasal region). The term *articulatory* is problematic when used in this context because it is not the only speech subsystem that contains an articulator (defined as a movable structure that contributes to the production of speech sounds); the larynx also acts as an articulator (see Chapters 3 and 5), as does the velopharynx (see Chapter 4). Similarly, the term *resonatory* is problematic because the resonators (defined as parts of an acoustic system that emphasize certain sound frequencies and reject others) are not found exclusively in the velopharyngeal and nasal regions; the lower pharynx and the oral cavities also serve as acoustic resonators. Also, it is important to acknowledge that these anatomical regions are not used exclusively for articulating or resonating but also serve other functions, such as swallowing. For all these reasons, we have adopted an anatomical approach to naming the speech subsystems.

In this book, we divide the speech system into four subsystems, as depicted in Figure 1–1: *respiratory, laryngeal, velopharyngeal-nasal,* and *pharyngeal-oral.*

The respiratory subsystem consists of the pulmonary apparatus (lungs and lower airways) and the chest wall that surrounds it (rib cage, diaphragm, abdomen and its contents). The laryngeal subsystem includes a set of structures that are located at the exit of the respiratory subsystem. The *velopharyngeal-nasal* subsystem includes both the velopharynx and the nasal airways and associated structures. The nasal portion is included because it is critical to understanding the aeromechanic and acoustic functions of this part of the speech system. The *pharyngeal-oral* subsystem includes the middle and lower pharynx and the oral cavity and associated structures. Inclusion of the pharyngeal part of the apparatus reflects the fact that during speech production, this part of the pharynx acts as an articulator and resonator

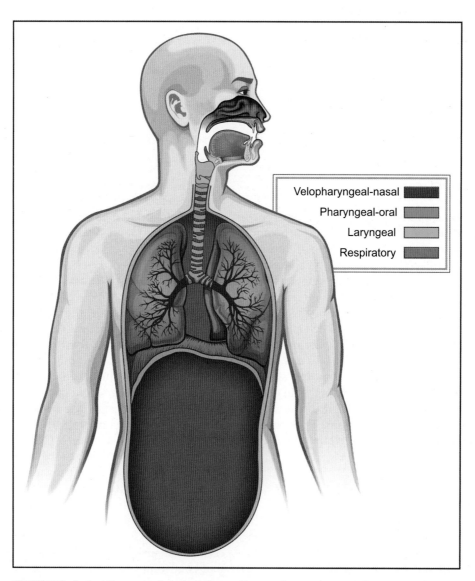

| Velopharyngeal-nasal |
| Pharyngeal-oral |
| Laryngeal |
| Respiratory |

FIGURE 1–1. The speech subsystems. Four subsystems are shown: respiratory (*orange*), laryngeal (*green*), velopharyngeal-nasal (*purple*), and pharyngeal-oral (*blue*).

along with its oral counterparts. It is also critical for swallowing.

The pharyngeal-oral and velopharyngeal-nasal subsystems form what is called the upper airway. In this book, the term *upper airway* is used in the context of the anatomy and physiology of this region to be consistent with terms such as *lower airways*, *laryngeal airway*, *velopharyngeal-nasal airway*, and *oral airway*. The term *vocal tract* also refers to the pharyngeal-oral regions but is used primarily when referring to their acoustic (sound) properties. Similarly, the term *nasal tract* is often used when discussing the acoustic properties of the nasal air spaces.

Hearing Subsystems

The hearing mechanism, like the speech mechanism, acts as an integrated system but is often divided into parts. The most conventional way to divide the hearing system, and the one that is adopted in this book, is into regions simply called the *outer ear*, *middle ear*, and *inner ear*, shown in Figure 1–2 with color-coding. It is

important to recognize that the inner ear contains both auditory (hearing) structures and vestibular (balance) structures. The major hearing structure of the inner ear is the part that looks like a snail's shell (called the cochlea), and the vestibular portion looks like a trio of loops (called semicircular canals). Figure 1–2 should give the reader an appreciation of the location of the auditory-vestibular system within the head, as well as how small it is relative to most of the other structures discussed in this book. More details are provided in Chapter 6.

DIRECTIONS AND PLANES

A special vocabulary is used when describing locations and orientations of anatomical structures. This vocabulary pertains to *directions* and *planes* and is generally discussed in the context of what is called the *anatomical position* of the body. This position is described as the body standing erect with the arms at the sides and the palms facing forward, as shown in Figure 1–3.

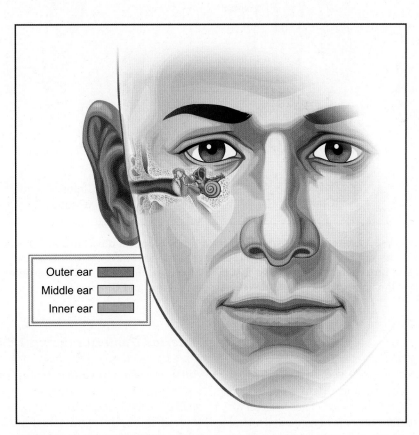

Outer ear
Middle ear
Inner ear

FIGURE 1–2. The hearing subsystems. Three subsystems are shown: outer ear (*brown*), middle ear (*yellow*), and inner ear (*pink*). Note that the inner ear also contains vestibular (balance) structures.

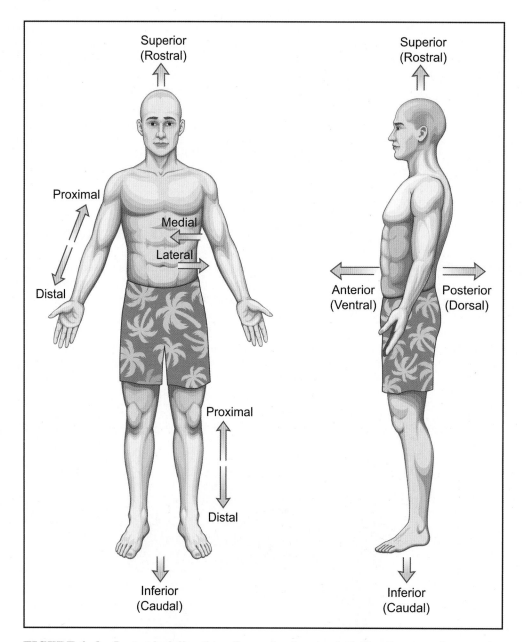

FIGURE 1–3. Anatomical directions. Four sets of anatomical directions are shown: anterior (ventral) and posterior (dorsal), superior (rostral) and inferior (caudal), medial and lateral, and proximal and distal. Note that the definitions of ventral and dorsal differ when applied to the upper part of the brain (see associated text and Chapter 8).

Directions

Several directional terms are used in this book to describe anatomical locations and orientations within the speech and hearing mechanisms. These terms are *anterior/posterior* (*ventral/dorsal*), *superior/inferior* (*rostral/caudal*), *medial/lateral*, *proximal/distal*, *external/internal* (*superficial/deep*), and *ipsilateral/contralateral*. The first three sets of terms are depicted in Figure 1–3.

Anterior/Posterior (Ventral/Dorsal)

Anterior means toward the front of the body and *posterior* means toward the back of the body. Similarly, *ventral* means toward the front of the body (literally, toward the belly), and *dorsal* means toward the back of the body. Thus, in many contexts, *anterior* and *ventral* can be used interchangeably, as can *posterior* and *dorsal*. Nevertheless, it is best to use them in their designated pairs (e.g., *anterior* and *posterior*) rather than mix them (e.g., *anterior* and *dorsal*). An example of how these terms are used is: The umbilicus (belly button) is anterior (ventral) to the spine and the spine is *posterior* (*dorsal*) to the umbilicus.

There is an important exception to how the terms *ventral* and *dorsal* are used. When applied to the upper region of the brain comprising the cerebral hemispheres, *ventral* means toward the bottom and *dorsal* means toward the top of the cerebral hemispheres. This is explained and illustrated more fully in Chapter 8.

Which Way Is Up?

Anatomy is hard enough to learn without having to learn that certain terms means different things in different contexts. It's just not fair. Why doesn't *ventral* just mean "toward the front" and *dorsal* just mean "toward the back"? Period. Why assign these terms different meanings when talking about the lower part of the brain versus the higher part? Believe it or not, it's simpler than you think. What may seem arbitrary at first glance is actually completely logical. Try this exercise: Ask your cat or dog or other four-legged pet to stand quietly while you view it from the side. Now ask yourself these questions: "Which direction is ventral? Which direction is dorsal?" It should be immediately apparent that ventral is toward the lower part of the brain (cerebral hemispheres) and dorsal the opposite. Clear as a bell. The confusion comes when the animal stands on its two back legs. If we humans had only stayed on all fours, learning the anatomical directions would have been so much easier!

Superior/Inferior (Rostral/Caudal)

Superior and *rostral* mean toward the head. Sometimes the term *cranial* is also used to mean toward the head. The terms *inferior* and *caudal* mean toward the tail or, in the case of the human, away from the head. For example, the brain is *superior* (*rostral*) to the spinal cord and the spinal cord is *inferior* (*caudal*) to the brain.

Medial/Lateral

Medial means toward the midline. *Lateral* means away from the midline or toward the side. For example, the nose is *medial* to the ear and the ear is *lateral* to the nose.

Proximal/Distal

Proximal means toward the body and *distal* means away from the body. These terms are usually applied to the limbs (arms and legs). For example, the fingers are *distal* to the wrist and the wrist is *proximal* to the fingers.

External/Internal (Superficial/Deep)

When something is closer to the outer surface of the body than something else, it is said to be *external* (or *superficial*) to it. Conversely, when something is farther away from the outer surface of the body than something else, it is said to be *internal* (or *deep*) to it. These terms are often used interchangeably. An example of their usage is: The skin is *external* (or *superficial*) to the muscle and the muscle is *internal* (or *deep*) to the skin.

Ipsilateral/Contralateral

Ipsilateral means the same side of the body. *Contralateral* means the opposite side of the body. For example, the right ear is *ipsilateral* to the right arm and *contralateral* to the left arm.

Planes

Many structures of the speech and hearing mechanisms (and all structures of the nervous system) are inside the body and can only be viewed when exposed by slicing open the body. An example of this is Figure 1–1, which depicts the cranial portion of the speech mechanism (velopharyngeal-nasal and pharyngeal-oral subsystems) as viewed with that part of the body sliced in half. These slices are called planes of reference, and three are commonly used in anatomy: sagittal, coronal (frontal), and horizontal (transverse or axial). These three planes are illustrated in the upper part of Figure 1–4.

Sagittal Plane

A *sagittal* plane divides the body into right and left parts. When the plane divides the body into halves (equal parts), it is called the *midsagittal* plane. Sagittal cuts away from the midline are called *parasagittal* planes. The lower left image in Figure 1–4 shows a magnetic resonance (MR) image of the head and neck of a young man in the midsagittal plane.

Coronal Plane

A *coronal* plane (also called a *frontal* plane) divides the front and back parts of the body. The *midcoronal* plane

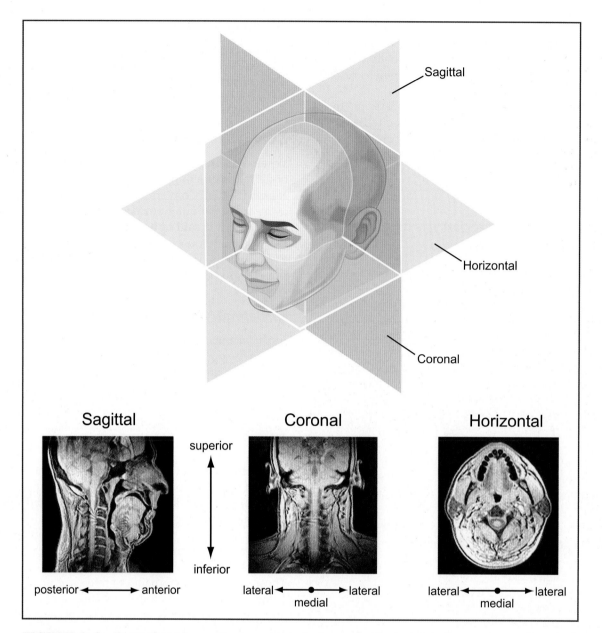

FIGURE 1–4. Anatomical planes. Three anatomical planes are illustrated in the upper panel: sagittal, coronal (also called frontal), and horizontal (also called transverse or axial). The lower panel contains magnetic resonance (MR) images of the head of a young man in the same three planes.

divides the front and back (anterior and posterior) parts of the body equally. The lower middle image in Figure 4–1 is a coronal MR image of the head and neck at the approximate location as the ears as viewed from the back (in a posterior-to-anterior direction).

Horizontal Plane

The *horizontal* plane is also called a *transverse* plane or *axial* plane. This plane divides the upper (superior or cranial) part of the body from the lower (inferior or

caudal) part of the body. Figure 1–4 shows an example of a horizontal MR image of the head located just below the ears.

TISSUE TYPES

The speech and hearing mechanisms are made up of cells. Cells, the basic living constituent of the human body, comprise a nucleus and the material that surrounds the nucleus, called the cytoplasm. The number of cells in the human body continues to be debated, but it is undoubtedly on the order of the tens of trillions. Cells come in many forms and are made up of a multitude of components.

Groups of similar cells that work together to perform a particular function are called *tissues*. There are four types of tissues: *epithelial tissue, connective tissue, muscle tissue,* and *nerve tissue*. The first three of these are discussed below; nerve tissue is discussed in Chapter 8.

Epithelial Tissue

Epithelial tissue consists of layers of cells that cover external and internal surfaces of the body. For example, epithelial tissue makes up the superficial layer of the skin (external) on the face and lines the inside of the oral cavity (internal). Epithelial tissue serves to protect deeper layers of tissue and perform other functions depending on the specific type of epithelial tissue. There are many types of epithelial tissue; only two types will be described and illustrated here.

One type of epithelial tissue is called stratified squamous epithelium, an example of which is shown in Figure 1–5 (left side). This is the type of epithelium that covers the anterior part of the vocal folds (further discussed in Chapter 3). Another type is pseudostratified columnar epithelium, which consists of a single layer of cells, although it can appear as if there are multiple layers (thus, the reason for the prefix *pseudo* before stratified). The example shown in Figure 1–5 (right side) also contains hair-like projections called cilia. This is the type of epithelium that covers the upper respiratory airways; the cilia move mucous away from the respiratory airways toward the pharynx.

Connective Tissue

As with epithelial tissue, there are many types of connective tissue. They can be divided into two general categories: connective tissue proper and supportive connective tissue. Included under connective tissue proper are tendons, aponeuroses, and ligaments; included under supportive connective tissue are cartilage and bone. All of these are shown in Figure 1–6. Note that this figure does not depict an actual anatomical system but rather presents a generic set of structures that are typical of each of these types of connective tissue.

Those tissues that belong in the connective tissue proper category are made up of collagen fibers (tissue fibers that are not stretchable). These fibers are arranged in patterns that make them resistant to traction (pulling) forces. Tendons are dense bundles of fibers that attach muscles to bones. Aponeuroses (singular is aponeurosis) are like tendons, except that they are broad and flat. Ligaments, like tendons, comprise bundles of fibers, the difference being that they attach bones to cartilages and bones to bones.

Muscle Tissue

Muscle tissue is made up of long, thin cells. There are three types of muscle tissue: *smooth, cardiac,* and *skeletal*. Smooth muscle is found in blood vessels, the gastrointestinal (digestive) tract, the urinary bladder, and other body organs, and cardiac muscle is found only in the heart. Both smooth and cardiac muscle are considered to be under involuntary (unconscious) control. In contrast, skeletal muscle is under voluntary (conscious) control. Skeletal muscles are found throughout the

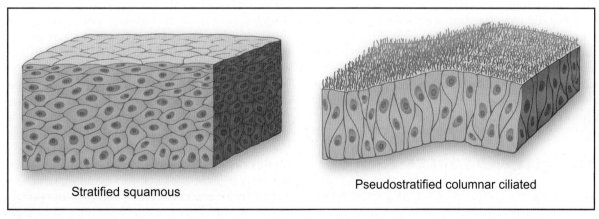

Stratified squamous

Pseudostratified columnar ciliated

FIGURE 1–5. Example of stratified squamous epithelium (*left*) and pseudostratified columnar epithelium (*right*).

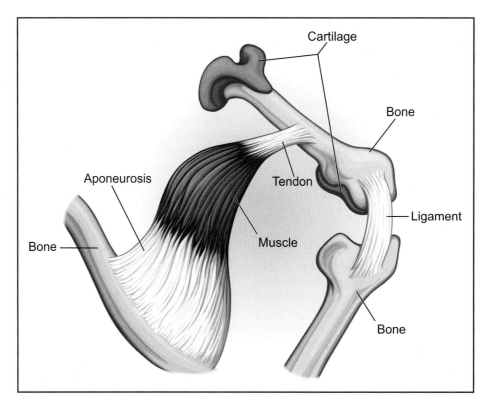

FIGURE 1–6. Examples of connective tissue proper (tendon, aponeurosis, and ligament) and supportive connective tissue (cartilage and bone). This figure is not meant to depict an actual set of anatomical structures.

body, usually directly or indirectly attached to bone; they make it possible for us to move and maintain posture. Although smooth and cardiac muscle tissue are critical to survival and to overall body function, skeletal muscle is most relevant to the understanding of speech and hearing anatomy and physiology and is the focus here.

A skeletal muscle is made up of cells called *muscle fibers* that run parallel to each other. Groups of muscle fibers are bundled together into what are called *fascicles* and surrounded by connective tissue, as illustrated in Figure 1–7. The muscle depicted in the figure is called the *masseter*, a strong muscle that participates in speaking and chewing (see Chapters 5 and 8). Skeletal muscles, such as the *masseter*, are responsible for many of the movements and forces discussed in this book.

MOVEMENTS AND FORCES

Movements and forces of speaking and swallowing result primarily from activation of skeletal muscles. In fact, it is said that we use over 100 skeletal muscles when we speak. The details of muscle physiology are complex and well described in other textbooks (e.g., Rizzo, 2016). A very simple explanation is provided here.

When muscles activate, they usually shorten. This shortening occurs because small protein filaments (thread-like structures) within the muscle fibers move past each other in such a way that the overall muscle becomes shorter than it was at rest. Muscles are activated by nerves, cable-like bundles of nerve fibers that travel from the brainstem or spinal cord out to the muscles. Nerves are described in much greater detail in other chapters (especially Chapter 8); however, a few basic concepts about the action of nerves on muscles are considered here.

The nerves that activate muscles are called peripheral nerves. A peripheral nerve activates a number of muscle fibers. This is illustrated in Figure 1–8, where the peripheral nerve is in contact with a few fibers of the *masseter* muscle. A signal is sent through the nerve (in this case, it is the trigeminal nerve that supplies the *masseter* muscle; see Chapters 5 and 8), which in turn causes those muscle fibers to contract. In reality, there are many such nerve fibers connecting to all the fibers throughout the muscle. Each nerve and its associated muscle fibers is called a *motor unit*. Some motor units

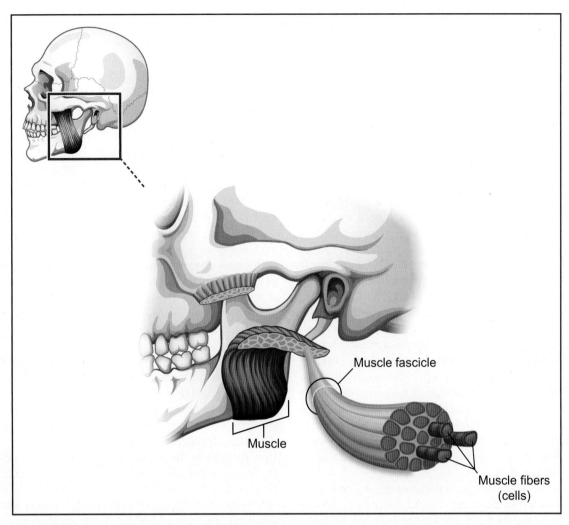

FIGURE 1-7. A speech muscle (masseter) that has been cut away and disassembled to depict a fascicle that contains many individual muscle fibers.

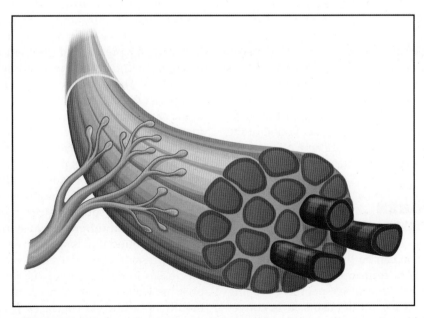

FIGURE 1-8. The terminal section of a peripheral nerve shown communicating with several muscle fibers.

include just a few muscle fibers (for example, fewer than 10), and others include many (perhaps hundreds). Another way to say this is that some motor units have small innervation ratios (that is, a nerve communicates with just a few muscle fibers) and some have large innervation ratios (that is, a nerve communicates with many muscle fibers). Muscles that generate small and precise movements and forces require small innervation ratios. Thus, it is not surprising that many of the muscles involved in speaking, hearing, and swallowing have small innervation ratios, allowing them to exert finely graded control over movements and forces.

When a muscle is activated by the peripheral nerves that innervate its fibers, the muscle produces force. If there are no other influences acting on the muscle, this activation will result in a shortening of the muscle. This is called a *concentric* contraction. But muscles do not always shorten. Sometimes a muscle is held in place by the activation of other surrounding muscles so that when it activates, it does not change length. This is called an *isometric* contraction. It is even possible for a muscle to be activated and lengthen at the same time; this can occur if other muscles are acting in ways that counteract and overpower the activation of the target muscle. A lengthening contraction is referred to as an *eccentric* contraction.

Thus, muscle contraction generates a force and that force may produce a movement. Taking the *masseter* muscle as an example (see Figure 1–7), a concentric contraction causes the jaw to move upward so that the teeth are brought together. This contraction also creates a force that can be felt as pressure being exerted on the teeth. When the *masseter* is contracted very forcefully, the muscle shortens so much that it actually bulges, something that can be detected by placing your hands on the face where the *masseter* is located. The *masseter* can also undergo eccentric contraction. This occurs when the *masseter* is activated and, at the same time, other muscles that exert force in the opposite direction are activated even more forcefully. In this case, the jaw moves downward despite the activation of the jaw-raising *masseter* muscle because activation of the opposing muscles overpowered it.

STAGES OF SPOKEN COMMUNICATION

Spoken communication can be thought of as the process of conveying ideas from one person's brain to the brain(s) of one or more other people by using our speaking and hearing mechanisms. It is convenient to describe spoken communication as a linear set of stages, such as those depicted in Figure 1–9 and described below. Nevertheless, this depiction is overly simplistic, and in fact, there are significant interactions among the processes involved at all these stages. Some of these interactions are explored in more detail in subsequent chapters.

The *neural* stage of spoken communication is carried out by the brain, spinal cord, and the peripheral nerves that serve the speech mechanism. This stage of spoken communication involves the neural processes that participate in conceptualization of the message, the planning and execution of the speech movements, and the processing of the sensory information that influences the ongoing control of speech production. Some neural processes are voluntary and some are automatic; some require awareness and some do not.

The nervous system communicates with muscles to initiate the *muscular* stage of spoken communication. Muscles are effectors that respond to signals from the nervous system to produce forces and movements. In the speech mechanism, it is often difficult to determine individual muscle contributions to forces and movements because they are usually accomplished by groups of muscles working together.

The *structural* stage of the speech communication process is the stage in which speech production becomes visible. Some movements of speech production, such as the movements of the vocal folds, are visible only with the aid of special viewing instruments, whereas other movements, such as the movements of the lips, are visible to the naked eye. Speech reading (lip reading) has its roots in the structural stage of speaking.

Movements of speech structures give rise to the *aeromechanical* (air motion) stage of the spoken communication process. Structural movements raise and lower the air pressure in different parts of the speech mechanism and cause the air to flow from one region to another. These air pressures and airflows are usually invisible, except in those who speak and smoke at the same time or in those who speak in subfreezing temperatures.

Next is the *acoustic* stage, the stage of the process in which speech is produced. Speech is the sound wave—the acoustic product—that results from the act of speaking. It is made up of sonorous, buzzing, hissing, and popping sounds caused by the speaker valving the airstream in different ways and at different locations. The sound that is speech is the rapid alternations of compressions (increases in density) and rarefactions (decreases in density) of air molecules that constitute pressure waves. These pressure waves radiate from the mouth, nose, and skin surfaces. It is this acoustic stage that makes it possible to communicate around corners, through obstacles, in the dark, and over long distances.

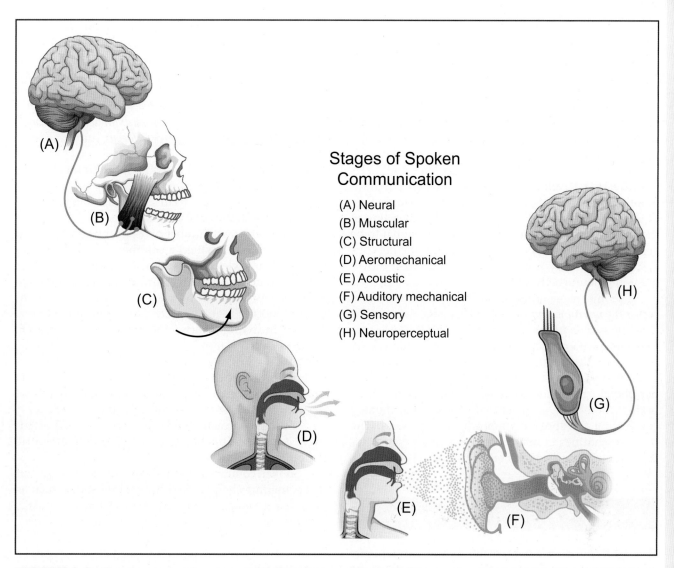

Stages of Spoken Communication

(A) Neural
(B) Muscular
(C) Structural
(D) Aeromechanical
(E) Acoustic
(F) Auditory mechanical
(G) Sensory
(H) Neuroperceptual

FIGURE 1–9. The stages of spoken communication shown as (A) neural, (B) muscular, (C) structural, (D) aeromechanical, (E) acoustic, (F) auditory mechanical, (G) sensory, and (H) neuroperceptual.

Air Travel

Students often find it hard to separate the aeromechanic from the acoustic stage of speech production, probably because they both involve air travel. An example may help clear things up. Try talking while holding your hand up to your mouth—you should feel air flowing into your hand. Now do that while talking to someone at least 6 feet away from you (something we've learned to do in the time of COVID-19). That person can hear you just fine, but they can't feel the air flowing from your mouth (hopefully). That's because the air flows from your mouth slowly and that flow only travels a short distance from your mouth. In contrast, the compressions and rarefactions created by air molecules bumping into each (while remaining more or less in place) move rapidly *through* the air and over long distances as a wave of energy. So think of the aeromechanic stage as transporting air molecules themselves from one place to another, whereas in the acoustic stage, the air molecules assist in moving energy from one place to another.

These acoustic pressure waves reach the ears of the listener and initiate the next stage of the spoken communication process: the ***auditory mechanical*** stage. It is during this stage that the acoustic pressure waves hit structures of the ear and cause them to move ever so slightly. These movements are transmitted from one structure to the next through various regions of the ear until they reach the auditory sensors that serve as the interface between sound and the nervous system.

The auditory sensors, which look like small hairs (and are, in fact, called hair cells), bend when a hydraulic pressure wave hits them. This is the ***sensory*** stage of the spoken communication process. The bending of these hair-like sensors causes an electrical signal to be generated, and that signal is sent through the nervous system. In this way, the sensors transduce their movement into neural activity.

The final stage of the spoken communication process is the ***neuroperceptual*** stage. This stage relies on the nervous system of the listener (although it is also true that the speaker's nervous system is simultaneously processing the acoustic speech signal). The signals generated in the ears' sensory cells are sent through peripheral nerves and routed to different parts of the brain, where they are eventually perceived, thereby completing the spoken communication process. The message that began in the speaker's brain completes its journey in the listener's brain.

REVIEW

This book covers the anatomy (structural components) and physiology (functions of those components) of the speech and hearing mechanisms.

The speech mechanism consists of the respiratory, laryngeal, velopharyngeal-nasal, and pharyngeal-oral subsystems.

The hearing (auditory) mechanism can be thought of as comprising the outer ear, middle ear, and inner ear.

Anatomical directions are often critical for being able to describe the relation of one part to another and include terms such as *anterior/posterior* (*ventral/dorsal*), *superior/inferior* (*rostral/caudal*), *medial/lateral*, *proximal/distal*, *external/internal* (*superficial/deep*), and *ipsilateral/contralateral*.

Anatomical planes are also important for describing the perspective from which a body part is being depicted and go by the terms *sagittal*, *coronal* (*frontal*), and *horizontal* (*transverse* or *axial*).

There are a vast number of tissue types in the body, including those classified as epithelial tissue, connective tissue, muscle tissue, and nerve tissue.

Movements and forces are primarily caused by activation of skeletal muscle by the nervous system through nerves that communicate with muscle fibers.

An individual nerve and its associated muscle fibers is called a motor unit, with small motor units (innervating just a few muscle fibers) serving muscles that perform precise movements and large motor units (innervating many muscle fibers) serving muscles that perform larger, less precise movements.

Muscle contractions can be concentric (shortening), isometric (unchanging length), and eccentric (lengthening).

Spoken communication is truly a fluid process, but it is sometimes helpful to divide it into stages such as neural, muscular, structural, aeromechanical, acoustic, auditory mechanical, sensory, and neuroperceptual.

REFERENCE

Rizzo, D. C. (2016). *Fundamentals of anatomy and physiology* (4th ed.). Independence, KY: Cengage.

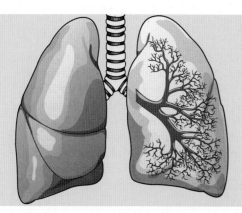

2

Respiratory Structure and Function

INTRODUCTION

The respiratory system operates somewhat like a pump, moving air into and out of the body for the purpose of sustaining life as well as for performing other important functions such as speaking, swallowing, and coughing. It includes an energy source (muscles) and passive components that couple this source to the air it moves.

This chapter begins with detailed consideration of respiratory anatomy, forces (including muscles) and movements of the respiratory system, respiratory control variables, neural substrates of respiratory control, and ventilation and gas exchange. The latter part of the chapter is dedicated to respiratory function during speech production, selected variables that influence it, and some clinical considerations. Respiratory function for swallowing is covered in Chapter 7.

RESPIRATORY ANATOMY

The respiratory system is located within the torso (body trunk) and comprises its skeletal framework and its subdivisions, which include the pulmonary apparatus (pulmonary airways and lungs) and chest wall (rib

Coming to Terms

Terms can either enlighten you or get you into verbal quagmires. Respiratory physiologists have gone out of their way to be precise in their use of terms. They've even held conventions to iron out their differences in language. It's a good idea to take a little extra time and care when reading the early sections of this chapter. Let the lexicon of the respiratory physiologist take firm root. Don't be tempted to skip over parts just because the words in the headings look familiar to you. You may be surprised to find that a term you thought you understood actually has an entirely different meaning to a respiratory physiologist.

cage wall, diaphragm, abdominal wall, and abdominal content). These are described in this section; the muscles of the chest wall are discussed in the next section (Forces of the Respiratory System). To view some of the anatomy of the respiratory system in a human cadaver, the reader is directed to watch Video 2–1 (Respiratory Anatomy).

Skeletal Framework

A skeleton of bone and cartilage forms the framework of the respiratory system. This framework is depicted in Figure 2–1. At the back of the torso, 34 irregularly shaped vertebrae (bones) form the vertebral column or backbone. The uppermost 7 of these vertebrae are termed cervical (neck), the next lower 12 are called thoracic (chest), and the next three lower groups of 5 each are referred to as lumbar, sacral, and coccygeal (collectively, abdominal). The vertebral column constitutes a back midline post for the torso.

The ribs comprise most of the upper skeletal framework. They are 12 flat, arch-shaped bones on each side of the body. The ribs slope downward from back to front along the sides of the torso, forming the rib cage and giving roundness to the upper framework. At the front, most of the ribs attach to bars of costal (rib) cartilage, which, in turn, attach to the sternum (breast-bone). The typical rib cage includes upper pairs of ribs attached to the sternum by their own costal cartilages, lower pairs that share cartilages, and the lowest two pairs that float without front attachments.

The remainder of the upper skeletal framework is formed by the pectoral girdle (shoulder girdle). This structure is near the top of the rib cage. The front of the pectoral girdle is formed by the two clavicles (collar bones), each of which is a strut extending from the sternum over the first rib toward the side and back of the rib cage. At the back, the clavicles attach to two triangularly shaped plates, the scapulae (shoulder blades). The scapulae cover most of the upper back portion of the rib cage.

Two large, irregularly shaped coxal (hip) bones are located in the lower part of the skeletal framework. These two bones, together with the sacral and coccygeal vertebrae, form the pelvic girdle (bony pelvis). The pelvic girdle comprises the base, lower back, and sides of the lower skeletal framework.

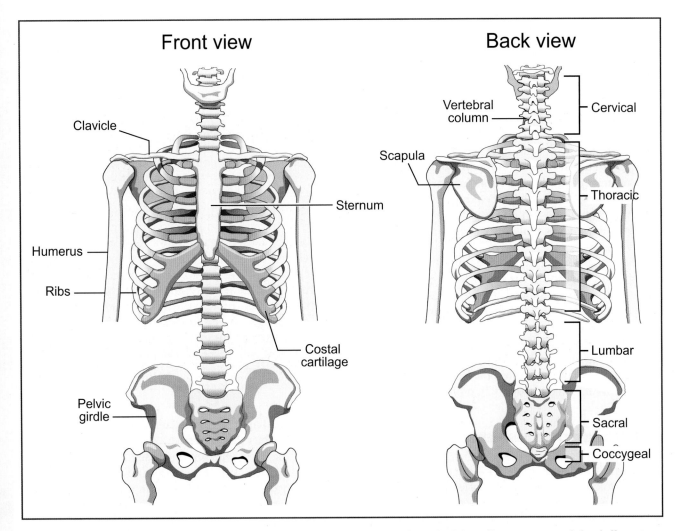

FIGURE 2–1. Skeletal framework of the respiratory system consisting of the clavicles, ribs, sternum, pelvic girdle, scapulae, and vertebral column.

Respiratory System Subdivisions

The respiratory system and its subdivisions are depicted in Figure 2–2. The torso, which houses the apparatus, consists of upper and lower cavities that are partitioned by the diaphragm. The upper cavity is called the thorax (or colloquially the chest) and is almost totally filled with the heart and lungs; the lower cavity, called the abdomen (or colloquially the belly), contains much of the digestive system and other organs and glands. The structures of the respiratory system form two major subdivisions: the pulmonary apparatus and chest wall. These subdivisions are concentrically arranged, with the chest wall surrounding the pulmonary apparatus.

Pulmonary Apparatus

The pulmonary apparatus, portrayed in Figure 2–3, is the air containing, air conducting, and gas exchanging part of the respiratory system. It provides oxygen to the cells of the body and removes carbon dioxide from them. The pulmonary apparatus can be subdivided into two components: the pulmonary airways and lungs.

Pulmonary Airways

The pulmonary (lower) airways constitute a complex network of flexible tubes through which air can be moved to and from the lungs and between different parts of the lungs. These tubes are arranged like the branches of an inverted deciduous tree. The network, in fact, is commonly referred to as the pulmonary tree.

The trunk of the pulmonary tree (the top part) is the trachea (windpipe). The trachea is a tube attached to the bottom of the larynx (voice box). It runs down through the neck into the torso. The trachea is composed of a series of C-shaped cartilages whose open ends face toward the back where the structure is completed by a flexible wall shared with the esophagus (the muscular tube leading to the stomach). At its lower end, the trachea divides into two smaller tubes, one running to the left lung and one running to the right lung. These two tubes, called the main-stem bronchi, branch into what are called lobar bronchi, tubes that run to the five lobes of the lungs (two lobes on the left and three on the right). The five lobar bronchi each branch and their offspring also branch, and so on, through more than 20 generations. Each successive branching leads to smaller and less rigid structures. These include, in

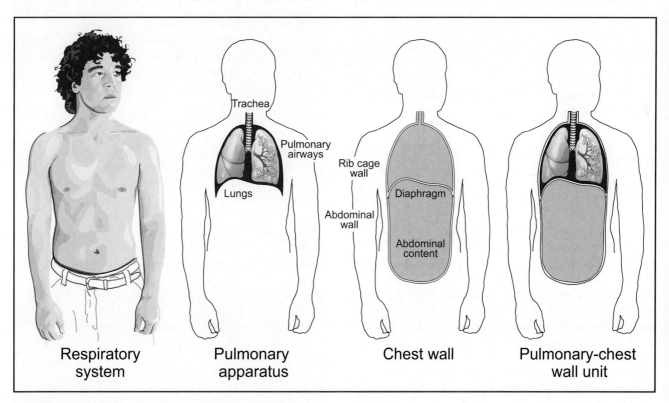

FIGURE 2–2. Respiratory system and its subdivisions: the pulmonary apparatus (lungs and airways) and the chest wall (rib cage wall, diaphragm, abdominal wall, and abdominal content). From *Evaluation and Management of Speech Breathing Disorders: Principles and Methods* (p. 13), by T. Hixon and J. Hoit, 2005, Tucson, AZ: Redington Brown. Copyright 2005 by Thomas J. Hixon and Jeannette D. Hoit. Modified and reproduced with permission.

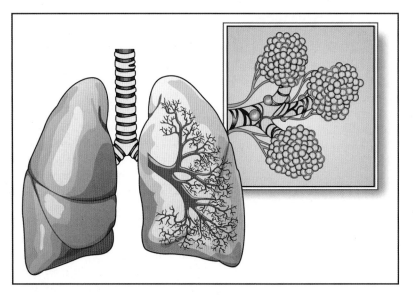

FIGURE 2–3. The pulmonary apparatus. It consists of the airways (trachea, main-stem bronchi, lobar bronchi, segmental bronchi, subsegmental bronchi, small bronchi, terminal bronchi, bronchioles, terminal bronchioles, respiratory bronchioles, alveolar ducts, alveolar sacs, and alveoli) and lungs (spongy structures that surround the pulmonary airways).

succession, segmental bronchi, subsegmental bronchi, small bronchi, terminal bronchi, bronchioles, terminal bronchioles, respiratory bronchioles, alveolar ducts, alveolar sacs, and alveoli. The last of these, the alveoli, are extremely small cul-de-sacs filled with air. They number more than 300 million and are the sites where oxygen and carbon dioxide are exchanged. The total surface area of the alveoli, if laid out flat, is said to approximate the size of a tennis court.

Lungs

The lungs are the organs of breathing. They are a pair of cone-shaped structures that are porous and spongy. Each lung contains an abundance of resilient elastic fibers and behaves like a stretchable bag. The outer surfaces of the lungs are covered with a thin airtight membrane, called the visceral pleura. A similar membrane, the parietal pleura, covers the inner surface of the chest wall where it contacts the lungs. Together, these two membranes form a double-walled sac that encases the lungs. Both walls of this sac are covered with a thin layer of liquid that lubricates them and enables them to move easily upon one another. The same layer of liquid links the visceral and parietal membranes together, in the way a film of water holds two glass plates together. This is called *pleural linkage*. Thus, the lungs and chest wall tend to move as a unit—where one goes the other follows.

Passive Elastic

Something that is elastic returns to its original shape following deformation. Take, for example, a rubber ball. Drop it on the floor and the ball's shape will deform, producing internal forces that launch it upward and return it to its original shape. Now consider a ball of clay. Drop it on the floor and what happens? Thud! Deformation occurs just like the rubber ball, but there are no internal forces generated to return the ball to its original shape and no bounce to return it upward. Elastic objects have what is called elastic potential energy. This energy increases as the object is deformed or stretched. Take, for example, the lungs. Stretch them by filling them with air and the elastic potential energy increases until the lungs are full—this is energy that can be used to deflate the lungs. You can simulate this with a balloon: Blow it up all the way, then let go and watch it deflate to its original size. You can watch a demonstration of this in Video 2–2 (Balloon Analogy). Elastic energy of the lungs contributes to what is called the "passive" force of the respiratory system. Passive force may not sound important, but it has a lot to do with how the respiratory system behaves.

Chest Wall

The chest wall encases the pulmonary apparatus. There are four parts to the chest wall: the rib cage wall, diaphragm, abdominal wall, and abdominal content.

Rib Cage Wall

The rib cage wall surrounds the lungs and is shaped like a barrel. The rib cage framework includes the thoracic segments of the vertebral column, the ribs, the costal cartilages, the sternum, and the pectoral girdle. The remainder of the rib cage wall is formed by muscular and nonmuscular tissues that fill the spaces between the ribs and cover their inner and outer surfaces.

Diaphragm

The diaphragm forms the convex floor of the thorax (upper cavity of the respiratory system) and the concave roof of the abdomen. The diaphragm separates the thorax and abdomen and, thus, gets its name—diaphragm meaning *the fence between*. The diaphragm is dome shaped, like an inverted bowl. The left side of the diaphragm is positioned slightly lower than the right (to accommodate the heart above and the liver below). At its center, the diaphragm consists of a tough sheet of inelastic tissue, called the central tendon. The remainder of the structure is formed by a sheet of muscle that rises as a broad rim from all around the lower portion

of the inside of the rib cage and extends upward to the edges of the central tendon.

Abdominal Wall

The abdominal wall provides a casing for the lower half of the torso. This casing is shaped like an oblong tube and runs all the way around the torso. The lower portion of the skeletal framework of the torso forms the structure around which the abdominal wall is built. This includes a back post of 15 vertebrae (lumbar, sacral, and coccygeal) that extends from near the bottom of the rib cage to the tailbone and pelvic girdle. Much of the abdominal wall consists of two broad sheets of connective tissue and several large muscles. The two sheets of connective tissue cover the front and back of the abdominal wall and are called the abdominal aponeurosis (similar to a broad flat tendon) and lumbodorsal fascia (an encasing connective tissue), respectively. Muscles are located all around the abdominal wall—front, back, and flanks (sides)—and combine with the abdominal aponeurosis, lumbodorsal fascia, vertebral column, and pelvic girdle to form its casing.

Abdominal Content

The abdominal content is everything in the abdominal cavity. This includes the stomach, intestines, and various other internal structures. This content is close to unit density (the density of water). Its mass is suspended from above by a suction force at the undersurface of the diaphragm and is held in place circumferentially and at its base by the casing of the abdominal wall. Together, the abdominal cavity and the abdominal content can be thought of as the mechanical equivalent of an elastic bag filled with water.

Pulmonary Apparatus–Chest Wall Unit

The pulmonary apparatus and chest wall are linked by pleural membranes (this is called pleural linkage) to form a single functional unit. As illustrated in Figure 2–4, the resting positions (sizes) of the pulmonary apparatus and chest wall, when linked as a unit, are different from their individual resting positions. When the pulmonary apparatus is removed from the chest wall, it collapses to a small size and contains very little air. This is represented as a collapsed spring in the figure (lower left). In contrast, the chest wall expands when the pulmonary apparatus is removed, as represented by the stretched spring in the figure (lower middle). With the pulmonary apparatus and chest wall held together by pleural linkage, the respiratory

---

Ribbit, Ribbit

Ever watch a frog breathe? Did you notice how its cheeks moved? Frogs don't have a diaphragm to pull air into their lungs. They push the air in using their mouths like pistons. Frogs are positive pressure breathers. People are negative pressure breathers. A frog doesn't have the ability to emulate us (except, perhaps, Kermit) if its positive pressure pump fails. But we have the ability to emulate the frog if our negative pressure pump fails by doing what is called glossopharyngeal breathing. And what would you suppose is the common name for such breathing? Well, it's "frog breathing." In frog breathing, the tongue and throat are used to pump air into the lungs. Air is gulped in small portions (mouthfuls), each held in place by closing the larynx as a one-way valve. Frog breathing isn't difficult to learn and, once mastered, can be used to fill the lungs in a stepwise fashion all the way to the top.

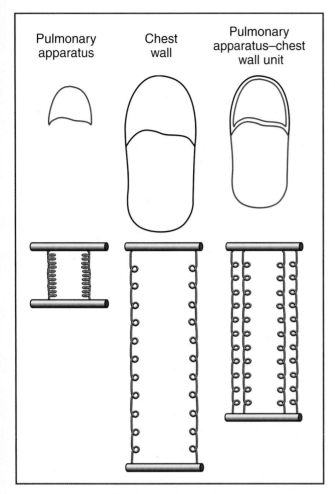

FIGURE 2–4. Resting positions of the pulmonary apparatus, chest wall, and pulmonary apparatus–chest wall unit (respiratory system). Note that when the pulmonary apparatus and chest wall are linked (*right side of figure*), the resting size of the pulmonary apparatus is larger and the resting size of the chest wall is smaller than when they are separated. When linked, the forces of the pulmonary apparatus and chest wall are equal and opposite and the pulmonary–chest wall unit assumes a mechanically neutral (balanced) state.

system assumes an intermediate size. This resting position of the linked pulmonary apparatus–chest wall unit is a mechanically neutral or balanced state in which the force of the pulmonary apparatus to collapse is opposed by an equal and opposite force of the chest wall to expand. The linked pulmonary apparatus–chest wall unit (respiratory system) is represented as a combined spring in the Figure 2–4 (lower right).

FORCES OF THE RESPIRATORY SYSTEM

Both passive and active forces operate on the respiratory system. Passive force is inherent and always present. Active force, in contrast, is applied willfully by skeletal (voluntary) muscles.

Passive Force

The passive force acting on the respiratory system is substantial, primarily because the respiratory system is so massive. Passive force comes from (a) the natural recoil of muscles, cartilages, ligaments, and lung tissue; (b) the surface tension of alveoli; and (c) the pull of gravity. It is passive force that causes the respiratory system to behave like a coil spring (like that illustrated in Figure 2–4), which, when stretched or compressed, tends to recoil toward its resting size.

The sign (inspiratory or expiratory) and magnitude (strength) of passive force depends on the amount of air contained within the respiratory system. When the respiratory system contains more air than it does at rest, it recoils toward a smaller size (expires), like the release of a stretched spring. The more air it contains, the greater the recoil force to expire. In contrast, when the respiratory system contains less air than it does at rest, it recoils toward a larger size (inspires),

---

Laundry Starch

The stiffness of the respiratory system changes across life. The term that pertains to this is *compliance*, and it refers to the tendency to yield to an applied force. In the lexicon of the respiratory physiologist, compliance is quantified in terms of how much volume is displaced for the pressure applied. We are reminded of laundry starch when we think of this concept. You get a little more starch in the "fabric" of your respiratory system as time

goes by. The compliance of the respiratory system of a newborn is relatively high and somewhat like that of a dishrag. In contrast, the compliance of the respiratory system of a senescent adult is relatively low and somewhat like that of a plastic garbage can lid. Thus, we start out being relatively floppy and end up life being relatively stiff (no pun intended on the stiff part, honestly).

like the release of a compressed spring. The less air it contains, the greater the recoil force to inspire. Thus, like a coil spring, the more the respiratory system is deformed from its resting size, whether in the inspiratory (stretched) or expiratory (compressed) direction, the greater the passive recoil force it generates.

Active Force

Active force comes from the actions of muscles of the chest wall. The sign (inspiratory or expiratory) and magnitude of this force depend on which muscles are active and in what combinations. Active force also depends on the amount of air contained in the respiratory system. The more air it contains, the greater the active force that can be generated to expire, and the less air it contains, the greater the active force that can be generated to inspire.

The roles of individual muscles in generating active force are described below for the rib cage wall, diaphragm, and abdominal wall. These descriptions assume that only the muscle under consideration is active and that it is shortening during contraction. It should be noted, however, that several factors might influence the contribution of an individual muscle, including the actions of other muscles, the mechanical status of different parts of the chest wall, and the activity being performed. All respiratory muscles and sets of muscles are paired, being located on the left and right sides of the body.

Muscles of the Rib Cage Wall

The muscles of the rib cage wall are defined to include muscles of the neck and rib cage. These muscles are depicted in different views in Figure 2–5.

The *sternocleidomastoid* muscle is a broad, thick structure positioned on the front and side of the neck. It originates in two subdivisions, one at the top and front of the sternum and the other at the top of the sternal end of the clavicle. Fibers from these subdivisions pass upward and backward and insert into the bony skull behind the ear. When the head is fixed in position, contraction of the *sternocleidomastoid* muscle results in elevation of the sternum and clavicle. The force generated is transmitted to the ribs through their connections to the sternum and clavicle. Consequently, the ribs are also elevated.

The *scalenus anterior*, *scalenus medius*, and *scalenus posterior* muscles are three separate muscles that form a functional group. These are positioned on the side of the neck. The *scalenus anterior* muscle originates from the third through sixth cervical vertebrae and runs downward and toward the side to insert along the inner border of the top of the first rib. The *scalenus medius* muscle arises from the lower six cervical vertebrae and descends along the side of the vertebral column to insert into the first rib behind the point of insertion of the *scalenus anterior* muscle. And the *scalenus posterior* muscle originates from the lower two or three cervical vertebrae and passes downward and toward the side to attach to the outer surface of the second rib. When the head is fixed in position, contraction of the *scalenus anterior* and/or *scalenus medius* muscles results in elevation of the first rib, whereas contraction of the *scalenus posterior* muscle results in elevation of the second rib.

The *pectoralis major* muscle is a broad, fan-shaped muscle positioned on the upper front wall of the rib cage. This muscle has a complex origin that includes the front surface of the upper costal cartilages, sternum, and inner half of the clavicle. Fibers run across the front of the rib cage wall and converge to insert into the humerus (the major bone of the upper arm). When the humerus is held in position, contraction of the *pectoralis major* muscle pulls the sternum and ribs upward.

Rib Torque

Sounds like leftovers. Actually, it refers to rotational stress produced when one end of a rib is twisted out of line with the other. Some have suggested that when the ribs are elevated during resting tidal inspiration, they're twisted outward (placed under positive torque) and store energy, which is then supposedly released during expiration. Not so. The ribs are actually twisted inward (are under negative torque) at the resting tidal end-expiratory level (bottom of a resting tidal breath) because the lungs are pulling inward on the rib cage wall at that level. The ribs untwist during resting tidal inspiration but do not reach neutral (zero torque) until the 60% VC (percent vital capacity) level is attained (when in an upright body position). Because resting tidal inspiration involves only about a 10% increase in vital capacity, rib torque actually opposes resting tidal expiration rather than assists it. The only thing left over about rib torque in this context is the folklore.

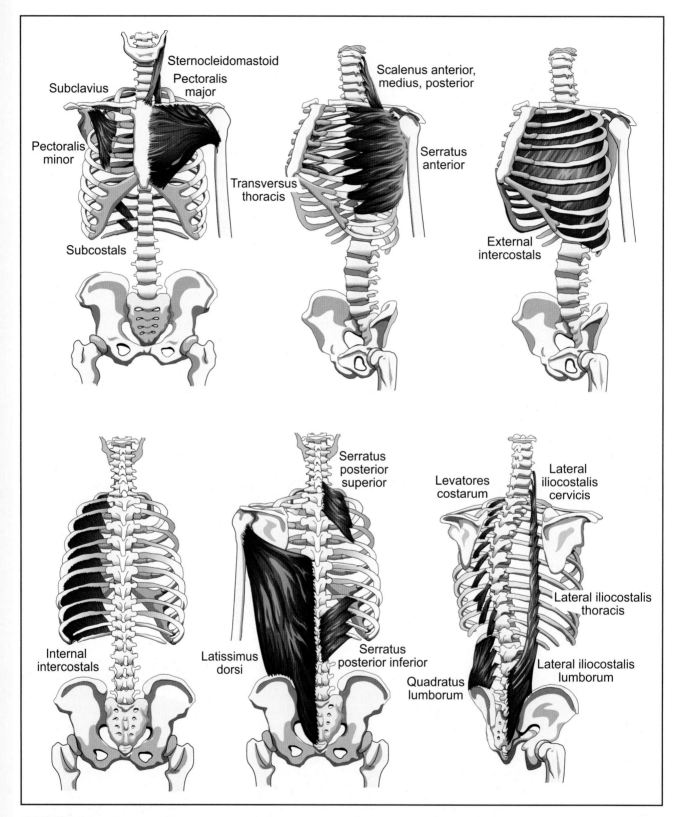

FIGURE 2–5. Muscles of the rib cage wall. From *Evaluation and Management of Speech Breathing Disorders: Principles and Methods* (pp. 19–20), by T. Hixon and J. Hoit, 2005, Tucson, AZ: Redington Brown. Copyright 2005 by Thomas J. Hixon and Jeannette D. Hoit. Modified and reproduced with permission.

The *pectoralis minor* muscle is a relatively large, thin muscle that lies underneath the *pectoralis major* muscle. Its fibers originate from the second through fifth ribs near their cartilages. From there, they extend upward and toward the side, where they insert into the front surface of the scapula. When the scapula is fixed in position, contraction of the *pectoralis minor* muscle elevates the second through fifth ribs.

The *subclavius* muscle is a small muscle that originates from the undersurface of the clavicle. It runs slightly downward and toward the midline, where it attaches at the junction of the first rib and its cartilage. When the clavicle is braced, contraction of the *subclavius* muscle elevates the first rib.

The *serratus anterior* muscle is a large muscle positioned on the side of the rib cage wall. It originates from the outer surfaces of the upper eight or nine ribs. Fibers pass backward around the side of the rib cage, where they converge and insert into the front of the scapula. When the scapula is fixed in position, contraction of the *serratus anterior* muscle results in elevation of the upper ribs.

The *external intercostal* muscles are 11 muscles that fill the outer (external) portions of the rib interspaces. Each is a thin layer of muscle that runs between adjacent ribs. The fibers of the muscles are oriented forward and downward. Together, the 11 muscles form a large sheet of muscle that links the ribs to one another. This sheet of muscle is anchored from above to the first rib, the cervical vertebrae, and the base of the skull. When the muscle in any rib interspace contracts, it elevates the rib immediately below and, perhaps, other ribs below through their linkage to the sheet of muscle. The *external intercostal* muscles may activate individually in different rib interspaces or they may activate collectively. En masse activation causes the ribs to move upward as a unit. Muscle activation also stiffens the tissue-filled rib interspaces. This prevents them from being sucked inward and pushed outward as internal pressure is lowered and raised, respectively.

The *internal intercostal* muscles are 11 muscles that lie in the inner (internal) portions of the rib interspaces. They are located underneath the *external intercostal* muscles and extend from around the sides of the rib cage to the sternum. The *internal intercostal* muscles do not fill the rib interspaces at the back of the rib age. Fibers of the *internal intercostal* muscles run downward and backward and at a right angle to those of the *external intercostal* muscles. The *internal intercostal* muscles form a large sheet of muscle that links the ribs to one another and to the pelvic girdle through other muscles, especially those of the abdominal wall. When muscle in a rib interspace contracts, it pulls downward on the rib immediately above and, perhaps, on other ribs above through the linkage created by the muscle sheet. The *internal intercostal* muscles may activate individually in any rib interspace or they may activate collectively. When they activate collectively, the ribs tend to move downward as a unit. Muscle contraction stiffens the tissue-filled rib interspaces and prevents them from being sucked inward and bulged outward with changes in internal pressure.

The portion of the *internal intercostal* muscles that lies between the costal cartilages (the *intercartilaginous internal intercostal* muscles) is arranged such that the muscle tissue exerts an upward pull on the rib cage wall rather than the downward pull exerted by the portion of the muscle that lies between the bony ribs (the *interosseous internal intercostal* muscles). Thus, the *internal intercostal* muscles play a functional role in the intercartilaginous region that is similar to that played by their companion *external intercostal* muscles throughout the rib cage wall. Stated otherwise, the two layers of *intercostal* muscles (external and internal) function similarly toward the front of the rib cage but dissimilarly at other locations.

The *transversus thoracis* muscle is a fan-shaped structure located on the inside, front wall of the rib cage. It originates at the midline on the inner surface of the lower sternum and fourth or fifth through seventh costal cartilages. From there, it fans out across the rib cage and inserts into the inner surface of the costal cartilages and bony ends of the second through sixth ribs. The upper fibers of the muscle run nearly vertically, whereas the intermediate and lower fibers course at other angles. When the *transversus thoracis* muscle contracts, it exerts a downward pull on the second through sixth ribs.

The *latissimus dorsi* muscle is a large muscle positioned on the back of the body. It has a complex origin from the lower six thoracic, lumbar, and sacral vertebrae, along with the back surfaces of the lower three or four ribs. Fibers run upward across the back of the lower torso at different angles to insert into the humerus. When the humerus is fixed in position, contraction of the fibers of the *latissimus dorsi* muscle that insert into the lower ribs will elevate them. Contraction of the muscle as a whole, in contrast, compresses the lower portion of the rib cage wall. Thus, the *latissimus dorsi* muscle is capable of generating active force of different signs (inspiratory and expiratory).

The *serratus posterior superior* muscle is located on the upper back portion of the rib cage wall. It is a thin muscle that originates from the back of the vertebral column. Points of origin include the seventh cervical and first three or four thoracic vertebrae. Fibers course downward across the back of the rib cage and insert into the second through fifth ribs. When the *serratus posterior superior* muscle contracts, it pulls upward on the second through fifth ribs.

The *serratus posterior inferior* muscle is a thin muscle positioned on the lower back portion of the rib cage wall. It arises from the lower two thoracic and upper two or three lumbar vertebrae and slants upward across the back of the rib cage where it inserts into the lower borders of the lower four ribs. Contraction of the *serratus posterior inferior* muscle results in a downward pull on the lower four ribs.

The *lateral iliocostalis* muscle group includes three muscles located on the back of the torso. These are positioned to the side of the vertebral column and extend between the cervical and lumbar regions. The *lateral iliocostalis cervicis* muscle originates from the outer surfaces of the third through sixth ribs and courses upward and toward the midline to insert into the fourth through sixth cervical vertebrae. The *lateral iliocostalis thoracis* muscle arises from the upper edges of the lower six ribs and courses upward to insert into the lower edges of the upper six ribs. And the *lateral iliocostalis lumborum* muscle originates from the lumbodorsal fascia, lumbar vertebrae, and back surface of the coxal bone. It courses upward and toward the side to insert into the lower edges of the lower six ribs. Contraction of the *lateral iliocostalis cervicis* muscle causes elevation of the third through sixth ribs, whereas contraction of the *lateral iliocostalis lumborum* muscle results in depression of the lower six ribs. Contraction of the *lateral iliocostalis thoracis* muscle stabilizes large segments of the back of the rib cage wall and makes them move in concert with either the rib elevation or depression caused by the cervical and lumbar elements of the muscle group, respectively.

The *levatores costarum* muscles are 12 small muscles positioned on the back of the rib cage wall. Their origin is from the seventh cervical and upper 11 thoracic vertebrae and they extend downward and slightly outward to insert into the back surface of the rib immediately below the vertebra of origin. When an individual muscle of the *levatores costarum* muscle group contracts, it elevates the ribs into which it inserts. When the muscle group contracts collectively, its action is similar to that effected by collective contraction of the *external intercostal* muscles (the ribs elevate as a unit).

The *quadratus lumborum* muscle is a flat, quadrilateral sheet of muscle located on the back of the torso. It arises from the top of the coxal bone and runs upward and toward the midline where it inserts into the first four lumbar vertebrae and lower border of the inner half of the lowest rib. When the *quadratus lumborum* muscle contracts, it pulls downward on the lowest rib.

The *subcostal* muscles comprise a group of thin muscles located on the inside back wall of the rib cage. They differ in number from person to person and are most often located and best developed in the lower portion of the rib cage wall. The *subcostal* muscles originate near the vertebral column on the inner surfaces of ribs and course upward and toward the side where they insert into the inner surfaces of ribs immediately above or skip a rib or two and insert into higher ribs. When the *subcostal* muscles contract, they pull downward on the ribs into which they are inserted.

Muscle of the Diaphragm

The muscular features of the diaphragm are portrayed in Figure 2–6. The *diaphragm* muscle is a large, complex muscle that subdivides the torso into two compartments: the thorax (upper cavity) and abdomen. It originates around the internal circumference of the lower rib cage, including the bottom of the sternum, the lower six ribs and their cartilages, and the first three or four lumbar vertebrae. From this internal rim, muscle fibers radiate upward to insert into the circumference of the central tendon, a broad sheet of inelastic tissue that forms the central portion of the diaphragm.

When the *diaphragm* muscle contracts, it can generate two actions. One of these is to pull the central tendon downward and forward, thus enlarging the thorax vertically; the other is to enlarge the thorax circumferentially through elevation of the lower six ribs. The actions of lowering the base of the thorax and expanding its circumference occur in patterns that depend on the relative stiffness (compliance) of the rib cage wall and abdominal wall.

Muscles of the Abdominal Wall

The muscles of the abdominal wall are depicted in Figure 2–7. They are located on the front and sides of the abdominal wall.

The *rectus abdominis* muscle is a ribbon-like structure located on the front of the lower rib cage wall and abdominal wall just off the midline. It arises from the upper, front edge of the coxal bone and runs upward vertically to insert into the outer surfaces of the fifth, sixth, and seventh costal cartilages and lower sternum. The *rectus abdominis* muscle is compartmentalized into four or five short segments by tendinous breaks. The entire muscle is encased in a fibrous sheath formed by the abdominal aponeurosis. The muscle and sheath form a central post along the front of the abdominal wall that is a continuation of the front post formed by the sternum on the rib cage wall. When the *rectus abdominis* muscle contracts, it pulls the lower ribs and

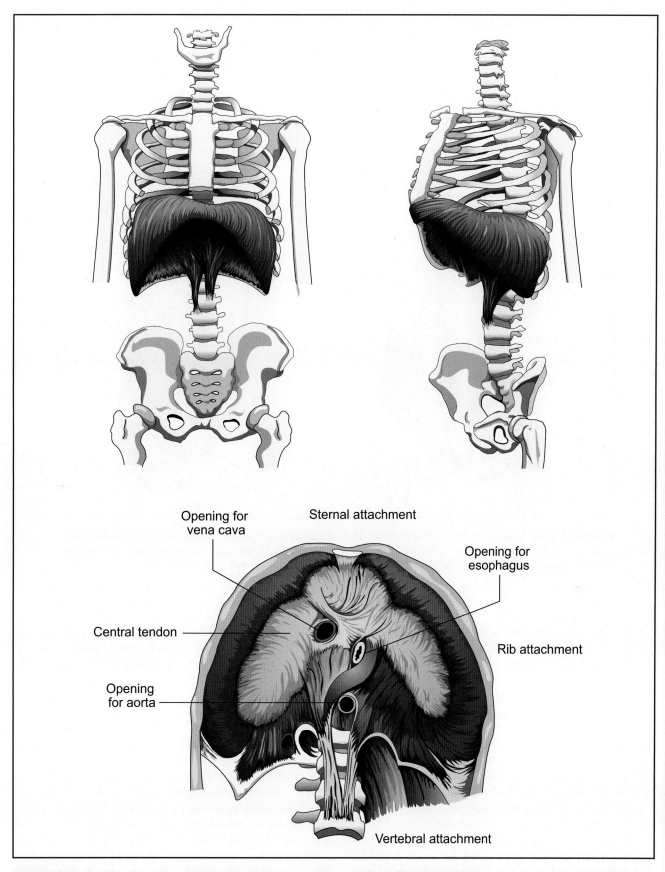

FIGURE 2–6. Muscle of the *diaphragm* shown from different views. Upper panels are views from the front (*left*) and side (*right*). Lower panel is a view of the diaphragm from below. Upper panels from *Evaluation and Management of Speech Breathing Disorders: Principles and Methods* (p. 25), by T. Hixon and J. Hoit, 2005, Tucson, AZ: Redington Brown. Copyright 2005 by Thomas J. Hixon and Jeannette D. Hoit. Modified and reproduced with permission.

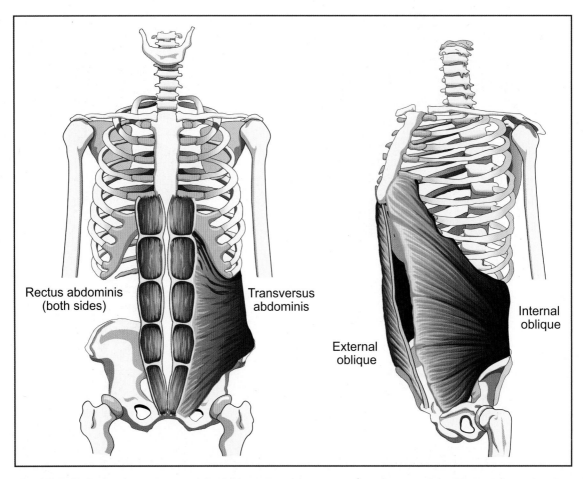

FIGURE 2–7. Muscles of the abdominal wall. From *Evaluation and Management of Speech Breathing Disorders: Principles and Methods* (p. 26), by T. Hixon and J. Hoit, 2005, Tucson, AZ: Redington Brown. Copyright 2005 by Thomas J. Hixon and Jeannette D. Hoit. Modified and reproduced with permission.

sternum downward and forces the front of the abdominal wall inward. The compartmentalized segments of the muscle are also capable of independent contraction.

The *external oblique* muscle is a broad structure located on the side and front of the lower rib cage wall and abdominal wall. It originates from the upper surface of the coxal bone and abdominal aponeurosis near the midline. Fibers course upward across the abdominal wall at various angles. The most prominent course is upward and toward the side, with insertions being on the outer surfaces and lower borders of the lower eight ribs. When the *external oblique* muscle contracts, it pulls the lower ribs downward and forces the front and side of the abdominal wall inward.

The *internal oblique* muscle is a large muscle positioned on the side and front of the lower rib cage wall and abdominal wall. It lies underneath the *external oblique* muscle. The *internal oblique* muscle originates from the upper surface of the coxal bone and lumbodorsal fascia. Its fibers fan out across the abdominal wall to insert into the abdominal aponeurosis and

the lower borders of the costal cartilages of the lower three or four ribs. The fibers of the *internal oblique* muscle run at a right angle to those of the *external oblique* muscle. When the *internal oblique* muscle contracts, it pulls the lower ribs downward and forces the front and side of the abdominal wall inward. Thus, its functional potential is similar to that of the *external oblique* muscle.

The *transversus abdominis* muscle is a broad structure located on the front and side of the abdominal wall. It lies underneath the *internal oblique* muscle. The *transversus abdominis* muscle has a complex origin that includes the upper surface of the coxal bone, lumbodorsal fascia, and inner surfaces of the costal cartilages of ribs 7 through 12. Fibers of the muscle run horizontally around the abdominal wall and insert at the front into the abdominal aponeurosis. The paired left and right *transversus abdominis* muscles encircle the abdominal wall. When the *transversus abdominis* muscle contracts, it forces the front and side of the abdominal wall inward.

The four muscles just described—*rectus abdominis, external oblique, internal oblique,* and *transverse abdominis* muscles—are routinely referred to as "the abdominal muscles." However, the abdominal wall runs all the way around the torso and includes more than just its front and sides. Three other muscles traverse the abdominal wall at the back and are as much a part of the abdominal wall as the muscles just discussed. These are the *latissimus dorsi, lateral iliocostalis lumborum,* and *quadratus lumborum* muscles, described above in the context of the rib cage wall muscles. Actions of these muscles do not produce major displacements of the abdominal wall; rather, they brace the abdominal wall at the back and alter its stiffness.

Summary of Passive and Active Forces

The respiratory system can exert passive and active forces that are both inspiratory and expiratory. The pulmonary apparatus only exerts passive force (it contains no muscles) and only in the expiratory direction (when it recoils toward a smaller size). The chest wall can exert both passive and active force. At large chest wall sizes, it recoils (passively) inward (expiratory), and at small sizes, it recoils outward (inspiratory). Muscles of the chest wall can generate active force to either inspire or expire the respiratory system at any chest wall size. Muscles that can produce inspiratory force are located in the rib cage wall and diaphragm, and muscles that can produce expiratory force are located in the rib cage wall and abdominal wall.

The chest wall muscles that exert active force on the respiratory system are summarized in Table 2–1. Activation of these muscles can change the volume (size) of the pulmonary apparatus (pulmonary airways and lungs) by increasing or decreasing the circumference of the thorax, increasing or decreasing the vertical length of the thorax (by lowering or raising its floor), or both. Increasing thoracic size (and, thus, increasing the volume of the pulmonary apparatus) is an *inspiratory* action, and decreasing thoracic size is an *expiratory* action.

TABLE 2–1. Muscles of the Chest Wall and Their Potential Actions on the Thorax

Circumference Increasers	Circumference Decreasers
Sternocleidomastoid	*Internal intercostal* (interosseus)
Scalenes (anterior, medius, posterior)	*Transverse thoracis*
Pectoralis major	*Latissimus dorsi*
Pectoralis minor	*Serratus posterior inferior*
Subclavius	*Lateral iliocostalis lumborum*
Serratus anterior	*Lateral iliocostalis thoracis*
External intercostal	*Quadratus lumborum*
Internal intercostal (intercartilaginous)	*Subcostal*
Latissimus dorsi	*Rectus abdominis*
Serratus posterior superior	*External oblique abdominis*
Lateral iliocostalis cervicis	*Internal oblique abdominis*
Lateral iliocostalis thoracis	
Levatores costarum	
Diaphragm	
Vertical Length Increaser	**Vertical Length Decreasers**
Diaphragm	*Rectus abdominis*
	External oblique abdominis
	Internal oblique abdominis
	Transverse abdominis

Note. Those muscles that increase the circumference or increase the vertical length of the thorax are considered *inspiratory* muscles and those that decrease the circumference or decrease the vertical length of the thorax are considered *expiratory* muscles.

Realization of Passive and Active Forces

Forces of breathing are realized in two ways. One way is through pulls on structures and the other way is through pressures developed at various locations within the respiratory system. Pulling forces are distributed in a complex fashion. Fortunately, they are uniformly distributed at certain points where they manifest as pressures. The locations of the most important of these pressures are shown in Figure 2–8.

Included among these pressures are alveolar pressure, pleural pressure, abdominal pressure, and transdiaphragmatic pressure. Alveolar pressure is the pressure inside the lungs, pleural pressure is the pressure inside the thorax but outside the lungs (between the pleural membranes), abdominal pressure is the pressure inside the abdominal cavity, and transdiaphragmatic pressure is the difference in pressure across the diaphragm (the difference between pleural pressure and abdominal pressure). The most important pressure for understanding of speech production is alveolar pressure. A reasonably good estimate of alveolar pressure during speech production can be obtained by measuring the pressure in the trachea.

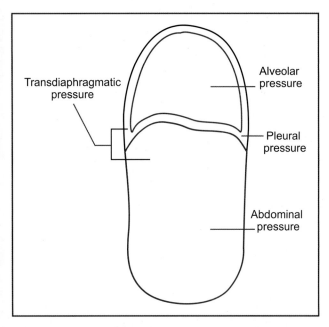

FIGURE 2–8. Important pressures of the respiratory system. Alveolar pressure is the pressure inside the lungs and is the most important pressure for speech production. Pleural pressure is the pressure between the pleural (visceral and parietal) membranes. Abdominal pressure is the pressure inside the abdomen. Transdiaphragmatic pressure (meaning the pressure across the diaphragm) is the difference between the pleural and abdominal pressures.

Needling the Teacher

One way to tap tracheal pressure is to puncture the trachea with a hypodermic needle. We know someone whose tracheal pressure was studied this way. The physician inserted the needle (attached to a syringe) but had difficulty on the first attempt. He withdrew the needle and made a successful second insertion. After the study, the subject went off to teach. Shortly into the lecture, a pea-size bump rose on his neck. As the lecture continued, the bump enlarged to walnut size. Seeing it continue to grow, a student told the teacher what was happening. In the emergency room, it was discovered that the teacher had emphysema (air inflation) within the interstices (spaces) inside his neck. Some air had apparently been pumped into the interstices during attempts at needle insertion. When the teacher raised his internal pressures to speak, this air was forced to the surface and made his neck balloon. Never again did he allow himself to be needled.

MOVEMENTS OF THE RESPIRATORY SYSTEM

Breathing, speaking, and other activities carried out by the respiratory system are accomplished through movements of the rib cage wall, diaphragm, and abdominal wall. These movements can be described for each part individually, as they are below. Nevertheless, the forces that underlie these movements are not necessarily easy to determine. This is because the interactions among the different parts of chest wall are quite complex.

Movements of Rib Cage Wall

The rib cage wall is able to move because it includes two sets of joints, those between the ribs and sternum (costosternal joints) and those between the ribs and the vertebral column (costovertebral joints). Actual movement differs somewhat from rib to rib, owing to differences in the lengths and shapes of individual ribs. Nevertheless, two types of rib movements are typical; these are illustrated in Figure 2–9. One type of rib movement is a vertical excursion of its front (sternal) end and is either upward and forward or downward and backward, resulting in an increase or decrease,

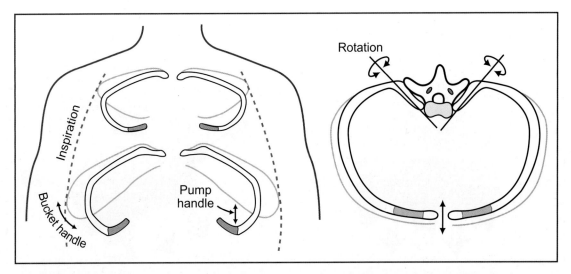

FIGURE 2–9. Two types of rib movements. They are (1) upward and forward/downward and backward (like the handle on a water pump) and (2) upward and outward/downward and inward (like a bucket handle).

respectively, in the front-to-back diameter of the rib cage. Each rib rotates through the axis of its neck (at the back near the vertebral column) in a movement pattern that resembles the raising and lowering of the handle on a water pump.

Not Doing What Comes Naturally

The initiation and execution of voluntary breathing movements comes naturally for most of us. But, for some individuals with maldeveloped or damaged brains, these may not be easy, or even possible, to do. Their problem is praxis or action. They have dyspraxia when they have difficulty with action and apraxia when they are unable to carry out action at all. One of the most perplexing clients we ever encountered was a young man who showed difficulties with breathing actions following a traumatic brain injury. When he attempted to initiate voluntary inspirations or expirations on command, he often became frozen in position. Occasionally, his attempt resulted in movement in the opposite direction (he breathed in when trying to breathe out). He knew exactly what he wanted to do but just couldn't do it. Imagine the depth of his frustration.

The other type of rib movement is vertical excursion along the side of the rib cage that involves a rotation of the rib around an axis extending between its two ends. The rotation is either upward and outward or downward and inward, the result being an increase or decrease, respectively, in the side-to-side (transverse) diameter of the rib cage. Such movement is similar to the raising and lowering of the handle on a water bucket.

These two types of rib movement occur together and in phase. Thus, the circumference of the rib cage wall increases and decreases along with simultaneous increases and decreases in its two diameters (front-to-back and side-to-side).

Movements of the Diaphragm

The diaphragm can enlarge the thorax vertically by pulling down on the central tendon or it can enlarge the thorax circumferentially by elevating the lower ribs. It can also do both simultaneously, as depicted in Figure 2–10.

The actions of the diaphragm (Figure 2–10), as well as the actions of the rib cage wall and abdominal wall, can change the configuration of the diaphragm such that it can flatten or become more highly domed, as illustrated in Figure 2–11. Flattening is accompanied by descent of the central tendon and/or elevation of the lower ribs; doming of the diaphragm is accompanied by elevation of the central tendon and/or descent of the lower ribs. In general, the more highly domed the diaphragm, the more active (inspiratory) force it is able to exert. This is because its muscle fibers are stretched and are on more favorable portions of their length-force characteristics.

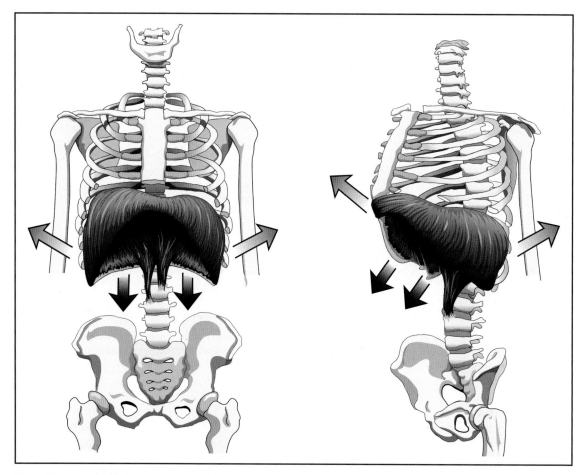

FIGURE 2–10. Actions of the diaphragm. The diaphragm can enlarge the thorax vertically by pulling the central tendon downward and forward (*downward pointing arrows*) and it can expand the thorax circumferentially by lifting the lower ribs (*upward pointing arrows*). Structural features from *Evaluation and Management of Speech Breathing Disorders: Principles and Methods* (p. 25), by T. Hixon and J. Hoit, 2005, Tucson, AZ: Redington Brown. Copyright 2005 by Thomas J. Hixon and Jeannette D. Hoit. Modified and reproduced with permission.

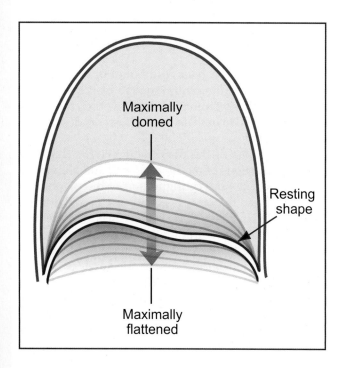

FIGURE 2–11. Configurations of the diaphragm. The diaphragm can assume a flattened configuration by descent of the central tendon and/or lifting of the lower ribs, and a domed configuration by elevation of the central tendon and/or descent of the lower ribs.

Movements of the diaphragm are hidden from view and usually must be inferred from movements of more superficial structures of the chest wall. (For an "inside" view of diaphragm movement, see Video 2–3.) Diaphragm movements are manifested in changes in the radius of its curvature and depend on the relative fixation of the lower ribs and central tendon. When the rib cage is fixed in position, the movement of the diaphragm is reflected superficially in movement of the abdominal wall; when the central tendon is fixed in position, the movement of the diaphragm is reflected in movement of the rib cage wall.

Movements of the Abdominal Wall

When at rest in an upright position, the lower abdominal wall is distended somewhat because the pressure inside the abdomen is greater near the bottom than near the undersurface of the diaphragm. This pressure pushes the lower abdominal wall outward. Inward movement flattens the abdominal wall and outward movement increases the degree to which the abdominal wall is protruded. Most movement occurs in the anteroposterior dimension, as depicted in Figure 2–12.

Relative Movements of the Rib Cage Wall and Diaphragm-Abdominal Wall

The rib cage wall contacts about three-fourths of the surface of the pulmonary apparatus, whereas the diaphragm-abdominal wall unit contacts only about one fourth of the surface area. This means that a small

movement of the rib cage wall can move a substantial amount of air into or out of the pulmonary apparatus or cause a large change in pressure within the pulmonary apparatus. In contrast, the diaphragm-abdominal wall unit must move a much greater distance to displace (move) the same amount of air or create the same alveolar pressure change. The relative consequences of rib cage wall movement versus diaphragm-abdominal wall movement on pulmonary volume and pressure are illustrated in Figure 2–13.

Forces Underlying Movements

Movements of the respiratory system can look deceptively simple, but they are not. A couple of examples will demonstrate the complexities of determining what forces underlie respiratory movements. Take the example of the rib cage wall moving outward. It might be assumed that this movement was produced by activation of inspiratory rib cage wall muscles, and this might be correct, but it might also be incorrect. It is also possible that the abdominal muscles activated and pushed the rib cage wall outward through its structural attachments and through the raising of abdominal pressure. Consider another example wherein the abdominal wall moves outward. It is clear in this case that the abdominal wall did not move itself outward because the abdominal wall contains no inspiratory muscles. Therefore, it must have been moved outward by some other part of the chest wall. Which part is not obvious, however, because either (or both) the diaphragm and the rib cage wall can generate forces that could move the abdominal wall outward. Thus, a good rule of thumb is to recognize that just because a particular respiratory structure moved does not mean that it necessarily moved itself.

RESPIRATORY CONTROL VARIABLES

The respiratory system controls a number of variables, some of which are particularly important to speech production. These variables are lung volume, alveolar pressure, and chest wall shape.

Lung Volume

Volume is defined as the size of a three-dimensional object or space. The volume of interest here is the volume of air inside the pulmonary apparatus. This volume is called the lung volume, and it reflects the size of the respiratory system. Movements of

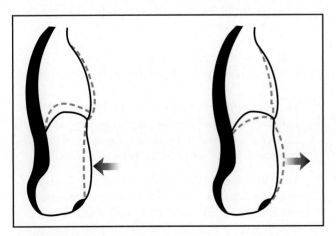

FIGURE 2–12. Inward and outward movements of the abdominal wall.

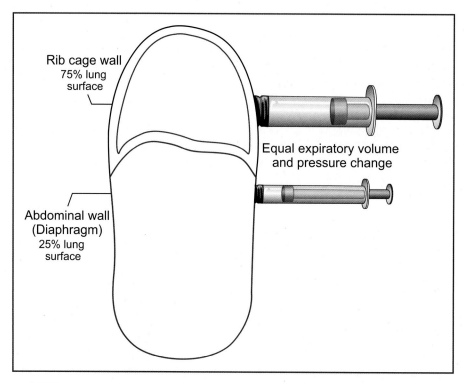

FIGURE 2–13. Relative movements of the rib cage wall and diaphragm-abdominal wall. The different-sized plungers represent the fact that a small movement of the rib cage wall can cause a large volume or pressure change within the pulmonary apparatus when compared to the same movement of the diaphragm-abdominal wall. This is because the rib cage wall covers approximately three times as much surface area of the pulmonary apparatus compared to the diaphragm-abdominal wall.

the respiratory system can change lung volume by moving air into or out of the pulmonary apparatus. Such movement, sometimes called volume displacement, can occur only if the larynx and upper airway are open.

The volume variable can be partitioned into what are called lung volumes and lung capacities. As shown in Figure 2–14, volume can be displayed in a spirogram, a record of lung volume change over time obtained from a spirometer (a device that records volume displacement).

There are four lung volumes. Each covers a portion of the lung volume range that is mutually exclusive of the others.

The *tidal volume* (TV) is the volume of air inspired or expired during the breathing cycle. When recorded in the resting individual, this volume is termed the *resting tidal volume.*

The *inspiratory reserve volume* (IRV) is the maximum volume of air that can be inspired from the tidal end-inspiratory level (the peak of the tidal volume cycle).

The *expiratory reserve volume* (ERV) is the maximum volume of air that can be expired from the tidal end-expiratory level (the trough of the tidal volume cycle).

The *residual volume* (RV) is the volume of air remaining in the pulmonary apparatus at the end of a maximum voluntary expiration. This volume cannot be measured directly.

There are four lung capacities. Each capacity includes two or more of the lung volumes defined above.

The *inspiratory capacity* (IC) is the maximum volume of air that can be inspired from the resting tidal end-expiratory level. It is the sum of the tidal volume and the inspiratory reserve volume.

The *vital capacity* (VC) is the maximum volume of air that can be expired following a maximum inspiration (or inspired following a maximum expiration). It includes the inspiratory reserve volume, the tidal volume, and the expiratory reserve volume.

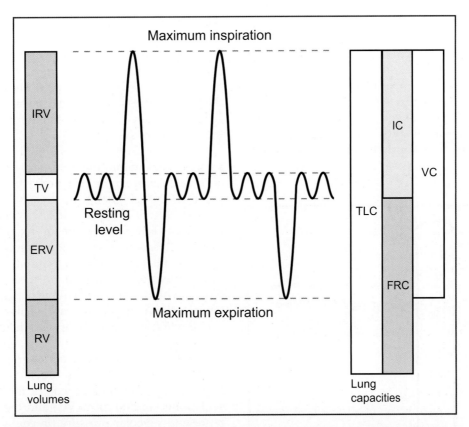

FIGURE 2–14. A spirogram showing lung volumes and lung capacities. The lung volumes are tidal volume (TV), inspiratory reserve volume (IRV), expiratory reserve volume (ERV), and residual volume (RV). The lung capacities are inspiratory capacity (IC), vital capacity (VC), functional residual capacity (FRC), and total lung capacity (TLC). From *Evaluation and Management of Speech Breathing Disorders: Principles and Methods* (p. 36), by T. Hixon and J. Hoit, 2005, Tucson, AZ: Redington Brown. Copyright 2005 by Thomas J. Hixon and Jeannette D. Hoit. Modified and reproduced with permission.

The *functional residual capacity* (FRC) is the volume of air in the pulmonary apparatus at the resting tidal end-expiratory level. This capacity includes the expiratory reserve volume and the residual volume. Because this includes the residual volume, it cannot be measured directly.

The *total lung capacity* (TLC) is the volume of air in the pulmonary apparatus at the end of a maximum inspiration. It includes the inspiratory reserve volume, the tidal volume, the expiratory reserve volume, and the residual volume. This lung capacity cannot be measured directly because it includes the residual volume.

Where Did That Come From?

We have seen many young children with cerebral palsy and breathing disorders. Many of these children, especially those who are quadriplegic and show major signs of spasticity, seem almost to have a governor on them that limits the degree to which they can willfully adjust the respiratory system. For example, when asked to perform an inspiratory capacity maneuver ("Take in all the air you can"), they may only be able to inspire to their resting tidal end-inspiratory level. Try it over and over again and the same thing happens. Then, out of the blue, the child shows you a gaping yawn of boredom and takes in an enormous breath. The breath may actually be several times the size the child could generate during voluntary inspiration. Now, you're faced with a dilemma. What do you record as the child's inspiratory capacity? Think about it, carefully.

The lung volumes used in a number of everyday breathing activities are shown in Figure 2–15. Here, lung volume is expressed in percent vital capacity (% VC), a common way of expressing breathing events because it allows for comparisons across people of different sizes. Note that in this figure, the volume of the respiratory system at the end of a resting tidal expiration is shown as 40% VC. This is a typical resting level for someone in an upright (sitting or standing) body position.

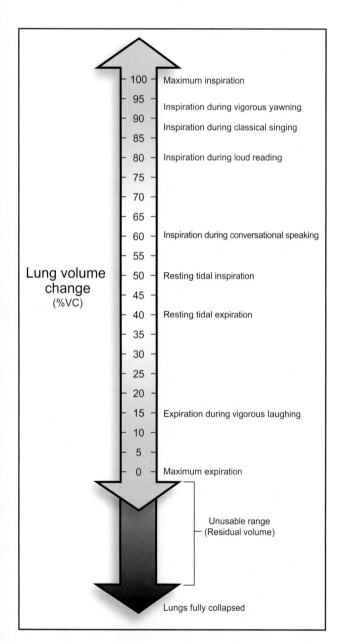

FIGURE 2–15. Lung volumes used in some everyday activities expressed in percent vital capacity (% VC) and performed in an upright body position. Some of these volumes shift when performed in other body positions.

Alveolar Pressure

Pressure is defined as a force distributed over a surface (pressure = force/area). The most important pressure for present purposes is the pressure inside the lungs, the alveolar pressure. Alveolar pressure represents the sum of all the passive and active forces operating on the respiratory system.

Alveolar pressure is generated by the collision of air molecules within the pulmonary apparatus. When air molecules are more crowded, more collisions occur and pressure is higher. In contrast, when air molecules are less crowded, fewer collisions occur and alveolar pressure is lower. When the larynx and/or upper airway are closed, lung volume and alveolar pressure are inversely related. That is, in a closed system, a halving of volume causes a doubling of pressure, and a doubling of volume causes a halving of pressure (provided temperature remains constant). This is called Boyle's law. Boyle's law does not apply when the larynx and upper airway are open.

One way to display alveolar pressure is in a volume-pressure diagram, such as that shown in Figure 2–16. The vertical axis of the diagram represents lung volume (in % VC) and the horizontal axis represents alveolar pressure (in centimeters of water, cmH$_2$O). The light horizontal line represents the resting level of the respiratory system (resting end-expiration), shown to be 40% VC in this diagram. The light vertical

Always Under Pressure

The zero pressure seen on breathing diagrams really doesn't mean zero. It actually represents atmospheric pressure, the pressure we are under all the time. Far from zero, atmospheric pressure has a magnitude of 1.01325×10^5 newtons per square meter (N/m^2). That's roughly 1,000 centimeters of water (cmH$_2$O), a unit of pressure measurement often used by respiratory physiologists. When we blow our hardest, we might (on a good day) develop 225 cmH$_2$O of alveolar pressure. That's interesting. We blow as hard as we possibly can, and we can only increase our alveolar pressure to about one-fourth the magnitude of the pressure that is operating on us as we just sit there. Because it acts on us from all directions, we aren't even aware that we have 1,000 cmH$_2$O of pressure continuously trying to squash us. But, in fact, we're always under pressure.

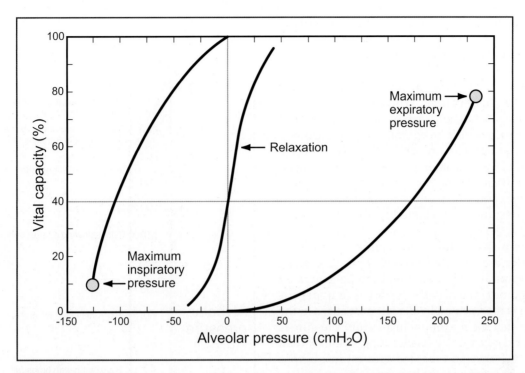

FIGURE 2-16. Volume-pressure diagram (for an upright body position). Volume is shown on the vertical axis (in percent vital capacity, % VC) ranging from 0% to 100%. Alveolar pressure is on the horizontal axis (in centimeters of water, cmH₂O) ranging from negative to positive pressures. Alveolar pressure is 0 (atmospheric) at 40% VC in this diagram. Relaxation pressure *(curved line in the middle of the diagram)* is the passive pressure generated in the absence of active muscular pressure and is negative (inspiratory) at small lung volumes (smaller than 40% VC in this diagram) and positive (expiratory) at large lung volumes (larger than 40% VC in this diagram). Maximum inspiratory pressure is generated with passive plus maximum active inspiratory muscular pressure at the prevailing lung volume and is represented by the curved line to the left of the Relaxation line. The lower left circle represents the greatest negative (inspiratory) pressure achievable. Maximum expiratory pressure is generated with passive plus maximum active expiratory muscular pressure at the prevailing lung volume and is represented by the curved line to the right of the Relaxation line. The upper right circle represents the greatest positive (expiratory) pressure achievable. Modified from *Evaluation and Management of Speech Breathing Disorders: Principles and Methods* (p. 38), by T. Hixon and J. Hoit, 2005, Tucson, AZ: Redington Brown. Copyright 2005 by Thomas J. Hixon and Jeannette D. Hoit. Modified and reproduced with permission.

line represents atmospheric pressure (zero, by convention). Points to the left of this line represent pressures that are below atmospheric (negative, by convention) and points to the right of this line represent pressures that are above atmospheric (positive, by convention). The middle, curved line labeled "Relaxation" represents the volume-pressure relation when the muscles of the respiratory system are completely quiescent and the larynx or upper airway is closed.

The relaxation pressure is the pressure produced entirely by the passive force of the respiratory system. As shown in Figure 2–16, the relaxation pressure varies with lung volume. Relaxation pressure is positive at lung volumes larger than the resting level of the respi-

ratory system (40% VC in the figure) and negative at lung volumes smaller than the resting level. The greatest positive relaxation pressure is generated at the largest lung volume, and the greatest negative relaxation pressure is generated at the smallest lung volume. In the midrange of the vital capacity, the relaxation pressure changes nearly in direct proportion to lung volume change, whereas at the extremes of the vital capacity, pressure changes more abruptly with volume change. This is because the respiratory system is stiffer at very large and very small lung volumes.

Departures from the relaxation pressure require active muscular pressure. A net inspiratory muscular pressure is needed to generate pressure that is lower than the relaxation pressure (to the left of the volume-pressure relaxation curve) at the prevailing lung volume. In contrast, a net expiratory muscular pressure is needed to generate pressure that is higher than the relaxation pressure (to the right of the relaxation curve) at the prevailing lung volume. When net is specified, as it is here, it means that both inspiratory and expiratory muscular pressures may be operating simultaneously, but one or the other is predominating. When pressure is equal to the relaxation pressure, this may mean that all the muscles of the chest wall are relaxed, or it may mean that equal inspiratory and expiratory muscular pressures are being exerted so that they cancel one another.

Maximum inspiratory and expiratory pressure characteristics are also depicted in Figure 2–16. The maximum inspiratory pressure that can be generated by the respiratory system (with the larynx or upper airway closed) is represented by the leftmost curve in the figure. Note that the maximum inspiratory pressure is greater (more negative) at smaller lung volumes than larger lung volumes and that the greatest inspiratory pressure is generated near the bottom of the vital capacity (see the circle labeled "Maximum inspiratory pressure"). This is because negative relaxation pressure is more forceful at smaller lung volumes and because the inspiratory muscles are operating under more favorable length-force conditions at smaller lung volumes.

The maximum expiratory pressure that can be generated by the respiratory system (with the larynx or upper airway closed) is represented by the rightmost curve in Figure 2–16. The maximum expiratory pressure is greater (more positive) at larger lung volumes than smaller lung volumes, and the greatest expiratory pressure is generated at near the top of the vital capacity (see the circle labeled "Maximum expiratory pressure"). This is because positive relaxation pressure is more forceful at larger lung volumes and because the expiratory muscles are operating under more favorable length-force conditions at larger lung volumes.

Figure 2–17 shows the range of alveolar pressures (in cmH$_2$O) that might be generated by a healthy young man. Shown along the pressure scale is a list of activities and typical alveolar pressures associated with those activities.

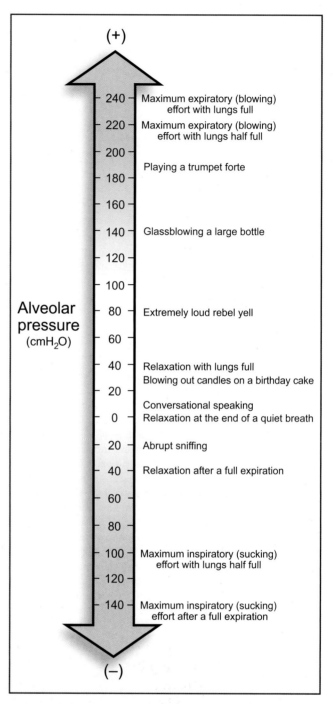

FIGURE 2–17. Alveolar pressures (in cmH$_2$O) used for different activities. The range of values shown here approximate those of a healthy young man.

Chest Wall Shape

Shape is the configuration of an object, independent of its volume (size). The shape of interest in the present context is the shape of the chest wall. Chest wall shape refers to the surface configuration of the rib cage wall and abdominal wall, the two parts of the chest wall that can be observed externally. Shape is important because it provides information about the prevailing mechanical advantages of different parts of the chest wall and clues about what muscle groups might be activated.

One convention for illustrating shape is to display the relative sizes of the rib cage wall and abdominal wall against one another, as portrayed in Figure 2–18. In this figure, the size of the rib cage wall is on the vertical axis, increasing upward, and the size of the abdominal wall is on the horizontal axis, increasing rightward. The actual size measurement may be a circumference or anteroposterior diameter, depending on the type of instrumentation used.

The dashed line in Figure 2–18 represents the relaxation characteristic of the chest wall. This is the shape assumed by the chest wall at different lung volumes when the breathing muscles are completely relaxed. The open circle at the top of the relaxation characteristic represents the total lung capacity, and the open circle at the bottom of the characteristic represents the residual volume. The filled circle represents the resting level of the respiratory system (recall the resting spring analogy represented in Figure 2–4, bottom right). The circumscribed area in the diagram depicts the full range of shapes that the chest wall can assume. Each point within the circumscribed area represents a unique combination of chest wall shape and lung volume.

Figure 2–19 shows the range of achievable chest wall shapes (in relative terms) and activities associated with those shapes. A chest wall shape near the bottom of the arrow is characterized by a larger-than-relaxed abdominal wall and a smaller-than-relaxed rib cage wall; this shape would be represented to the right of the relaxation characteristic in Figure 2–18. Conversely, a chest wall shape characterized by a smaller-than-relaxed abdominal wall and a larger-than-relaxed rib cage wall (upper part of arrow in Figure 2–19) would be represented to the left of the relaxation characteristic in Figure 2–18.

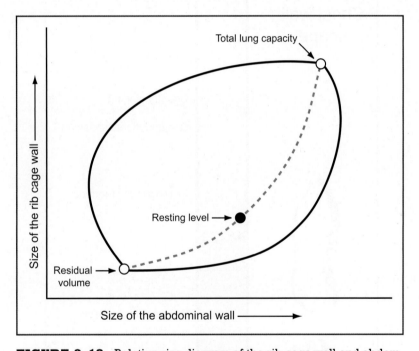

FIGURE 2–18. Relative size diagram of the rib cage wall and abdominal wall to represent chest wall shape. Rib cage wall size is shown as increasing upward on the vertical axis and abdominal wall size is shown as increasing rightward on the horizontal axis. The dashed line represents the continuum of chest wall shapes assumed during relaxation (no muscle activity) throughout the vital capacity. The solid lines represent the most extreme chest wall shapes that can be assumed (using muscle activity) throughout the vital capacity (from residual volume to total lung capacity). The resting level of the lung volume (resting end expiration) is shown as a filled circle at approximately 40% VC in this figure (as is typical in upright body positions). Modified from *Evaluation and Management of Speech Breathing Disorders: Principles and Methods* (p. 41), by T. Hixon and J. Hoit, 2005, Tucson, AZ: Redington Brown. Copyright 2005 by Thomas J. Hixon and Jeannette D. Hoit. Modified and reproduced with permission.

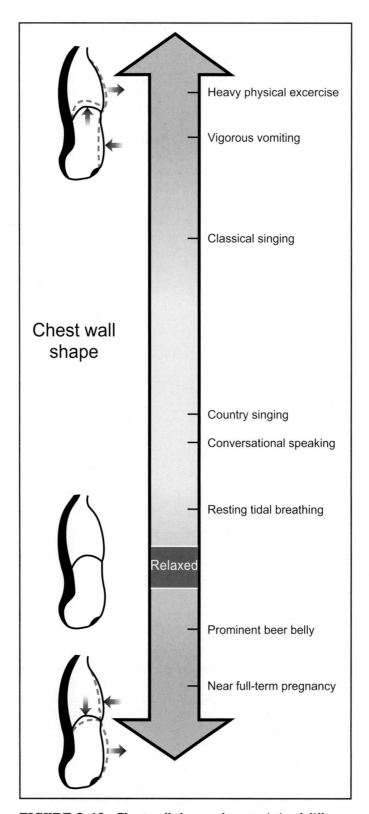

FIGURE 2–19. Chest wall shapes characteristic of different events and conditions. Shapes range from a larger-than-relaxed abdominal wall and a smaller-than-relaxed rib cage wall (*bottom part of arrow*) to a smaller-than-relaxed abdominal wall and a larger-than-relaxed rib cage wall (*upper part of arrow*).

NEURAL SUBSTRATES OF RESPIRATORY CONTROL

The respiratory system is controlled by the central nervous system (brain and spinal cord) and selected nerves within the peripheral nervous system (cranial and spinal nerves), as illustrated very simply in Figure 2–20. The brainstem (lower part of the brain) is responsible for the control of tidal breathing, and higher brain centers are responsible for controlling special acts of breathing. Control of all respiratory activities is played out through peripheral nerves (including spinal nerves and some cranial nerves). Much more

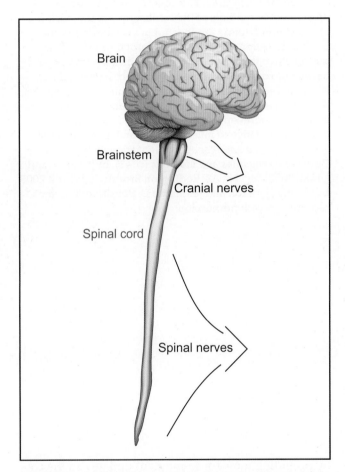

FIGURE 2–20. The central nervous system (brain and spinal cord) and peripheral nervous system (cranial and spinal nerves). Control of tidal breathing is vested in the brainstem and control of special acts of breathing is vested in higher brain centers. Control commands are sent to muscles through peripheral nerves. From *Evaluation and Management of Speech Breathing Disorders: Principles and Methods* (p. 43), by T. Hixon and J. Hoit, 2005, Tucson, AZ: Redington Brown. Copyright 2005 by Thomas J. Hixon and Jeannette D. Hoit. Modified and reproduced with permission.

information is provided about the nervous system and its role in speech production in Chapter 8.

Control of Tidal Breathing

Tidal breathing, the most common form of breathing, is sometimes called automatic breathing, metabolic breathing, or involuntary breathing. The control of tidal breathing is vested in the brainstem, primarily in structures located in the medulla, the lowest region of the brainstem that is contiguous with the spinal cord. These structures contain a network of neurons (nerve cells) that generate a rhythmic pattern of breathing and regulate gas levels (oxygen and carbon dioxide) in arterial blood by adjusting ventilation (the amount of air inspired or expired). This network is often called the central pattern generator for breathing. It can run breathing on its own automatically without input from higher brain centers.

Signals from the brainstem travel via peripheral nerves to reach the muscles of the chest wall. For example, signals from the brainstem reach the *diaphragm* muscle via the phrenic nerve and cause its fibers to contract for inspiration. Signals may also travel via other spinal nerves to the *external intercostal* muscles, causing them either to stiffen the rib cage wall (during resting tidal inspiration) or to assist the diaphragm as a supplemental prime mover (during more forceful tidal inspiration). Signals are sent simultaneously through cranial nerves to enlarge the laryngeal airway and stiffen the tissues of the upper airway to make it less likely that the airways will be sucked inward during inspiration.

The breathing pattern generated by the brainstem is strongly conditioned by afferent (incoming) information from a variety of sources. Most of the time, this afferent information is received and processed unconsciously. Sometimes, however, afferent information is processed to a level of awareness (sensation) or to a level of meaning and association (perception). At such times, individuals may begin to consciously attend to their breathing and to develop breathing-related perceptions having to do with forces, movements, and feelings of breathing comfort or discomfort.

The most important afferent information comes from chemoreceptors and mechanoreceptors. Chemoreceptors are sensitive to chemical status, and those most relevant to breathing are called central and peripheral chemoreceptors. As illustrated in Figure 2–21, central chemoreceptors are located on the front and side surfaces of the medulla, and peripheral chemoreceptors are located in what are called the carotid bodies at the bifurcation of the common carotid arter-

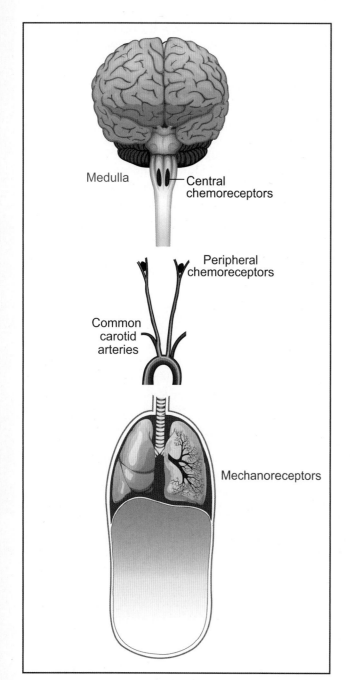

Medulla

Central chemoreceptors

Peripheral chemoreceptors

Common carotid arteries

Mechanoreceptors

FIGURE 2–21. Central and peripheral chemoreceptors and mechanoreceptors. The central chemoreceptors are located in the medulla of the brainstem and the peripheral chemoreceptors are located in the carotid bodies at the bifurcation of the common carotid arteries. They are sensitive to changes in gas composition (oxygen and carbon dioxide) in the blood and cerebral spinal fluid. Mechanoreceptors are found in the pulmonary apparatus; these are sensitive to stretch, irritants, and alveolar distortion. Mechanoreceptors are also found in the chest wall; these are sensitive to muscle length and force changes. From *Evaluation and Management of Speech Breathing Disorders: Principles and Methods* (p. 43), by T. Hixon and J. Hoit, 2005, Tucson, AZ: Redington Brown. Copyright 2005 by Thomas J. Hixon and Jeannette D. Hoit. Modified and reproduced with permission.

ies, near the major blood supply to the brain. Central chemoreceptors respond primarily to changes in the amount of carbon dioxide in cerebral spinal fluid (fluid that surrounds the brain and spinal cord), and peripheral chemoreceptors are the primary oxygen sensors for the body, although they also respond to changes in the level of carbon dioxide and acidity-alkalinity (pH, potential of hydrogen) balance in arterial blood. Central and peripheral chemoreceptors generally act synergistically to stimulate adjustments in breathing by providing moment-to-moment updates on the concentration of gas in the blood. For example, an increase in carbon dioxide or a decrease in oxygen stimulates the brainstem to send signals through the peripheral nerves to the chest wall muscles to increase breathing.

Mechanoreceptors are sensitive to mechanical changes, and those of special importance to the control of tidal breathing are located in the pulmonary apparatus and chest wall. Those in the pulmonary apparatus respond to stimuli such as the stretching of smooth muscles (such as occurs with an increase in lung volume), airway irritants (such as smoke, dust, chemicals, or cold air), and distortions of the alveolar wall (such as might occur when excess fluid surrounds the alveoli). Signals from these pulmonary mechanoreceptors reach the central nervous system by way of cranial nerve X (vagus). Mechanoreceptors in the chest wall respond to changes in muscle length (such as occur with changes in rib cage wall or abdominal wall volume) or changes in force (such as occur with changes in inspiratory or expiratory muscular efforts). Their afferent signals reach the central nervous system via spinal nerves.

Other afferent input can also influence tidal breathing. For example, afferent signals from mechanoreceptors located in the larynx or upper airway and signals from cranial nerves that transmit visual and auditory information (cranial nerves II and VIII, respectively) can affect breathing. Thus, tidal breathing can be altered by the presence of an irritant in the larynx or upper airway, by images in an action-packed movie, or by musical rhythms (Shea, Walter, Pelley, Murphy, & Guz, 1987; Wyke, 1974).

Tidal breathing can also be influenced by internally generated activity from brain areas outside the brainstem (Mador & Tobin, 1991; Shea, 1996; Shea, Murphy, Hamilton, Benchetrit, & Guz, 1988; Western & Patrick, 1988). For example, cognitive activity (originating from cortical areas), such as that associated with the performance of mental arithmetic, can change tidal breathing. In fact, merely being consciously aware of breathing can change its pattern. Emotional influences (originating from limbic areas) can also have a profound influence on tidal breathing. Feelings of excitement, anger, or fear, for example, can be associated with hyperventilation, breath holding, or erratic breathing. Changes in tidal breathing can even be a primary sign (and feelings of breathlessness a primary symptom) of certain psychogenic disorders, such as anxiety disorder or panic disorder. These types of disorders have been so strongly linked to breathing that they are sometimes classified as hyperventilation disorders (Gardner, 1996).

Control of Special Acts of Breathing

Special acts of breathing can be defined as acts of breathing that are not carried out for the primary purpose of maintaining homeostasis of arterial blood gases (Shea, 1996). They are controlled by higher brain centers that either override or bypass activity of the lower (brainstem) center for breathing (Corfield, Murphy, & Guz, 1998). Special acts of breathing can be vol-

untary (highly conscious), such as breath holding or performing a guided breathing exercise. Or, they can be learned, well practiced, and require little conscious control of breathing—for example, breathing associated with glass blowing, wind instrument playing, singing, or speaking.

It is common for the nervous system to manage multiple breathing-related drives simultaneously, and often these drives compete with one another. Voluntary breath holding is one example. Breath holding is controlled by the cerebral cortex and is a clear demonstration of the ability of the cortex to override the brainstem's control of breathing. Nevertheless, cortical control must eventually give way to brainstem control as danger signals from chemoreceptors make it impossible to continue to inhibit inspiration. Less dramatic examples of competing drives occur frequently and include situations such as attempting to speak while exercising or playing a wind instrument while experiencing stage fright.

Breathing as a Laughing Matter

Breathing plays a huge role in laughter. Much of laughter, especially the hearty type, goes on within the expiratory reserve volume. Laughter also often involves large movements of the abdominal wall. This is probably the reason our folk language is riddled with statements like "I busted a gut laughing," "He kept me in stitches with his jokes," and "We laughed 'til our sides hurt." The neural mechanisms that underlie laughter are different from those that underlie speech breathing. This is illustrated dramatically in persons who can't move the abdominal wall on command or use it for speech production but show vigorous movement of the wall during involuntary laughter. Thus, even if someone appears to be paralyzed, it's always wise to ask the question, "Paralyzed for what activity?"

Peripheral Nerves of Breathing

The peripheral nervous system connects the central nervous system with different parts of the respiratory system via cranial and spinal nerves. Four cranial nerves participate in the control of breathing: Cranial nerves IX (glossopharyngeal), X (vagus), and XII (hypoglossal) innervate muscles that dilate the larynx and stiffen the upper airway during inspiration, and cranial nerve XI (accessory) innervates the *sternocleidomastoid* muscle that elevates the sternum, clavicle, and rib cage.

Twenty-two spinal nerves contribute to the control of breathing. These are listed in Table 2–2 along with the muscles they innervate. As shown there, the spinal nerves relevant to breathing include the 8 cervical (C) nerves, the 12 thoracic (T) nerves, and the first 2 lumbar (L) nerves. Successively lower spinal nerves generally provide motor nerve supply to successively lower regions of the respiratory system. An exception is the diaphragm, which derives its motor nerve supply from C3 to C5, a collection of motor nerves designated as the phrenic nerve. Table 2–2 lists only the motor nerve supply to the chest wall muscles. The sensory nerve supply to the chest wall is generally similar in pattern to its motor nerve supply, a notable exception being that the sensory supply of the diaphragm is vested in the phrenic nerve and lower thoracic nerves.

The Young(er) and the Reckless

Young men contribute mightily to the statistics on spinal cord injury. They tend to engage in activities that involve fast movement and in which collision may occur. And they are often less concerned about taking risks than are their opposite-sex counterparts or their elders. No wonder insurance companies charge them high premiums. There are about 300,000 people in the United States with spinal cord injury (a number equal to the population of St. Louis, Missouri). Each year, about 17,000 new cases are added to the roll. About 80% of people with spinal cord injury are men. Automobile crashes lead the way as the cause, followed by falls, violent acts (such as gunshot wounds), and sports injuries. Although several decades ago, the average age was 29 years, the average has now risen to over 40. It looks like the approach of middle age is no longer quelling the desire to engage in the risk-taking behaviors or that people are living longer after their spinal cord injury.

VENTILATION AND GAS EXCHANGE DURING TIDAL BREATHING

Tidal breathing is the most common type of breathing. Its name comes from the ebb and flow of air that resembles the ebb and flow of an ocean tide. Tidal breathing

TABLE 2–2. Summary of the Segmental Origins of the Motor Nerve Supply to the Muscles of the Chest Wall

Muscle	Spinal Nerve
Rib Cage Wall	
Sternocleidomastoid[a]	C1–C5
Scalenus group	C2–C8
Pectoralis major	C5–C8
Pectoralis minor	C5–C8
Subclavius	C5–C6
Serratus anterior	C5–C7, T2–T3
External intercostals	T1–T11
Internal intercostals	T1–T11
Transversus thoracis	T2–T6
Latissimus dorsi	C6–C8
Serratus posterior superior	T2–T3
Serratus posterior inferior	T9–T12
Lateral iliocostals group	C4–T6, T1–T11, T7–L2
Levatores costarum	C8–T11
Quadratus lumborum	T12–L2
Subcostals	T1–T11
Diaphragm	
Diaphragm	C3–C5
Abdominal Wall	
Rectus abdominis	T7–T12
External oblique	T8–L1
Internal oblique	T8–L1
Transversus abdominis	T7–T12
Latissimus dorsi	See above
Lateral iliocostal lumborum	See above
Quadratus lumborum	See above

Note. C = cervical; T = thoracic; L = lumbar.

[a]Innervation of the **sternocleidomastoid** muscle comes from the spinal portion of the spinal accessory nerve, which is considered a cranial nerve (cranial nerve XI; see Chapter 8). The spinal accessory nerve also innervates the **trapezius** muscle; however, this muscle is not included in this chapter because it does not have a breathing function.

Source: Based on Dickson and Maue-Dickson (1982).

is driven by the need to ventilate (to move air in and out of the pulmonary apparatus) for the purpose of gas exchange (to deliver oxygen, O_2, to the body and remove carbon dioxide, CO_2, from it).

Pink Puffers and Blue Bloaters

No, we're not talking about exotic tropical fish. Pink puffers and blue bloaters are terms that refer to people with chronic obstructive pulmonary disease. Pink puffers suffer mainly from emphysema. Their blood is relatively well saturated with oxygen, making their complexion pink. The puffer part comes from their compensatory expiration through pursed lips. They have decreased lung recoil, decreased vital capacity, increased residual volume, and increased total lung capacity. Blue bloaters suffer mainly from chronic bronchitis. They have associated heart problems with cyanosis and edema. Thus, their bodies turn blue and become bloated. They show decreased vital capacity and increased residual volume. Chronic obstructive pulmonary disease can be nasty and debilitating. Bronchitis may be reversible. Emphysema usually is not.

Figure 2–22 depicts the process of gas exchange. Air, which consists of approximately 21% oxygen, enters the alveoli during tidal breathing. Oxygen then leaves the alveoli and enters the bloodstream to travel to tissues throughout the body. Tissues absorb oxygen from the blood and return carbon dioxide (a by-product of metabolism) to the blood. The carbon dioxide then travels through the bloodstream and eventually reaches the alveoli, where it is released. When metabolic demand increases, as with increased physical or mental activity, more oxygen is consumed and more carbon dioxide is produced. Appropriate levels of oxygen and carbon dioxide are maintained by adjusting ventilation; for example, when metabolic demand is higher, ventilation increases, and when metabolic demand is lower, ventilation decreases. Ventilation can be adjusted by increasing the rate of breathing, increasing the volume of air inspired, or both, as demonstrated in Video 2–4 (Ventilation).

Tidal breathing at rest is associated with a relatively regular inspiration-expiration pattern, as shown in the top panel of Figure 2–23. A tidal breath begins and ends at the resting size of the respiratory system (shown as "0" lung volume in the figure). During inspiration, the chest wall expands, causing the lungs to expand and alveolar pressure to fall. This creates a pressure gradient, with the pressure inside the pulmonary apparatus being lower than that outside the apparatus (see bottom panel of Figure 2–23). As a result, air flows into the pulmonary apparatus and lung volume increases. When equilibration is reached (the pressure outside and inside the pulmonary apparatus is equal), inspiratory airflow ceases (where the dashed line intersects both the upper and lower panels of Figure 2–23).

Expiration begins as the lungs compress and alveolar pressure becomes slightly positive (relative to atmosphere). Expiration continues until the resting level of the respiratory system is reached and alveolar pressure returns to 0 cmH$_2$O (atmospheric). These patterns of lung volume and alveolar pressure change are

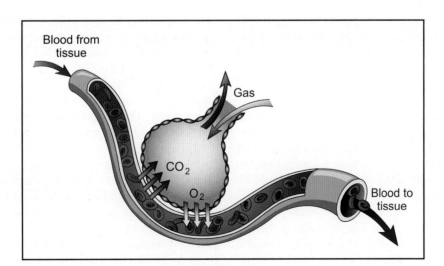

FIGURE 2–22. Gas exchange during tidal breathing. Oxygen is delivered to the blood and carbon dioxide is removed from the blood via the alveoli.

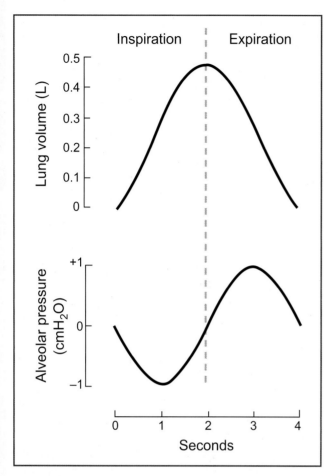

FIGURE 2–23. Pattern of lung volume change (in liters, L) and alveolar pressure change (in cmH₂O) during a single resting tidal breath.

when the diaphragm contracts. Abdominal wall muscle activity usually causes the abdominal wall to move inward slightly. When the abdominal wall moves inward, the rib cage wall is lifted slightly and the diaphragm is pushed slightly headward. This stretches the fibers of the diaphragm so that they are placed on more favorable portions of their length-force characteristics for contraction. In the supine body position, as in the upright body position, the rib cage wall muscles are slightly active to stiffen the rib cage wall. However, in contrast to upright body positions, the abdominal wall muscles are relaxed. This is because the abdominal wall is already pulled inward and the diaphragm is already pushed headward by the force of gravity in supine.

During resting tidal expiration, the passive (recoil) pressure of the respiratory system moves the rib cage wall and abdominal wall inward. Thus, resting tidal expiration is primarily a passive event. Nevertheless, in the upright body position, the abdominal wall muscles remain active throughout the resting tidal breathing cycle.

Although resting tidal breathing shares general features across individuals, its specific details differ from person to person. In fact, each person has what might be thought of as a signature resting tidal breathing pattern that remains relatively unchanged over the years (Benchetrit et al., 1989; Dejours, 1996; Shea & Guz, 1992; Shea, Horner, Benchetrit, & Guz, 1990; Shea, Walter, Murphy, & Guz, 1987).

RESPIRATORY FUNCTION AND SPEECH PRODUCTION

The respiratory system provides the driving forces that generate speech and contribute substantially to the control of speech intensity (loudness), linguistic stress (emphasis), and the segmentation (division) of speech into units (syllables, words, phrases). At the same time that it performs these speech-related functions, the respiratory system continues to serve its primary functions of ventilation and gas exchange.

This section describes two forms of speech breathing—extended steady utterances and running speech activities—as performed in an upright body position (standing or seated erect). These are based on the conceptualizations and elaborations of others (Hixon, 1973; Hixon et al., 1973; Hixon, Mead, & Goldman, 1976; Weismer, 1985). More detailed information can be found elsewhere (Hixon & Hoit, 2005; Hixon, Weismer, & Hoit, 2020).

generally the same across body positions, except that the absolute lung volume range differs with body position. For example, resting tidal breathing ranges from about 40% to 50% VC in upright body positions and from about 20% to 30% VC in the supine (lying on one's back, facing upward) body position.

Resting tidal breathing is driven by a combination of passive and active forces that are somewhat dependent on body position. These forces are summarized graphically in Figure 2–24 for two body positions: upright and supine. During inspiration, essentially all of the active force comes from the diaphragm. This is true for all body positions. In the upright body position, some other chest wall muscles are also active during inspiration (Hixon, Goldman, & Mead, 1973; Loring & Mead, 1982). Rib cage wall muscle activity stiffens the rib cage wall to prevent it from being sucked inward

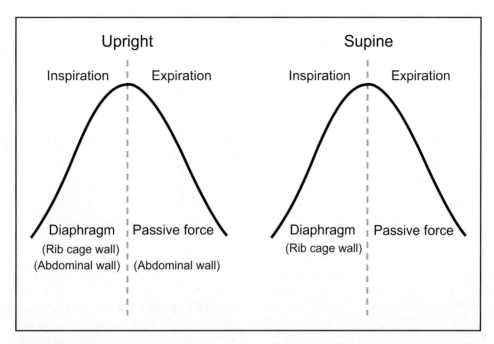

FIGURE 2–24. Passive and active forces of resting tidal breathing in upright and supine body positions. In both body positions, the diaphragm is the primary muscle of inspiration. In upright, the rib cage wall and abdominal wall muscles are also tonically (continuously) active, but only to enhance the mechanical conditions for diaphragm contraction. In supine, the force of gravity supplants the need for the abdominal wall muscles to activate. Expiration is driven by passive force (recoil of the respiratory system) in both body positions, though the abdominal muscles usually remain active during expiration in upright.

Thomas J. Hixon (1940–2009)

Tom was a mentor to all three of us and the lead author of our *Preclincal* textbook. He was also the speech scientist who put *speech breathing* on the map. At age 25, Tom burst on the scene, having already completed his master's degree (in 1 year) and his PhD (in 2 years!) from the University of Iowa. His intense fascination of speech breathing led him to Harvard, where, under the tutelage of Jere Mead, Tom learned about respiratory mechanics. He spent hours each day in Countway Library poring over articles on respiratory physiology and then more hours poring over data in the laboratory. He immersed himself for years, doing the experiment again and again, until he understood beyond doubt exactly how the respiratory system works for speech production. He completely revolutionized our understanding of this complicated system and then presented it with elegant simplicity in his textbook writings. You can thank Tom for everything you know about speech breathing.

Extended Steady Utterances

An extended steady utterance is one that is produced throughout most of the vital capacity. It begins after taking the deepest inspiration possible and continues until the air supply is depleted. Such an utterance might be a sustained vowel, a sung note, or a series of repeated syllables.

Figure 2–25 shows the lung volume and alveolar pressure events associated with a sustained vowel produced at a usual and steady loudness and voice quality. As can be seen in the figure, lung volume decreases at a

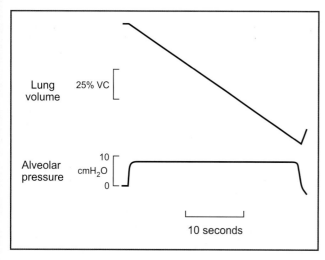

FIGURE 2–25. Lung volume (in % VC) and alveolar pressure (in cmH_2O) events for an extended steady utterance (sustained vowel). Only expiration (vowel production) is represented. From *Evaluation and Management of Speech Breathing Disorders: Principles and Methods* (p. 57), by T. Hixon and J. Hoit, 2005, Tucson, AZ: Redington Brown. Copyright 2005 by Thomas J. Hixon and Jeannette D. Hoit. Modified and reproduced with permission.

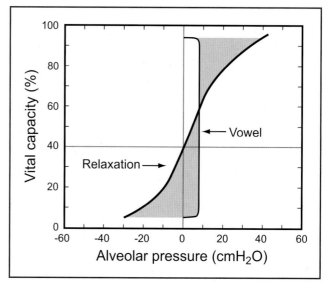

FIGURE 2–26. Volume-pressure diagram illustrating sustained vowel production in the upright body position. The graph depicts the relaxation pressure (*curved line*) and the target alveolar pressure (8 cmH_2O) for the vowel. The horizontal line at 40% VC represents the resting level of the respiratory system. Only expiration (vowel production) is represented. To produce the target alveolar pressure, inspiratory braking (primarily by the inspiratory rib cage wall muscles) is required at the beginning of the vowel. As the vowel proceeds, the need for inspiratory muscle activation ceases and expiratory muscle activation begins. Expiratory muscular pressure (exerted by the expiratory rib cage wall and abdominal wall muscles) becomes increasingly more forceful as the vowel production proceeds into the expiratory reserve volume. From *Evaluation and Management of Speech Breathing Disorders: Principles and Methods* (p. 59), by T. Hixon and J. Hoit, 2005, Tucson, AZ: Redington Brown. Copyright 2005 by Thomas J. Hixon and Jeannette D. Hoit. Modified and reproduced with permission.

constant rate throughout the vital capacity as the utterance progresses. In contrast, alveolar pressure rises abruptly at the beginning of the utterance, remains steady at about 8 cmH_2O throughout the utterance, and falls abruptly as the utterance ends. To watch how lung volume and alveolar pressure change over time during vowel production, see Video 2–5 (Sustained Vowel—Volume and Pressure).

Both relaxation (passive) pressure and active muscular pressure contribute to extended steady utterance production. This is illustrated in Figure 2–26 for the same sustained vowel as that depicted in Figure 2–25. In this graph, the alveolar pressure for the sustained vowel is plotted vertically (rather than horizontally), and time progresses from the top of the graph to the bottom (instead of horizontally left to right), showing lung volume to decrease with utterance production. Lung volume (in % VC) is plotted on the vertical axis, with 40% VC representing the resting level of the respiratory system. Recall that the resting level (size) is that at which the respiratory system is in a mechanically neutral position and alveolar pressure is the same as atmospheric pressure (zero).

At the beginning of the sustained vowel (top of the vowel tracing), the relaxation pressure is a very high positive (expiratory) pressure. In fact, it is much higher than the positive alveolar pressure being targeted for the vowel (approximately 8 cmH_2O). This means that to generate the target alveolar pressure, *inspiratory* muscles must be activated to "hold back" the high expiratory relaxation pressure. This inspiratory braking action (sometimes called checking) is accomplished primarily by the inspiratory rib cage wall muscles, along with a brief activation of the diaphragm.[1] As the utterance proceeds into the midrange of the vital capacity, the relaxation pressure eventually drops below 8 cmH_2O and *expiratory* muscles must be engaged to maintain the target alveolar pressure. These expiratory muscles include both rib cage wall and abdominal wall muscles. As the utterance continues into the expiratory

---

[1]Interestingly, the abdominal muscles are active from the beginning to the end of the sustained utterance. Thus, at the beginning of the utterance, both inspiratory (rib cage wall and diaphragm) and expiratory (abdominal wall muscles) are active, although the net effect is inspiratory.

reserve volume (below the 40% resting level), the expiratory muscles of the rib cage wall and abdominal wall must become increasingly more active to maintain the target alveolar pressure.

Thus, extended steady utterance is produced using a continuously changing combination of relaxation pressure and muscular pressure, and a continuously changing activation of different chest wall muscles. Relaxation pressure goes from substantially positive (expiratory) to substantially negative (inspiratory). Muscular pressure follows an opposite pattern, going from substantially negative (inspiratory) to substantially positive (expiratory) so as to counteract the relaxation pressure and maintain the target alveolar pressure. The inspiratory muscles of the rib cage wall do nearly all of the inspiratory work at large lung volumes (with some help from the diaphragm), and the expiratory muscles of the rib cage wall and abdominal wall muscles do all of the expiratory work.

Running Speech Activities

Running speech activities present different demands and require a different set of muscular strategies than extended steady utterances. Running speech activities include reading aloud, extemporaneous speaking, conversational speaking, and other activities that demand relatively continual utterance production.

Respiratory events associated with running speech activities are much more varied than those associated with extended steady utterances. This is because running speech production is characterized by variations in phonetic content (sounds that differ in voicing and manner of production), prosody (utterances that differ in rate, intonation, loudness variation, and linguistic stress), and voice quality (utterances that differ in breathiness).

Volume events during running speech activities usually occur in the midrange of the vital capacity. As illustrated in the upper part of Figure 2–27, running speech production generally starts at about twice resting tidal breathing depth (or less) and continues to near the resting level of the respiratory system, although at times it may encroach upon the expiratory reserve volume. There are mechanical advantages to speaking in this mid-lung volume range. To begin, the respiratory system is less stiff and the relaxation pressure is not as extreme as at very large and very small lung volumes. Furthermore, the relaxation pressure is positive for most running speech production (because relaxation pressure is positive at lung volumes that are larger than the resting level), and this positive pressure is used to supplement the positive muscular pressure required to achieve the target alveolar pressure. When speech production encroaches upon the expiratory reserve volume, expiratory muscular pressure must be exerted against a negative (inspiratory) relaxation pressure.

Volume change during inspiration is much quicker (that is, airflow is much faster) during running speech breathing than during resting tidal breathing. This is represented in Figure 2–27 (top panel) as a steeper inspiratory (upward) volume slope. In contrast, volume change during expiration is slower than during resting tidal breathing, as indicated by a shallower downward slope. The slower average expiratory airflow can be explained by the valving of the airstream by the larynx and the upper airway articulators that create the sounds of speech.

Alveolar pressure during running speech breathing, shown in the bottom panel of Figure 2–27, is negative during inspiration and positive during expiration. During speaking (expiration), alveolar pressure varies somewhat (in contrast to extended steady vowel production during which loudness is meant to remain constant). Specifically, alveolar pressure often increases momentarily to produce stressed (relatively more prominent) syllables and may decline somewhat near the end of breath groups (thus loudness declines). To watch how lung volume and alveolar pressure change over time during running speech production, see Video 2–6 (Running Speech—Volume and Pressure).

Both relaxation pressure and muscular pressure contribute to the production of running speech breathing, as illustrated in the volume-pressure diagram con-

---

What's Your Sign?

Speech is usually produced on expiration. But it's possible to produce it on inspiration. Try it. It's a bit awkward and difficult at first and your voice may sound higher in pitch and be more harsh than usual. But you should be able to produce quite intelligible speech during inspiration, especially if you whisper. Once in a while, a person is encountered who uses inspiratory speech production. For example, we've seen people who produce voice more easily on inspiration than expiration following surgical reconstruction of a damaged larynx. Some people become so proficient at inspiratory speech production that you can be tricked into believing you're hearing expiratory speech production (with a voice quality disorder). Never take a speaker's sign for granted.

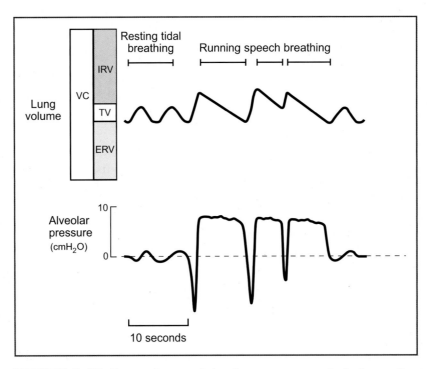

FIGURE 2-27. Lung volume and alveolar pressure events during resting tidal breathing and running speech breathing (such as conversational speaking or reading aloud). Running speech breathing occurs in the midrange of the vital capacity, ranging from about twice resting tidal volume and to near the resting level (note that the resting level is at about 40% of the vital capacity in this figure). Inspirations are faster (steeper volume slope), requiring a larger negative alveolar pressure, and expirations are slower (shallower volume slope), requiring a larger positive alveolar pressure compared to resting tidal breathing. Expiratory volume and duration vary from breath to breath, depending on the length of the phrase. Alveolar pressure during speaking varies slightly depending on variations in linguistic stress and loudness. VC = vital capacity; IRV = inspiratory reserve volume; TV = tidal volume; ERV = expiratory reserve volume.

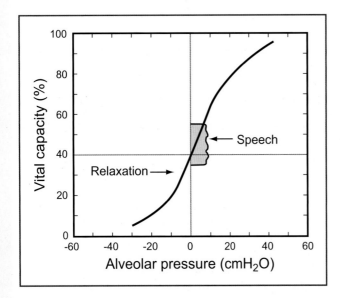

FIGURE 2-28. Volume-pressure diagram illustrating running speech production in the upright body position. The graph depicts the relaxation pressure and the target alveolar pressure (averaging around 8 cmH$_2$O) for one breath group (an expiration containing speech). Relaxation pressure is positive throughout most of the breath group but not positive enough to achieve the target alveolar pressure. Thus, expiratory rib cage and abdominal muscles generate the remaining pressure (with the abdominal muscles predominating). There is *no* inspiratory braking during running speech production. The alveolar pressure varies slightly where certain syllables are stressed.

tained in Figure 2–28. This figure shows a single breath group (meaning an expiration containing speech) of conversational speech. Comparison of the relaxation and speech lines indicates that the target alveolar pressure (averaging around 8 cmH$_2$O) is usually higher (more positive) than the prevailing relaxation pressure. Therefore, positive muscular pressure must be added to the relaxation pressure throughout the breath group. To maintain the target alveolar pressure, the magnitude of the positive muscular pressure increases as the breath group proceeds because the relaxation pressure becomes increasingly less positive and, in fact, becomes negative (inspiratory) as the breath group continues into the expiratory reserve volume (that is, below the resting level of the respiratory system). Note that conversational speaking is produced within a lung volume range that does *not* require inspiratory braking.

The alveolar pressure varies slightly throughout the breath group. This is because alveolar pressure increases (moves farther to the right on the graph) slightly when a syllable is stressed, an adjustment that increases the magnitude of the sound (and causes it to be perceived as louder to the listener). For running speech that is louder overall, the target alveolar pressures are higher on average; conversely, softer speech is produced with lower average alveolar pressure. Thus, louder speech requires higher-than-usual muscular pressure, and softer speech requires lower-than-usual muscular pressure at the prevailing lung volume. Another strategy for producing louder speech is to speak at larger lung volumes where the prevailing relaxation pressure is greater (not shown in the figure).

Expiratory muscles in both the rib cage wall and abdominal wall are active during running speech production in an upright body position, with the abdominal wall muscles contributing a greater proportion of the overall expiratory muscular pressure. The inspiratory phase of the running speech breathing cycle (not included in the figure) is driven by the diaphragm. Interestingly, expiratory muscles of the rib cage wall and abdominal wall maintain a low level of activity during inspiration. This enables them to be in a state of readiness to begin driving expiration (speech production) as soon as inspiration has ended.

The abdominal wall plays an important role in running speech breathing in upright body positions. As mentioned, it generates most of the expiratory muscular pressure during speech production. It is also responsible for imposing the general background configuration assumed by the chest wall throughout the speech breathing cycle (that of a smaller than relaxed abdominal wall and larger than relaxed rib cage wall).

As it turns out, there are important advantages to having the abdominal wall play such a prominent role in running speech breathing.

Figure 2–29 depicts the shape of the chest wall used for running speech activities in the upright body position. This shape is created by inward displacement of the abdominal wall (by its own muscular action). This inward displacement of the abdominal wall has important and beneficial consequences for the diaphragm and rib cage wall. As the abdominal wall moves inward, the diaphragm is pushed headward so that it becomes more domed and its principal muscle fibers elongate. This positions the diaphragm so that it can produce the quick and powerful inspirations that are critical for minimizing interruptions during running speech activities. Inward displacement of the abdominal wall also lifts the rib cage wall. This stretches the expiratory muscles of the rib cage wall, thereby increasing their potential for generating the quick expiratory pulses needed to produce linguistic stress and loudness change. Also, with the abdominal wall held firmly inward, expiratory efforts by the rib cage wall can be fully resolved into pressure change. If the abdominal wall were not held firmly in place, expiratory efforts

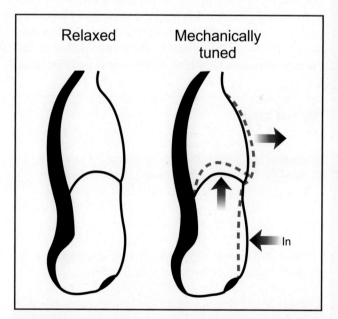

FIGURE 2–29. Shape of the chest wall for running speech activities in an upright body position. This chest wall shape is characterized by an inwardly displaced abdominal wall that causes the diaphragm to move headward and the rib cage wall to lift. This shape "tunes" the diaphragm to produce quick inspirations between breath groups and the expiratory rib cage wall muscles to generate quick expiratory pressure changes during speech production.

of the rib cage wall would move the abdominal wall outward before alveolar pressure could increase. Thus, the activation of abdominal wall muscles and the resultant inward displacement serve to "mechanically tune" the respiratory system for both inspiration and expiration during running speech breathing.

VARIABLES THAT INFLUENCE RESPIRATORY STRUCTURE AND FUNCTION

The previous section describes speech breathing produced in an upright body position by a typical young adult and contains the most important foundational concepts for understanding speech breathing. Nevertheless, several variables that influence speech breathing may be relevant to clinical and research applications. These include body position, body type, age, sex, ventilation and drive to breathe, and cognitive-linguistic and social variables.

Body Position

A change in body position alters the behavior of the respiratory system, primarily because gravity has such a strong influence on this massive structure. Thus, with each new body position, a new muscular solution may need to be found. Most of this section is devoted to discussion of speech breathing in the supine body position (as contrasted to the upright body position discussed above), but other body positions are considered as well.

Figure 2–30 depicts the influence of gravity on the chest wall when moving from upright to supine. When in supine, gravity pulls down on both the rib cage wall and abdominal wall and causes them to move inward. Inward displacement of the abdominal wall pushes the diaphragm toward the head. These actions reduce the size of the resting respiratory system, causing some air to move out of the pulmonary apparatus, usually about 20% VC. Thus, the resting level of the respiratory system decreases from its upright value of about 40% VC to about 20% VC in supine.

Another way to illustrate the effects of moving from upright to supine is with a volume-pressure diagram, such as that shown in Figure 2–31. This figure contains the relaxation characteristic already seen in previous figures (Figures 2–16, 2–26, and 2–28) for the upright body position (shown as a solid curved line). To the right of the upright relaxation characteristic is the relaxation characteristic for supine. Note that the alveolar pressure at any given lung volume is more positive in supine than upright (more rightward along the horizontal axis). Note also that the relaxation characteristic crosses the zero alveolar pressure (vertical) line at 40% VC in upright and at 20% VC in supine.

Now consider Figure 2–32, which contains a volume-pressure diagram containing a single breath group of running speech produced in the supine body position. This shows that speech is produced around the resting level (volume) of the respiratory system,

Flat Out

Two terms that get more than their fair share of misuse are *supine* and *prone*. Supine means lying on your back (usually face up). The easy way to remember this is to consider the spelling of supine. Take out its second letter and you have *spine*. On your spine is on your back. So-called couch potatoes spend a lot of supine time in front of their television sets or smartphones. Prone, also called procumbent, means lying on your front (usually face down). Take its first three letters and you have the first three letters of the word *prostrate* (as in face-down submission or adoration). Certain yoga poses, such as the sphinx pose, begin by assuming a prone position. The confusion encountered when using the terms *supine* and *prone* arises because both involve being flat out. The memory devices suggested here should make it easy to keep the two body positions straight (pun intended).

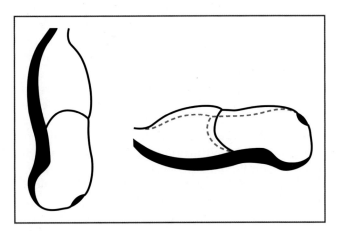

FIGURE 2–30. Gravitational effects on the respiratory system. When moving from upright (*left torso*) to supine (*right torso*), the resting respiratory system becomes smaller because gravity pulls downward on the rib cage wall and abdominal wall and moves the diaphragm headward (shown by the dashed lines). These actions make the thorax smaller and result in some air moving out of the pulmonary apparatus (about 20% VC).

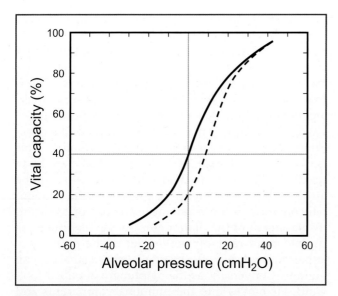

FIGURE 2–31. Gravitational effects on the volume-pressure relaxation characteristic of the respiratory system. When moving from upright (*solid curved line*) to supine (*dashed curved line*), the relaxation characteristic moves to the right. This means that the relaxation (passive) pressure at a given lung volume is more positive in supine than upright. It also means that the resting size (lung volume) of the respiratory system is smaller (by about 20% VC) in supine.

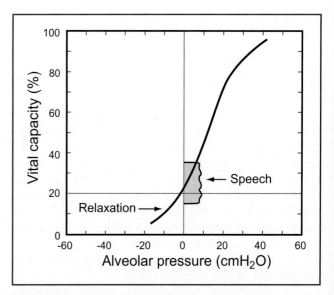

FIGURE 2–32. Volume-pressure diagram illustrating one breath group of running speech production in the supine body position. The diagram depicts the relaxation pressure (*curved line*) and target alveolar pressure (averaging about 8 cmH$_2$O). Note that speech is produced near the resting level (volume) of the respiratory system, which in supine is 20% VC.

even though it has shifted downward (become smaller) by 20% VC. Stated differently, lung volume events for speaking range from about 40% to 20% VC in supine compared to about 60% to 40% VC in upright.

Not shown in the volume-pressure diagram in Figure 2–32 is the fact that the respiratory muscles responsible for producing speech in supine are somewhat different from those used in upright body positions. In supine, expiratory muscular pressure is provided primarily by activation of rib cage wall expiratory muscles. This is in contrast to upright body positions in which the abdominal wall muscles also participate (even more so than the expiratory rib cage wall muscles). Only when loud speech is produced or when speech is produced within the expiratory reserve volume do abdominal wall muscles also become active in supine. Inspiration during running speech breathing is driven by the diaphragm, just as it is in the upright body position.

A major difference in the muscular strategy used for upright and that used for supine is that the role of the abdominal wall is quite different for the two body positions. Recall that in upright, abdominal wall muscle activation plays a critical role during speech production (expiration) as well as during inspiration. In contrast, it plays little or no role for running speech produced in the supine body position. This is because

in supine, gravity does what the abdominal wall muscles do in upright; that is, gravity drives the abdominal content and diaphragm headward, stretching the muscle fibers of the diaphragm and positioning them to be able to generate forceful and rapid inspirations. Gravity also forces the rib cage wall somewhat headward and positions its expiratory muscles for quicker actions. Because the respiratory system is mechanically tuned by gravity in supine, the expiratory rib cage wall muscles are generally sufficient to produce the required muscular pressures for speaking.

To summarize, some important differences (and similarities) between upright and supine running speech breathing are as follows:

(a) Although the size of breath groups is the same in the two body positions (about 20% VC on average), lung volume events occur at smaller lung volumes in supine (40% to 20% VC) than in upright (60% to 40% VC). This is because the resting lung volume level of the respiratory system is smaller in supine and speech breathing tends to follow the resting level.

(b) Alveolar pressure is the same in the two body positions for speech of normal loudness and is generally in the range of 5 to 10 cmH$_2$O.

(c) In upright, the chest wall assumes a shape of an inwardly displaced abdominal wall and outwardly displaced rib cage wall, a shape that "tunes" the diaphragm for producing quick inspirations and the expiratory rib cage muscles for producing quick expiratory pressure changes. In supine, gravity displaces the abdomen inward passively so that the abdominal muscles can remain quiescent.

(d) In upright, speech is produced with a combination of expiratory rib cage wall muscular pressure and abdominal wall muscular pressure, with the latter predominating. In contrast, supine running speech is usually produced with only expiratory rib cage wall muscular pressure. There are times when abdominal muscular pressure may also contribute to the generation of alveolar pressure, such as during loud speaking or speaking at small lung volumes.

(e) Inspiration is driven by the diaphragm in both upright and supine body positions.

Discussion thus far has focused on contrasting speech breathing in the upright (seated and standing) and supine body positions because these are two commonly encountered body positions, and they provide examples of two different mechanical and muscular solutions. It would be impossible (and boring) to cover the details of the limitless number of body positions that are possible. Nevertheless, there are some overarching principles that apply across body positions.

One principle is that the resting level of the respiratory system changes as body position changes. This is illustrated in Figure 2–33 for several different body positions. Much of the change in resting level can be attributed to the influence of gravity on the abdominal content and the resultant headward or footward displacement of the diaphragm. As the diaphragm is pushed headward, air moves out of the pulmonary apparatus and shifts the resting level to a smaller lung volume. Conversely, as the diaphragm is pulled footward, air moves into the pulmonary apparatus and shifts the resting level to a larger lung volume. Of particular importance in the present context is that lung

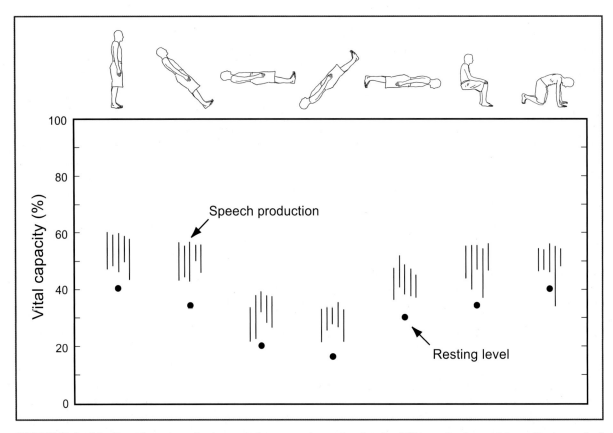

FIGURE 2–33. Breath groups during running speech production in different body positions. Each vertical line represents a single breath group (expiration containing speech). Note that breath groups are produced just above the resting level of the respiratory system (*represented by filled dots*) in all body positions. From *Evaluation and Management of Speech Breathing Disorders: Principles and Methods* (p. 77), by T. Hixon and J. Hoit, 2005, Tucson, AZ: Redington Brown. Copyright 2005 by Thomas J. Hixon and Jeannette D. Hoit. Modified and reproduced with permission.

volume events for running speech production are determined primarily by the resting level of the respiratory system (as shown by the several sets of vertical lines in Figure 2–33, each line representing a single breath group).

A second principle is that the relaxation pressure for any given lung volume increases as the body is tilted from upright toward supine. This means that a different muscular pressure is required to achieve a given alveolar pressure target at a specified lung volume.

A third principle is that the chest wall muscles assume different roles in generating muscular pressure as body position changes. In particular, the abdominal wall muscles are highly active during speaking in more upright body positions, whereas they are increasingly less active as the body is tilted toward supine.

The fourth principle is that the expiratory rib cage muscles almost always participate in running speech production, regardless of body position. The rib cage wall has the mechanical advantage of covering a much larger area of the lungs than does the diaphragm-abdominal wall (recall Figure 2–13) and of containing small and fast-acting muscles. These features make the rib cage wall well suited for generating muscular pressure change for speech production in all body positions.

Body Type

People come in many different sizes, shapes, and compositions, or so-called body types. Because the respiratory system makes up a large portion of the body, it is not surprising that those differences might influence the way the respiratory system functions for speaking.

Figure 2–34 illustrates men with three very different body types (from left to right): highly endomorphic (high in relative fatness), highly mesomorphic (high in musculoskeletal development), and highly ectomorphic (high in relative linearity). Differences in speech breathing are most striking when comparing endomorphic and ectomorphic body types: Endomorphic men tend to pull the abdominal wall inward farther and move it a greater distance during speaking than ectomorphic men (Hoit & Hixon, 1986). This is probably because the diaphragm is flattened by the downward pull of the large abdominal mass in an endomorphic person (when in an upright body position). By actively moving the abdominal wall inward, the diaphragm can assume a more domed configuration and produce more forceful inspirations, such as those required during speech breathing. The ectomorphic person, with his flat abdominal wall, already has a well-positioned diaphragm and has no need to move the abdominal wall during speech breathing.

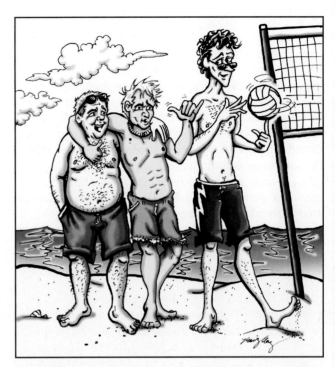

FIGURE 2–34. Cartoon of three teammates of different body types. The endomorph (*left*) is high in relative fatness, the mesomorph (*middle*) is particularly muscular, and the ectomorph (*right*) is lean and linear with little fat and muscle.

Age

Thus far, this chapter has discussed the respiratory system and speech breathing from the perspective of a young adult (fully mature) system. However, structure and function of the respiratory system change over the course of a lifetime. Changes during the developmental years are the most obvious and involve increases in the size of the respiratory system and alterations in its musculoskeletal geometry, chest wall compliance, pressure generation capability, neural control, and many other factors. Modifications during adulthood are more gradual and less obvious but nonetheless important.

Developmental trends in speech breathing have been identified for early infancy through the mid-teenage years (Boliek, Hixon, Watson, & Jones, 2009; Boliek, Hixon, Watson, & Morgan, 1996, 1997; Connaghan, Moore, & Higashakawa, 2004; Hoit, Hixon, Watson, & Morgan, 1990; Moore, Caulfield, & Green, 2001; Parham, Buder, Oller, & Boliek, 2011). The most salient trends are that (a) the amount of air expired per breath becomes increasingly larger as the child becomes larger, and (b) speech breathing starts out quite variable and becomes increasingly less variable as the child grows older. Unlike adults, who tend to be rather consistent in their speech breathing across time, infants and toddlers seem to use a different strategy for each vocalization (different lung volumes and different chest wall shapes and patterns of chest wall shape change) as if they are experimenting with the respiratory system to see what works best. Other speech breathing features seem to be nearly adult-like from the beginning. For example, infants and toddlers, whether 5 weeks or 3 years of age, usually initiate their vocalizations (or speech) within the midrange of the vital capacity, just like adults do. Also, as early as 18 months of age, inspirations preceding vocalization are quicker than inspirations associated with tidal breathing.

Rock-a-Bye Baby

Lullabies tend to put infants to sleep and change their breathing patterns. A supine infant who is awake breathes with in-phase movements of the rib cage wall and abdominal wall. The two structures rise and fall together in a gentle rhythm. But, if the same infant falls asleep, there may be an abrupt change in breathing pattern. During rapid eye movement sleep, for example, the pattern may change to out-of-phase movements of the rib cage wall and abdominal wall. One structure rises while the other falls. The reason is that, during sleep, structures in the pharyngeal-oral airway relax and the tongue falls toward the back of the infant's throat. This increases the airway resistance through which the respiratory system must work. One consequence is that pleural pressure must be lowered more during each inspiration, causing the floppy rib cage wall to be sucked inward. So, it's rock-a-bye baby, but bye-bye in-phase movements.

When volume measures are normalized to take into account age-related size differences (for example, by expressing them as % VC), speech breathing is essentially adult-like in most features by 10 years of age (before puberty). The only major difference seen beyond age 10 years is an increase in the amount of speech per breath group, reflecting changes in linguistic skill and sophistication. Also, young children tend to use relatively high alveolar pressures when speaking (Bernthal & Beukelman, 1979; Netsell, Lotz, Peters, & Schulte, 1994; Stathopoulos & Sapienza, 1993, 1997; Stathopoulos & Weismer, 1985), a behavior that gradually reduces over time.

Speech breathing remains relative stable throughout adulthood until the seventh or eighth decade of life, and then it begins to change (Hoit & Hixon, 1987; Hoit, Hixon, Altman, & Morgan, 1989; Huber, 2008; Huber, Darling, Francis, & Zhang, 2012; Huber & Darling-White, 2017; Sperry & Klich, 1992). In a senescent person, breath groups tend to start from larger lung volumes, contain less speech, and encompass more of the vital capacity when compared to breath groups of a younger adult. This means that senescent speakers tend to take deeper breaths before speaking, probably in anticipation of the increased air loss, and expend more air per syllable. This air loss appears to be due to uneconomical valving by the larynx. In men, air wastage has been attributed to an age-related decrease in laryngeal airway resistance during phonation (Melcon, Hoit, & Hixon, 1989), whereas in women, the air wastage appears to be related to nonspeech expirations before or after spoken utterances (Hoit & Hixon, 1992; Sperry & Klich, 1992). Of course, it is possible that age-related changes in speech breathing and laryngeal function are more tightly linked to biological age (health status and physical fitness) than to chronological age.

Sex

There is a pervasive myth that males and females breathe differently. This myth might also be applied to speech breathing, except that there is substantial evidence that contradicts it (Boliek et al., 1996, 1997, 2009; Hodge & Rochet, 1989; Hoit et al., 1989, 1990). From infancy through senescence, speech breathing is generally the same in the two sexes. The one exception is that, after puberty, the absolute lung volumes associated with speech breathing are generally larger in boys than girls (and men than women) because boys are generally taller and, therefore, have larger airways. Nevertheless, when volume measures are normalized to take into account differences in size, there are no sex-related differences in speech breathing to be found.

Ventilation and Drive to Breathe

Most of the time, ventilation (the rate at which air moves in and out of the respiratory system) matches the gas exchange (metabolic) needs of the body. For example, ventilation is lower when sleeping (low metabolic need) than when exercising (high metabolic need). Sometimes, however, ventilation is higher or lower than the metabolic need, resulting in hyperventilation or hypoventilation, respectively.

Under normal circumstances, speech breathing is associated with hyperventilation (Abel, Mottau, Klubendorf, & Koepchen, 1987; Bunn & Mead, 1971; Hoit & Lohmeier, 2000; Meanock & Nicholls, 1982; Warner, Waggener, & Kronauer, 1983). That is, ventilation is greater (as reflected, in part, by lower-than-usual carbon dioxide levels in the blood) when we speak than when we sit quietly. The degree of hyperventilation is dictated, in part, by the nature of the speaking activity. Ventilation is greater during continuous speaking (such as lecturing) than during intermittent speaking (such as conversing, wherein both speaking and listening occur). In addition, ventilation is greater when the speech sample is heavily loaded with high-flow sounds (such as voiceless consonants) than if the sample contains all-voiced sounds.

When the drive to breathe is strong, such as at a high elevation or during vigorous exercise, speaking can become a struggle (Figure 2–35), and there arises an awareness of having to balance the need to breathe with the desire to speak. Speaking under conditions of high drive differs substantially from speaking under usual (resting) conditions. Speaking in high drive has been studied using two general approaches: One is to have people speak while exercising (walking on a treadmill or riding a stationary bicycle) and the other is to alter the gas composition of the blood, usually by having people breathe air containing high con-

centrations of carbon dioxide (Bailey & Hoit, 2002; Baker, Hipp, & Alessio, 2008; Bunn & Mead, 1971; Doust & Patrick, 1981; Hale & Patrick, 1987; Hoit, Lansing, & Perona, 2007; Meanock & Nicholls, 1982; Otis & Clark, 1968; Phillipson, McClean, Sullivan, & Zamel, 1978).

The most robust characteristic of speech breathing in high drive is perhaps the least surprising: Ventilation increases with the magnitude of the stimulus (exercise or carbon dioxide levels). Ventilation increases during speaking are accomplished by larger tidal volumes, faster breathing frequencies, or both. To help maximize ventilation, people tend to produce less speech per breath group when speaking under high drive. This is done using two commonly adopted strategies. The first is to blow off air. When people use this strategy, they may produce a few syllables and then expire the remainder of the breath without speaking, or they may expire at the beginning of the breath group and then speak. The second strategy for increasing ventilation is to produce breathy speech. When people use this strategy, they use high airflow while speaking so that air is expired more quickly. Often, people use a combination of these two strategies.

When speaking under high drive, people tend to adjust the size and shape of the respiratory system. Specifically, they tend to begin and end breath groups at larger-than-usual lung volumes, so that the respiratory

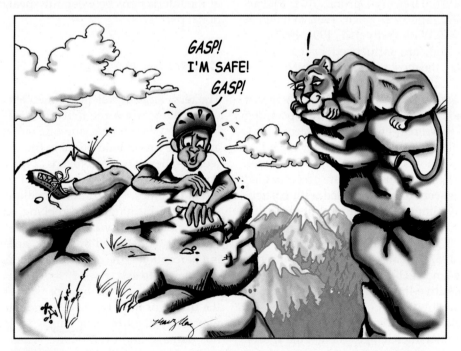

FIGURE 2–35. Cartoon depicting elevation, exercise, and speaking as a triple challenge to ventilation.

system is larger overall than it is when they are speaking under usual conditions. They also make large and fast chest wall shape changes when speaking in high drive. These adjustments in size and shape may reflect physiological strategies to help relieve the discomfort (dyspnea) that accompanies a high drive to breathe.

Cognitive-Linguistic and Social Variables

Cognitive-linguistic demands differ widely, depending on whether one recites a well-memorized poem, reads aloud a simple paragraph, converses with a friend, or delivers an extemporaneous speech on a complex topic. Cognitive-linguistic variables affect certain details of speech breathing. For example, inspirations are most likely to occur at linguistic structural boundaries (sentence, clause, and phrase boundaries), especially during reading aloud and, to a lesser degree, when speaking extemporaneously (Bailey & Hoit, 2002; Conrad, Thalacker, & Schönle, 1983; Grosjean & Collins, 1979; Henderson, Goldman-Eisler, & Skarbek, 1965; Hixon et al., 1973; Sugito, Ohyama, & Hirose, 1990; Wang, Green, Nip, Kent, & Kent, 2010; Winkworth, Davis, Adams, & Ellis, 1995; Winkworth, Davis, Ellis, & Adams, 1994). Also, inspirations tend to be larger (deeper) when followed by longer breath groups and smaller (shallower) when followed by shorter breath groups (Denny, 2000; Horii & Cooke, 1978; Huber & Darling, 2011; McFarland & Smith, 1992; Sperry & Klich, 1992; Whalen & Kinsella-Shaw, 1997; Winkworth et al., 1994, 1995).

Expirations, too, are influenced by cognitive-linguistic variables, the most powerful of which relates to silent pausing. Silent pauses (moments of silence that last at least 200 to 250 milliseconds) are believed to reflect the time needed to formulate the upcoming spoken message (Goldman-Eisler, 1956; Greene, 1984; Greene & Cappella, 1986; Henderson et al., 1965; Lay & Paivio, 1969; Reynolds & Paivio, 1968; Rochester, 1973; Taylor, 1969). Silent pauses that are accompanied by breath holding seem to be associated with particularly high cognitive-linguistic demands, but those that are accompanied by nonspeech expirations are more common (Mitchell, Hoit, & Watson, 1996; Webb, Williams, & Minifie, 1967). Because nonspeech expirations "waste air," there tends to be less speech produced per breath when cognitive-linguistic demands are high than when they are low.

Social variables may also come into play, especially during conversational interchange wherein the speech breathing patterns, or rhythms, of one conversational partner may influence the behavior of the other conversational partner. There is substantial evidence that people tend to entrain their intrinsic biological and behavioral rhythms with people with whom they are interacting and that the most enjoyable interactions are those in which individual rhythms entrain easily to one another (Chapple, 1970).

Different types of rhythms have been identified in conversational speech breathing (McFarland, 2001; Warner et al., 1983). Long-term rhythms (oscillations), ranging from as short as a minute to as long as several minutes, have been identified in which ventilation and speaking activity wax and wane relatively cyclically during conversation (Warner et al., 1983). Short-term rhythms (oscillations) are characterized by synchrony between the breathing movements of conversational partners in which the breathing movements during listening resemble the speech breathing movements of the conversational partner. For example, when listening to the speech of a conversation partner, inspiratory movements are quicker and expiratory movements are slower (more like speech breathing) than when not listening to someone speak (McFarland, 2001; Rochet-Capellan & Fuchs, 2014). Respiratory synchronies have even been identified in infants less than a year of age as they interact with their mothers (McFarland, Fortin, & Polka, 2020).

Thus, speech breathing produced in the context of conversational interchange appears to have emergent properties. Its nature is complex and determined by the speaker, the conversational partner(s), and the nature of the interactions between the speaker and conversational partner(s).

CLINICAL NOTES

The term *dyspnea* was mentioned above in the context of speaking when the drive to breathe is high, as it might be when hiking one of Colorado's 14ers (these are the 50+ mountain peaks in the state that are 14,000 feet or taller). Dyspnea means "breathing discomfort" and, like pain, can be experienced in the form of different qualities. For example, qualities of pain include sharp, dull, burning, and throbbing, among others; similarly, qualities of dyspnea include air hunger, effortful breathing, constricted breathing, and others. Dyspnea is a perception—the only way to know if someone feels dyspneic is to ask.

Currently (at the time of this writing), we are in the throes of the COVID-19 pandemic. This virus can wreak havoc on the respiratory system, causing serious damage and even death. When a person arrives at the emergency department with COVID-19, it is not unusual to find that their oxygen saturation is low, as indicated by the readout on a pulse oximeter, such as that shown in Figure 2–36. The oxygen saturation displayed in the pulse oximeter in the figure is 65%, which means that 65% of the red blood cells are saturated with oxygen. In a healthy person, oxygen saturation (abbreviated SpO$_2$ when measured with a pulse oximeter) should be in the 95% to 100% range. An SpO$_2$ value of 65% is clearly in the danger zone, and it is typically associated with dyspnea—for example, a patient might say, "I am short of breath," or "I feel like I'm gasping for air." In the case of COVID-19, however, there have been patients who have presented with dangerously low SpO$_2$ readings and report that their breathing feels entirely comfortable. This unexpected presentation of dangerously low SpO$_2$ and no dyspnea has perplexed physicians and spawned the term *happy hypoxia* (although a more accurate term would be *silent hypoxemia* because the patients are not happy and because hypoxia refers to reduced oxygen levels in tissues, whereas hypoxemia refers to reduced oxygen levels in blood). But they should not be perplexed; the explanation for this phenomenon has been understood for many years (Moosavi et al., 2003). Without getting too technical, what may have been forgotten is that the chemoreceptors (particularly the central chemoreceptors) are very sensitive to levels of carbon dioxide in the blood, and it is the presence of abnormally high levels of carbon dioxide that is a particularly strong stimulus for dyspnea, even more so than low levels of oxygen. There are additional explanations for the "happy hypoxia" phenomenon (Tobin, Laghi, & Jubran, 2020), but this one is key to understanding basic respiratory physiology.

Is any of this relevant to speech breathing? Yes. As mentioned above, when the drive to breathe is high, it is natural to change our speech breathing behavior. But even more important is the interaction of dyspnea and speech breathing in people who live day in and day out with chronic breathing discomfort, people such as those with pulmonary conditions, heart disease, or disorders of the nervous system that cause chest wall weakness or other abnormalities. From what little is known about dyspnea and speech breathing, it appears that the act of speaking exacerbates breathing discomfort in people with chronic conditions and may cause them to avoid social situations that require that they speak (Hoit, Lansing, Brown, & Nitido, in press; Hoit, Lansing, Dean, Yarkosky, & Lederle, 2011). This has serious implications for quality of life.

REVIEW

The respiratory system behaves like a mechanical pump that moves air in and out for the purpose of sustaining life as well as serving other functions such as speaking.

The respiratory system is formed around a skeletal framework and consists of the pulmonary apparatus

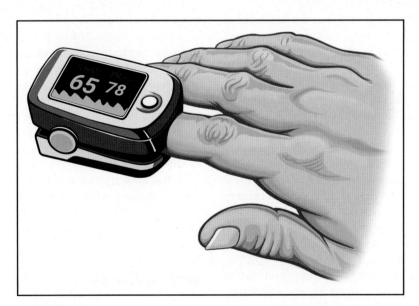

FIGURE 2–36. Pulse oximeter showing abnormally low oxygen saturation level. The number on the left (65) reflects the percentage of red blood cells that is saturated with oxygen. In healthy people, this number is typically at least 95%. The number on the right is the pulse rate (number of beats per minute).

and chest wall (linked together as a unit), the former including the pulmonary airways and lungs and the latter including the rib cage wall, diaphragm, abdominal wall, and abdominal content.

The forces of breathing are passive and active, the former arising from the natural recoil of tissues, surface tension within alveoli, and gravity, and the latter being vested in more than 20 muscles of the chest wall.

Muscles of the rib cage wall include the *sternocleidomastoid, scalenus anterior, scalenus medius, scalenus posterior, pectoralis major, pectoralis minor, subclavius, serratus anterior, external intercostal, internal intercostal, transversus thoracis, latissimus dorsi, serratus posterior superior, serratus posterior inferior, lateral iliocostalis cervicis, lateral iliocostalis thoracis, lateral iliocostalis lumborum, levatores costarum, quadratus lumborum*, and *subcostal*.

The *diaphragm* muscle divides the torso into two compartments: the thorax (upper cavity) and abdomen.

Muscles of the abdominal wall include the *rectus abdominis, external oblique, internal oblique*, and *transversus abdominis* at the front and the *latissimus dorsi, lateral iliocostalis lumborum*, and *quadratus lumborum* at the back.

The forces of the respiratory system are realized as pulls on structures and pressures developed at various locations, with the most important pressure for speech production being alveolar pressure.

The movements of breathing occur within the rib cage wall, diaphragm, and abdominal wall, with each part having its own movement capabilities.

Movement of the rib cage wall has the potential to create greater volume and pressure change than movement of the abdominal wall because it covers a greater surface area of the pulmonary apparatus.

Movements of the respiratory system are caused by passive and active forces that come from different parts of the system, making it difficult to specify what forces are responsible for any given movement.

The respiratory control variables of interest are lung volume, alveolar pressure, and chest wall shape.

The nervous system controls different respiratory acts through groups of lower and higher brain centers that mediate breathing movements and related perceptions during tidal breathing and special acts of breathing, and that control is sent to the respiratory system through peripheral nerves.

Ventilation (the movement of air into and out of the pulmonary apparatus) supports the life-sustaining process of oxygen and carbon dioxide exchange.

Speech breathing is the process by which driving forces are supplied to generate the sounds of speech, while simultaneously serving the functions of ventilation and gas exchange.

Speech breathing, whether it be during extended steady utterance or during running speech activities, is achieved through the combining of relaxation pressure and muscular pressure, the muscular pressure required at any moment depending on the relaxation pressure available at the prevailing lung volume and the target alveolar pressure of the utterance.

The activity of individual parts of the chest wall (rib cage wall, diaphragm, and abdominal wall) may differ for the generation of utterances involving different alveolar pressures at different lung volumes.

The control strategy for running speech activities is distinct from that for other forms of breathing and serves to enhance function during both the inspiratory and expiratory phases of the speech breathing cycle.

Speech breathing is influenced by body position, mainly because gravity affects relaxation pressure, the resting level of the respiratory system, and the mechanical advantages of different parts of the chest wall.

Body type affects speech breathing, with the most dramatic contrasts existing between people who are endomorphic and ectomorphic, the former showing a much higher degree of abdominal wall participation.

Speech breathing develops during childhood, becoming adult-like in many ways by 10 years of age, and then changes again around the seventh or eighth decade of life, due, at least in part, to factors believed to be related to laryngeal valving economy and air wastage.

Despite the pervasive myth that the two sexes breathe differently, there is no evidence to support this notion and, in the case of speech breathing, substantial evidence to contradict it.

People naturally hyperventilate during speaking and reorganize their speech breathing behaviors under conditions of high drive so as to relieve breathing discomfort.

Cognitive-linguistic factors influence both the inspiratory and expiratory phases of speech breathing, as do social interactions between conversational partners.

Dyspnea is a perception that can be manifested in different qualities (such as air hunger and effort to breathe) and may or may not be reflected in physiological measures but appears to have an influence on speech breathing behavior and the willingness to participate in social situations.

REFERENCES

Abel, H., Mottau, B., Klubendorf, D., & Koepchen, H. (1987). Pattern of different components of the respiratory cycle and autonomic parameters during speech. In G. Sieck, S. Gandevia, & W. Cameron (Eds.), *Respiratory muscles and their neuromotor control* (pp. 109–113). New York, NY: Alan R. Liss.

Bailey, E., & Hoit, J. (2002). Speaking and breathing in high respiratory drive. *Journal of Speech, Language, and Hearing Research, 45,* 89–99.

Baker, S., Hipp, J., & Alessio, H. (2008). Ventilation and speech characteristics during submaximal aerobic exercise. *Journal of Speech, Language, and Hearing Research, 51,* 1203–1214.

Benchetrit, G., Shea, S., Pham Dinh, T., Bodocco, S., Baconnier, P., & Guz, A. (1989). Individuality of breathing patterns in adults assessed over time. *Respiration Physiology, 75,* 199–210.

Bernthal, J., & Beukelman, D. (1978). Intraoral air pressure during the production of /p/ and /b/ by children, youths, and adults. *Journal of Speech and Hearing Research, 21,* 361–371.

Boliek, C., Hixon, T., Watson, P., & Jones, P. (2009). Refinement of speech breathing in healthy 4- to 6-year-old children. *Journal of Speech, Language, and Hearing Research, 52,* 990–1007.

Boliek, C., Hixon, T., Watson, P., & Morgan, W. (1996). Vocalization and breathing during the first year of life. *Journal of Voice, 10,* 1–22.

Boliek, C., Hixon, T., Watson, P., & Morgan, W. (1997). Vocalization and breathing during the second and third years of life. *Journal of Voice, 11,* 373–390.

Bunn, J., & Mead, J. (1971). Control of ventilation during speech. *Journal of Applied Physiology, 31,* 870–872.

Chapple, E. (1970). *Culture and biological man.* New York, NY: Holt, Rinehart, and Winston.

Connaghan, K., Moore, C., & Hagashakawa, M. (2004). Respiratory kinematics during vocalization and nonspeech respiration in children from 9 to 48 months. *Journal of Speech, Language, and Hearing Research, 47,* 70–84.

Conrad, B., Thalacker, S., & Schönle, P. (1983). Speech respiration as an indicator of integrative contextual processing. *Folia Phoniatrica, 35,* 220–225.

Corfield, D., Murphy, K., & Guz, A. (1998). Does the motor cortical control of the diaphragm "bypass" the brain stem respiratory centres in man? *Respiratory Physiology, 114,* 109–117.

Dejours, P. (1996). *Respiration.* New York, NY: Oxford University Press.

Denny, M. (2000). Periodic variation in inspiratory volume characterizes speech as well as inspiration. *Journal of Voice, 10,* 23–38.

Doust, J., & Patrick, J. (1981). The limitation of exercise ventilation during speech. *Respiration Physiology, 46,* 137–147.

Gardner, W. (1996). The pathophysiology of hyperventilation disorders. *Chest, 109,* 516–534.

Goldman-Eisler, F. (1956). The determinants of the rate of speech output and their mutual relations. *Journal of Psychosomatic Research, 1,* 137–143.

Greene, J. (1984). Speech preparation processes and verbal fluency. *Human Communication Research, 11,* 61–84.

Greene, J., & Cappella, J. (1986). Cognition and talk: The relationship of semantic units to temporal patterns of fluency in spontaneous speech. *Language and Speech, 29,* 141–157.

Grosjean, F., & Collins, M. (1979). Breathing, pausing, and reading. *Phonetica, 36,* 98–114.

Hale, M., & Patrick, J. (1987). Ventilatory patterns during human speech in progressive hypercapnia. *Journal of Physiology, 394,* 60P.

Henderson, A., Goldman-Eisler, F., & Skarbek, A. (1965). Temporal patterns of cognitive activity and breath control in speech. *Language and Speech, 8,* 236–242.

Hixon, T. (1973). Respiratory function in speech. In F. Minifie, T. Hixon, & F. Williams (Eds.), *Normal aspects of speech, hearing, and language* (pp. 75–125). Englewood Cliffs, NJ: Prentice-Hall.

Hixon, T., Goldman, M., & Mead, J. (1973). Kinematics of the chest wall during speech production: Volume displacements of the rib cage, abdomen, and lung. *Journal of Speech and Hearing Research, 16,* 78–115.

Hixon, T., & Hoit, J. (2005). *Evaluation and management of speech breathing disorders: Principles and methods.* Tucson, AZ: Redington Brown.

Hixon, T., Mead, J., & Goldman, M. (1976). Dynamics of the chest wall during speech production: Function of the thorax, rib cage, diaphragm, and abdomen. *Journal of Speech and Hearing Research, 19,* 297–356.

Hixon, T., Weismer, G., & Hoit, J. (2020). *Preclinical speech science: Anatomy, physiology, acoustics, and perception.* San Diego, CA: Plural Publishing.

Hodge, M., & Rochet, A. (1989). Characteristics of speech breathing in young women. *Journal of Speech and Hearing Research, 32,* 466–480.

Hoit, J., & Hixon, T. (1986). Body type and speech breathing. *Journal of Speech and Hearing Research, 29,* 313–324.

Hoit, J., & Hixon, T. (1987). Age and speech breathing. *Journal of Speech and Hearing Research, 30,* 351–366.

Hoit, J., & Hixon, T. (1992). Age and laryngeal airway resistance during vowel production in women. *Journal of Speech and Hearing Research, 35,* 309–313.

Hoit, J., Hixon, T., Altman, M., & Morgan, W. (1989). Speech breathing in women. *Journal of Speech and Hearing Research, 32,* 353–365.

Hoit, J., Hixon, T., Watson, P., & Morgan, W. (1990). Speech breathing in children and adolescents. *Journal of Speech and Hearing Research, 33,* 51–69.

Hoit, J. D., Lansing, R. W., Brown, V. P., & Nitido, H. (in press). Speaking dyspnea in Parkinson's disease. *Journal of Communication Disorders.*

Hoit, J., Lansing, R., Dean, K., Yarkosky, M., & Lederle, A. (2011). Nature and evaluation of dyspnea in speaking and swallowing. *Seminars in Speech and Language, 32,* 5–20.

Hoit, J., Lansing, R., & Perona, G. (2007). Speaking-related dyspnea in healthy adults. *Journal of Speech, Language, and Hearing Research, 50,* 361–374.

Hoit, J., & Lohmeier, H. (2000). Influence of continuous speaking on ventilation. *Journal of Speech, Language, and Hearing Research, 43,* 1240–1251.

Horii, Y., & Cooke, P. (1978). Some airflow, volume, and duration characteristics of oral reading. *Journal of Speech and Hearing Research, 21,* 470–481.

Huber, J. (2008). Effects of utterance length and vocal loudness on speech breathing in older adults. *Respiratory Physiology and Neurobiology, 164,* 323–330.

Huber, J., & Darling, M. (2011). Effect of Parkinson's disease on the production of structured and unstructured speaking tasks: Respiratory physiologic and linguistic considerations. *Journal of Speech, Language, and Hearing Research, 54,* 33–46.

Huber, J., Darling, M., Francis, E., & Zhang, D. (2012). Impact of typical aging and Parkinson's disease on the relationship among breath pausing, syntax, and punctuation. *American Journal of Speech-Language Pathology, 21*, 368–379.

Huber, J., & Darling-White, M. (2017). Longitudinal changes in speech breathing in older adults with and without Parkinson's disease. *Seminars in Speech and Language, 38*, 200–209.

Lay, C., & Paivio, A. (1969). The effects of task difficulty and anxiety on hesitations in speech. *Canadian Journal of Behavioral Sciences, 1*, 25–37.

Loring, S., & Mead, J. (1982). Abdominal muscle use during quiet breathing and hyperpnea in uninformed subjects. *Journal of Applied Physiology, 52*, 700–704.

Mador, J., & Tobin, M. (1991). Effect of alterations in mental activity on the breathing pattern in healthy subjects. *American Review of Respiratory Disease, 144*, 481–487.

McFarland, D. (2001). Respiratory markers of conversational interaction. *Journal of Speech, Language, and Hearing Research, 44*, 128–143.

McFarland, D., Fortin, A., & Polka, L. (2020). Physiological measures of mother-infant interactional synchrony. *Developmental Psychobiology, 62*, 50–61.

McFarland, D., & Smith, A. (1992). Effect of vocal task and respiratory phase on prephonatory chest wall movements. *Journal of Speech and Hearing Research, 35*, 971–982.

Meanock, C., & Nicholls, A. (1982). The effect of speech on the ventilatory response to carbon dioxide or to exercise. *Journal of Physiology, 325*, 16P–17P.

Melcon, M., Hoit, J., & Hixon, T. (1989). Age and laryngeal airway resistance during vowel production. *Journal of Speech and Hearing Disorders, 54*, 282–286.

Mitchell, H., Hoit, J., & Watson, P. (1996). Cognitive-linguistic demands and speech breathing. *Journal of Speech and Hearing Research, 39*, 93–104.

Moore, C., Caulfield, T., & Green, J. (2001). Relative kinematics of the rib cage and abdomen during speech and nonspeech behaviors of 15-month-old children. *Journal of Speech, Language, and Hearing Research, 44*, 80–94.

Moosavi, S., Golestanian, E., Binks, A., Lansing, R., Brown, R., & Banzett, R. (2003). Hypoxic and hypercapnic drives to breathe generate equivalent levels of air hunger in humans. *Journal of Applied Physiology, 94*, 141–154.

Netsell, R., Lotz, W., Peters, J., & Schulte, L. (1994). Developmental patterns of laryngeal and respiratory function for speech production. *Journal of Voice, 8*, 123–131.

Otis, A., & Clark, R. (1968). Ventilatory implications of phonation and phonatory implications of ventilation. In A. Bouhuys (Ed.), *Sound production in man* (pp. 122–128). New York, NY: Annals of the New York Academy of Sciences.

Parham, D., Buder, E., Oller, D. K., & Boliek, C. (2011). Syllable-related breathing in infants in the second year of life. *Journal of Speech, Language, and Hearing Research, 54*, 1039–1050.

Phillipson, E., McClean, P., Sullivan, C., & Zamel, N. (1978). Interaction of metabolic and behavioral respiratory control during hypercapnia and speech. *American Review of Respiratory Disease, 117*, 903–909.

Reynolds, A., & Paivio, A. (1968). Cognitive and emotional determinants of speech. *Canadian Journal of Psychology, 22*, 164–175.

Rochester, S. (1973). The significance of pauses in spontaneous speech. *Journal of Psycholinguistic Research, 2*, 51–81.

Rochet-Capellan, A., & Fuchs, S. (2014). Take a breath and take the turn: How breathing meets turns in spontaneous dialogue. *Philosophical Transactions of the Royal Society B, 369*, 20130399.

Shea, S. (1996). Behavioural and arousal-related influences on breathing in humans. *Experimental Physiology, 81*, 1–26.

Shea, S., & Guz, A. (1992). Personnalite ventilatoire: An overview. *Respiration Physiology, 52*, 275–291.

Shea, S., Horner, R., Benchetrit, G., & Guz, A. (1990). The persistence of a respiratory "personality" into Stage IV sleep in man. *Respiration Physiology, 80*, 33–44.

Shea, S., Murphy, K., Hamilton, R., Benchetrit, G., & Guz, A. (1988). Do the changes in respiratory pattern and ventilation seen with different behavioural situations reflect metabolic demands? In C. von Euler & M. Katz-Salamon (Eds.), *Respiratory psychophysiology* (pp. 21–28). Basingstoke, UK: Macmillan Press.

Shea, S., Walter, J., Murphy, K., & Guz, A. (1987). Evidence for individuality of breathing patterns in resting healthy men. *Respiration Physiology, 68*, 331–344.

Shea, S., Walter, J., Pelley, C., Murphy, K., & Guz, A. (1987). The effect of visual and auditory stimuli upon resting ventilation in man. *Respiration Physiology, 68*, 345–357.

Sperry, E., & Klich, R. (1992). Speech breathing in senescent and younger women during oral reading. *Journal of Speech and Hearing Research, 35*, 1246–1255.

Stathopoulos, E., & Sapienza, C. (1993). Respiratory and laryngeal measures of children during vocal intensity variation. *Journal of the Acoustical Society of America, 94*, 2531–2543.

Stathopoulos, E., & Sapienza, C. (1997). Developmental changes in laryngeal and respiratory function with variations in sound pressure level. *Journal of Speech, Language, and Hearing Research, 40*, 595–614.

Stathopoulos, E., & Weismer, G. (1985). Oral airflow and air pressure during speech production: A comparative study of children, youths, and adults. *Folia Phoniatrica, 37*, 152–159.

Sugito, M., Ohyama, G., & Hirose, H. (1990). A preliminary study on pauses and breaths in reading speech materials. *Annual Bulletin of the Research Institute of Logopedics and Phoniatrics, 24*, 121–130.

Taylor, I. (1969). Content and structure in sentence production. *Journal of Verbal Learning and Verbal Behavior, 8*, 170–175.

Tobin, M., Laghi, F., & Jubran, A. (2020). Why COVID-19 silent hypoxemia is baffling to physicians. *American Journal of Respiratory and Critical Care Medicine, 202*, 356–360.

Wang, Y.-T., Green, J., Nip, I., Kent, R., & Kent, J. (2010). Breath group analysis for reading and spontaneous speech in healthy adults. *Folia Phoniatrica et Logopaedica, 62*, 297–302.

Warner, R., Waggener, T., & Kronauer, R. (1983). Synchronized cycles in ventilation and vocal activity during spontaneous conversational speech. *Journal of Applied Physiology, 54*, 309–317.

Webb, R., Williams, F., & Minifie, F. (1967). Effects of verbal decision behavior upon respiration during speech production. *Journal of Speech and Hearing Research, 10*, 49–56.

Weismer, G. (1985). Speech breathing: Contemporary views and findings. In R. Daniloff (Ed.), *Speech science* (pp. 47–72). San Diego, CA: College-Hill Press.

Western, P., & Patrick, J. (1988). Effects of focusing attention on breathing with and without apparatus on the face. *Respiration Physiology, 72*, 123–130.

Whalen, D., & Kinsella-Shaw, J. (1997). Exploring the relationship of inspiration duration to utterance duration. *Phonetica, 54*, 138–152.

Winkworth, A., Davis, P., Adams, R., & Ellis, E. (1995). Breathing patterns during spontaneous speech. *Journal of Speech and Hearing Research, 38*, 124–144.

Winkworth, A., Davis, P., Ellis, E., & Adams, R. (1994). Variability and consistency in speech breathing during reading: Lung volumes, speech intensity, and linguistic factors. *Journal of Speech and Hearing Research, 37*, 535–556.

Wyke, B. (1974). Respiratory activity of intrinsic laryngeal muscles: An experimental study. In B. Wyke (Ed.), *Ventilatory and phonatory control systems* (pp. 408–429). New York, NY: Oxford University Press.

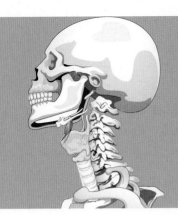

3

Laryngeal Structure and Function

INTRODUCTION

The larynx is an air valve located within the front of the neck. This valve is positioned between the trachea (windpipe) and pharynx (throat) and can be adjusted to vary the amount of coupling between the two. The larynx serves a variety of functions, including the critical role of voice production.

This chapter begins with a description of laryngeal anatomy, followed by discussion of the forces and movements of the larynx, control variables and neural substrates, and laryngeal function for speech production. The chapter ends with some clinical notes. Laryngeal function during swallowing is covered in Chapter 7.

LARYNGEAL ANATOMY

The skeletal framework of the larynx, its joints, and its internal topography are considered in this section. The laryngeal muscles are discussed in the next section on Forces of the Larynx.

Skeletal Framework

The skeletal framework of the larynx is depicted in Figure 3–1. This framework consists of five cartilages

(two of which are paired), a bone, ligaments, and tendons. Its flexibility changes with age, being soft and pliable in childhood and hard and more rigid in adulthood.

Sizing Things Up

There's a tendency to overestimate the size of things when looking at drawings, photographs, and video images of the larynx. The glottis seems to be a big, triangular space. The vocal folds appear to be massive lip-like structures. The vocal ligaments look as large as pencils. And the vibratory movements of the vocal folds (when slowed down) give the impression of a flag blowing in the breeze. Some calibration may be helpful. Your wide-open glottis is about the size of a dime. Your vocal folds have a surface area about the size of your thumbnail (well trimmed). The vocal ligaments are about as thick as wooden matchsticks. And your vocal folds only move about the length of the cuticle on your thumbnail. If you're like us, you'll find this to be surprisingly small. Yes?

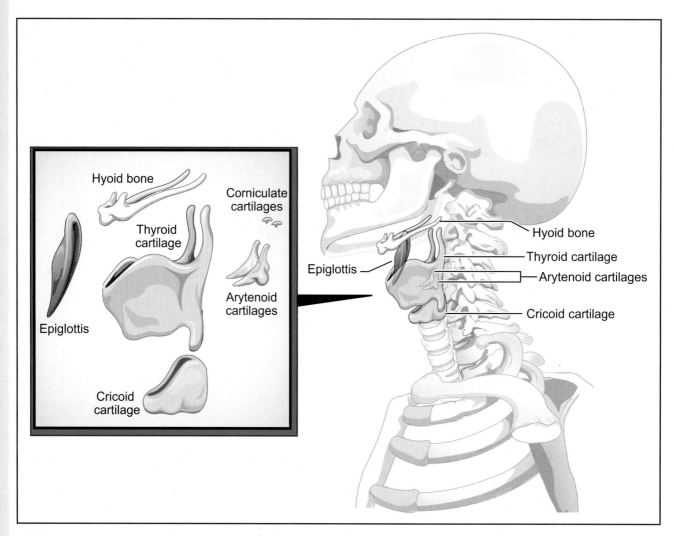

FIGURE 3–1. Skeletal framework of the larynx. This framework is composed of two paired cartilages (arytenoid cartilages and corniculate cartilages), three unpaired cartilages (thyroid cartilage, cricoid cartilage, and epiglottis), and one bone (hyoid bone).

Thyroid Cartilage

The thyroid cartilage is the largest of the laryngeal cartilages and forms most of the front and sides of the laryngeal skeleton. This cartilage provides a shield-like housing for the larynx and offers protection for many of its structures.

Figure 3–2 shows the thyroid cartilage from four different views. Two quadrilateral plates, called the thyroid laminae, are fused together at the front of the thyroid cartilage and diverge widely (more so in women than in men) toward the back. The shape of the two thyroid laminae resembles the bow of a ship. The line of fusion between the two plates is called the angle of the thyroid. The upper part of the structure contains a prominent V-shaped depression, called the thyroid notch, that can be palpated (examined by touch) at the

front of the neck. This notch is located just above the most forward projection of the cartilage, an outward jutting called the thyroid prominence or Adam's apple.

The back edges of the thyroid laminae extend upward into two long horns and downward into two short horns. The upper horns, called the superior cornua, are coupled to the hyoid bone. The lower horns, termed the inferior cornua, have facets (areas where other structures join) on their lower inside surfaces. These facets help form joints with the cricoid cartilage. The inferior cornua straddle the cricoid cartilage like a pair of legs (see Figure 3–1).

Cricoid Cartilage

The cricoid cartilage forms the lowest part of the laryngeal skeleton. It is a ring-shaped structure located

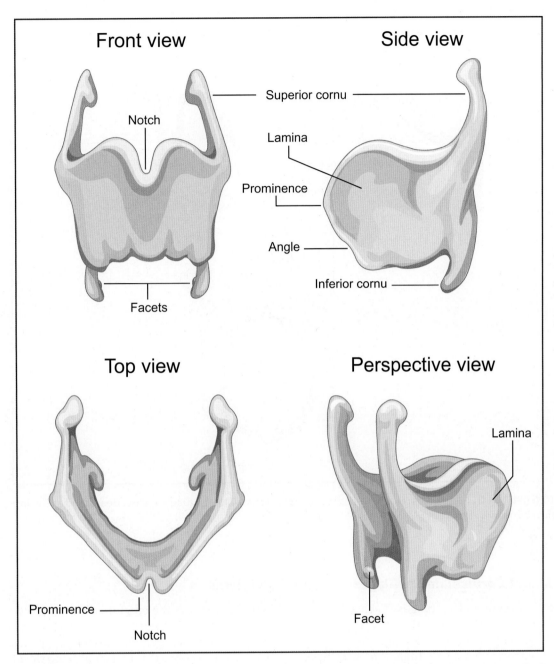

FIGURE 3–2. Thyroid cartilage from four different views. The thyroid prominence is also called the Adam's apple.

above the trachea. As shown in Figure 3–3, the cricoid cartilage has a thick plate at the back, the posterior quadrate lamina, which resembles a signet on a finger ring. A semicircular structure, called the anterior arch, forms the front of the cricoid cartilage and is akin to the band of a finger ring.

The cricoid cartilage has four facets. The lower two facets, one on each side at the same level, are positioned near the junction of the posterior quadrate lamina and anterior arch. Each of these facets articulates with a facet on one of the inferior cornua of the thyroid cartilage. The upper two facets of the cricoid cartilage, one on each side at the same level, are located on the sloping rim of the posterior quadrate lamina. Each of these facets articulates with a facet on the undersurface of one of the arytenoid cartilages.

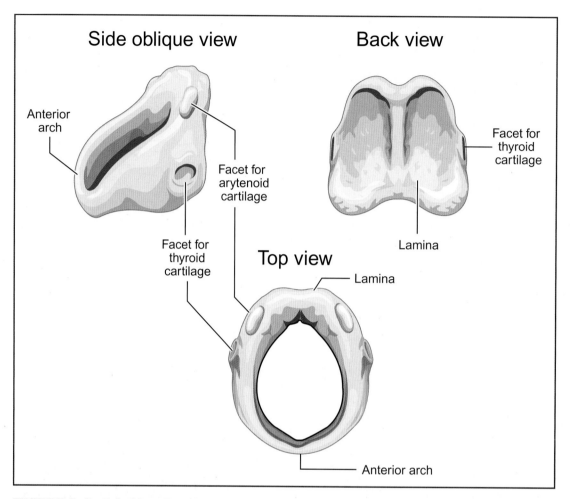

Side oblique view

Anterior arch

Facet for arytenoid cartilage

Facet for thyroid cartilage

Back view

Facet for thyroid cartilage

Lamina

Top view

Lamina

Anterior arch

FIGURE 3–3. Cricoid cartilage from three different views. This cartilage is often described as having the shape of a signet ring.

Arytenoid and Corniculate Cartilages

There are two arytenoid cartilages. Each is located atop one side of the sloping rim of the posterior quadrate lamina of the cricoid cartilage. As shown in Figure 3–4, each arytenoid cartilage has a complex shape that includes an apex, a base, and three sides. The apex of each cartilage is capped with another small cone-shaped cartilage called a corniculate cartilage that is often fused to the arytenoid cartilage. The base of each arytenoid cartilage has a flexible pointed projection that extends toward the front and is designated the vocal process. The base also includes a rounded stubby projection that extends toward the back and side and is referred to as the muscular process. The undersurface of each muscular process has a facet that articulates with one of the upper facets of the cricoid cartilage.

Epiglottis

Figure 3–5 shows the epiglottis. The epiglottis is a single cartilage that is positioned behind the hyoid bone and root of the tongue. The upper part of the epiglottis, its body, is broad and resembles the distal end of a forward-curving shoehorn. The front and back surfaces of this part of the structure are referred to as its lingual (tongue) and laryngeal (larynx) surfaces, respectively. The lingual surface attaches to the hyoid bone. The lower part of the cartilage tapers downward into a stalk called the petiolus (little leg) and attaches to the inside of the thyroid cartilage just below the thyroid notch.

Hyoid Bone

The hyoid bone (tongue bone) is shown in Figure 3–6. Technically, the hyoid bone is not a part of the larynx.

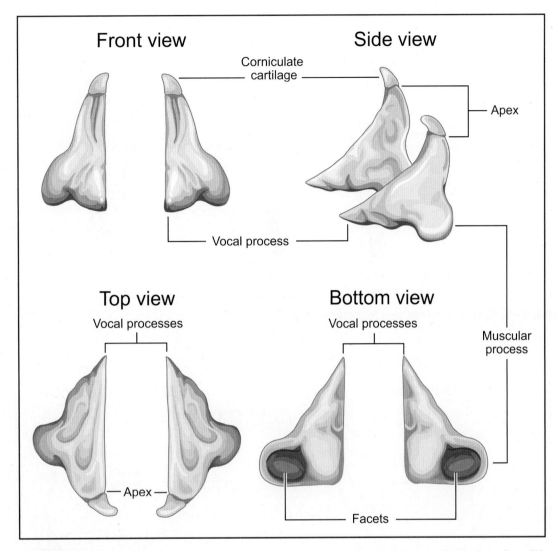

FIGURE 3-4. Arytenoid and corniculate cartilages, both paired cartilages, shown from four different views.

Nevertheless, it serves as an integral component in many laryngeal functions and is commonly afforded a prominent place in discussion of the laryngeal skeleton.

The hyoid bone is free-floating in the sense that it is not attached to any other bone. It is a U-shaped structure that is positioned horizontally within the neck with its open end facing toward the back. The hyoid bone consists of a body and two pairs of greater and lesser horns (cornua) that project upward. The greater cornua are located toward the back of the structure and join with the superior cornua of the thyroid cartilage. The lesser cornua are small eminences (protruberances) that extend from the body of the hyoid. The hyoid bone is positioned at the top of the larynx and connects to it through muscles and other structures.

Laryngeal Joints

There are two pairs of joints in the larynx. One pair is between the cricoid and thyroid cartilages, and the other is between the cricoid and arytenoid cartilages. Movements at these joints are conditioned by the nature of the facets on their articulating cartilages and the arrangement of surrounding ligaments.

Cricothyroid Joints

The cricothyroid joints are illustrated in Figure 3–7. These joints are positioned on the right and left sides of the larynx and involve articulations between facets on the inner surfaces of the inferior cornua of the thyroid

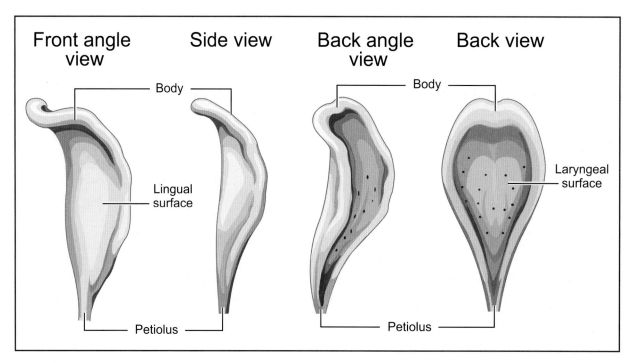

FIGURE 3–5. Epiglottis shown from four different views.

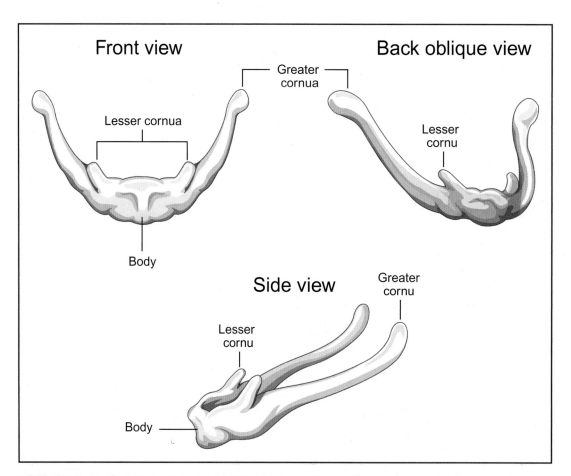

FIGURE 3–6. Hyoid bone from three different views. The hyoid bone, often described as horseshoe shaped, has the special status of being the only free-floating bone in the body, meaning that it does not directly articulate with any other bones. The hyoid bone is not technically part of the larynx.

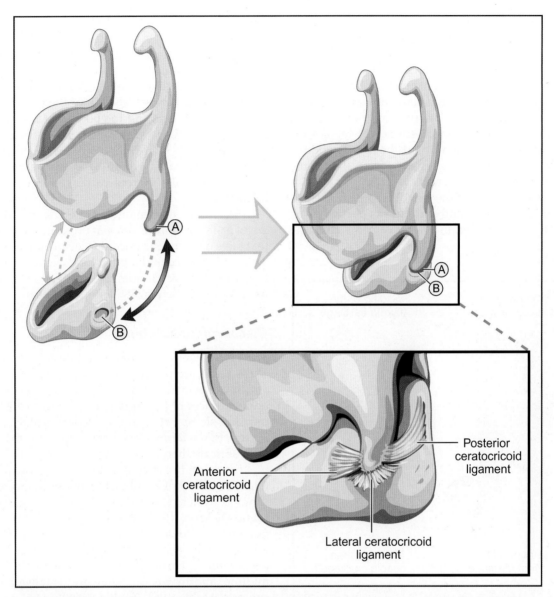

FIGURE 3–7. Cricothyroid joints. These two joints, one on each side, are created by articulations between convex facets on the inner surface of the inferior cornu of the thyroid cartilage (A) and concave facets on the outer surface of the cricoid cartilage (B). The anterior, lateral, and posterior ceratocricoid ligaments secure the joints and restrict their movements.

cartilage (see A in the figure) and the outer surfaces of the lower part of the cricoid cartilage (see B in the figure). The cricothyroid joints are encapsulated by membranes that secrete fluid (called synovial fluid), which serves as a lubricant.

Facets on the cricoid and thyroid cartilages vary from larynx to larynx and from side to side within the same larynx (Dickson & Maue-Dickson, 1982). Those on the cricoid cartilage generally face upward, toward the side, and backward. They are usually round or oval in shape and are concave. Facets on the thyroid cartilage typically face downward, toward the midline, and forward. They are usually round and convex. Occasionally, a larynx will have cricothyroid joint facets that are rudimentary. Then the articulation between the cricoid and thyroid surfaces is formed by fibrous connective tissue (Zemlin, 1998).

Three ligaments extend between the side and back surfaces of the cricoid cartilage and the lower outside surfaces of the inferior cornu of the thyroid cartilage on each side. These three ligaments encircle most of the corresponding cricothyroid joint and are referred to as the anterior, lateral, and posterior ceratocricoid (cerato meaning horn) ligaments. The anterior ligament extends backward into the front surface of the inferior cornu. The lateral ligament extends upward into the lower surface of the cornu. And the posterior ligament extends forward into the back surface of the cornu. Together, the three ligaments bind the corresponding cricothyroid joint and place restrictions on the movements of the cricoid and thyroid cartilages.

The movements at the cricothyroid joints are of two types—rotating and sliding—as portrayed in Figure 3–8. The most significant movements are rota-

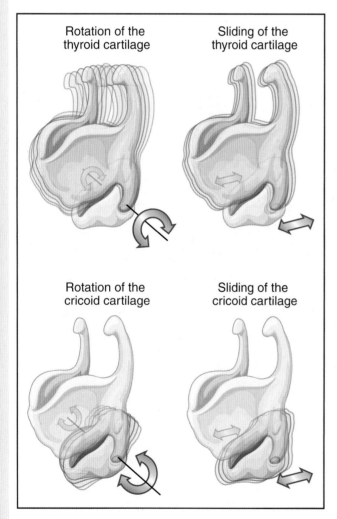

FIGURE 3–8. Cricothyroid joint movements. These movements are primarily rotational, with the thyroid cartilage rocking on the cricoid cartilage (*upper left*) or the cricoid rocking on the thyroid (*lower left*). They can also be of a sliding nature (*upper and lower right*).

tional and occur about a lateral axis extending through the two joints. Either or both the cricoid and thyroid cartilages can rotate about this axis (Mayet & Muendnich, 1958; Takano & Honda, 2005; Vennard, 1967; Zemlin, 1998). One consequence of rotation is a change in the distance between the top of the anterior arch of the cricoid cartilage and the bottom of the laminae of the thyroid cartilage at the front. This is analogous to rotating the chin guard (representing the anterior arch of the cricoid cartilage) and the visor (representing the laminae of the thyroid cartilage) on a motorcycle helmet.

Secondary movements at the cricothyroid joints are of a sliding nature and can occur in those larynges that have oval-shaped cricoid facets. These movements are small and occur along the long axes of the cricoids facets (Takano & Honda, 2005; Titze, 1994; van den Berg, Vennard, Berger, & Shervanian, 1960).

Cricoarytenoid Joints

The cricoarytenoid joints are shown in Figure 3–9. These joints are positioned near the top of the larynx and involve articulations between the facets on the undersurfaces of the arytenoid cartilages (A in the figure) and sloping rims of the cricoid cartilage (B in the figure). Synovial membranes encapsulate these joints and lubricate them.

Facets on the cricoid and arytenoid cartilages are relatively uniform in characteristics from larynx to larynx and from side to side within a larynx (Dickson & Maue-Dickson, 1982). Facets on the cricoid cartilage face upward, toward the side, and forward. These facets are usually oval in shape and are convex. Facets on the arytenoid cartilages face downward, toward the midline, and backward. They are usually round and concave (Frable, 1961; Zemlin, 1998).

Two ligaments, the anterior and posterior cricoarytenoid ligaments, influence the function of each cricoarytenoid joint by binding it and restricting its movements. The anterior cricoarytenoid ligament extends from the side of the cricoid cartilage to the front and side of the arytenoid cartilage. The ligament runs upward and backward and limits the degree to which the arytenoid cartilage can be moved backward. The posterior cricoarytenoid ligament extends upward and toward the side from the back of the cricoid cartilage to the back of the arytenoid cartilage. This ligament limits the degree to which the arytenoid cartilage can be moved forward.

The movements at the cricoarytenoid joints are portrayed in Figure 3–10. Movements at these joints can be of two types: rocking and sliding. The most sig-

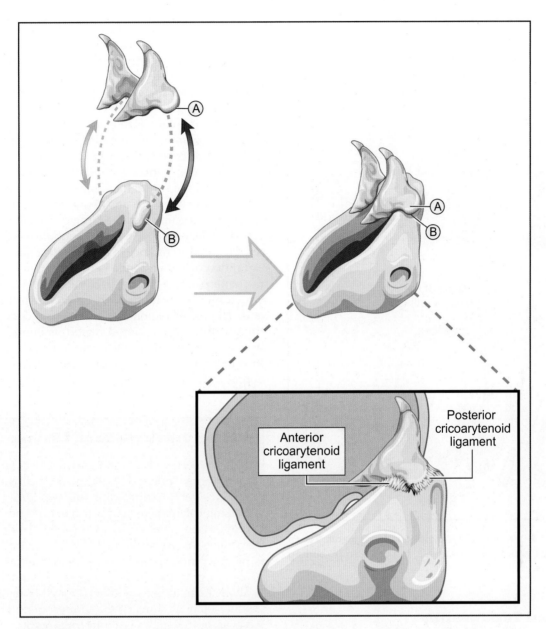

FIGURE 3-9. Cricoarytenoid joints. These two joints, one on each side, are created by articulations between concave facets on the arytenoid cartilages (A) and convex facets on the cricoid cartilage (B). The anterior and posterior cricoarytenoid ligaments secure the joints and restrict their movements.

nificant movements are of a rocking nature in which the arytenoid cartilages move at right angles to the long axes of their articulating cricoid facets (Ardran & Kemp, 1966; Selbie, Zhang, Levine, & Ludlow, 1998; Sellars & Keen, 1978; Sonesson, 1959; von Leden & Moore, 1961). The long axes of interest slope downward and toward the sides of the cricoid cartilage. This means that as the arytenoid cartilages rock on the cricoid car-

tilage, their vocal processes move either upward and outward or downward and inward.

Limited sliding movements can also occur along the cricoid facets. These movements involve small upward and inward or downward and outward adjustments of the arytenoid cartilages that follow the long axes of the cricoid facets (Fink, Basek, & Epanchin, 1956; Pressman, 1942; von Leden & Moore, 1961; Wang, 1998).

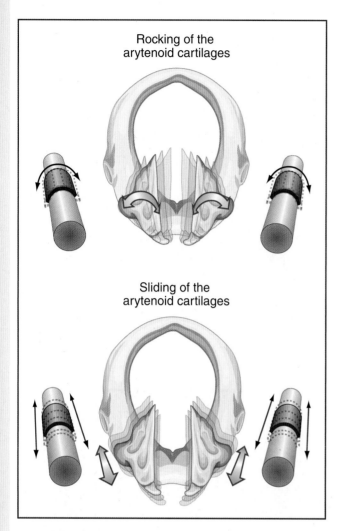

Rocking of the
arytenoid cartilages

Sliding of the
arytenoid cartilages

FIGURE 3–10. Cricoarytenoid joint movements. These are primarily rocking movements, but can also be sliding movements.

Internal Topography

The interior of the larynx defines the boundaries of the laryngeal airway. Figure 3–11 depicts the structures that form these boundaries and lie immediately deep to them. These structures include the laryngeal cavity, vocal folds, ventricular folds, laryngeal ventricles, and an assortment of ligaments and membranes.

Laryngeal Cavity

The laryngeal cavity extends from a lower opening formed by the base of the cricoid cartilage to an upper opening called the laryngeal aditus (aditus means an opening to an interior space or cavity). The laryngeal aditus forms a collar at the top of the larynx. The rim

of this collar comprises the tops of the arytenoid cartilages (and corniculate cartilages), sides of the epiglottis, and the aryepiglottic folds. The aryepiglottic folds run between the arytenoid cartilages and the epiglottis and envelop the *aryepiglottic* muscles (discussed below) and a pair of small cuneiform (wedge-shaped) cartilages. The cuneiform cartilages stiffen the aryepiglottic folds and help to maintain the upper opening (collar entrance) into the larynx.

The upper region of the laryngeal cavity (sometimes called the supraglottal region) is bounded below by the ventricular folds and above by the laryngeal aditus (upper opening into the larynx). This region is also called the laryngeal vestibule (vestibule means a space or cavity at the entrance to another structure). The configuration of the vestibule is roughly that of a funnel, the lumen (lumen means space within a hollow tubular structure) of which increases in size toward its upper end. The lower region of the laryngeal cavity (sometimes called the subglottal region) is bounded below by the lower margin of the cricoid cartilage and above by the vocal folds. This region is cone shaped and converges toward the undersurface of the vocal folds.

Being One With Your Larynx

Many aspects of laryngeal measurement show an uncanny "oneness" with the metric system. As Titze (1994) pointed out, this is helpful when making calculations off the top of your head without references at hand. A partial listing of items that he recommends be committed to memory are that (a) the mass of a vocal fold is about 1 g, (b) the length of a vibrating vocal fold is about 1 cm, (c) the excursion of a vibrating vocal fold is about 1 mm, (d) the shortest period of vocal fold vibration is about 1 ms, (e) the surface wave velocity on a vibrating vocal fold is about 1 m/s, (f) the maximum peak-to-peak airflow through a vibrating larynx is about 1 L/s, and (g) the maximum aerodynamic power generated by a vibrating larynx is about 1 J/s. We suggest you memorize these before you go to sleep tonight.

Vocal Folds

The vocal folds are two prominent shelf-like structures that extend from the sidewalls of the laryngeal cavity into the laryngeal airway. Each vocal fold has a front attachment near the midline of the thyroid cartilage

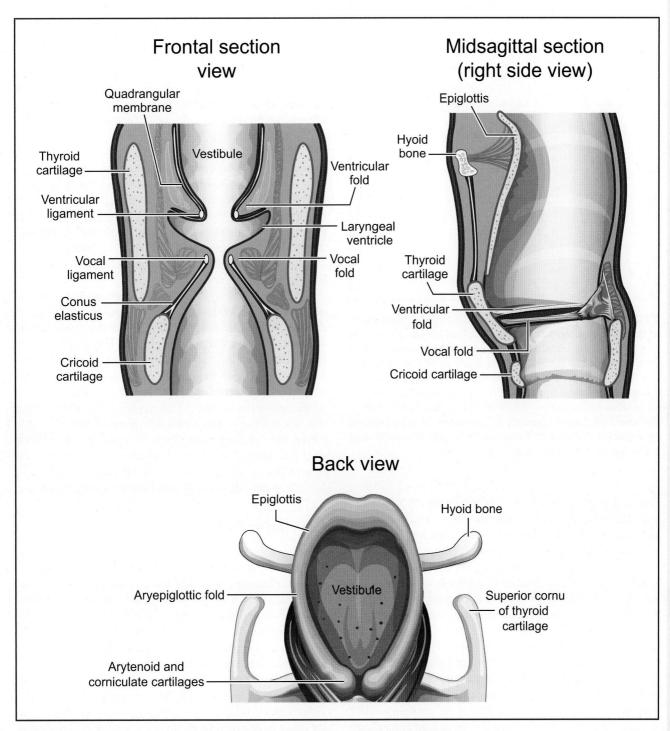

FIGURE 3–11. Structures of the interior of the larynx from three different views.

and a rear attachment to the vocal process of the arytenoid cartilage on the same side.

The vocal folds are made up of muscle covered by different layers of tissue. Figure 3–12 shows a coronal section through the mid-length of an adult vocal fold

that exemplifies this characteristic layering. Up to five layers are recognized (Hirano, 1974; Hirano & Sato, 1993) and include (starting with the outer layer and moving inward) (a) a thin stiff capsule of squamous epithelium that determines the outer shape of the vocal

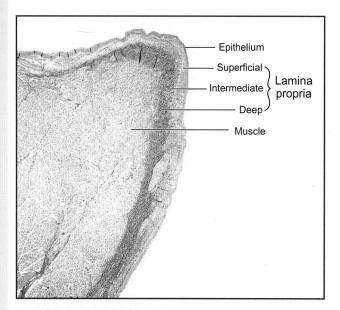

FIGURE 3–12. Coronal section through the mid-length of the membranous adult vocal fold. This section shows the five layers of the vocal folds. The epithelium and the superficial layer of the lamina propria make up the mucosa and the intermediate, and deep layers of the lamina propria make up the vocal ligament. From *Histological Color Atlas of the Human Larynx* (p. 45), by M. Hirano and K. Sato, 1993, Belmont, CA: Delmar Learning. Copyright 1993 by Delmar Learning, a division of Thomson Learning. Modified and reproduced with permission.

fold, (b) a superficial layer of lamina propria (subflooring) that consists of loose fibrous matrix and resembles soft gelatin and is anchored to the epithelium through a region called the basement membrane zone, (c) an intermediate layer of lamina propria that contains elastic fibers and is likened to a bundle of soft rubber bands, (d) a deep layer of lamina propria that contains collagen fibers and bears a resemblance to a bundle of cotton thread, and (e) muscle fibers that form the inner vocal fold and are the mechanical equivalent of a bundle of stiff rubber bands. The combined epithelium and superficial layer of the lamina propria make up what is called the mucosa. The combined intermediate and deep layers of the lamina propria make up what is called the vocal ligament, a ligament that runs along the inner edge of the vocal folds from front to back.

Although the layering in Figure 3–12 is typical at the mid-length of the vocal folds, it may be quite different at other locations because the layers of the lamina propria change in their relative proportions along the length of the vocal fold. For example, toward the ends of each vocal fold, elastic fibers and then collagenous fibers predominate. These masses of elastic and collag-

enous fibers act to cushion and protect those areas of the vocal folds from stresses. There are also differences in the cellular structure and concentration of other constituents at other locations within the lamina propria (Catten, Gray, Hammond, Zhou, & Hammond, 1998; de Melo et al., 2003; Ishii, Zhai, Akita, & Hirose, 1996; Obrebowski, Wojnowski, & Obrebowski-Karsznia, 2006; Strocchi et al., 1992).

The five layers of the vocal folds are often subgrouped into a so-called body and cover. The vocal fold body comprises muscle fibers and the deep layer of the lamina propria; the vocal fold cover comprises the intermediate and superficial layers of the lamina propria and the epithelium. This two-layered scheme, depicted in two views in Figure 3–13, helps explain certain aspects of the mechanical behavior of the vocal folds during phonation.

When viewed from above, the medial borders of the vocal folds diverge from front, as illustrated in Figure 3–14. Between the vocal folds is a triangularly shaped opening called the glottis. The front part of the glottis is called the membranous glottis and occupies about 60% of the length of the vocal folds. It lies between the thyroid cartilage and the tips of the vocal processes of the arytenoid cartilages and courses along the vocal ligaments. The back part of the glottis is called the cartilaginous glottis. It occupies about 40% of the length of the vocal folds and lies between the tips of the vocal processes of the arytenoid cartilages and the most rearward points on their medial surfaces.

Ventricular Folds

As shown in Figure 3–11 (upper images), another set of shelf-like structures also extends from the sidewalls of the laryngeal cavity into the laryngeal airway. These structures lie above the vocal folds but are less prominent. They are referred to as the ventricular folds or false vocal folds. These folds attach to the front of the thyroid cartilage and to the fronts and sides of the arytenoid cartilages at the back. Each fold contains a ventricular ligament that runs from front to back near its medial edge. Muscular tissue is sparse within the ventricular folds. The opening between the ventricular folds is referred to as the false glottis and is nearly always wider than the glottis between the vocal folds.

Laryngeal Ventricles

The vocal folds and ventricular folds have a sinus (depression) between them (Figure 3–11, upper left image). This sinus is called the laryngeal ventricle and constitutes a horizontal pouch in each sidewall of the

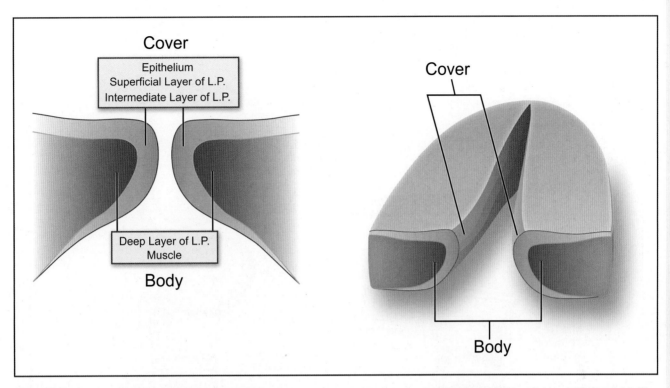

FIGURE 3–13. Subgroupings of the five layers of the vocal folds into the body (*dark pink*) and cover (*light pink*). The body consists of the muscle and deep layer of the lamina propria (L.P.) and the cover consists of the intermediate and deep layers of the lamina propria and the epithelium. The body and cover are shown in coronal view (*left*) and full view from above and behind (*right*).

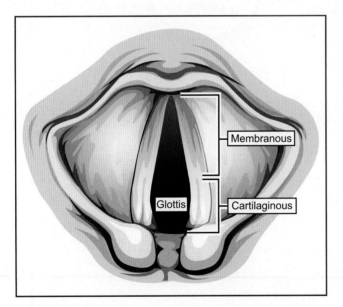

FIGURE 3–14. The vocal folds as viewed from above with the front of the larynx at the top. The glottis (opening between the vocal folds) is bounded in the front by the membranous vocal folds and in the back by the vocal processes of the arytenoid cartilages.

laryngeal tube. The laryngeal ventricles extend most of the length of the vocal folds. Toward the front of the larynx, they course upward into saccules that are richly endowed with mucous glands. These glands contain mucus that lubricates the vocal folds.

Ligaments and Membranes

Ligaments and membranes help to bind the laryngeal structures to one another and to structures outside the larynx. The ligaments that bind the joints of the larynx are discussed above and depicted in Figures 3–7 and 3–9. These are the anterior, lateral, and posterior ceratocricoid ligaments, for the cricothyroid joints, and the anterior and posterior cricoarytenoid ligaments, for the cricoarytenoid joints. Most of the other intrinsic and extrinsic ligaments and membranes are depicted in Figure 3–15 and discussed below.

Intrinsic Ligaments and Membranes

The intrinsic ligaments and membranes of the larynx (Figure 3–15, left side) are those that connect laryngeal

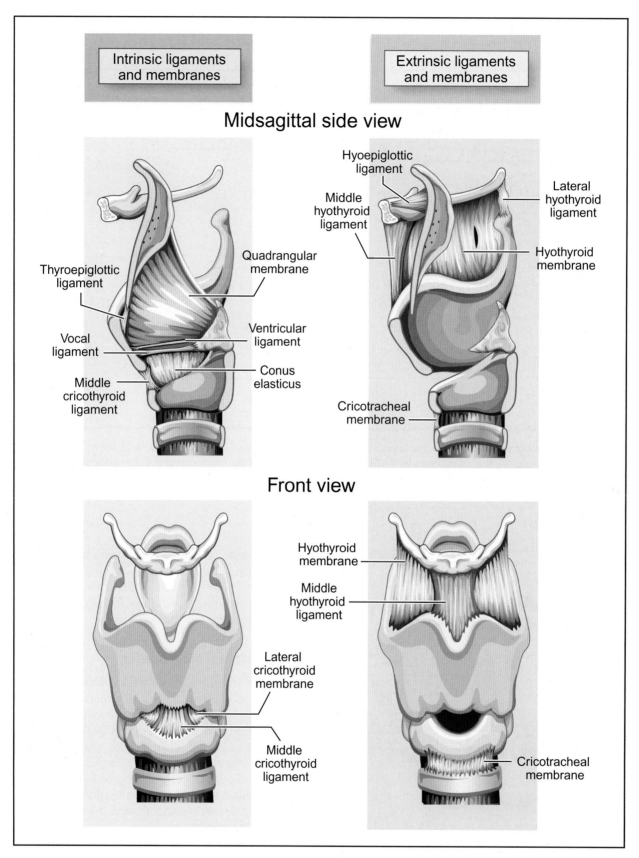

FIGURE 3–15. Intrinsic and extrinsic laryngeal ligaments and membranes. The intrinsic ligaments (middle cricothyroid, vocal, ventricular, and thyroepiglottic ligaments) and membranes (conus elasticus, lateral cricothyroid, and quadrangular membranes) connect laryngeal cartilages to one another. Extrinsic ligaments (hyoepiglottic and middle and lateral hyothyroid ligaments) and membranes (cricotracheal and hyothyroid membranes) connect laryngeal cartilages to structures outside the larynx. Mucous membrane (not shown) lines the entire laryngeal cavity.

cartilages to one another. These ligaments and membranes are important in regulating the extent and direction of movement of the laryngeal cartilages in relation to one another. Most of the intrinsic ligaments and membranes of the larynx arise from a common sheet of connective tissue called the elastic membrane. This sheet lines the entire laryngeal airway, except for the part that lies between the vocal ligaments and ventricular ligaments on each side. This discontinuity in the membrane enables the mucous glands in the laryngeal saccules to be expressed into the laryngeal cavity and lubricate the vocal folds.

The part of the elastic membrane that lines the region between the lower margin of the cricoid cartilage and the vocal folds is called the conus elasticus. The conus elasticus connects the cricoid, arytenoid, and thyroid cartilages to one another and gives rise to a middle cricothyroid ligament, two lateral cricothyroid membranes, and two vocal ligaments. The middle cricothyroid ligament extends between the top of the anterior arch of the cricoid cartilage and the bottom of the thyroid cartilage in the region of the angle of the thyroid cartilage. This ligament limits the degree to which the cricoid cartilage and thyroid cartilage can be separated vertically at the front. The two lateral cricothyroid membranes are thinner than the middle cricothyroid ligament and extend upward from the upper border of the anterior arch of the cricoid cartilage at the sides. They, like the middle cricothyroid ligament, restrict the separation of the cricoid and thyroid cartilages toward the front. The lateral cricothyroid membranes thicken significantly toward the top of the conus elasticus and are continuous with the paired vocal ligaments. The vocal ligaments extend between the angle of the thyroid cartilage and the vocal processes of the arytenoid cartilages and lie near the free margins of the vocal folds. These ligaments restrict the degree to which the thyroid and arytenoid cartilages can be separated from front to back.

The part of the elastic membrane that lines the region from the ventricular folds to the laryngeal aditus is referred to as the quadrangular membrane. The quadrangular membrane connects the epiglottis, thyroid cartilage, arytenoid cartilages, and corniculate cartilages to one another. This membrane is paired left and right and thickens significantly toward the bottom to form the ventricular (false vocal fold) ligaments. These ligaments extend the length of the ventricular folds near their free margins and attach to the thyroid and arytenoid cartilages. The ventricular ligaments place limits on the degree to which the thyroid and arytenoid cartilages can be separated from front to back. The remaining intrinsic ligament of the larynx is the thyroepiglottic ligament. This ligament extends between the bottom of the epiglottis and the inside of the angle of the thyroid cartilage, just beneath the thyroid notch, and functions as a fastener.

Extrinsic Ligaments and Membranes

Extrinsic ligaments and membranes of the larynx (Figure 3–15, right side) connect laryngeal cartilages to structures outside the larynx and provide support and stability for the laryngeal housing (the rigid structures that encase more pliable laryngeal structures). The cricotracheal membrane (sometimes called the cricotracheal ligament) comprises the lowermost extrinsic connection to the larynx. This membrane extends around the bottom of the larynx between the first tracheal ring and the lower margin of the cricoid cartilage. The cricotracheal membrane is somewhat more extensive than the connective tissue between successive tracheal rings, the first tracheal ring being somewhat larger than the rest. The hyoepiglottic ligament extends between the upper back surface of the body of the hyoid bone and the lingual surface of the epiglottis. This ligament limits the degree to which these two structures can be separated from front to back. The hyothyroid (also called the thyrohyoid) ligaments and membrane form a large interconnection between the hyoid bone and the upper margin of the thyroid cartilage of the larynx. This interconnection gives the appearance that the laryngeal housing proper is suspended from the hyoid bone. The hyothyroid membrane thickens toward the midline of the larynx at the front and is designated in that location as the middle hyothyroid ligament. The same membrane also thickens toward the back in the space between the greater cornua of the hyoid bone and the superior cornua of the thyroid cartilage. These thickenings are referred to as the lateral hyothyroid ligaments. Often embedded within each of these lateral ligaments is a small tritcial cartilage (so called because it resembles a grain of wheat).

Mucous Membrane

The entire internal laryngeal cavity is lined by a mucous membrane, like the trachea below it and the pharynx above it. This lining is covered by columnar epithelium, except for the inner edges of the vocal folds and ventricular folds and the upper half of the epiglottis, which are covered with squamous epithelium (see Figure 1–5).

FORCES OF THE LARYNX

Two types of force operate on the larynx: passive and active. Passive force is inherent within the larynx and comes from several sources. These include the natural

Motorboat

As a child, you may have played "motor boat" with friends by rapidly pounding your fists on their chests or backs while they sustained "ah." The loudness variations that sounded to you like an idling motorboat were caused by rapid changes in alveolar pressure. Pound on someone's chest or back and with each blow their lungs compress a small amount and the air pressure inside them goes up momentarily. Pound at different rates and you change the perceived speed of your imaginary motor noise. The basis of all this fun is that the larynx and the voice are sensitive to adjustments in the respiratory system. You don't necessarily need to have a friend pounding on you to appreciate this sensitivity. Try to talk while driving a car down a cross-rutted dirt road or while sitting atop a trotting horse. The road and the horse will effectively do the pounding for you by bouncing your gut up and down and changing your alveolar pressure.

recoil of muscles, cartilages, and connective tissues (ligaments and membranes); the surface tension between structures in apposition; and the pull of gravity. The distribution, sign (direction), and magnitude of passive force depend on the mechanical context, including the positions, deformations, and levels of muscle activity (if applicable) of different parts of the larynx.

Active force results from activation of laryngeal muscles. Laryngeal muscles can be categorized as intrinsic, extrinsic, or supplementary. Intrinsic muscles have both ends attached within the larynx, whereas extrinsic muscles have one end attached within the larynx and one end attached outside the larynx. Muscles categorized as supplementary do not attach to the larynx directly but influence it by way of attachments to the neighboring hyoid bone. The function described below for individual muscles assumes that the muscles of interest are engaged in concentric (shortening) contractions and that no other muscles are active, unless otherwise specified.

Intrinsic Laryngeal Muscles

The intrinsic muscles of the larynx are depicted in Figure 3–16. They are the *thyroarytenoid, posterior cricoarytenoid, lateral cricoarytenoid, arytenoid*, and *cricothyroid* muscles.

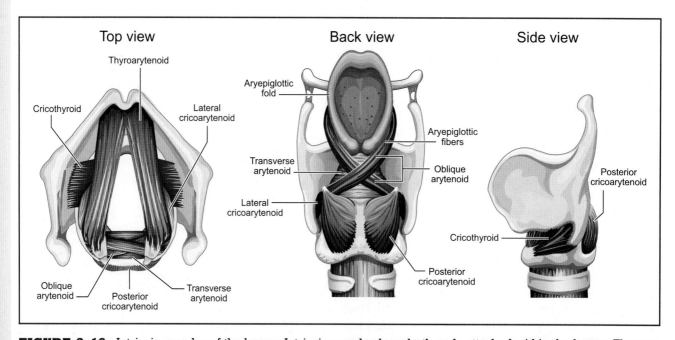

FIGURE 3–16. Intrinsic muscles of the larynx. Intrinsic muscles have both ends attached within the larynx. They are the ***thyroarytenoid***, ***posterior cricoarytenoid***, ***lateral cricoarytenoid***, ***arytenoid*** (***transverse*** and ***oblique***), and ***cricothyroid*** muscles.

The *thyroarytenoid* muscle forms most of each vocal fold. This muscle extends between the inside surface of the thyroid cartilage (near the angle) and the arytenoid cartilage on the corresponding side. The front attachment of the muscle lies to the side of the front attachment of the corresponding vocal ligament. Fibers run generally parallel to the vocal ligament to insert on the front and outer sides of the arytenoid cartilage. Upper fibers run a straight course from front to back, whereas lower fibers twist in their course and swing off in an outward, backward, and upward direction (Broad, 1973; Zemlin, 1998). A small number of fibers located toward the side of the muscle depart from the predominant front-to-back orientation of the others and course upward to the aryepiglottic fold, the side of the epiglottis, and into the region of the ventricular fold on the same side (Zemlin, 1998). The effects of contraction of different parts of the *thyroarytenoid* muscle are portrayed in Figure 3–17. Concentric contraction of its longitudinal fibers shortens it and reduces the distance between the thyroid and arytenoid cartilages. The reduction in distance between the two cartilages is typically effected as a forward pull on the arytenoid cartilage that rocks it toward the midline. Fixed-length (isometric) or lengthening (eccentric) contractions of the *thyroarytenoid* muscle (with other intrinsic mus-

cles opposing) increase its internal tension (force per unit length). Contraction of vertical fibers of the *thyroarytenoid* muscle near the sidewall of the larynx may have an influence on the position and configuration of the corresponding ventricular fold (Reidenbach, 1998; not illustrated in Figure 3–17).

The *thyroarytenoid* muscle is sometimes described as having two distinct parts (Dickson & Maue-Dickson, 1982; van den Berg & Moll, 1955; Wustrow, 1953): the *thyromuscularis* muscle (sometimes called the *external thyroarytenoid*) and *thyrovocalis* or *vocalis* muscle (sometimes called the *internal thyroarytenoid*). As depicted schematically in Figure 3–18, the *thyromuscularis* muscle lies nearest the laryngeal wall and to the side of the *thyrovocalis* muscle. The notion of a two-part *thyroarytenoid* muscle, although not universally accepted, has implications for voice production (discussed below in another section).

The *thyrovocalis* muscle and the vocal ligament are sometimes referred to as the vocal cord, as distinguished from the vocal fold (which also includes the *thyromuscularis* muscle); however, the terms *vocal cord* and *vocal fold* are also used interchangeably. The term *vocal fold* is more descriptive of the entire shelf-like structure and is generally preferred (Hall, Cobb, Kapoor, Kuchai, & Sandhu, 2017).

The *posterior cricoarytenoid* muscle is a fan-shaped muscle located on the back surface of the cricoid cartilage. The muscle originates on the cricoid lamina and courses upward and toward the side in a converging pattern to insert on the upper and back

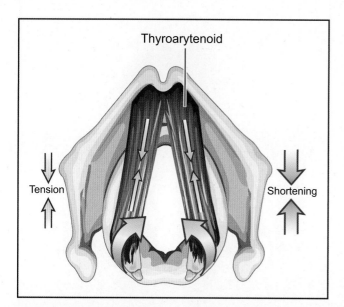

FIGURE 3–17. Effects of contractions of different parts of the *thyroarytenoid* muscles. Contraction of the longitudinal fibers shortens the muscle (*straight green arrows*) and reduces the distance between the thyroid and arytenoid cartilages. This contraction also rocks the arytenoid cartilages toward the midline (*curved green arrows*). If the contraction is isometric (fixed length) and is opposed by other muscle forces, the internal tension of the muscle increases (*yellow arrows*).

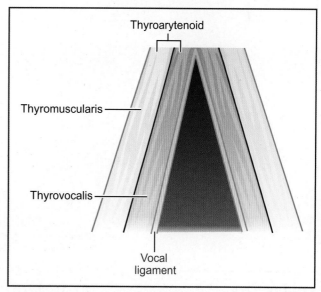

FIGURE 3–18. *Thyromuscularis* and *thyrovocalis* (or *vocalis*) subdivisions of the *thyroarytenoid* muscles. The vocal ligament runs along the internal edge of the *thyrovocalis* muscle.

surfaces of the muscular process of the arytenoid cartilage. As illustrated in Figure 3–19, contraction of the *posterior cricoarytenoid* muscle rocks the arytenoid cartilage away from the midline (thereby separating the vocal folds, which contain the *thyroarytenoid* muscles). This rocking is effected mainly by fibers located laterally within the muscle and that insert on the upper surface of the muscular process. Forceful contraction of these fibers may also slide the arytenoid cartilage upward and backward along the sloping rim of the cricoid cartilage. Fibers in the medial part of the *posterior cricoarytenoid* muscle insert on the back surface of the muscular process and contract to stabilize the arytenoid cartilage against other forces that are directed forward (Zemlin, Davis, & Gaza, 1984).

The *lateral cricoarytenoid* is a small fan-shaped muscle that originates from the upper rim of the cricoid cartilage. Fibers of this muscle extend upward and backward to insert on the muscular process and front surface of the arytenoid cartilage. As depicted in Figure 3–20, contraction of the *lateral cricoarytenoid* muscle rocks the arytenoid cartilage toward the midline (and also moves the vocal folds toward the midline).

Activation of the *lateral cricoarytenoid* muscle may also slide the arytenoid cartilage forward and toward the side along the downward sloping path of the long axis of the cricoid facet of the cricoarytenoid joint.

The *arytenoid* (also called the *interarytenoid*) muscle extends from the back surface of one arytenoid cartilage to the back surface of the other arytenoid cartilage. The *arytenoid* muscle is a complex structure that is considered to have two distinct and separate subdivisions: the *transverse arytenoid* muscle and the *oblique arytenoid* muscle. The *transverse arytenoid* muscle arises from the back surface and side of one arytenoid cartilage and courses horizontally to insert on the back surface and side of the other arytenoid cartilage. Those muscle fibers that insert on the sides of the arytenoid cartilages interdigitate with fibers of the *thyroarytenoid* muscles. The *oblique arytenoid* muscle overlies the transverse component of the muscle and diagonally crosses the back surface of the two arytenoid cartilages. The muscle originates from the back and side surface and muscular process of one arytenoid cartilage and courses upward to insert near the apex of the other arytenoid cartilage. Some muscle fibers of the *oblique ary-*

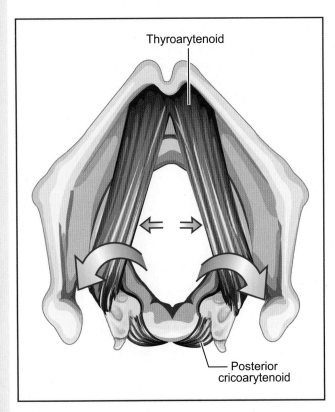

FIGURE 3–19. Effects of contraction of the *posterior cricoarytenoid* muscles. Their contraction rocks the arytenoid cartilages away from the midline and also moves the vocal folds (which contain the *thyroarytenoid* muscles) away from the midline.

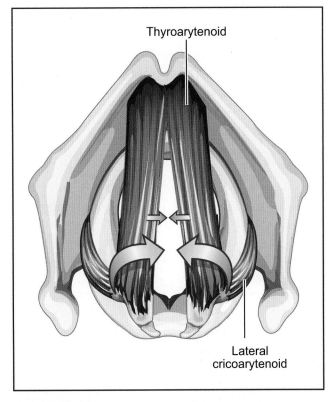

FIGURE 3–20. Effects of contraction of the *lateral cricoarytenoid* muscles. Their contraction rocks the arytenoid cartilages toward the midline and moves the vocal folds (which contain the *thyroarytenoid* muscles) toward the midline.

tenoid muscle extend around the side of the apex of the arytenoid cartilage and course upward and forward to insert into the side of the epiglottis. This part of the muscle is given its own name, the ***aryepiglottic*** mus-

cle. As illustrated in Figure 3–21, contraction of different components of the ***arytenoid*** muscle has different effects. Contraction of the ***transverse arytenoid*** muscle pulls the arytenoid cartilages toward one another. This

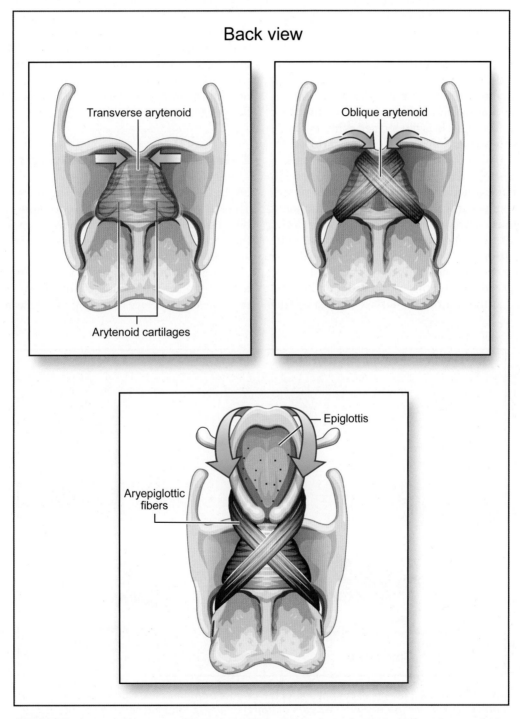

FIGURE 3–21. Effects of contractions of different parts of the ***arytenoid*** muscles. Contraction of the ***transverse arytenoid*** muscle pulls the arytenoid cartilages toward one another. Contraction of the ***oblique arytenoid*** muscle tips the arytenoid cartilages toward one another. Contraction of the ***aryepiglottic*** muscle (an extension of the ***oblique arytenoid*** muscle) pulls the epiglottis backward and downward.

is manifested through an upward, inward, and backward sliding movement along the long axis of each cricoarytenoid joint. Contraction of the *oblique arytenoid* muscle pulls one arytenoid cartilage toward the other in a tipping action that occurs in accordance with the movement permitted at the cricoarytenoid joint. And contraction of the *aryepiglottic* muscle pulls the epiglottis backward and downward to cover the upper opening into the larynx.

The *cricothyroid* muscle extends between the outer front and side of the anterior arch of the cricoid cartilage and the outer front and side of the lower border of the lamina and inferior cornu of the thyroid cartilage. The muscle is fan shaped with its fibers diverging as they course from the cricoid cartilage to the thyroid cartilage. Two subdivisions of the muscle are most often recognized, a vertical component toward the front, called the *par rectus*, and an upward sloping component toward the back, called the *pars oblique* (Zemlin, 1998). As illustrated in Figure 3–22, contraction of the *cricothyroid* muscle increases the distance between the thyroid and arytenoid cartilages and decreases the distance between the upper border of the cricoid cartilage and the lower border of the thyroid cartilage at the front of the larynx (decreases the visor angle formed between the two cartilages). These distance changes result from a rotation of the thyroid cartilage on the cricoid cartilage and/or a rotation of the cricoid cartilage on the thyroid cartilage. Rotation is effected through activation of both the *pars rectus* and *pars oblique* components of the *cricothyroid* muscle. Activation of the *pars oblique* component also results in a secondary movement that increases the distance between the thyroid and arytenoid cartilages. This movement causes a limited forward sliding of the thyroid cartilage, backward sliding of the cricoid cartilage, or both (Arnold, 1961; Takano & Honda, 2005; van den Berg et al., 1960).

Extrinsic Laryngeal Muscles

Figure 3–23 depicts the extrinsic muscles of the larynx. The extrinsic muscles have a role in supporting and stabilizing the larynx and in changing its position within the neck. They include the *sternothyroid, thyrohyoid*, and *inferior constrictor* muscles.

The *sternothyroid* muscle is a long muscle located toward the front and side of the larynx. It originates from the back surface of the top of the sternum (breast-

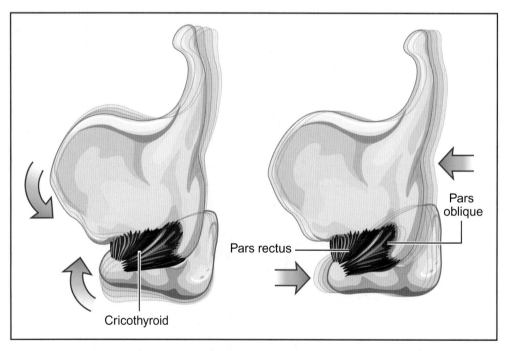

FIGURE 3–22. Effects of contraction of the *cricothyroid* muscles. Contraction of the *cricothyroid* muscles (*pars rectus* and *pars oblique*) rotates the thyroid cartilage on the cricoid cartilage (or vice versa). This rotation increases the distance between the thyroid and arytenoid cartilages at the back and decreases the distance between the thyroid and cricoid cartilages at the front. The *pars oblique* component can also cause the thyroid cartilage to slide forward and/or the cricoid cartilage to slide backward.

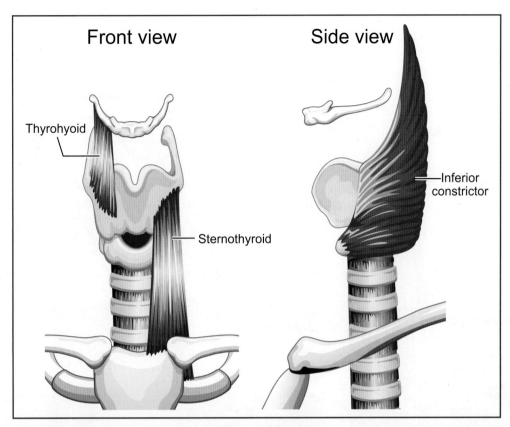

FIGURE 3–23. Extrinsic muscles of the larynx. Extrinsic muscles have one attachment inside the larynx and one attachment outside the larynx. The extrinsic laryngeal muscles are the **sternothyroid**, **thyrohyoid**, and **inferior constrictor** muscles.

bone) and the first costal (rib) cartilage. Fibers of the muscle course upward and slightly toward the side to insert on the outer surface of the thyroid cartilage. Contraction of the **sternothyroid** muscle pulls the thyroid cartilage downward. This action may also enlarge the pharynx (throat) by drawing the larynx forward and downward (Zemlin, 1998).

The **thyrohyoid** muscle is located on the front and side of the larynx. It extends between the outer surface of the thyroid cartilage and the lower edge of the greater cornu of the hyoid bone. The course of its fibers is essentially vertical. Contraction of the **thyrohyoid** muscle decreases the distance between the thyroid cartilage and the hyoid bone. Relative fixation of the thyroid cartilage and hyoid bone determines the extent to which the structures may move toward one another.

The **inferior constrictor** muscle (discussed in more detail in Chapter 4) is the lowest of the group of three muscles that forms the back and sidewalls of the pharynx. Fibers of the **inferior constrictor** muscle extend forward from the median raphe (seam) at the back of the pharynx to insert on the sides of the cricoid and thyroid cartilages. Contraction of the **inferior constric-**

tor muscle moves the sidewall of the lower pharynx inward and decreases the size of the pharyngeal lumen (tubular cavity). Its activation also serves to stabilize the position of the laryngeal housing.

Supplementary Muscles

Some muscles do not attach to the larynx but are nonetheless important in influencing its position and stability. These muscles, depicted in Figure 3–24, are referred to as supplementary muscles of the larynx. Most of them attach to the hyoid bone and are subdivided into those that originate below the hyoid bone, the so-called infrahyoid muscles, and those that originate above the hyoid bone, the so-called suprahyoid muscles.

Infrahyoid Muscles

The infrahyoid muscles include the **sternohyoid** and **omohyoid** muscles. These two muscles apply forces that can influence the positioning of the hyoid bone from below.

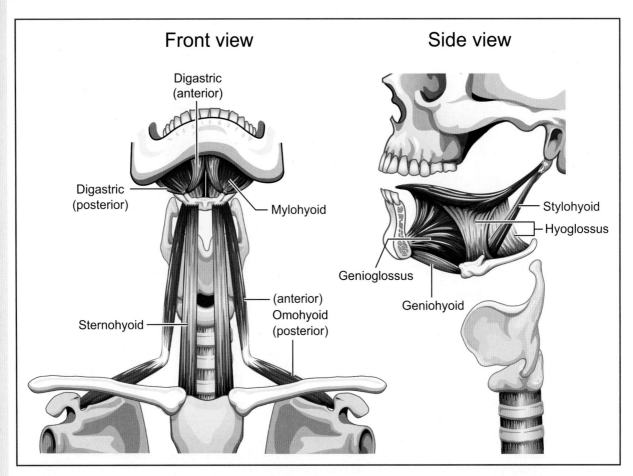

Front view

Digastric (anterior)

Digastric (posterior)

Mylohyoid

Sternohyoid

(anterior) Omohyoid (posterior)

Side view

Stylohyoid

Hyoglossus

Genioglossus

Geniohyoid

FIGURE 3–24. Supplementary muscles of the larynx. Supplementary muscles do not attach directly to the larynx but exert indirect influences through attachments to the hyoid bone. Infrahyoid muscles (*sternohyoid* and *omohyoid* muscles) originate below the hyoid bone, and suprahyoid muscles (*digastric*, *stylohyoid*, *mylohyoid*, *geniohyoid*, *hyoglossus*, and *genioglossus* muscles) originate above the hyoid bone.

The *sternohyoid* muscle is a flat structure that courses vertically along the front surface of the neck and overlies the *sternothyroid* muscle (an extrinsic laryngeal muscle). The *sternohyoid* muscle originates from the back surface of the top of the sternum and the inner end of the clavicle (collar bone). Fibers course upward and insert on the lower edge of the body of the hyoid bone. Contraction of the *sternohyoid* muscle places a downward pull on the hyoid bone. This downward pull lowers the hyoid bone, or it can anchor the hyoid bone in position if the downward pull is counterbalanced by other forces.

The *omohyoid* (shoulder-to-hyoid bone) muscle is located on the front and side of the neck. It is a narrow muscle that has two long bellies. The *posterior* (lower) belly arises from the upper edge of the scapula (shoulder blade) and courses horizontally inward and forward to attach to an intermediate tendon near the sternum. The *anterior* (upper) belly arises from the

opposite end of the same intermediate tendon and runs vertically and toward the midline to attach to the lower edge of the greater cornu of the hyoid bone. Contraction of the *omohyoid* muscle places a downward and backward pull on the hyoid bone.

Suprahyoid Muscles

The suprahyoid muscles apply forces that can influence the positioning of the hyoid bone from above. They are the *digastric, stylohyoid, mylohyoid, geniohyoid, hyoglossus,* and *genioglossus* muscles.

The *digastric* muscle is a two-bellied sling of muscle in which the two bellies are joined end-to-end by an intermediate tendon that attaches to the top of the hyoid bone. The *anterior* belly originates inside the lower border of the mandible (jaw) and courses downward and backward to the intermediate tendon. The *posterior* belly originates from the mastoid process of

They Didn't Quite Get It

She had a beautiful coloratura soprano voice and, after years of formal training, was just about to begin an operatic career. It ended abruptly on a ski slope when a careless youngster crashed into her and slammed her headfirst into a tree. She suffered facial lacerations, blunt trauma to the larynx, and temporomandibular joint damage. She never again had full singing ability. Jaw movement was especially a problem and very painful. She could no longer meet the demands of operatic roles. Forensic testimony concluded that she was 100% impaired because she could not perform a full operatic role. The career for which she had prepared was lost. The jury decided otherwise and awarded her little more than her medical expenses. The twisted logic was revealed in an interview with the foreman of the jury following the trial. "We didn't see why she couldn't just sing country songs instead. They're short and not as demanding." They didn't quite get it.

the temporal bone of the skull and courses downward and forward to the intermediate tendon. Contraction of the *digastric* muscle pulls upward on the hyoid bone and/or downward on the mandible. The relative movement of the hyoid bone and mandible is dependent on the degree to which the two structures are fixed in position by other muscles. Of interest here are influences on the hyoid bone. Contraction of the *anterior* belly of the muscle moves the hyoid bone upward and forward, whereas contraction of the *posterior* belly of the muscle moves the hyoid bone upward and backward. Contraction of the two bellies of the *digastric* muscle at the same time pulls the hyoid bone upward and forward or upward and backward at any angle, depending on the forces exerted by the two bellies.

The *stylohyoid* muscle runs a course somewhat parallel to the *posterior* belly of the *digastric* muscle. The *stylohyoid* muscle originates from the back and side surfaces of the styloid process of the temporal bone of the skull and courses downward and forward to the hyoid bone. The muscle divides into two bundles that pass on either side of the intermediate tendon of the *digastric* muscle before inserting at the junction of the body and greater cornu of the hyoid bone. Contraction of the *stylohyoid* muscle places an upward and backward pull on the hyoid bone. The action is similar to that which results from contraction of the *posterior* belly of the *digastric* muscle.

The *mylohyoid* muscle contributes to the formation of the floor of the oral cavity. Fibers of this muscle originate along much of the inner surface of the body of the mandible and course inward, backward, and downward. They join with fibers of their paired mate of the opposite side at a tendinous midline raphe (running down the center of the floor of the oral cavity). Fibers toward the rear of the oral cavity attach directly into the front surface of the body of the hyoid bone. Contraction of the *mylohyoid* muscle results in an upward and forward pull on the hyoid bone. Contraction can also result in elevation of the floor of the oral cavity and tongue. With the hyoid bone fixed in position, contraction of the *mylohyoid* muscle may lower the mandible.

The *geniohyoid* muscle is a cylindrical muscle that lies above the *mylohyoid* muscle. This muscle extends from the inner surface of the front of the mandible to the front surface of the body of the hyoid bone. Its fibers extend backward and downward in a diverging pattern. The muscle bundle runs above and nearly parallel to the fiber course of the *anterior* belly of the *digastric* muscle. Contraction of the *geniohyoid* muscle pulls the hyoid bone upward and forward. Its functional potential is similar to that of the *anterior* belly of the *digastric* muscle.

The *hyoglossus* muscle is an extrinsic muscle of the tongue (having attachments within and outside the tongue) that has the potential to exert force on the hyoid bone and move the housing of the larynx. Fibers of the muscle course vertically and extend between the side of the tongue toward the back and the body and greater cornu of the hyoid bone. When the *hyoglossus* muscle contracts, it retracts and depresses the tongue and/or elevates the hyoid bone. If the tongue is relatively more fixed than the hyoid bone, the hyoid bone will rise within the neck.

The *genioglossus* muscle is the largest and strongest of the extrinsic muscles of the tongue. This muscle has the potential to exert force on both the tongue and hyoid bone. Fibers of the *genioglossus* muscle extend from the inner surface of the mandible and course complexly to insert into the entire undersurface of the tongue and body of the hyoid bone. Contraction of the *genioglossus* muscle can have a variety of influences on the positioning of the tongue and/or hyoid bone. Its major influence on the hyoid bone is to draw it upward and forward.

Summary of the Laryngeal Muscles

The laryngeal muscles are categorized as intrinsic, extrinsic, and supplemental, depending on the locations of their attachments (inside or outside the larynx).

Actions of the intrinsic laryngeal muscles (those with both attachments inside the larynx) have a direct and profound influence on the vocal folds. Specifically, they can abduct (move apart), adduct (move together), shorten, lengthen, and tense the vocal folds. Actions of the extrinsic and supplemental laryngeal muscles (those with at least one attachment outside the larynx) serve to stabilize the larynx and can change its position within the neck. In general, contractions of muscles with attachments below the larynx can lower the larynx, and contractions of those with attachments above the larynx can raise the larynx. These laryngeal movements and their associated forces are detailed in the next two sections.

Donation and a Growing Cause

Two interesting developments hold promise for those with severe laryngeal injury or disease. One is laryngeal transplantation in which a donor larynx from another individual is transferred to an individual whose larynx is no longer viable. The results of initial efforts in transplantation are somewhat encouraging, although only two laryngeal transplants have been reported in the medical literature to date. More promising is the regeneration and reconstruction of new laryngeal tissue through the use of tissue engineering. Tissue engineering has advanced to the stage where successful growth of new laryngeal tissue has been accomplished in humans. New cell therapies combined with new techniques for scaffold construction, such as three-dimensional printing, hold great promise for those with damaged or diseased larynges (Hertegård, 2016).

MOVEMENTS OF THE LARYNX

Movements of the larynx include those of the vocal folds, ventricular folds, epiglottis, and laryngeal housing. These movements allow the larynx to act as a valve at multiple levels and to perform a variety of functions.

Movements of the Vocal Folds

The vocal folds are movable and flexible. Their movements can change their vertical position, lateral (side-to-side) position, shape, and length.

Vertical and side-to-side position changes of each vocal fold can occur as its corresponding arytenoid cartilage rocks at a right angle to the long axis of its associated cricoid facet. When the rocking movement is downward and inward, the back end of the vocal fold moves downward and toward the midline. When rocking movement is upward and outward, the back end of the vocal fold moves upward and toward the side. Under normal circumstances, the two arytenoid cartilages move simultaneously and similarly so that the two vocal folds move in similar trajectories.

Changes in shape mainly constitute a thinning or thickening of the vocal fold toward its free margin such that the free margin may be relatively sharp or blunt in cross section toward the airway. The vocal fold may also appear to be somewhat tilted.

The vocal folds can be lengthened or shortened considerably. Lengthening is limited by the degree to which the covering tissue of the vocal fold, vocal ligament, and different parts of the *thyroarytenoid* muscle are distensible. Lengthening of the vocal folds occurs when either or both the thyroid and cricoid cartilages are moved away from one another. Shortening of the vocal folds results when either or both the thyroid and cricoid cartilages are drawn toward one another.

These movements are important in speech production. Of particular relevance are the movements that result in vocal fold abduction, adduction, and length change.

Vocal Fold Abduction

Vocal fold abduction is the movement of a vocal fold away from the midline. Abduction is normally simultaneous and symmetric in the two vocal folds. As the vocal folds move toward the side, the glottis (space between them) increases in size. As portrayed in Figure 3–25, full abduction of the vocal folds results in a wide glottis and the condition in which air flows most freely in and out of the pulmonary system. It is the vocal folds that abduct, not the glottis.

Abduction of the vocal folds and concomitant enlargement of the glottis are caused primarily by contractions of the *posterior cricoarytenoid* muscles. These muscles pull on the muscular processes of the arytenoid cartilages to swing the vocal folds upward and outward. Vocal fold abduction can also result from a downward pull on the larynx, which places a downward pull on the conus elasticus (lower elastic lining of the larynx). Such a pull tends to tug the free margin of the vocal fold downward and toward the side, thus dilating the laryngeal airway (Zenker, 1964). This is called tracheal tug and can happen when the diaphragm contracts footward and pulls downward on the trachea. The contribution of the *posterior cricoarytenoid* muscles to vocal fold abduction is much greater than that of tracheal tug.

Vocal Fold Adduction

Vocal fold adduction is the movement of a vocal fold toward the midline. During adduction, the two vocal folds usually follow similar movement pathways and the glottis decreases in size. As illustrated in Figure 3–26, movement toward the midline may be sufficient to approximate (bring together) the entire free margins of the two vocal folds and close the laryngeal airway. Alternatively, movement toward the midline may be limited to the membranous part of the vocal folds (front 60%), resulting in closure of only that portion

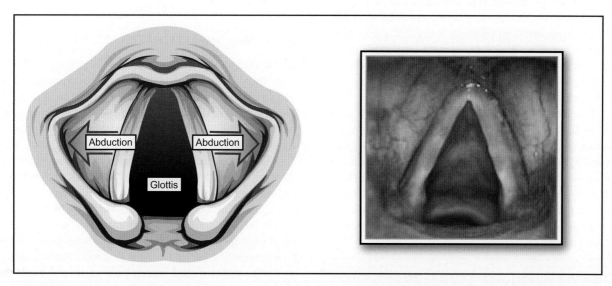

FIGURE 3–25. Vocal fold abduction and widening of the glottis. Vocal fold abduction is accomplished primarily by contraction of the paired *posterior cricoarytenoid* muscles. A downward force exerted on the larynx can also abduct the vocal folds. The image on the right is a photograph of an author's vocal folds (courtesy of Robin Samlan).

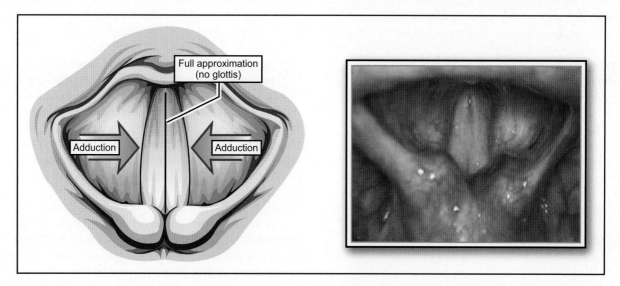

FIGURE 3–26. Vocal fold adduction. The *lateral cricoarytenoid* muscles adduct the front (membranous) portion of the vocal folds and the *arytenoid* muscles adduct the back (cartilaginous) portion of the vocal folds. The amount of vocal fold contact in the vertical dimension can be adjusted by bulging of the medial surfaces through contraction of the *thyrovocalis* muscles. The image on the right is a photograph of an author's vocal folds (courtesy of Robin Samlan).

of the airway, while leaving the cartilaginous portion (back 40%) of the vocal folds abducted.

Adduction resulting in full approximation of the two vocal folds is caused by the combined contraction of the *lateral cricoarytenoid* muscles and *arytenoid* muscles (*transverse* and *oblique* components); adduction resulting in approximation of only the membranous (front) portions of the vocal folds is caused by contraction of the *lateral cricoarytenoid* muscles alone. Action of the *lateral cricoarytenoid* muscles pulls forward on the muscular processes of the arytenoid cartilages, rocking them over the cricoid cartilage and swinging the vocal folds downward and inward. Action of the *arytenoid* muscles pulls the arytenoid cartilages toward the midline and approximates the cartilaginous (back) portion of the vocal folds.

Once the vocal folds are approximated (fully adducted), the vertical extent of their approximation (amount of contact) and the compressive force (force of contact) can be adjusted. The amount of contact of the cross-sectional thickness through the approximated vocal fold surfaces can be adjusted by contracting the *thyrovocalis* portion of the *thyroarytenoid* muscle. Contraction of the *thyrovocalis* muscle bulges the

Daniel R. Boone (1927–2018)

The Daniel Boone you've heard of may or may not be this one. Both are pioneers. This one wrote a clinical textbook that represented the first comprehensive approach to the topic of voice disorders. He proposed a large series of facilitating techniques that were widely adopted by speech-language pathologists; these remain in use today throughout the world. Boone was a master clinician and an outstanding teacher. He had a knack for cutting to the heart of clinical matters quickly, and few equaled him in his compassion for people with serious voice disorders. Boone was a past president of the American Speech-Language-Hearing Association (ASHA) and was instrumental in guiding ASHA to prominence. Boone had a wonderful sense of humor and a passion for the card game Hearts. He retired and lived in Tucson, Arizona, where he continued an active professional and personal life. During his final days, at the age of almost 91, he attended one author's birthday party, wrapped up details for his new book, and flew off to Texas to help give a workshop on voice therapy.

medial surfaces of the vocal folds toward the midline. The force of contact is adjusted by actions of the *lateral cricoarytenoid* muscles and the *arytenoid* muscles that squeeze the vocal folds together. The squeezing force exerted between the vocal processes of the arytenoid cartilages by the *lateral cricoarytenoid* muscles has been called medial compression (van den Berg et al., 1960). Medial compression can be applied even when the vocal folds are separated along their cartilaginous length.

Vocal Fold Length Change

The length of the vocal folds can be changed through a variety of external and internal adjustments. The length changes that are most important to speech production are mediated through the cricothyroid joints. Length changes can also be mediated through the cricoarytenoid joints.

The vocal fold length changes that are mediated through the cricothyroid joints are best understood in the context of approximated vocal folds, as illustrated in Figure 3–27. Vocal fold lengthening (upper images in Figure 3–27) is achieved by forward directed forces pulling on the front ends of the vocal folds at their points of attachment to the inside of the thyroid cartilage and/or by backward directed forces pulling on the back ends of the vocal folds at their points of attachment to the vocal processes of the arytenoid cartilages. Forward directed forces result from contraction of the *cricothyroid* muscles, which place pulls on the front ends of the thyroid and cricoid cartilages that tend to close the visor angle of the larynx by rocking the thyroid cartilage on the cricoid cartilage and/or rocking the cricoid cartilage on the thyroid cartilage. The consequence of any combination of rocking of the front ends of these two cartilages toward one another is an increase in the distance between the front of the thyroid cartilage and the vocal processes of the arytenoid cartilages and a stretching of the vocal folds. Actions of the *cricothyroid* muscles (especially the *pars oblique* portions) can also cause a sliding movement at the cricothyroid joints that can contribute to vocal fold lengthening by increasing the distance between the front of the thyroid cartilage and the vocal processes of the arytenoid cartilages.

Actions of the *posterior cricoarytenoid* muscles counteract those of the *cricothyroid* muscles and serve to anchor the arytenoid cartilages and their vocal processes from tilting forward and sliding during contractions of the *cricothyroid* muscles. The *posterior cricoarytenoid* muscles may also lengthen the vocal folds somewhat by pulling the arytenoid cartilages backward and upward along the facets on the slope

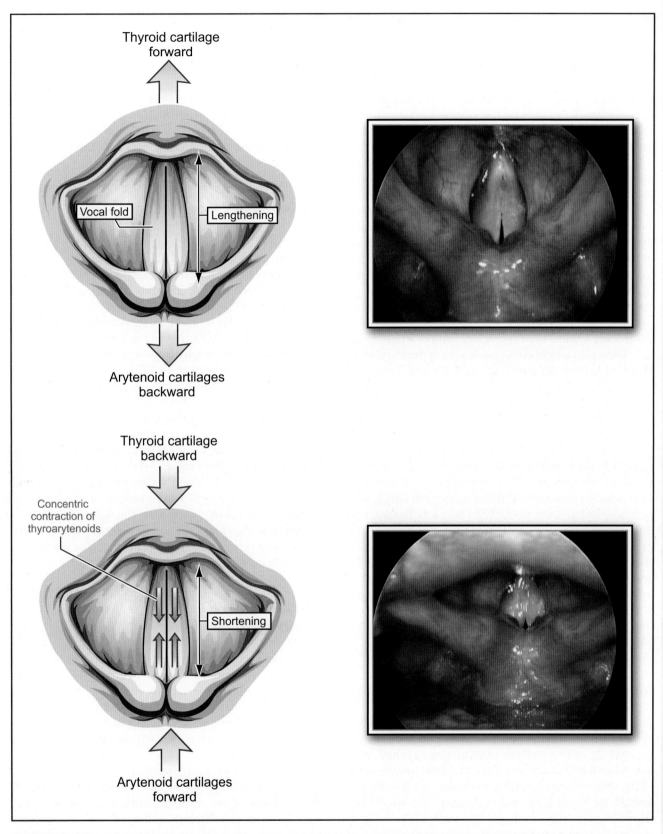

FIGURE 3–27. Vocal fold length changes mediated through the cricothyroid joints. Active vocal fold lengthening (*upper images*) is accomplished primarily by forward directed forces through contraction of the ***cricothyroid*** muscles (with possibly backward-directed forces exerted by the ***posterior cricoarytenoid*** muscles). Active vocal fold shortening (*lower images*) is accomplished primarily by contraction of the ***thyroarytenoid*** muscles. The images on the right are photographs of actual vocal folds (courtesy of Robin Samlan).

of the cricoid rim. Thus, the *cricothyroid* muscles are responsible for stretching the vocal folds to a greater length in a forward direction, whereas the *posterior cricoarytenoid* muscles are responsible for securing the back ends of the vocal folds or for stretching them to a greater length in a rearward direction.

Shortening of the vocal folds (lower images in Figure 3–27) results from relaxation of the external distending muscles just discussed (*cricothyroid* and *posterior cricoarytenoid* muscles) or from concentric (shortening) contractions of the *thyroarytenoid* muscles. Because the *thyroarytenoid* muscles constitute the main mass of the vocal folds, their contraction shortens the vocal folds and their internal fibers. If unopposed by actions of other muscles of the larynx, *thyroarytenoid* muscle contractions serve to draw the thyroid and arytenoid cartilages toward one another (pull the two ends of the vocal folds toward their respective centers lengthwise).

Vocal fold length changes also occur during abduction and adduction (see Figures 3–25 and 3–26) and are mediated through the cricoarytenoid joints. These length changes are the result of rocking and sliding of the arytenoid cartilages on the cricoid cartilage, which carries the tips of the vocal processes of the arytenoid cartilages upward, backward, and outward or downward, forward, and inward. Upward, backward, and outward movement of the vocal processes, as mediated through activation of the *posterior cricoarytenoid* muscles, abducts the vocal folds and lengthens them; downward, forward, and inward movement of the processes, as mediated through activation of the *lateral cricoarytenoid* muscles, adducts the vocal folds and shortens them. To gain a clearer understanding of how the vocal folds move, videos are provided that use a model of the vocal folds to illustrate selected vocal fold actions: see Videos 3–1 (Vocal Fold Model) and 3–2 (Abduction, Adduction, Length Change).

Movements of the Ventricular Folds

The ventricular (false) folds can also move and change shape. Although the ventricular folds tend to be widely separated, under certain circumstances, they may extend well into the airway to form a roof over the vocal folds. The ventricular folds may also tilt downward toward the vocal folds and even come in contact with them. Figure 3–28 illustrates the ventricular folds at rest and widely separated and substantially adducted in both schematic form and in actual photographs.

The muscular mechanisms underlying ventricular fold movements are not well understood. One suggestion is that the actions of other muscles in the vicinity of the ventricular folds combine to cause sphincter-like

folding and unfolding of the interior of the larynx that moves and shapes the passive ventricular folds (Fink, 1975; Zemlin, 1998). Fibers of the *thyromuscularis* portions of *thyroarytenoid* muscles that course upward along the sidewalls of the larynx above the vocal folds may contribute to the folding action of the ventricular folds (Reidenbach, 1998).

Movements of the Epiglottis

The epiglottis is usually oriented upright. From this position, it can be moved backward and downward to horizontal or beyond and thereby cover the laryngeal aditus (upper opening into the larynx). This is illustrated in Figure 3–29. Downward movement of the epiglottis can also be segmental, such that just the upper third is folded backward over the laryngeal aditus.

The epiglottis is cartilage only and has no motive force other than its own recoil properties and gravity; therefore, its movements and shape changes are effected by external mechanisms. One mechanism is contraction of the *aryepiglottic* muscles, which can lower the epiglottis and/or alter its configuration by folding it inward upon itself from top to bottom and/or across. The other mechanism is elevation of the laryngeal housing, which forces the front of the epiglottis against the base of the tongue, compressing it backward and downward over the upper opening to the larynx. This action helps to protect the laryngeal airway and prevent the aspiration of food or liquid into the lower airways and lungs during swallowing.

Movements of the Laryngeal Housing

The housing of the larynx (the interconnected rigid structures surrounding the more pliable laryngeal structures) can move within the neck. Although it can move in nearly all directions, its most important movement is vertical. The laryngeal housing can also be shifted forward or backward within the neck from its resting position.

Extrinsic and supplementary laryngeal muscles are responsible for moving and stabilizing the laryngeal housing. These muscles act by direct pulls on the larynx as well as indirect pulls through insertions on the hyoid bone. These actions are illustrated in Figure 3–30.

Upward movements of the laryngeal housing can be brought about by activation of one or a combination of muscles that includes the *thyrohyoid*, *digastric* (*anterior* and *posterior* bellies), *stylohyoid*, *mylohyoid*, *geniohyoid*, *hyoglossus*, and *genioglossus* muscles, and

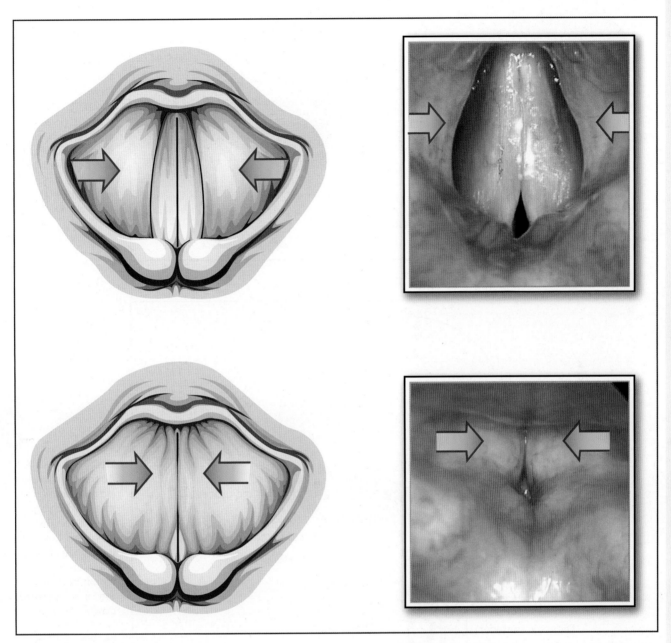

FIGURE 3–28. The ventricular folds at rest (*top*) and almost fully adducted (*bottom*). When at rest, the ventricular folds are far apart from one another and may be difficult to distinguish from the laryngeal walls. During effortful activities, the ventricular folds on both sides may move inward toward the midline and may even come into full contact with each other. (Photographs courtesy of Robin Samlan).

downward movements can result from activation of one or a combination of muscles that includes the *sternothyroid, sternohyoid,* and *omohyoid* (*anterior* and *posterior* bellies) muscles. Forward movements of the laryngeal housing can result from activation of one or a combination of muscles that includes the *sternothyroid, digastric* (*anterior* belly), *mylohyoid, geniohyoid,* and *genioglossus* muscles, and backward movements of the housing can be brought about through activa-

tion of one or a combination of muscles that includes the *omohyoid* (*anterior* and *posterior* bellies), *digastric* (*posterior* belly), and *stylohyoid* muscles.

The larynx can also be fixed in position through different combinations of counteractive forces exerted by the muscles listed above. Fixation may also include activation of the *inferior constrictor* muscle of the pharynx, which can stabilize the larynx against forward directed forces.

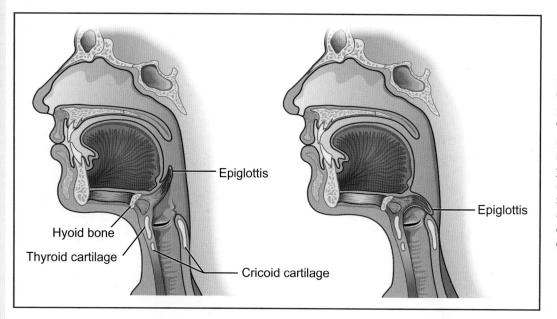

FIGURE 3–29.
The epiglottis in two positions. The epiglottis is shown in its usual standing (rest) position (*left*) and after it has been moved backward and downward to cover the laryngeal aditus (*right*).

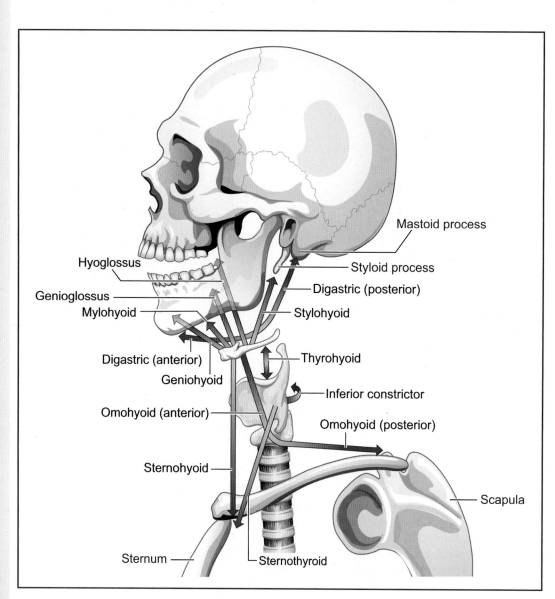

FIGURE 3–30.
Actions of extrinsic and supplementary laryngeal muscles on the laryngeal housing. These actions, alone or in combination, can move the larynx upward, downward, forward, and/or backward. They can also fix the larynx in position through counteractive forces.

Harry Hollien

Hollien has been a champion of the study of laryngeal function in the context of experimental phonetics for half a century. He pioneered the quantification of vocal fold correlates of voice fundamental frequency change, one of his most clever endeavors being his work on strobo-scopic laminagraphy (phase-advanced frontal x-rays). He also contributed significantly to our understanding of factors influencing speech intelligibility in deep-water divers. Well known for his forensic studies on speaker identification, he may be the most celebrated expert witness in the world in matters involving the use of voice in the commission of crime. Hollien founded the American Association of Phonetic Sciences, published extensively (over 400 research articles, over 60 chapters, and 1 book), and has fostered the careers of many outstanding speech and voice scientists. A colorful and outspoken advocate for his professional passions, Hollien is one of the key figures in the history of experimental phonetics.

LARYNGEAL CONTROL VARIABLES

The forces and movements of the larynx make it possible to breathe, speak, sing, laugh, whistle, cough, and swallow. Such activities require that certain laryngeal variables be controlled. Those of interest here are (a) laryngeal opposing pressure, (b) laryngeal airway resistance, (c) glottal size and configuration, (d) stiffness of the vocal folds, and (e) effective mass of the vocal folds. The relevance of a particular control variable depends on the activity being performed. For example, during singing, stiffness of the vocal folds is critical for adjusting fundamental frequency (pitch) of the voice, but it is inconsequential during whistling, an activity that does not involve direct participation of the vocal folds.

Laryngeal Opposing Pressure

Laryngeal opposing pressure is a measure of the opposition provided by the larynx to translaryngeal air pressure (the air pressure difference between the trachea and pharynx) when the larynx is closed airtight (Hixon & Minifie, 1972). This opposition is the pressure (force

over an area) provided by the larynx to maintain it in a closed configuration when positive (or negative) aero-mechanical forces would otherwise blow (or suck) it open. As illustrated in Figure 3–31, laryngeal opposing pressure is the net opposing pressure (meaning the sum of all the pressures) being exerted, and it has three components: (a) compressive muscular pressure that squeezes the vocal folds together, (b) surface tension between the apposed surfaces of the moist vocal folds that helps hold them together, and (c) gravity that weighs down the vocal folds and influences them differently depending on body position (or gravity field). Of these three, compressive muscular pressure is by far the greatest contributor to laryngeal opposing pressure. The laryngeal opposing pressure required to maintain airtight closure of the larynx can range from low to high, depending on the activity.

Laryngeal Airway Resistance

Laryngeal airway resistance is a measure of the opposition provided by the larynx to airflow through it.

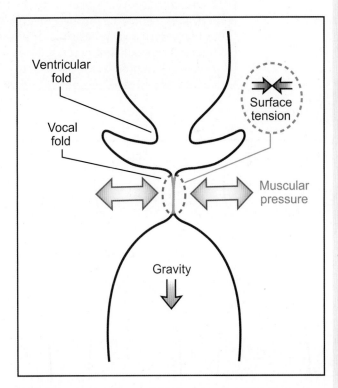

FIGURE 3–31. Laryngeal opposing pressure has three components. These are muscular pressure (the greatest contributor to laryngeal opposing pressure), surface tension between the surfaces of the moist vocal folds, and gravity.

Because the main constriction within the larynx is at the level of the vocal folds, this region of the larynx is the foremost contributor to laryngeal airway resistance. The ventricular folds may be a secondary contributor. Thus, by adjusting the cross-sectional area and/or length of the internal larynx in the region of the vocal folds and ventricular folds, the laryngeal airway resistance will likely change. Resistance increases with increasing constriction and length of constriction. It is important to note that laryngeal airway resistance is airflow dependent. This means that even at fixed cross-sectional areas and/or lengths of the laryngeal airway, the resistance is influenced by how fast air is moving through it (van den Berg, Zantema, & Doornenbal, 1957). Laryngeal airway resistance cannot be measured directly; instead, it is estimated by determining the quotient of translaryngeal air pressure to translaryngeal airflow (the rate at which air is flowing through the larynx). Laryngeal airway resistance can range from very low (wide open airway with low airflow) to infinite (airtight closure of the airway), as illustrated in Figure 3–32.

Opposition to Certain Terms of Opposition

Laryngeal airway resistance, discussed in the text, is opposition to the movement of air through the laryngeal airway. This resistance is often mistakenly labeled as vocal fold resistance, glottal resistance, or laryngeal resistance. It's none of these. It's not a measure of the mechanical status of the vocal folds or a measure of the size of the hole designated as the glottis. Laryngeal airway resistance is a property of the airway itself. To gain a more concrete understanding (pun intended), think of a plaster cast of the inside of a larynx. Nothing in the plaster cast is adjustable. Everything is dead-stiff rigid. Yet, resistance to the flow of air through the cast is airflow dependent. Force air through the cast in either direction and you'll find that laryngeal airway resistance goes up and down as airflow goes up and down. Laryngeal airway resistance isn't something you can look at and measure. It's something you have to calculate.

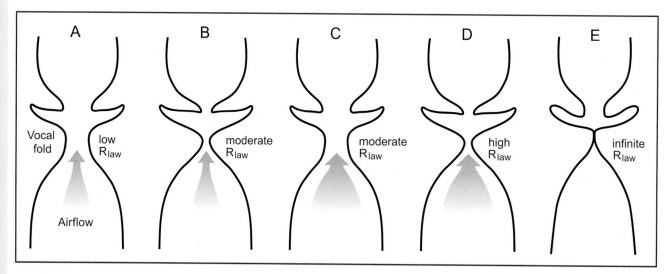

FIGURE 3–32. Laryngeal airway resistance (R_{law}), a calculated quantity that reflects the opposition provided by the larynx to airflow through it. It can range from low (A) to moderate (B and C) to high (D) to infinite (E). Laryngeal airway resistance can increase by a narrowing and/or lengthening of the airway (compare A to B) and/or by increasing airflow (compare A to C).

Glottal Size and Configuration

The glottis can be adjusted in length, diameter, area, and shape, as shown in Figure 3–33. Maximum glottal size (A in the figure) can be achieved during a very deep inspiration following panting (Sekizawa, Sasaki, & Takishima, 1985) and is accomplished mainly from contraction of the *posterior cricoarytenoid* muscles. A glottis of medium size (B in the figure) might be associated with resting tidal breathing. A small glottis may result from simultaneous contraction of the *lateral cricoarytenoid* muscles and *arytenoid* muscles (*transverse* and *oblique* subdivisions) to form a narrow opening along the length of the vocal folds (C in the figure). Alternatively, a small glottis can be in the form of a gap at the posterior part of the larynx (D in the figure) if just the *lateral cricoarytenoid* muscles are activated. Stronger activation of the *lateral cricoarytenoid* and *arytenoid* muscles can bring the vocal folds in full contact with one another so that the airway is closed airtight and there is no glottis (E in the figure).

Stiffness of the Vocal Folds

Stiffness of the vocal folds is an indication of their rigidity or tautness. Stiffness is the reciprocal of compliance (floppiness). In physical terms, this refers to how much the vocal folds move for a given force applied to them. Stiffness may differ somewhat from one region to another within the vocal folds. For example, the folds may be stiffer nearer their points of attachment to the thyroid and arytenoid cartilages than at their midpoints.

Vocal fold stiffness is adjusted primarily by lengthening the vocal folds (Titze, 1994). Vocal fold lengthening, accomplished primarily by contracting the *cricothyroid* muscles, increases their longitudinal tension (like stretching a rubber band), as illustrated on the left side of Figure 3–34. The tensile strength of the vocal ligaments along the medial edges of the vocal folds is the limiting factor as to how much the vocal folds can be stretched and how much longitudinal tension can be applied.

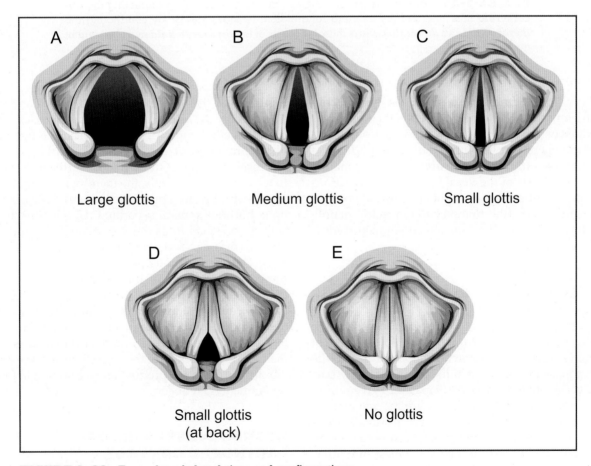

A Large glottis

B Medium glottis

C Small glottis

D Small glottis (at back)

E No glottis

FIGURE 3–33. Examples of glottal sizes and configurations.

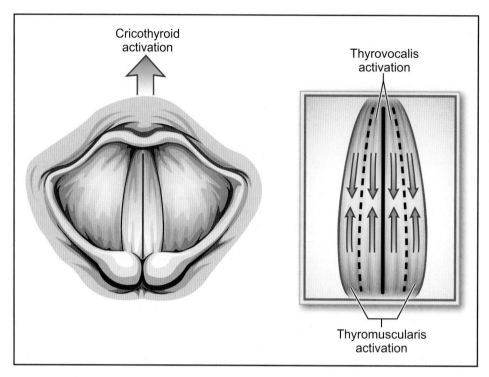

FIGURE 3–34. Vocal fold stiffness. Stiffness can be increased by contracting the *cricothyroid* muscles (thereby exerting longitudinal tension) and/or by contracting the *thyrovocalis* and *thyromuscularis* muscles (parts of the *thyroarytenoid* muscles) within the vocal folds.

Vocal fold stiffness can also be changed by contracting muscles within the vocal folds themselves, as illustrated on the right side of Figure 3–34. Contraction of muscle fibers that lie within the lateral portions of the vocal folds (the *thyromuscularis* muscles) mainly stiffen those parts of the vocal folds, and contractions of the muscle fibers that lie within the medial portions of the vocal folds (the *thyrovocalis* muscles) mainly affect those portions. The more forceful the contraction, the greater stiffness.

Effective Mass of the Vocal Folds

Although the overall mass of the vocal folds (i.e., the quantity of matter making up the vocal folds) does not change (at least on a moment-to-moment basis), the *effective* mass may change in the sense that only part of the vocal fold mass may participate in a given activity. Full mass and effective mass are the same when the vocal folds are fully abducted, are maximally elongated, and have unencumbered free margins along their lengths. Full mass and effective mass are different, however, when the vocal folds are partitioned by some action that encumbers them at some intermediate point along their lengths. An example can be seen in

Figure 3–35 in which the vocal folds have been adducted by the *lateral cricoarytenoid* muscles, resulting in "medial compression" between the tips of the vocal processes of the arytenoid cartilages. When the vocal processes of the arytenoid cartilages are made to toe inward sufficiently, the membranous portions of the vocal folds are approximated and their cartilaginous portions remain separated. Under this circumstance, the vocal folds are partitioned longitudinally into two masses having very different functional potentials. The membranous portion of the configuration impedes the flow of air through the larynx, whereas the cartilaginous portion allows air to pass freely. As medial compression increases (via increased activation of the *lateral cricoarytenoid* muscles), there may be a concomitant decrease in the effective mass of the membranous portions of the vocal folds that are able to vibrate during voice production (see section below on Fundamental Frequency).

NEURAL SUBSTRATES OF LARYNGEAL CONTROL

Laryngeal movement is controlled by the nervous system. The nature of the movement and its neural con-

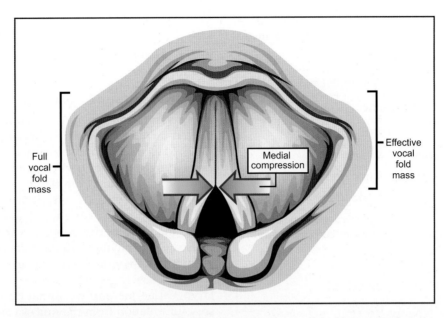

FIGURE 3–35. Effective vocal fold mass. Forceful medial compression by contraction of the *lateral cricoarytenoid* muscles can reduce the effective mass of the membranous portions of the vocal folds for an activity such as vocal fold vibration.

trol are different for different activities (for example, coughing, throat clearing, crying, singing, speaking, and swallowing).

All control commands are sent to the larynx through cranial nerves that originate in the brainstem and through cervical spinal nerves that originate in the uppermost segments of the spinal cord. These nerves provide motor innervation to the intrinsic, extrinsic, and supplementary muscles of the larynx. As shown in Table 3–1, motor innervation to the larynx is supplied by cranial nerves V (trigeminal), VII (facial), X (vagus), and XII (hypoglossal) and cervical spinal nerves C1, C2, and C3.

Innervation to the five intrinsic muscles of the larynx is through cranial nerve X, also called the vagus nerve. As cranial nerve X leaves the brainstem and descends in the neck, it gives off two main branches to innervate intrinsic laryngeal muscles. These are the superior laryngeal nerve and the recurrent laryngeal nerve. The recurrent laryngeal nerve (also called the inferior laryngeal branch) provides motor supply to four intrinsic muscles: the *thyroarytenoid, posterior cricoarytenoid, lateral cricoarytenoid*, and *arytenoid* muscles. The *cricothyroid* muscle receives its motor supply from the external branch of the superior laryngeal nerve. There is variation among larynges in the way specific nerves branch on their way to the larynx and how they interconnect with other nerves (Sanders, Wu, Mu, & Biller, 1993; Sanudo et al., 1999). For example, the recurrent laryngeal nerve has been shown to bifurcate or trifurcate before entering into the left or

right sides of the larynx in more than a third of larynges studied (Beneragama & Serpell, 2006).

Innervation of the three extrinsic muscles of the larynx is provided by cervical spinal nerves for the *sternothyroid* (C1, C2, and C3) and *thyrohyoid* (C1 and C2) muscles, whereas the *inferior constrictor* muscle of the pharynx is supplied by branches of cranial nerve X. The eight supplementary muscles of the larynx receive their motor innervation in various combinations through cranial nerves V, VII, and XII and cervical spinal nerves C1, C2, and C3. The *sternohyoid* and *omohyoid* muscles receive motor supply from C1, C2, and C3; the *geniohyoid* muscle from C1; and the *hyoglossus* and *genioglossus* muscles by cranial nerve XII. The remaining three supplementary muscles are innervated by cranial nerves V and/or VII. The *digastric* muscle receives motor innervation from both cranial nerves, its *anterior* belly from cranial nerve V and its *posterior* belly from cranial nerve VII (Dickson & Maue-Dickson, 1982). The *stylohyoid* and *mylohyoid* muscles receive motor innervation from cranial nerves VII and V, respectively.

Laryngeal movements are not executed without information about their consequences. Sensory information is critical to the control of laryngeal movements, especially the rapid and precise movements that are characteristic of the vocal folds. This information comes from several sources, the relative importance of which depends on the activity being performed. These sources have in common some type of mechanoreceptor that converts a mechanical event into a neural

TABLE 3–1. Summary of the Cranial and Segmental Origins of the Motor Nerve Supply to the Muscles of the Larynx

MUSCLE	INNERVATION
INTRINSIC	
Thyroarytenoid	X (recurrent)
Posterior cricoarytenoid	X (recurrent)
Lateral cricoarytenoid	X (recurrent)
Arytenoid	X (recurrent)
Cricothyroid	X (external branch of superior laryngeal nerve)
EXTRINSIC	
Sternothyroid	C1, C2, C3
Thyrohyoid	C1, C2
Inferior constrictor	X
SUPPLEMENTARY	
Sternohyoid	C1, C2, C3
Omohyoid	C1, C2, C3
Digastric	V, VII
Stylohyoid	VII
Mylohyoid	V
Geniohyoid	C1
Hyoglossus	XII
Genioglossus	XII

Note. Cranial nerves include V (trigeminal), VII (facial), X (vagus), and XII (hypoglossal). Spinal nerves include the first three cervical spinal nerves (C1, C2, C3). Cranial nerve X includes a recurrent laryngeal nerve and a superior laryngeal nerve. Muscles are categorized as intrinsic, extrinsic, or supplementary.

signal that is then transmitted along a sensory nerve to the central nervous system.

Mechanoreceptors are distributed throughout the larynx in its muscles, joints, and mucosal coverings. Included among these are receptors that provide information about muscle lengths and their rates of change (Konig & von Leden, 1961b; Okamura & Katto, 1988; Sanders, Han, Wang, & Biller, 1998), joint movements (Jankovskaya, 1959; Kirchner & Wyke, 1965), and mucosal deformations (Kirchner & Suzuki, 1968; Konig & von Leden, 1961a; Sampson & Eyzaguirre, 1964). Such information is used to determine the mechanical status of the larynx and to elicit certain reflexive behaviors. For laryngeal adjustments that target sound production, such a system would also have to take into account information provided by another type of mechanoreceptor, hair cells within the cochlea of the auditory system (via cranial nerve VIII).

Less than full agreement exists about which cranial and spinal nerves and branches convey sensory information from different structures of the larynx to the central nervous system (Dickson & Maue-Dickson, 1982). Most agree that the internal branch of the superior laryngeal nerve (part of cranial nerve X) carries sensory information from the mucosa that covers the region of the laryngeal cavity above the glottis, including the base of the tongue, epiglottis, aryepiglottic folds, and backs of the arytenoid cartilages. This nerve is also believed to transmit information from mechanoreceptors in the muscles of the larynx that respond to stretch. There is general agreement that the recurrent laryngeal nerve (part of cranial nerve X) carries sensory information from the mucosa and structures that are located below the vocal folds. Sensory information from the extrinsic and supplementary muscles travels via several different nerves. For example, the *mylohyoid* and *stylohyoid* muscles are served by sensory components of cranial nerves V and VII, respectively, whereas the *digastric* muscle is served by sensory components of both cranial nerves V and VII.

LARYNGEAL FUNCTION AND SPEECH PRODUCTION

The larynx performs a variety of functions, including those related to breathing, airway protection, containment of pulmonary air, and speech production. It is interesting to note that all of these functions include an interaction between the larynx and the respiratory system. The focus of this section is speech production; however, brief consideration of the other three laryngeal functions is provided first.

During breathing, the larynx remains open so that air can move easily to and from the lungs where some of it reaches the alveoli and participates in gas exchange. When breathing at rest, the glottis is generally midsized (see Figure 3–33B) and air flows relatively slowly through it. Interestingly, the size of the glottis fluctuates ever so slightly in synchrony with the breathing cycle: The glottis widens slightly during inspiration and narrows slightly during expiration. Stated another way, the vocal folds abduct slightly as air flows toward the lungs and adduct slightly as the air flows out. These subtle changes in glottal size serve to lower the airway resistance during inspiration (to make inspiration easier) and raise the resistance during expiration (to improve gas exchange). When breathing during physical exercise, the glottis enlarges substantially to lower the resistance for the much higher airflows.

Protection of the pulmonary airways is a critical function of the larynx. The larynx, being positioned at the juncture between the pulmonary airways and the upper airway (pharyngeal cavity, oral cavity, nasal cavities), is strategically located to protect the pulmonary airways from the invasion of foreign matter. Its role is particularly important during swallowing, given that the main food channel (from the mouth to the esophagus) and the main air channel (from the nose and mouth to the larynx) cross paths just above the larynx. Thus, during swallowing, the laryngeal airway must be closed to prevent food or liquid from entering the trachea. This closure is accomplished by approximation of the vocal folds and other laryngeal structures and includes a brief period of apnea (breath holding). This is described in detail in Chapter 7.

Closure of the laryngeal valve is also important to seal off the pulmonary air supply for activities that require the generation of high pressures at different locations within the torso (abdominal, pleural, alveolar, tracheal) and/or the fixation of structures of the torso (rib cage wall, diaphragm, abdominal wall). For example, closure of the laryngeal valve to raise internal pressure is critical to forceful acts such as defecation, parturition (childbirth), and lifting heavy objects and is considered a modification of the original Valsalva maneuver (see sidetrack on Ear Pop). Laryngeal closure is also a key element for producing a strong cough, an act that requires a rapid rise in tracheal pressure and a rapid expelling of air as the larynx blows open.

Ear Pop

A technique for raising internal pressure was developed by the physician-scientist Antonio Maria Valsalva, who lived in the 1600s. With a particular interest in the human ear, he wanted to find a way to treat middle ear infections. He found that by attempting to expire forcefully while closing the mouth and pinching the nostrils, air pressure would build in the upper airway and enter the middle ear via the eustachian tube, a small canal that interconnects the middle ear and oral cavity. In this way, pressure in the middle ear could increase and force out the pus. This came to be called the Valsalva maneuver and continues to be used today for the diagnosis and treatment of certain heart abnormalities. But most of us know it as a convenient way to "pop" our ears.

Get Thee Out

Reflexive coughing is our friend. It serves to clear the breathing airway via a powerful and violent explosion or series of such explosions. Your own experience with uncontrollable coughing is evidence of just how dedicated the larynx is to keeping things out of your lungs. Enormous air pressures and airflows are generated during reflexive coughing that cause violent movements of the vocal folds. Excessive coughing, whether reflexive or voluntary, can be abusive to the larynx, lead to unpleasant symptoms, and result in voice disorders. Then there is the equally notorious family cousin, the bad habit of continual throat clearing. Less outgoing than its other two relatives (pun intended), frequent throat clearing can be grating on the vocal folds. Abuse not thy larynx.

Laryngeal function in speech production is complex and takes many forms. The sounds generated by the larynx can be transient (popping) sounds (in which the airstream is momentarily obstructed and then abruptly released), turbulence (hissing) sounds (in which air is forced through a narrowed airway), and quasi-periodic (buzzing) sounds (in which the vocal folds are forced into vibration and move rapidly to and fro to interrupt the airstream repeatedly). The last of these generates voice and is what gives the larynx its popular designation as the "voice box."

Transient Utterances

A transient (very brief) utterance can be produced at the level of the larynx in the form of a sudden explosive burst. This is called a glottal stop-plosive and is analogous to the way voiceless stop-plosives consonants (/p/, /t/, and /k/) are produced. As depicted in Figure 3–36, glottal stop-plosive production requires blocking the airstream by full adduction of the vocal folds. Air pressure then builds up within the tracheal space. This is followed by an abrupt release of the vocal fold adductory force and a simultaneous abrupt release of the pent-up air (Rothenberg, 1968; Stevens, 2000).

The speed with which air flows through the rapidly opening laryngeal airway is very high and gives rise to a brief burst of noise that excites the pharyngeal-oral airway. The sudden release of pent-up air creates an impulse-like popping sound at the glottis (Broad, 1973) and bears analogy to the discharge of an electrical

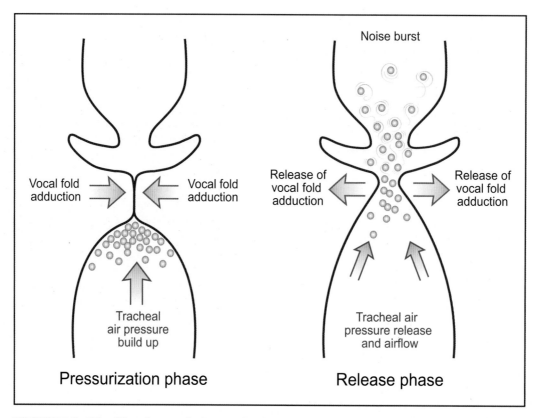

FIGURE 3–36. Glottal stop-plosive production. Production begins with full adduction of the vocal folds and buildup of tracheal air pressure followed by an abrupt release of the vocal fold adductory force and simultaneous release of tracheal air.

capacitor through a time-varying resistance (Fant, 1960). The noise excitation during the release causes the pharyngeal-oral airway to vibrate throughout its entire length and to produce a plosive sound that is distinctly lower in pitch than the pitches associated with other stop-plosives generated by the tongue and lips.

Sustained Turbulence Noise Production

When an airway is constricted and air is forced through it, the air flow will become turbulent. This means that air tumbles on itself, forming eddies (back flows), burbles (bubbles), and other irregularities. This agitation of air results in turbulence (friction) noise that contains a broad range of frequencies. The specific spectrum (frequency and sound pressure level content) of this noise depends on the nature of the interaction between the airstream and the constriction (Fant, 1960; Hixon, 1966; Minifie, 1973; Stevens, 2000).

Sustained noise can be produced by constriction of the laryngeal airway, typically at the level of the vocal folds. A common example is the production of the glottal fricative /h/, as illustrated in Figure 3–37. Glottal fricative production can be achieved by positioning the vocal folds well inward to form a long slit-like constriction.

Another example of sustained noise production is whispering. Whispering can be accomplished with a long slit-like constriction but is often accompanied by other glottal configurations. One of the most frequent of these is a rearward-facing Y configuration in which the membranous front parts of the vocal folds are firmly approximated (as in Figure 3–33D), loosely approximated, or not approximated at all and the cartilaginous rear parts of the vocal folds are relatively far apart (Monoson & Zemlin, 1984; Rubin, Praneetvataku, Gherson, & Moyer, 2006; Solomon, McCall, Trosset, & Gray, 1989; Zemlin, 1998). This configuration is achieved by contracting the *lateral cricoarytenoid* muscles so that the vocal processes of the arytenoid cartilages toe inward, while leaving the *arytenoid* muscles less active or inactive. Glottal configuration during whispering does not appear to change with changes in loudness (Solomon et al., 1989). This suggests that it may be the size of the glottis, rather than its specific configuration, that is the more important variable.

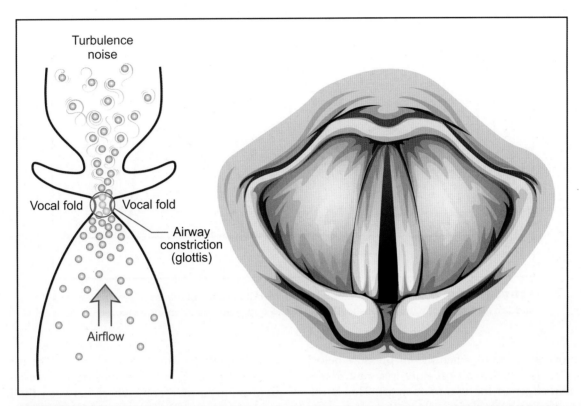

FIGURE 3–37. Glottal voiceless fricative production. Air is forced through a small laryngeal constriction, causing the air molecules to tumble on themselves and create turbulence noise. This form of noise is associated with production of the glottal fricative /h/ and whispering.

 A demonstration of how the vocal folds participate in turbulence noise production is provided in Video 3–3 (Glottal Fricative and Whisper).

Sustained Voice Production

Voice (the acoustic product of voice production) results from vibration of the vocal folds. Such vibration modulates (chops up) the airstream into a series of air puffs. As depicted in Figure 3–38, the repeated, sudden decreases in airflow are what acoustically excite the pharyngeal, oral, and nasal cavities during voice production (Gauffin & Sundberg, 1989; Rothenberg, 1983). This section discusses the nature of vocal fold vibration during sustained voice production. It also touches on other aspects of voice, including fundamental frequency, sound pressure level, fundamental frequency–sound pressure level profiles, spectrum, and registers.

Vocal Fold Vibration

Once vocal fold vibration is established, it proceeds in a relatively steady quasiperiodic fashion. Each vibration consists of lateral and medial excursions of the vocal folds that rapidly and repeatedly valve the expiratory airstream.

Individual vocal fold vibrations are *not* caused by individual muscular contractions that pull them apart and force them back together again. Rather, movements of the vocal folds are passive and can be compared to the movements of the lips when air is blown between them. (Try it. Moisten your lips, pucker up slightly, gently blow air through them, and feel them vibrate.) Muscular forces are important, but only in the sense that they set the vocal folds (or lips) in position to be moved passively to and fro primarily by aeromechanical forces. Thus, a key element of the laryngeal adjustment for sustained vocal fold vibration is to position and hold the vocal folds in the airway so that vibration can be established and maintained by air pressures and airflows acting on the vocal folds (van den Berg, 1958). The conditions needed to sustain vocal fold vibration, once established, are a steady source of energy from the respiratory system and some form of nonlinear interaction with the structures being vibrated, namely, the vocal folds.

A single cycle of vocal fold vibration is depicted in Figure 3–39. Taking closure of the larynx (full approximation of the edges of the vocal folds) as a starting

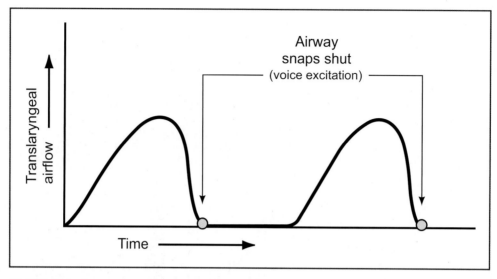

FIGURE 3–38. Voice source generation. The abrupt closures of the laryngeal airway and sudden airflow declination acoustically excite the upper airway to create voice.

point, movement begins when the air pressure below the vocal folds (tracheal air pressure) rises and forces the bottom edges of the two folds apart. This is followed by forcing apart the middle and upper parts of the folds. This pattern of lateral excursion of the vocal folds exhibits a so-called *vertical phase difference* in which lower points on the medial surfaces of the vocal folds are displaced earlier than points above them. A vertical phase difference is also manifested as the vocal folds move back together again. That is, lower points on the medial surfaces of the vocal folds move together before points on the upper surfaces move together (Hirano, Yoshida, & Tanaka, 1991; Schonharl, 1960; Timcke, von Leden, & Moore, 1958). These movements of the medial surfaces of the vocal folds occur because the covers of the vocal folds (consisting of the intermediate and superficial layer of the lamina propria and the epithelium; see Figure 3–13) are relatively loosely coupled to their muscular bodies (Story & Titze, 1995). Such movements have been described as vertically propagating *mucosal waves* (like surface waves on water) that progress within the covers of the vocal folds and whose rippling effects can be seen on the top surfaces of the vocal folds (Berke & Gerratt, 1993; Hirano, Kakita, Kawasaki, Gould, & Lambiase, 1981). The mucosal wave can be somewhat appreciated in the sequence of video frames shown in Figure 3–40 that depict a single cycle of vocal fold vibration as viewed from above.

The vertical phase difference of vocal fold vibration has also been conceptualized as two primary modes of movement, one translational and one rotational (Berry & Titze, 1996; Story, 2002). The translational mode is the lateral movement of the vocal folds

away from the midline and back again. The rotational mode is the rotation of the vocal fold cover around a pivot point located somewhere between the bottom and top of the medial surface (the location of the pivot point depends on factors such as muscle activation levels and hydration of the tissue). This is illustrated schematically in Figure 3–41.

Figure 3–42 offers an even more detailed look at a single cycle of vocal fold vibration. When tracheal pressure is high enough to push the lower portion of the vocal folds apart, a convergent-shaped glottis is created (that is, wider at the bottom than the top), as illustrated in (A) in the figure. At this point in the vibratory cycle, the intraglottal air pressure (the pressure within the glottis) is relatively high, higher than the opposing recoil force being exerted by the vocal fold tissues. The intraglottal pressure pushes the vocal folds away from the midline until the restoring force exerted by the vocal folds exceeds the force exerted by the intraglottal pressure. At this point, the vocal folds begin to move inward, back toward the midline, starting from the bottom and rotating into a divergent-shaped glottis (narrower at the bottom than the top), as shown in (B) in Figure 3–42. As this divergent-shaped glottis is created, intraglottal pressure decreases rapidly because the air column above the vocal folds is continuing to flow toward the airway opening, leaving fewer air molecules within the glottis and just above it. This drop in intraglottal pressure, along with the inward-directed recoil force of the vocal fold tissue, causes the vocal folds to move medially toward each other relatively rapidly (see Titze, 2006, for a more detailed explanation).

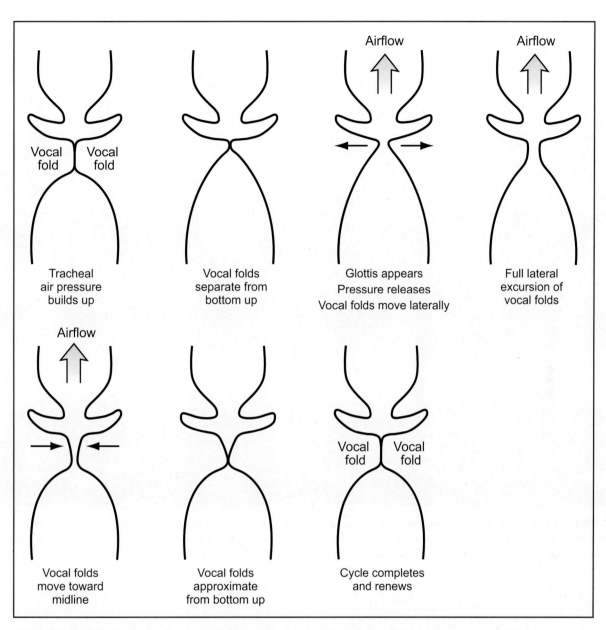

FIGURE 3–39. Vertical phase difference of the vocal folds during voice production. This figure represents a single vocal fold vibration cycle, beginning with the vocal folds approximated. The vocal folds are separated from bottom to top by air pressure until a glottis appears. Next, the vocal folds move laterally and then back toward the midline until they approximate again from bottom to top.

For many decades, the predominant belief was that the vibration of the vocal folds was sustained by the Bernoulli effect. Stated simply, the Bernoulli effect (or Bernoulli principle) describes the observation that as fluid (such as air) velocity increases, pressure decreases until it produces a force that tends to "suck" the medial vocal fold surfaces toward each other. It is now known that the Bernoulli effect has almost no influence on vocal fold vibration. Instead, vocal fold vibration is self-sustained because of the combined contributions of the changing glottal geometry (convergent to divergent and back again) and the changes in airflow and air pressure just above of the glottis. Although the air pressure within the glottis rises and falls, and may even become negative (that is, lower than atmospheric pressure) for short periods just prior to glottal closure, the Bernoulli effect is not the mechanism that sustains vibration. A simulation of vocal fold vibration can be viewed in Video 3–4 (Vocal Fold Vibration).

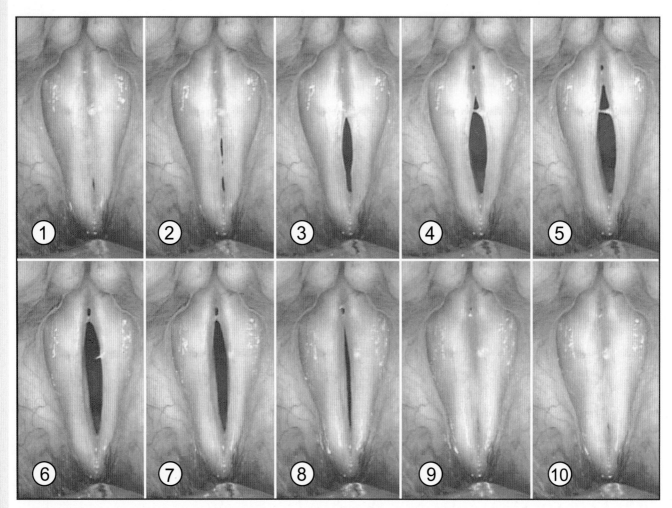

FIGURE 3–40. Successive images from one complete cycle of vocal fold vibration as viewed from above. The cycle begins with the vocal folds approximated (Image 1). The vocal folds begin to separate (Image 2) until they reach maximum separation (Images 5–6) and then return to midline again (Images 7–10). Images provided courtesy of KayPENTAX, Montvale, NJ. Reproduced with permission.

Every Which Way

Despite current understanding of how the vocal folds vibrate to produce voice, it was only within the earlier part of the past century that scholars were unenlightened about many aspects of the process. Some scholars argued that voice resulted from up and down movements of the two vocal folds in opposite directions. Others believed that vocal fold movements during voice production were strictly horizontal and akin to stiff shutters that slid together and apart repeatedly. These incorrect guesses about how the vocal folds functioned during voice production were dispelled by data obtained with high-speed motion picture filming of the larynx. This technology enabled the study of the rapid movements of the vocal folds in precise detail. Thus, what earlier in the past century seemed to be "every which way" of vocal fold movement during voice production has settled down to the way it is described in the adjacent text.

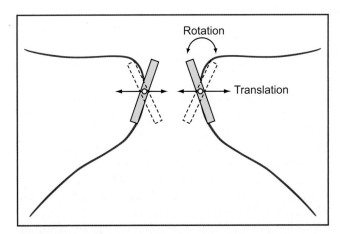

FIGURE 3–41. Two primary modes of vocal fold vibration. The translational mode constitutes the lateral movement of the vocal folds and the rotational mode is the rotation of the vocal fold cover around a pivot point (open circle). Modified after Story (2002).

Fundamental Frequency

The fundamental frequency is the rate at which the vocal folds vibrate. Fundamental frequency can be changed over a very wide range, typically about three octaves (an octave is a doubling or a halving of frequency) for a young adult (Fairbanks, 1960). Fundamental frequency is usually expressed on a continuum in units of cycles per second or hertz (abbreviated Hz). It can also be expressed on a musical scale in semitones (the interval between two adjacent keys on a keyboard instrument). The average fundamental frequency of the human voice depends in large part on the size of the larynx and the sex of the individual, with men having lower average fundamental frequencies than women and women having lower average fundamental frequencies than children. The vocal folds are primarily responsible for changing fundamental frequency. The respiratory system serves a supporting role in fundamental frequency control.

The strongest auditory-perceptual correlate of fundamental frequency is the pitch of the voice. Pitch is the subjective impression of the relative position of a sound along a musical scale. For the most part, a higher fundamental frequency is associated with a higher pitch and a lower fundamental frequency is associated with a lower pitch.

Vocal fold adjustments that influence fundamental frequency (and pitch) are those that determine the stiffness of the vocal folds and their effective vibrating mass, with stiffness generally considered the more important of the two factors (Stevens, 2000). The most important mechanisms for increasing vocal fold stiff-

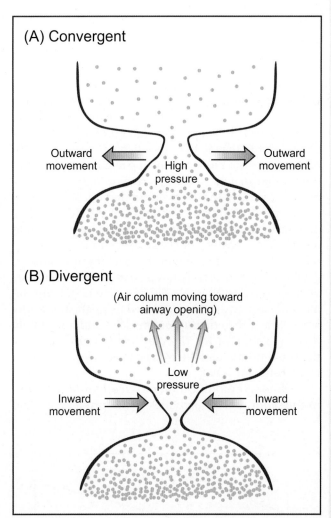

FIGURE 3–42. Convergent (A) and divergent (B) glottal shapes and associated intraglottal air pressure (the air pressure within the glottis) and vocal fold movements during a single vibration. When the glottis is in a convergent shape, intraglottal air pressure is high enough to overcome the tissue recoil forces and pushes the vocal folds away from each other. When the glottis is in a divergent shape, intraglottal pressure lowers and tissue recoil pressure moves the vocal folds back together.

ness operate through external force exerted by the *cricothyroid* muscles and internal force exerted through the *thyroarytenoid* muscles. As discussed above and illustrated in Figure 3–34, contraction of the *cricothyroid* muscles tends to stretch the vocal folds and increase the force per unit length along them, whereas activation of the *thyroarytenoid* muscles (particularly the *thyrovocalis* part) tends to increase the stiffness of the muscular part of the vibrating vocal folds. It is the combined activities of these two pairs of muscles that are primarily responsible for setting the effective stiffness of the vocal folds and for controlling the fundamental frequency (Shipp & McGlone, 1971; Titze, 1994; Titze, Jiang, & Drucker, 1988; Titze, Luschei, & Hirano, 1989).

The relative activations of the *cricothyroid* and *thyroarytenoid* muscles can vary substantially for the production of a given fundamental frequency (Titze & Story, 2002). This is represented in graphic form in Figure 3–43, with the relative activation of the *cricothyroid* muscle increasing upward and the relative activation of the *thyroarytenoid* muscle increasing rightward. This graph illustrates that a given fundamental frequency can be produced by a continuum of different combinations of muscular activities. For example, a fundamental frequency of 120 Hz can be produced by using relatively high activation of the *cricothyroid* muscles combined with relatively low activation of the *thyroarytenoid* muscles; alternatively, the same 120-Hz fundamental frequency can be produced using relatively low activation of the *cricothyroid* muscles and a relatively high activation of the *thyroarytenoid* muscles. Thus, the same fundamental frequency can be produced in many different ways.

Although modification of *cricothyroid* and *thyroarytenoid* muscle activities is the primary mecha-

nism for changing fundamental frequency, it is not the only one. The mechanism of medial compression can also effect changes in the fundamental frequency of the voice. This is done through actions of the *lateral cricoarytenoid* muscles that can adjust the medial compression of the vocal folds in the area of approximation of the tips of the vocal processes (illustrated in Figure 3–35). Studies of air-driven excised larynges, in which medial compression was experimentally manipulated, have shown that increases in medial compression result in increases in fundamental frequency (van den Berg & Tan, 1959; van den Berg et al., 1960). The suspected mechanism is a decrease in the effective vibrating mass of the vocal folds caused by stopping their vibration in the region of the tips of the arytenoid processes (Honda, 1995). This mechanism has been likened to the pressing of a guitar string against a fret so that only the part of the string nearer the sounding box of the guitar is permitted to vibrate (Broad, 1973). Medial compression is considered a secondary or ancillary mechanism of fundamental frequency control.

Still another mechanism that can influence the fundamental frequency of the voice relates to the elevation of the larynx (sometimes referred to as its vertical height). When high fundamental frequencies are generated, there is a tendency for the larynx to rise in the neck, especially near the upper extreme of the fundamental frequency range. This elevation is probably accomplished by activation of the *thyrohyoid* muscles (Faaborg-Andersen & Sonninen, 1960; Sonninen, 1968). Elevation of the larynx is believed to further increase the stiffness of the vocal folds once major effort has been exerted to increase stiffness through activation of the *thyroarytenoid* and *cricothyroid* muscles. Elevation of the larynx results in a downward pull on the undersurface of the vocal folds mediated through the conus elasticus. This pull stiffens the covers of the vocal folds (especially at the free margins of the vocal folds) by placing a vertical tug on them and thereby increases the rate at which the vocal folds vibrate (Ohala, 1972). This mechanism is usually the last biomechanical adjustment invoked to reach the highest fundamental frequencies possible. Laryngeal elevation is considered a secondary or ancillary mechanism of fundamental frequency control.

Although nearly all fundamental frequency control is vested in the larynx, increases in tracheal pressure can raise fundamental frequency slightly (Rubin, 1963; van den Berg, 1957); however, typical magnitudes of change are only 2 to 4 Hz in fundamental frequency per cmH_2O of air pressure (Hixon, Klatt, & Mead, 1971; Titze, 1989). Changes in tracheal pressure can have a more significant effect on fundamental frequency in the loft register (discussed below).

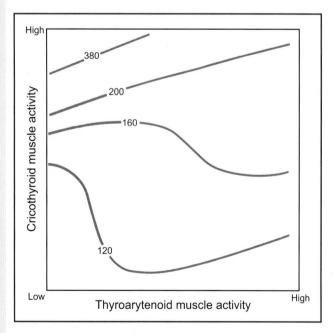

FIGURE 3–43. Continuum of *cricothyroid* and *thyroarytenoid* muscle activations for the production of selected fundamental frequencies (based on modeling data from Titze and Story [2002]). This graph illustrates that a single fundamental frequency can be produced using a wide range of combinations of relative activations of the *cricothyroid* and *thyroarytenoid* muscles.

To lower fundamental frequency from a high value to its usual value, muscle activations may reduce to decrease vocal fold stiffness and/or tracheal air pressure. To lower fundamental frequency below its usual value, other mechanisms may come into play. One mechanism is to reduce vocal fold stiffness by contraction of the *thyromuscularis* (lateral) portions of the *thyroarytenoid* muscles. This contraction shortens the vocal folds and causes a slackening of the vocal ligaments and the *thyrovocalis* (medial) portions of the *thyroarytenoid* muscles (Zemlin, 1998). Another frequency-lowering mechanism is to lower the larynx within the neck, which decreases the stiffness of the vocal folds by removing some of the usual traction placed on their undersurfaces. This is brought about through activation of the *sternothyroid* and *sternohyoid* muscles, which pull downward on the laryngeal housing (Atkinson, 1978; Honda, 1995; Ohala, 1972; Ohala & Hirose, 1970; Zemlin, 1998).

Sound Pressure Level

The sound pressure level (abbreviated as SPL) of speech (the acoustic signal) is a measure of its physical magnitude. This magnitude is related to the amplitude of the sound emanating from the mouth and nose and is generically referred to as the intensity of the signal (although technically sound pressure level and intensity are different quantities and the latter is more difficult to measure). The sound pressure level of speech is expressed on a continuum in ratio units of decibels (dB) and can be changed over a wide range, typically by about 40 dB for a young adult (Coleman, Mabis, & Hinson, 1977). A vowel produced at a usual loudness level and measured 30 cm from the lips (a standard distance) might be 65 dB, whereas a vowel produced at a shouting level might be in excess of 100 dB. Control of the sound pressure level of speech is vested primarily in adjustments of the respiratory system and the larynx and, to a lesser degree, the pharyngeal-oral component of the speech mechanism. These adjustments are usually executed simultaneously across these three subsystems.

The respiratory system influences sound pressure level of the voice through changes in tracheal air pressure (Cavagna & Margaria, 1965; Hixon & Minifie, 1972; Isshiki, 1964; Ladefoged & McKinney, 1963; Titze, 1994; van den Berg, 1956). For example, a doubling of tracheal air pressure for usual voice production might result in an increase in sound pressure level in the neighborhood of 8 to 12 dB (Broad, 1973; Daniloff, Shuckers, & Feth, 1980; Stevens, 2000).

The larynx also plays a role in changing sound pressure level. Specifically, higher sound pressure levels of the voice are produced with higher laryngeal opposing pressures (Isshiki, 1964; Kunze, 1962), brought about primarily by increasingly forceful contractions of the *lateral cricoarytenoid* and *arytenoid* muscles (*transverse* and *oblique* subdivisions). Higher laryngeal opposing pressures are needed to contain the increased tracheal air pressure and prevent it from escaping uselessly (Daniloff et al., 1980). The combined increase in tracheal pressure and the more forceful "squeezing" pressure by the larynx causes the vocal folds to separate faster, return to the midline faster, and remain in approximation for a longer period during each cycle of vocal fold vibration (Minifie, 1973).

Although the interaction between the respiratory system and the larynx contributes most to sound pressure level changes, the pharyngeal-oral mechanism also plays a role. In general, it tends to blossom open more and more with successive increases in sound pressure level, achieving an effect like a megaphone. The velum (soft palate and uvula) elevates, the mandible lowers, the tongue lowers, and the mouth opening increases (Netsell, 1973; Tucker, 1963), adjustments that lower the radiation impedance of the pharyngeal-oral mechanism so that the sound energy is transmitted more effectively to the atmosphere (Fant, 1960; Flanagan, 1972).

The strongest auditory-perceptual correlate of sound pressure level is loudness. Loudness is the subjective sensation of the relative magnitude of sound

---

Listen My Children and You Shall Hear

Some people are loud and then some people are really loud. The conversion of aerodynamic power to acoustic power is better in some than in others, and some of the best at it have been listed as celebrities in folk sources. Different hollering, yelling, screaming, shouting, and loud voice champions have been crowned around the world. The *Guinness Book of Records* (Folkard, 2006) lists Jill Drake as the reigning screaming champion at 129 dB (since 2000) and Annalisa Flanagan as the reigning shouting champion at 121.7 dB (since 1994). Alan Myatt, the town crier of Gloucester, England, once was touted in the *Guinness Book of Records* as having the world's loudest voice, an ear-piercing 112.8 dB. Had Paul Revere been so endowed as a town crier he wouldn't have had to knock on so many doors and he might have been able to awaken all of Lexington, Massachusetts, on a single breath. Well, maybe not all, but at least much of the South Side.

that relies mainly on sound pressure level. In general, the higher the sound pressure level, the greater the perceived loudness.

Fundamental Frequency–Sound Pressure Level Profiles

The term *voice range* is most often used when referring to the lowest and highest values that can be produced in either the fundamental frequency or sound pressure level of the voice. These two variables are not independent of one another; the fundamental frequency has a different set of lowest and highest values at different sound pressure levels, and sound pressure level has a different set of lowest and highest values at different fundamental frequencies (Fairbanks, 1960). These relations are illustrated in what are called fundamental frequency–sound pressure level profiles (Coleman et al., 1977; Damste, 1970; Gramming, 1991) or voice range profiles, such as that shown for an adult male in Figure 3–44.

Figure 3–44 depicts the lowest and highest fundamental frequencies and sound pressure levels attainable (and sustainable for brief durations) by a typical man across the ranges of fundamental frequency and sound pressure level. This figure illustrates that, in general, lower fundamental frequencies and sound pressure levels can be produced at lower values of the other

variable, whereas higher fundamental frequencies and sound pressure levels can be produced at higher values of the other variable. The fundamental frequency range of the voice is greatest in the midrange of sound pressure levels, and the sound pressure level range is greatest in the midrange of fundamental frequencies.

Spectrum

The spectrum of the sound generated by the vibrating larynx is complex and composed of a combination of different frequencies and sound pressure levels. The usual laryngeal source spectrum consists of a fundamental frequency and successive odd and even harmonics (whole-number multiples of the fundamental frequency) that decrease in sound pressure level with increasing harmonic number at a rate of about 12 dB per octave (each doubling of frequency) above 1000 Hz (Fant, 1960). The source spectrum can be changed by different respiratory and laryngeal adjustments.

The voice source spectrum changes with fundamental frequency because the spacing of the harmonics depends on the fundamental frequency (as fundamental frequency increases, the spacing between the harmonics increases). The spectrum also changes with sound pressure level (as sound pressure level increases, the energy in the higher-frequency region tends to increase). In addition, the spectral content of the voice source is influenced by changes in the vibratory pattern of the vocal folds (Stevens, 2000) and the degree to which the laryngeal airway is constricted. For example, a breathy voice (produced by allowing a continuous airflow between the vocal folds) contains less high-frequency energy (that is, the high-frequency harmonics are lower in sound pressure level) than a pressed voice (produced with the vocal folds forcefully approximated). The breathy voice also contains more noise (aperiodic sound) than its pressed counterpart.

The voice source generated at the laryngeal level constitutes the raw material of voice production and, when heard in the absence of an upper airway, it sounds like a coarse buzz (see sidetrack called The Cattle Are Lowing). To sound like a human voice, the voice source must be filtered by the air spaces above it (pharyngeal cavity, oral cavity, and, in some cases, nasal cavity).

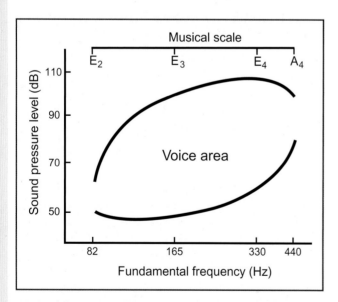

FIGURE 3–44. Fundamental frequency–sound pressure level profile (also called voice range profile) of an adult male. Note that the largest range of fundamental frequencies can be produced in the midrange of the sound pressure level range, and that the largest range of sound pressure levels can be produced in the midrange of the fundamental frequency range.

Voice Registers

The nature of vocal fold vibration is strongly conditioned by so-called voice registers. Voice registers reflect different modes of vocal fold vibration that result from different mechanical conditions (Titze, 1994) and that give rise to differences in perceived voice quality

The Cattle Are Lowing

An effective method for teaching certain principles of voice production involves the use of an excised cow larynx. The cow larynx is large compared to the human larynx and is different in some respects. The cow larynx does not have false vocal folds, nor is it richly endowed with mucous glands for lubricating the vocal folds. After all, cows don't produce voice for long periods like people do. A cow larynx can be made to vibrate by attaching the blower end of a vacuum cleaner to the tracheal end of the larynx—the vibration sounds like a coarse buzz. If you then manually stretch the vocal folds, change the medial compression, and make other adjustments, you can alter the fundamental frequency (pitch), sound pressure level (loudness), and source spectrum (voice quality). If you then place an inverted container (such as a small waste basket) above the larynx (roughly simulating the missing throat and mouth), the buzz can be transformed into something that almost sounds like a cow. When all is done right, the experience is both instructive and "moooooving" to students.

(Laver, 1991). Accordingly, a voice register can be defined perceptually as a series of consecutive utterances of similar voice quality produced along a pitch scale through application of similar mechanical principles.

The topic of voice registers is controversial, especially in singing pedagogy. The number and nature of voice registers is often argued in the singing literature, as are the mechanisms involved in their generation (sometimes taken to include laryngeal as well as pharyngeal, nasal, and oral adjustments). Far less controversy exists about the number and nature of voice registers in the speaking voice, and this section is limited to those.

There are three voice registers in the speaking voice. The general location of these along the fundamental frequency scale is illustrated for men and women in Figure 3–45. They are labeled as the pulse, modal, and loft voice registers and correspond to three different modes of vocal fold vibration encountered in sequence when speaking at an ascending fundamental frequency from the lowest to highest fundamental frequencies within the speaking range (Hollien, 1972, 1974). Each voice register is confined to a restricted range of fundamental frequencies, and within each register, a particular pattern of vocal fold vibration

prevails. The boundary between adjacent registers is determined by raising and lowering the fundamental frequency and noting where an abrupt change in voice quality occurs.

The modal voice register is the middle of the three speaking voice registers and gets its name from the statistical mode, the most often occurring event (in fundamental frequency). The modal register is characteristic of the type of vocal fold vibration described thus far in this chapter and is the voice register typically used during most conversational speech production.

The pulse voice register is the lowest of the three speaking voice registers and derives its name from the nature of its pulse-like voice source waveform. The voice quality produced in this register is sometimes referred to as vocal fry, glottal fry, or creaky voice and sounds like a string of tiny pops (like those that can be made by applying repeated bursts of pressure behind the lips when they are thickly puckered and gently held together). Pulse register usually occurs intermittently at the ends of breath groups when the voice trails off in sound pressure level and drops in fundamental frequency (comes to a growling halt). Fundamental frequency and sound pressure level tend to change together in the pulse register and do not have the relative independence found in modal voice register (Murry & Brown, 1971a, 1971b).

The loft voice register, also called the falsetto register, is the highest of the three speaking voice registers and gets its name from its high placement within the fundamental frequency range. The quality of the voice produced in this register is sometimes described as thin, flute-like, and breathy. In this register, excursions of the vocal folds are relatively small, the glottis is narrow, and there is little to no vertical phase difference. Rather, movements are mainly horizontal and confined to the vicinity of the free margins of the vocal folds. Such movements take on the appearance of vibrating strings alternately moving horizontally away from and toward one another. The vocal folds do not have to approximate for voice production in the loft register, and when they do, contact between them is usually light (low adductory forces).

Running Speech Activities

The larynx is a critical participant in running speech activities. During inspiration, the vocal folds abduct and dilate the laryngeal airway to allow air to flow freely into the pulmonary system. During expiration (speech production), the vocal folds are adducted and vibrate to produce the raw sound of the voice and intermittently abduct to allow air pressures and airflows to

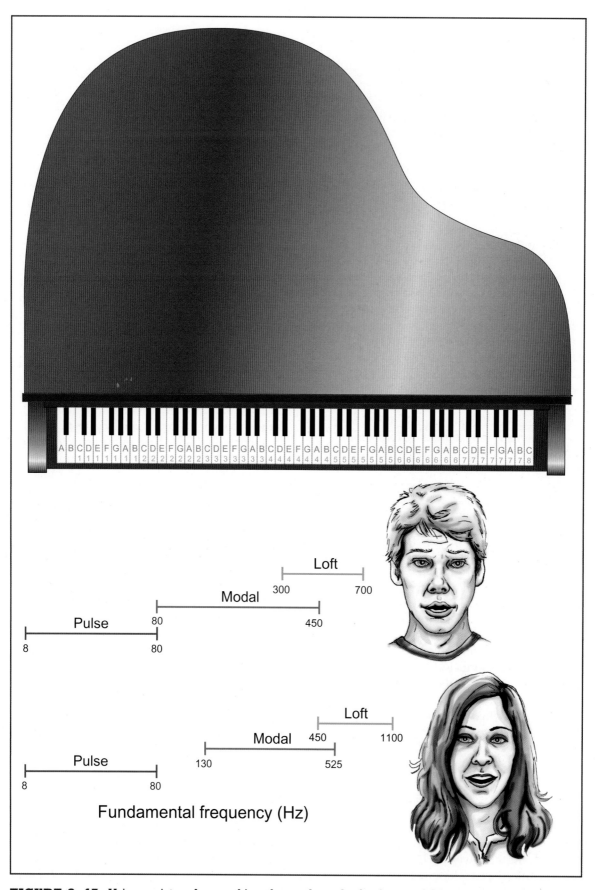

FIGURE 3–45. Voice registers for speaking shown along the fundamental frequency scale (and corresponding piano scale). The lowest register is pulse, the middle register is modal and the most often used register, and the highest register is loft.

reach downstream structures for voiceless oral consonant production.

The raw sound of the voice, sometimes called the laryngeal tone, is the carrier of speech and has an important influence on speech intelligibility. It also conveys information about the speaker's age, sex, physical stature, health status, emotional status, identity, and other factors. The laryngeal tone can be adjusted in fundamental frequency, sound pressure level, and spectrum to convey meaning, disambiguate certain aspects of the communication, emphasize certain parts of the flow of speech over others, provide information through different voice shadings and nuances, establish certain affects (impressions), and affirm roles in relationships. The larynx also plays an important role in articulation.

Fundamental Frequency

Fundamental frequency change is prominent during running speech activities and can range as much as two octaves (Fairbanks, 1960). Fundamental frequency is often displayed and measured in a tracing called a fundamental frequency contour, which tracks change in fundamental frequency over time. Such a contour is shown in Figure 3–46 for a spoken sentence.

Listening to fundamental frequency change in the voice evokes a perception of time-varying pitch change that is referred to as an intonation contour. The intonation contour underlies what the listener comes to consider as the melody or tunefulness of speech. This contour operates around the most often sensed pitch, which determines what the listener judges to be the characteristic (or habitual) pitch level of the voice.

Adjustments in fundamental frequency during running speech activities are vested mainly in laryngeal actions. These laryngeal actions rely, in large part, on interplay between contractions of the *cricothyroid* and *thyroarytenoid* muscles, along with bracing actions of the *posterior cricoarytenoid* muscles, which also adjust the stiffness of the vocal folds (Atkinson, 1978; Gay, Hirose, Strome, & Sawashima, 1972; Hirano, Ohala, & Vennard, 1969; Netsell, 1969). Actions of the *cricothyroid* muscles are more strongly correlated with the fundamental frequency of the voice than are the actions of other intrinsic muscles of the larynx, as long as the *cricothyroid* muscles are not functioning near their maximum output (Atkinson, 1978; Titze, 1994). Thus, as discussed above for sustained voice production, changes in the longitudinal tension of the vocal folds (via *cricothyroid* muscle activation) and change in internal stiffness of the vocal folds (via *thyroarytenoid* muscle activation) are of prime importance to the control of the fundamental frequency of the voice during running speech production.

Adjustments of the respiratory system in the form of changes in pressure and volume can also influence fundamental frequency. Although tracheal pressure remains relatively steady during running speech production, it does fluctuate slightly with linguistic stress. Pulsatile increases in tracheal pressure cause slight increases in the fundamental frequency of the voice (Hixon et al., 1971; Lester & Story, 2013; Titze, 1989), suggesting that pressure fluctuations associated with the production of stressed syllables may contribute to momentary increases in fundamental frequency. Although running speech is generally produced within the midrange of the vital capacity, when it is produced at higher than usual lung volumes, it may be associated with higher than usual fundamental frequencies (Watson, Ciccia, & Weismer, 2003). This may be due to higher tracheal pressure associated with higher expiratory recoil pressures at large lung volumes, or it may be due to a downward pull on the larynx (through its connections to the diaphragm) that could increase vocal fold tension, or both.

A summary of fundamental frequency and its control is provided in Video 3–5 (Fundamental Frequency). It concludes with an interesting look at the fundamental frequency contours of several TED Talks.

Sound Pressure Level

Like fundamental frequency, sound pressure level also changes continually during running speech activities. During a routine conversation, the sound pressure level might swing as much as 25 to 30 dB. The magnitude of sound pressure level and its directional changes can

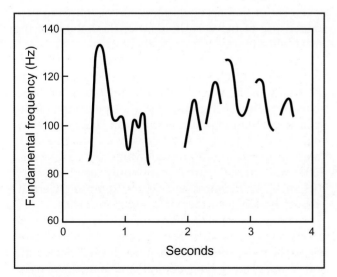

FIGURE 3–46. Fundamental frequency contour for a sentence spoken by an adult male.

be displayed and measured in a tracing referred to as a sound pressure level contour, one of which is shown for the production of a sentence in Figure 3–47.

Changes in sound pressure level over time give rise to a subjective impression of a loudness contour that embodies percepts of an average loudness and variations about it. Vowels are the main contributors to loudness judgments in running speech activities. Adjustment in vowel and consonant sound pressure levels, while usually moving in the same direction, find vowel sound pressure level to change more than consonant sound pressure level (Hixon, 1966; Stevens, 2000). This is due to a tendency to open up the pharyngeal-oral mechanism to increase sound pressure level for vowels and a tendency to constrict this part of the airway to increase sound pressure level for consonants. These two competing tendencies result in a trade-off in sound pressure level change, in which the vowel dominates because of its more prominent carrying power (Fairbanks & Miron, 1957).

Perceived loudness contours are strongly related to sound pressure level contours but do not bear a one-to-one correspondence to them. That is, although certain sounds have intrinsically higher or lower sound pressure levels, they may be perceived as being of equal loudness. For example, when counting from 1 to 10, the syllables tend to sound equally loud to the listener despite the differences in sound pressure levels across the different vowels in the series.

Sound pressure level for running speech activities is controlled by adjustments of the respiratory system, larynx, and pharyngeal-oral mechanism. The respiratory system is responsible for changing the magnitude of the average tracheal air pressure and with producing small increases in pressure to emphasize certain speech segments (Netsell, 1969). These background level and pulsatile tracheal air pressure events are the result of muscular pressure adjustments by the chest wall (Hixon, Mead, & Goldman, 1976).

Laryngeal participation in sound pressure level control for running speech activities usually involves heightened vocal fold adductory forces that manifest as increases in the laryngeal opposing pressure. These vocal fold adductory forces enable the buildup of tracheal air pressure and increase as speech becomes progressively louder or contrastive stress levels become greater from one syllable to another (Hirano et al., 1969; Netsell, 1969, 1973). The muscles implicated in heightening vocal fold adductory forces are primarily the *lateral cricoarytenoid* and *arytenoid* muscles, although the *thyroarytenoid* muscles also contribute by bulging the vocal folds toward the midline.

Pharyngeal-oral adjustments that change the acoustic radiation impedance are often associated with changes in the sound pressure level of running speech. That is, the pharyngeal-oral part of the speech mechanism tends to open more for high sound pressure level utterances as a way to enhance transmission of acoustic energy generated at the glottis (Daniloff et al., 1980; Netsell, 1973).

Spectrum

The spectrum of the laryngeal source (the distribution of energy as a function of frequency) changes rapidly and often during running speech activities as fundamental frequency, sound pressure level, and patterns of vocal fold vibration change. Slower changes in the spectrum of the laryngeal tone may result from prolonged use of the vocal folds, transient abuse of the vocal folds, illness, aging, or other factors.

Source spectrum changes may give rise to changes in voice quality, a perceptual attribute that pertains to the sound of the voice beyond its pitch and loudness characteristics (Behrman, 2007). Depending on the speaking situation, the spectrum can change in ways that cause the listener to perceive voice qualities that range from breathy to pressed (Minifie, 1973; Stevens, 2000) and include other commonly used descriptors such as roughness and strain (Kempster, Gerratt, Abbott, Barkmeier-Kraemer, & Hillman, 2009).

The spectrum of the human voice is not only influenced by the laryngeal source spectrum but also by the parts of the speech mechanism through which the sound travels (pharyngeal, oral, and sometimes nasal cavities). These air spaces are the resonating cavities that modify the laryngeal sound source in ways that

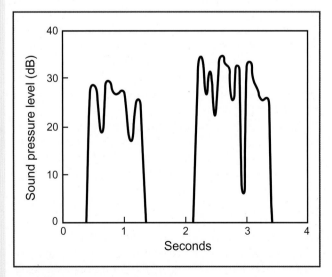

FIGURE 3–47. Sound pressure level contour for a sentence spoken by an adult male.

may create the vowel "oo" in one case and the vowel "ee" in another case, even when the laryngeal source is the same. Stated another way, the laryngeal sound source is shaped, or filtered, by air spaces (resonators) to create different speech sounds. Thus, speech is a product of the source plus the filter. This is demonstrated in Video 3–6 (Source-Filter).

Articulation

Although the larynx is most strongly associated with generating the voice source, it can also be thought of as an articulator (a movable structure that contributes to the production of speech sounds). The larynx, specifically the vocal folds, are the primary articulators for productions of what are called glottal sounds, which include the glottal stop-plosive consonant and the glottal fricative consonant /h/ (Hirose, 1977; Lofqvist & Yoshioka, 1984; Orlikoff & Kahane, 1996; Sawashima, Abramson, Cooper, & Lisker, 1970; see Figures 3–36 and 3–37). The vocal folds also abduct briefly to produce voiceless consonants such as /p/ or /s/. In the production of the word "pass," for example, the vocal folds abduct briefly during the /p/, adduct for the vowel, and abduct again for the /s/. The movements of the vocal folds toward and away from one another are rapid and precise in their timing, just as rapid and precise as other articulators found in the upper airway (tongue, lips, velum). Further consideration of the larynx as an articulator can be found in Chapter 5.

Tick Tock

Anyone who has played music to the beat of a metronome knows how maddening it can be. When just learning the music, it's a challenge to keep up. Then, once you have the music mastered, it seems like you have to slow down to be on pace. But something has to set the pace, like a conductor of an orchestra. The larynx usually does this during speech production. It's the metronome of the speech production mechanism. The movements of other speech structures are constrained by what the larynx does. It does no good to get to a position before the larynx because then you'll just have to wait. And, if you arrive at a position later than the time specified by the larynx, you have big problems. It's not quite as simple as we've portrayed, but it's close enough to give you the idea. Maybe you've heard the nursery rhyme "Hickory, dickory, dock, the voice box is the clock." Well, maybe not, because it was just written.

VARIABLES THAT INFLUENCE LARYNGEAL STRUCTURE AND FUNCTION

To this point in the chapter, discussion has focused on laryngeal structure and function as found in a typical adult. Nevertheless, the larynx changes across a life span, most dramatically during the first years of life and more gradually during adulthood. Once an individual reaches a certain age, important sex-related differences emerge in laryngeal structure and function. This section provides a brief overview of the influence of age and sex on the larynx.

Age

The larynx of the newborn is very different from that of the adult larynx. It rides high within the neck with the lower edge of the cricoid cartilage positioned between the third and fourth cervical vertebrae. The larynx descends gradually throughout the first two decades of life (Vorperian et al., 2009) until it reaches the region of the seventh cervical vertebra.

The framework of the infant larynx is destined to triple in size during the developmental period (Bosma, 1985). At the beginning of life, the laryngeal framework is soft and pliable, becoming firm and less flexible with age (Tucker & Tucker, 1979). The laminae of the thyroid cartilage are somewhat semicircular in the infant larynx and become more angular in the older child (Kahane, 1975).

The vocal folds double their length during childhood, and puberty adds another growth spurt to the vocal folds, especially in males (Dickson & Maue-Dickson, 1982; Kahane, 1978). The composition and resulting mechanical properties of the vocal folds also change significantly during development. The larynx of the newborn shows a homogeneous and undifferentiated lamina propria (Hirano & Sato, 1993) that is not adult-like until about 16 years of age (Kent, 1997). The difference in the lamina propria prevents the infant from achieving some of the subtle vocal fold adjustments that are a part of the adult repertoire (Fuamenya, Robb, & Wemke, 2015).

Perhaps the most obvious change in the voice during development is in its fundamental frequency. As portrayed in Figure 3–48, the fundamental frequency decreases from about 400 to 500 Hz (newborns) to about 200 to 300 Hz (10-year-olds) in both boys and girls, with much of the decrease occurring during the first 3 years (Kent, 1976). During and after puberty, fundamental frequency undergoes a large and rapid downward change in males and a much less precipitous

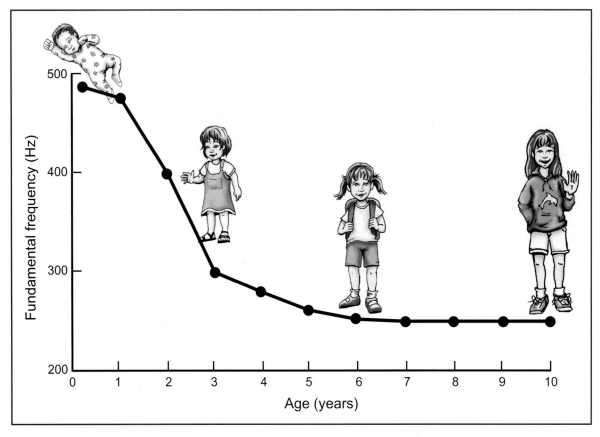

FIGURE 3–48. Fundamental frequency changes during the first decade of life. Based on data summarized in "Anatomical and Neuromuscular Maturation of the Speech Mechanism: Evidence From Acoustic Studies" (p. 423), by R. Kent, 1976, *Journal of Speech and Hearing Research, 19,* 421–447. Copyright 1976 by the American Speech and Hearing Association. Data summary reproduced with permission.

downward change in females. This is due to a greater growth spurt in both the length and thickness of the male vocal folds compared to the female vocal folds. The adolescent voice change that is perceptually prominent in males usually occurs between 12.5 and 14.5 years of age and may be accompanied by pitch breaks and other phenomena that reflect transient instability in the control of the voice (Hollien, Green, & Massey, 1994).

Donald Duck

Many of you who are reading this have breathed in from a helium-filled balloon and then tried to speak. The resulting sound makes people laugh because it reminds them of the voice of the cartoon character Donald Duck. What causes this? Helium is lighter than air, has a different kinematic viscosity, and effectively reduces the acoustic length of the upper airway. This makes the speech production mechanism behave acoustically as if it belonged to a smaller person. Helium results in resonances that are higher in frequency than expected. It's as if a child's upper airway were being excited by an adult's larynx. As utterance (expiration) proceeds, the inspired helium gives way to a mixture of helium and air and then just air. The sound of the voice gradually becomes less like a child's until it sounds like an adult again.

During the adult years, the larynx continues to lower slightly (Wind, 1970). Some of the cartilages of the larynx gradually ossify (turn to bone), whereas others gradually calcify (turn to salt), making the aging adult larynx increasingly stiff and brittle as time goes on (Zemlin, 1998). The arytenoid cartilages are unique as components of the laryngeal scaffolding because they are made of a hyaline matrix in some parts and an elastic matrix in other parts (Kahane, 1980, 1983; Sato, Kurita, Hirano, & Kiyokawa, 1990). Thus, the arytenoid cartilages are subjected to hardening twice during the aging process, early in adulthood by ossification and late in adulthood by calcification.

The joints of the larynx also change with advancing age in adulthood. The cricoarytenoid joints, for example, undergo modification in both their joint capsules and articular surfaces (Kahane & Hammons, 1987; Kahn & Kahane, 1986; Segre, 1971). Changes at the articular surfaces include abrasion, ossification, erosion, and deformation, all of which influence movements at the joints. Most important is that the movement of the arytenoid cartilages around the cricoarytenoid joints can be reduced in older individuals, which, in turn, can limit the degree to which the vocal folds can be approximated (Kahane, 1988).

The vocal folds undergo modification with advance age. Such modification includes nerve fiber loss and muscle atrophy that lead to losses in mass and muscle strength (Aronson, 1990; Cooper, 1990; Ferreri, 1959). Other changes include a reduction in tissue elasticity in the vocal folds, dehydration of the laryngeal mucosa, edema, and alteration in the density of different fibers constituting the structural matrices of the vocal folds (Aronson, 1990; Benjamin, 1988; Kahane & Beckford, 1991; Keleman & Pressman, 1955; Linville, 1995; Mueller, Sweeney, & Baribeau, 1985). Simultaneous age-related changes in the lamina propria may cause the vocal folds to take on a bowed configuration (Honjo & Isshiki, 1980; Mueller et al., 1985), develop surface irregularities along their free margins (Kahane, 1983), and stiffen (Kent, 1997). These age-related changes in vocal fold structure can have profound negative effects on vocal fold function and ultimately on quality of life (Mallick, Garas, & McGlashan, 2019; Rosow & Pan, 2019). Some of these are mentioned in the next section.

Sex

During infancy and early childhood, the structure and function of the larynx are relatively similar in boys and girls. Later in childhood, differences between the sexes start to emerge, especially during puberty, and are maintained throughout the life span.

Once fully mature, the most obvious difference between the male and female larynx is the overall size, with the typical male larynx being larger than the typical female larynx (Jotz et al., 2014). There is also a noticeable configuration difference, with the angle formed by the thyroid laminae being narrower in men than women (Glikson, Sagiv, Eyal, Wolf, & Primov-Fever, 2017; Kahane, 1978; Malinowski, 1967). This sharper angle accounts for the fact that men have a larger Adam's apple (thyroid prominence) than women.

Size and configuration differences between the male and female larynx are the primary contributors to sex-related differences in fundamental frequency. Following puberty, males have lower fundamental frequencies than females of similar age, as shown in Figure 3–49. Note that fundamental frequency tends to decrease with age in women; in contrast, fundamental frequency first decreases, then increases in men. In women, the decrease in fundamental frequency (very late in life) may have roots in an age-related increase in edema (Ferreri, 1959; Honjo & Isshiki, 1980). In men, the increase in fundamental frequency may have roots in muscle atrophy, thinning of the lamina propria, and general loss of mass (Hirano, Kurita, & Sakaguchi, 1989; Kahane, 1987; Segre, 1971). These age-related changes in fundamental frequency may help to explain why it may be difficult to tell whether the voice you hear on the telephone is that of a senescent man with a high pitch or a senescent woman with a low pitch.

In women, hormonal fluctuations appear to influence fundamental frequency. For example, there may be subtle changes in fundamental frequency (and intensity) associated with the menstrual cycle (Banal, 2017). The fundamental frequencies of women who have completed menopause are lower than those of women of the same age who have not completed menopause (Stoicheff, 1981). The effects of menopause on fundamental frequency appear to be offset somewhat by the use of hormone replacement therapy, as postmenopausal women who were using hormone replacement therapy have been found to have higher fundamental frequencies than those who were not (Hamdan et al., 2018).

Sex-related differences may also be seen in the way young adults approximate the vocal folds for voice production. As portrayed in Figure 3–50, many young women show an opening between the vocal folds during voicing, especially in the cartilaginous segment (Biever & Bless, 1989; Sodersten & Lindestad, 1990), whereas men do not. In contrast, men of all ages and older women more often exhibit either full vocal fold approximation or a spindle-shaped opening (Ahmad, Yan, & Bless, 2012; Biever & Bless, 1989; Linville, 1992; Pontes et al., 2006). Reasons for male-female differences in vocal fold approximation are speculative

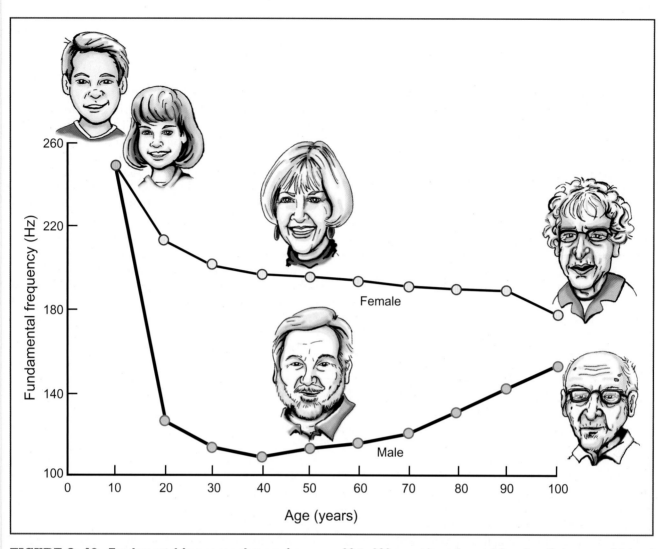

FIGURE 3–49. Fundamental frequency changes from ages 10 to 100 years in males and females. Data were obtained from cross-sectional studies and rounded to the nearest decade for each sex (Awan & Mueller, 1992; Benjamin, 1981; Eichhorn, Kent, Austin, & Vorperian, 2018; Hollien & Shipp, 1972; Honjo & Isshiki, 1980; Linville, 1987; Linville & Fisher, 1985; Mueller et al., 1985; Russell, Penny, & Pemberton, 1995; Stathopoulos, Huber, & Sussman, 2011; Stoicheff, 1981).

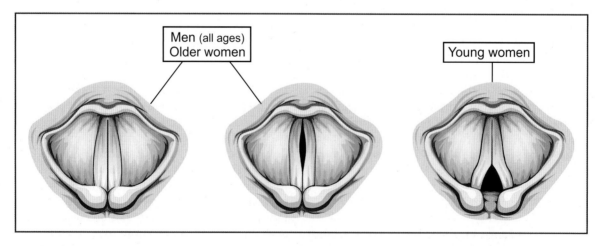

FIGURE 3–50. Vocal fold approximation during voice production in men and women. Whereas men of all ages and older women tend to either fully approximate the vocal folds or exhibit a spindle-shaped glottis during voice production, young women have a tendency to maintain a posterior glottis.

and include sex-related differences in the arrangement of the cricoarytenoid joints, muscle mass of the body of the vocal folds, and covers of the vocal folds (Hirano, Kiyokawa, & Kurita, 1988; Hirano, Kiyokawa, Kurita, & Sato, 1986). Cultural factors may also be at play, with a breathy voice quality being a more desirable characteristic of a female voice than a male voice (Linville, 1992).

Finding a New Voice

Male-female differences are inherently interesting. So are male-female differences in voice. Understanding these differences between male and female voices is particularly relevant to speech-language pathologists who work with transgender clients. The number of people who identify as transgender in the United States has substantially increased over the past decade (Flores, Herman, Gates, & Brown, 2016), and with this increase comes more and more people requesting clinical services to help their voices become gender congruent. Voice therapy with transgender clients typically focuses on modification of fundamental frequency and its variation, with trans women striving for a higher-pitched voice and greater pitch variability compared to their previous male voice. Voice quality is also a target of therapy, usually with a focus on increasing breathiness and changing resonance characteristics as a way to sound more feminine. Behavioral therapy to modify voice and communication style is considered the first line of treatment for transgender clients, sometimes followed by laryngeal surgery to help achieve optimal voice (Gray & Courey, 2019).

CLINICAL NOTES

The larynx is a particularly interesting speech subsystem, in part because so much can go wrong with it, and when it does, the consequences can be quite noticeable. Problems with the larynx are often manifested as voice disorders; these disorders can take many forms. One general form of voice disorder is classified as functional and refers to disorders that have no apparent physical cause. Functional voice disorders are sometimes the by-product of a serious psychogenic problem and may even be manifested as aphonia (the complete inability to produce voice). Functional disorders also include those that are caused by misuse or abuse of the voice that often result in abnormal vocal folds vibratory patterns and changes in voice quality. If the abuse is particularly extreme or long term (for example, repeated or prolonged periods of yelling or screaming), an organic voice disorder could emerge (one with a known physical basis). A common outcome of prolonged misuse or abuse is the development of nodules (callous-like lesions) on the vocal folds that can cause the voice to sound rough and breathy. Another category of voice disorders with known physical causes are those that accompany diseases or injuries of the nervous system. Some of these neural conditions affect all or most parts of the body—for example, amyotrophic lateral sclerosis. Specific to the larynx vocal fold paralysis is a condition caused by impairment of cranial nerve X (vagus), the peripheral nerve that is responsible for controlling the muscles of the vocal folds.

Vocal fold paralysis (inability to move) or paresis (weakness) resulting from damage to the vagus nerve can be unilateral or bilateral and may affect the ability to move one (unilateral) or both (bilateral) vocal folds. Unilateral vocal fold paralysis or paresis is often attributed to an accidental injury to the recurrent laryngeal nerve (a branch of the vagus) during thyroid or lung surgery. Some examples of the functional consequences of unilateral vocal fold paralysis or paresis are that one of the vocal folds may not be able to fully abduct, adduct, or both, depending on exactly which muscles are affected. An image of a paralyzed left vocal fold is shown in Figure 3–51 in which the individual is attempting to adduct the vocal folds. Note that the right vocal fold has approached the midline; however, the left vocal fold has remained in a lateral position. The result is that the vocal folds do not come close enough to each other to approximate and a large glottis remains. Clearly, this person would not be able to produce sound by setting the vocal folds into vibration and would only be left with the possibility of generating a whisper-like sound.

In some cases, vocal fold paralysis/paresis resolves on its own within a few months as the injured nerve heals. And sometimes voice therapy is recommended to help support the natural healing process. Nevertheless, there are cases in which the damage appears to be permanent and a more aggressive approach must be taken. One example of an intervention that can be very effective is for a laryngologist (a physician who specializes in the larynx and voice) to inject a gel-type substance into the impaired vocal fold. Bulking up the impaired vocal fold in this way can make it possible for the patient to produce voice again.

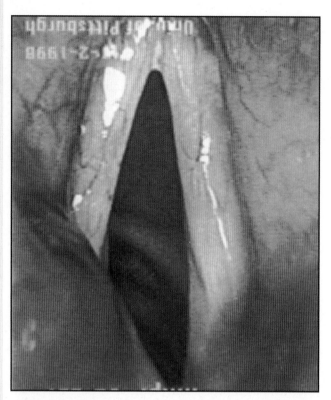

FIGURE 3–51. Unilateral (left) vocal fold paralysis. This is a view from above (the front of the larynx is at the top of the image) that shows an attempt to adduct the vocal folds. The left vocal fold does not approach the midline to the extent that the right vocal fold does. The consequence is that the vocal folds do not approximate and a rather large glottis remains. From *Atlas of Laryngoscopy, Third Edition* (p. 236), by Robert T. Sataloff, Mary J. Hawkshaw, Johnathan Brandon Sataloff, Rima A. DeFatta, and Robert Eller. Copyright © 2013 Plural Publishing. All rights reserved.

REVIEW

The larynx (voice box) is an air valve positioned between the trachea (windpipe) and the pharynx (throat) that can be adjusted to vary the amount of coupling between the two.

The skeleton of the larynx forms a framework consisting of bone, cartilages, ligaments, and tendons.

Major cartilages of the larynx include the thyroid, cricoid, arytenoids, and epiglottis, which function, along with the hyoid bone, as an integral unit.

Two pairs of joints mediate movements of the interior of the larynx, one between the cricoid and thyroid cartilages on each side, and one between the cricoid and arytenoid cartilages on each side.

Prominent structures within the larynx include the laryngeal cavity, vocal folds, ventricular folds (false vocal folds), laryngeal ventricles, and ligaments and membranes.

The most important laryngeal structures are the vocal folds, which have a muscular body at their core and an intricate outer covering with distinct layers.

Two types of forces operate on the larynx, one passive that includes the natural recoil of tissues, surface tension between structures in apposition, and the pull of gravity, and one active that includes intrinsic, extrinsic, and supplementary muscles that are nearly 20 in number.

Intrinsic muscles of the larynx include the ***thyroarytenoid***, ***posterior cricoarytenoid***, ***lateral cricoarytenoid***, ***arytenoid***, and ***cricothyroid***.

Extrinsic muscles of the larynx include the ***sternothyroid***, ***thyrohyoid***, and ***inferior constrictor***.

Supplementary muscles of the larynx are classified as infrahyoid muscles—***sternohyoid*** and ***omohyoid***—and suprahyoid muscles—***digastric***, ***stylohyoid***, ***mylohyoid***, ***geniohyoid***, ***hyoglossus***, and ***genioglossus***.

Movements of the larynx can result in changes in the positioning of the vocal folds (abduction, adduction, and changing length), ventricular folds, epiglottis, and laryngeal housing.

The control variables of laryngeal function include laryngeal opposing pressure, laryngeal airway resistance, glottal size and configuration, stiffness of the vocal folds, and effective mass of the vocal folds.

The neural substrates of laryngeal control are supported by cranial nerves V, VII, X, and XII and cervical spinal nerves C1, C2, and C3, which provide motor supply to the intrinsic, extrinsic, and supplementary muscles of the larynx and sensory supply that conveys information from mechanoreceptors about muscle lengths, rates of change in muscle length, joint movements, and mucosal deformations.

Laryngeal function is concerned mainly with protection of the pulmonary airways, containment of the pulmonary air supply, and sound generation.

Laryngeal function for speech production includes the generation of transient noise production (glottal stop-plosive), sustained noise production (glottal fricative or whisper), sustained voicing, and running speech activities.

Voice production relies on quasiperiodic vocal fold vibration that is governed by nonlinear interaction between an energy source (the respiratory system) and the structures being vibrated (the vocal folds).

Vocal fold vibration is self-sustaining because certain conditions exist, including alternations in the shape of the glottis (ranging from convergent to divergent), alternations in the intraglottal pressure (ranging from relatively high to relatively low), and the presence of vocal fold tissue recoil force (ranging from lower than intraglottal pressure to higher than the intraglottal pressure).

The fundamental frequency of the voice (correlated with the pitch of the voice) is the rate of vocal fold vibration and is controlled by primarily by the stiffness of the vocal folds as well as their mass.

Fundamental frequency is manipulated primarily by the *cricothyroid* and *thyroarytenoid* muscles, with additional contributions by other intrinsic, extrinsic, and supplementary laryngeal muscles.

The sound pressure level of the voice (correlated with the loudness of the voice) is controlled mainly by adjustments of the respiratory system (tracheal pressure) and the larynx (primarily laryngeal opposing pressure and laryngeal airflow declination rate) with somewhat less important adjustments of the pharyngeal-oral airway that alter the radiation impedance.

The lowest and highest values that can be produced in fundamental frequency and sound pressure level of the voice are not independent of one another, with the fundamental frequency range being greatest in the midrange of sound pressure levels and the sound pressure level range being greatest in the midrange of fundamental frequencies.

The voice source (tone produced at the larynx) is complex and has a spectrum (combination of frequencies and sound pressure levels) that bears some relation to the quality of the voice.

Pulse, *modal*, and *loft* are terms applied to three different voice registers that correspond to three different modes of vocal fold vibration and voice qualities encountered when speaking from the lowest to highest fundamental frequencies within the speaking range.

Laryngeal function during running speech activities is complex in that adjustments are made to control fundamental frequency, sound pressure level, and spectrum of the voice and to control actions of the larynx that constitute articulatory behaviors.

The larynx undergoes relocation and remodeling during a developmental period that extends into adolescence and is characterized by sexual dimorphism and a rapid growth spurt in males that lowers their fundamental frequency significantly in relation to females, whereas the mature larynx undergoes slower modification as a result of aging processes that stiffen it, degrade its joints, decrease its muscle mass, alter its composition, and otherwise make its function somewhat less efficient.

Males and females show laryngeal differences and voice production differences that have roots in structural and hormonal differences, different rates of ossification and calcification of laryngeal cartilages, different patterns of change in the covers of the vocal folds, and different patterns of valving by the vocal folds.

Disorders of the larynx can take many forms, some of which are caused by misuse or abuse of the voice and others that have physical causes, including vocal fold paralysis.

REFERENCES

Ahmad, K., Yan, Y., & Bless, D. (2012). Vocal fold vibratory characteristics of healthy geriatric females—Analysis of high-speed digital images. *Journal of Voice, 26,* 751–759.

Ardran, G., & Kemp, F. (1966). The mechanism of the larynx, I: The movements of the arytenoid and cricoids cartilages. *British Journal of Radiology, 39,* 641–654.

Arnold, G. (1961). Physiology and pathology of the cricothyroid muscle. *Laryngoscope, 71,* 687–753.

Aronson, A. (1990). *Clinical voice disorders: An interdisciplinary approach* (3rd ed.). New York, NY: Thieme.

Atkinson, J. (1978). Correlation analysis of the physiological factors controlling fundamental voice frequency. *Journal of the Acoustical Society of America, 63,* 211–222.

Awan, S., & Mueller, P. (1992). Speaking fundamental frequency characteristics of centenarian females. *Clinical Linguistics and Phonetics, 6,* 249–254.

Banal, I. (2017). Voice in different phases of menstrual cycle among naturally cycling women and users of hormonal contraceptives. *PLoS ONE, 12,* 1–13. https://doi.org/10.1371/journal.pone.0183462

Behrman, A. (2007). *Speech and voice science*. San Diego, CA: Plural Publishing.

Beneragama, T., & Serpell, J. (2006). Extralaryngeal bifurcation of the recurrent laryngeal nerve: A common variation. *ANZ Journal of Surgery, 76,* 928–931.

Benjamin, B. (1981). Frequency variability in the aged voice. *Journal of Gerontology, 36,* 722–736.

Benjamin, B. (1988). Changes in speech production and linguistic behaviors with aging. In B. Shadden (Ed.), *Communication behavior and aging: A sourcebook for clinicians* (pp. 162–181). Baltimore, MD: Williams & Wilkins.

Berke, G., & Gerratt, B. (1993). Laryngeal biomechanics: An overview of mucosal wave mechanics. *Journal of Voice, 7,* 123–128.

Berry, D., & Titze, I. (1996). Normal modes in a continuum model of vocal fold tissues. *Journal of the Acoustical Society of America, 100,* 3345–3354.

Biever, D., & Bless, D. (1989). Vibratory characteristics of the vocal folds in young adult and geriatric women. *Journal of Voice, 3,* 120–131.

Bosma, J. (1985). Postnatal ontogeny of performance of the pharynx, larynx, and mouth. *American Review of Respiratory Disease, 131,* 10–15.

Broad, D. (1973). Phonation. In F. Minifie, T. Hixon, & F. Williams (Eds.), *Normal aspects of speech, hearing, and language* (pp. 127–167). Englewood Cliffs, NJ: Prentice-Hall.

Catten, M., Gray, S., Hammond, T., Zhou, R., & Hammond, E. (1998). Analysis of cellular location and concentration in vocal fold lamina propria. *Otolaryngology-Head and Neck Surgery, 118,* 663–667.

Cavagna, G., & Margaria, R. (1965). An analysis of the mechanics of phonation. *Journal of Applied Physiology, 20,* 301–307.

Coleman, R., Mabis, J., & Hinson, J. (1977). Fundamental frequency—Sound pressure level profiles of adult male and female voices. *Journal of Speech and Hearing Research, 20,* 197–204.

Cooper, D. (1990). *Maturation, characteristics, and aging of laryngeal muscles.* Paper presented at the Pacific Voice Conference, San Francisco, CA.

Damste, H. (1970). The phonetogram. *Practica Oto-RhinoLaryngologica, 32,* 185–187.

Daniloff, R., Shuckers, G., & Feth, L. (1980). *The physiology of speech and hearing.* Englewood Cliffs, NJ: Prentice-Hall.

de Melo, E., Lemas, M., Filho, J., Sennes, L., Saldiva, P., & Tsuji, D. (2003). Distribution of collagen in the lamina propria of the human vocal fold. *Laryngoscope, 113,* 2187–2191.

Dickson, D., & Maue-Dickson, W. (1982). *Anatomical and physiological bases of speech.* Boston, MA: Little, Brown.

Eichhorn, J., Kent, R., Austin, D., & Vorperian, H. (2018). Effects of aging on vocal fundamental frequency and vowel formants in men and women. *Journal of Voice, 32,* 644.e1–644.e9.

Faaborg-Andersen, K., & Sonninen, A. (1960). The function of the extrinsic laryngeal muscles at different pitch: An electromyographic and roentgenologic investigation. *Acta Otolaryngologica, 51,* 89–93.

Fairbanks, G. (1960). *Voice and articulation drillbook.* New York, NY: Harper & Row.

Fairbanks, G., & Miron, M. (1957). Effect of vocal effort upon the consonant–vowel ratio within the syllable. *Journal of the Acoustical Society of America, 29,* 621–626.

Fant, G. (1960). *Acoustic theory of speech production.* Hague, Netherlands: Mouton.

Ferreri, G. (1959). Senescence of the larynx. *Italian General Review of Otorhinolaryngology, 1,* 640–709.

Fink, B. (1975). *The human larynx: A functional study.* New York, NY: Raven Press.

Fink, B., Basek, M., & Epanchin, V. (1956). The mechanism of opening of the human larynx. *Laryngoscope, 66,* 410–425.

Flanagan, J. (1972). *Speech analysis, synthesis, and perception.* New York, NY: Springer-Verlag.

Flores, A., Herman, J., Gates, G., & Brown, T. (2016). *How many adults identify as transgender in the United States?* Los Angeles, CA: The Williams Institute.

Folkard, C. (2006). *Guinness world records: 2006.* New York, NY: Bantam Books.

Frable, M. (1961). Computation of motion at the cricoarytenoid joint. *Archives of Otolaryngology, 73,* 551–556.

Fuamenya, N., Robb, M., & Wermke, K. (2015). Noisy but effective: Crying across the first 3 months of life. *Journal of Voice, 29,* 281–286.

Gauffin, J., & Sundberg, J. (1989). Spectral correlates of glottal voice source waveform characteristics. *Journal of Speech and Hearing Research, 32,* 556–565.

Gay, T., Hirose, H., Strome, M., & Sawashima, M. (1972). Electromyography of the intrinsic laryngeal muscles during phonation. *Annals of Otology, Rhinology, and Laryngology, 81,* 401–409.

Glikson, E., Sagiv, D., Eyal, A., Wolf, M., & Primov-Fever, A. (2017). The anatomical evolution of the thyroid cartilage from childhood to adulthood: A computed tomography evaluation. *Laryngoscope, 127,* E354–E358.

Gramming, P. (1991). Vocal loudness and frequency capabilities of the voice. *Journal of Voice, 5,* 144–157.

Gray, M. L., & Courey, M.S. (2019). Transgender voice and communication. *The Otolaryngologic Clinics of North America, 52,* 713–722.

Hall, A., Cobb, R., Kapoor, K., Kuchai, R., & Sandhu, G. (2017). The instrument of voice: The "true" vocal cord or vocal fold? *Journal of Voice, 31,* 133–134.

Hamdan, A.-L., Tabet, G., Fakhri, G., Sarieddine, D., Btaiche, R., & Seoud, M. (2018). Effect of hormonal replacement therapy on voice. *Journal of Voice, 32,* 116–121.

Hertegård, S. (2016). Tissue engineering in the larynx and airway. *Current Opinion in Otolaryngology Head and Neck Surgery, 24,* 469–476.

Hirano, M. (1974). Morphological structures of the vocal cord as a vibrator and its variations. *Folia Phoniatrica, 26,* 89–94.

Hirano, M., Kakita, Y., Kawasaki, H., Gould, W., & Lambiase, A. (1981). Data from high-speed motion picture studies. In K. Stevens & M. Hirano (Eds.), *Vocal fold physiology* (pp. 85–93). Tokyo, Japan: University of Tokyo Press.

Hirano, M., Kiyokawa, K., & Kurita, S. (1988). Laryngeal muscles and glottal shaping. In O. Fujimura (Ed.), *Vocal physiology: Voice production, mechanisms, and functions* (pp. 49–65). New York, NY: Raven Press.

Hirano, M., Kiyokawa, K., Kurita, S., & Sato, K. (1986). Posterior glottis: Morphological study in excised larynges. *Annals of Otology, Rhinology, and Laryngology, 95,* 576–581.

Hirano, M., Kurita, S., & Sagaguchi, S. (1989). Aging of the vibratory tissue of the human vocal folds. *Acta Otolaryngologica, 107,* 428–433.

Hirano, M., Ohala, J., & Vennard, W. (1969). The function of the laryngeal muscles in regulating fundamental frequency and intensity of phonation. *Journal of Speech and Hearing Research, 12,* 616–628.

Hirano, M., & Sato, K. (1993). *Histological color atlas of the human larynx.* San Diego, CA: Singular.

Hirano, M., Yoshida, T., & Tanaka, S. (1991). Vibratory behavior of human vocal folds viewed from below. In J. Gauffin & B. Hammarberg (Eds.), *Vocal fold physiology: Acoustic, perceptual, and physiological aspects of voice mechanisms* (pp. 1–6). San Diego, CA: Singular Publishing.

Hirose, H. (1977). Laryngeal adjustments in consonant production. *Phonetica, 34,* 289–294.

Hixon, T. (1966). Turbulent noise sources for speech. *Folia Phoniatrica, 18,* 168–182.

Hixon, T., Klatt, D., & Mead, J. (1971). Influence of forced transglottal pressure change on vocal fundamental frequency. *Journal of the Acoustical Society of America, 49,* 105.

Hixon, T., Mead, J., & Goldman, M. (1976). Dynamics of the chest wall during speech production: Function of the thorax, rib cage, diaphragm, and abdomen. *Journal of Speech and Hearing Research, 19,* 297–356.

Hixon, T., & Minifie, F. (1972, November). *Influence of forced transglottal pressure change on vocal sound pressure level.*

Paper presented at the Convention of the American Speech and Hearing Association, San Francisco, CA.

Hollien, H. (1972). Three major vocal registers: A proposal. In A. Rigault & R. Charbonneau (Eds.), *Proceedings of the Seventh International Congress of Phonetic Sciences* (pp. 320–331). Hague, Netherlands: Mouton.

Hollien, H. (1974). On vocal registers. *Journal of Phonetics, 2,* 125–143.

Hollien, H., Green, R., & Massey, K. (1994). Longitudinal research on adolescent voice change in males. *Journal of the Acoustical Society of America, 34,* 80–84.

Hollien, H., & Shipp, T. (1972). Speaking fundamental frequency and chronological age in males. *Journal of Speech and Hearing Research, 15,* 155–159.

Honda, K. (1995). Laryngeal and extra-laryngeal mechanisms of FO control. In F. Bell-Berti & L. Raphael (Eds.), *Producing speech: Contemporary issues—For Katherine Safford Harris* (pp. 215–245). New York, NY: American Institute of Physics.

Honjo, I., & Isshiki, N. (1980). Laryngoscopic and voice characteristics of aged persons. *Archives of Otolaryngology, 106,* 149–150.

Ishii, K., Zhai, W., Akita, M., & Hirose, H. (1996). Ultra-structure of the lamina propria of the human vocal fold. *Acta Otolaryngologica, 116,* 778–782.

Isshiki, N. (1964). Regulatory mechanism of voice intensity variation. *Journal of Speech and Hearing Research, 7,* 17–29.

Jankovskaya, N. (1959). The receptor innervation of the perichondrium of the laryngeal cartilages. *Arkhiv Anatomii, Gistologii l'Enbriologii, 37,* 70–75.

Jotz, G., Stefani, M., Pereira da Costa Filho, O., Malysz, T., Soster, P., & Leão, H. (2014). A morphometric study of the larynx. *Journal of Voice, 28,* 668–672.

Kahane, J. (1975). *The developmental anatomy of the human prepubertal and pubertal larynx* (Unpublished doctoral dissertation). University of Pittsburgh, Pittsburgh, PA.

Kahane, J. (1978). A morphological study of the human prepubertal and pubertal larynx. *American Journal of Anatomy, 151,* 11–20.

Kahane, J. (1980). Age-related histological changes in the human male and female laryngeal cartilages: Biological and functional implications. In V. Lawrence (Ed.), *Transcripts of the Ninth Symposium: Care of the professional voice, Part I* (pp. 11–20). New York, NY: The Voice Foundation.

Kahane, J. (1983). A survey of age-related changes in the connective tissue of the human adult larynx. In D. Bless & J. Abbs (Eds.), *Vocal fold physiology: Contemporary research and clinical issues* (pp. 44–49). San Diego, CA: College-Hill Press.

Kahane, J. (1987). Connective tissue changes in the larynx and their effects on voice. *Journal of Voice, 1,* 27–30.

Kahane, J. (1988). Age-related changes in the human cricoarytenoid joint. In O. Fujimura (Ed.), *Vocal physiology: Voice production, mechanisms, and functions* (pp. 145–157). New York, NY: Raven Press.

Kahane, J., & Beckford, N. (1991). The aging larynx and voice. In D. Ripich (Ed.), *Handbook of geriatric communication disorders* (pp. 165–186). Austin, TX: Pro-Ed.

Kahane, J., & Hammons, J. (1987). Developmental changes in the articular cartilage of the human cricoarytenoid joint. In T. Baer, C. Sasaki, & K. Harris (Eds.), *Laryngeal function in phonation and respiration* (pp. 14–28). San Diego, CA: College-Hill Press.

Kahn, A., & Kahane, J. (1986). India pin-prick experiments on surface organization of cricoarytenoid joints (CAJ) articular surfaces. *Journal of Speech and Hearing Research, 29,* 536–543.

Keleman, G., & Pressman, J. (1955). Physiology of the larynx. *Physiological Review, 35,* 506–554.

Kempster, G., Gerratt, B., Abbott, K., Barkmeier-Kraemer, J., & Hillman, R. (2009). Consensus auditory-perceptual evaluation of voice: Development of a standardized clinical protocol. *American Journal of Speech-Language Pathology, 18,* 124–132.

Kent, R. (1976). Anatomical and neuromuscular maturation of the speech mechanism: Evidence from acoustic studies. *Journal of Speech and Hearing Research, 19,* 421–447.

Kent, R. (1997). *The speech sciences.* San Diego, CA: Singular Publishing.

Kirchner, J., & Suzuki, M. (1968). Laryngeal reflexes and voice production. *Annals of the New York Academy of Sciences, 155,* 98–109.

Kirchner, J., & Wyke, B. (1965). Articular reflex mechanisms in the larynx. *Annals of Otology, Rhinology, and Laryngology, 74,* 749–768.

Konig, W., & von Leden, H. (1961a). The peripheral nervous system of the human larynx, 1: The mucous membrane. *Archives of Otolaryngology, 73,* 1–14.

Konig, W., & von Leden, H. (1961b). The peripheral nervous system of the human larynx, 2: The thyroarytenoid (vocalis) muscle. *Archives of Otolaryngology, 74,* 153–163.

Kunze, L. (1962). *An investigation of changes in sub-glottal air pressure and rate of air flow accompanying changes in fundamental frequency, intensity, vowels, and voice registers in adult male speakers* (Unpublished doctoral dissertation). University of Iowa, Iowa City.

Ladefoged, P., & McKinney, N. (1963). Loudness, sound pressure, and subglottal pressure in speech. *Journal of the Acoustical Society of America, 35,* 454–460.

Laver, J. (1991). *The gift of speech: Papers in the analysis of speech and voice.* Edinburgh, Scotland: Edinburgh University Press.

Lester, R., & Story, B. (2013). Acoustic characteristics of simulated respiratory-induced vocal tremor. *American Journal of Speech-Language Pathology, 22,* 205–211.

Linville, S. (1987). Maximum phonational frequency range capabilities of women's voices with advancing age. *Folia Phoniatrica, 39,* 297–301.

Linville, S. (1992). Glottal gap configurations in two age groups of women. *Journal of Speech and Hearing Research, 35,* 1209–1215.

Linville, S. (1995). Vocal aging. *Current Opinion in Otolaryngology and Head and Neck Surgery, 3,* 183–187.

Linville, S., & Fisher, H. (1985). Acoustic characteristics of perceived versus actual age in controlled phonation by adult females. *Journal of the Acoustical Society of America, 78,* 40–48.

Lofqvist, A., & Yoshioka, H. (1984). Intrasegmental timing: Laryngeal-oral coordination in voiceless consonant production. *Speech Communication, 3,* 279–289.

Malinowski, A. (1967). Shape, dimensions, and process of calcification of the cartilaginous framework of the larynx in relation to age and sex in the Polish population. *Folia Morphologica, 26,* 118–128.

Mallick, A. S., Garas, G., & McGlashan, J. (2019). Presbylaryngis: A state-of-the-art review. *Current Opinion in Otolaryngology & Head and Neck Surgery, 27,* 168-177.

Mayet, A., & Muendnich, K. (1958). Beitrag zur anatomie und zur funktion des m. cricothyroideus und der cricothyreiodgelenke. *Acta Anatomica, 33,* 273–288.

Minifie, F. (1973). Speech acoustics. In F. Minifie, T. Hixon, & F. Williams (Eds.), *Normal aspects of speech, hearing, and language* (pp. 236–284). Englewood Cliffs, NJ: Prentice-Hall.

Monoson, P., & Zemlin, W. (1984). Quantitative study of whisper. *Folia Phoniatrica, 36,* 53–65.

Mueller, P., Sweeney, R., & Baribeau, L. (1985). Acoustic and morphologic study of the senescent voice. *Ear, Nose, and Throat Journal, 63,* 71–75.

Murry, T., & Brown, W. (1971a). Regulation of vocal intensity in vocal fry phonation. *Journal of the Acoustical Society of America, 49,* 1905–1907.

Murry, T., & Brown, W. (1971b). Subglottal air pressure during two types of vocal activity: Vocal fry and modal phonation. *Folia Phoniatrica, 23,* 440–449.

Netsell, R. (1969). *A perceptual-acoustic physiological study of syllable stress* (Unpublished doctoral dissertation). University of Iowa, Iowa City.

Netsell, R. (1973). Speech physiology. In F. Minifie, T. Hixon, & F. Williams (Eds.), *Normal aspects of speech, hearing, and language* (pp. 211–234). Englewood Cliffs, NJ: Prentice-Hall.

Obrebowski, A., Wojnowski, W., & Obrebowski-Karsznia, Z. (2006). The characteristics of vocal fold molecular structure. *Otolaryngologia Polska, 60,* 9–14.

Ohala, J. (1972, April). *How is pitch lowered?* Paper presented at the Spring Meeting of the Acoustical Society of America, Buffalo, NY.

Ohala, J., & Hirose, H. (1970). The function of the sternohyoid muscle in speech. *Annual Report of the Institute of Logopedics and Phoniatrics, 4,* 41–44.

Okamura, H., & Katto, Y. (1988). Fine structure of muscle spindle in interarytenoid muscle of the human larynx. In O. Fujimura (Ed.), *Vocal fold physiology: Voice production, mechanisms, and functions* (pp. 135–143). New York, NY: Raven Press.

Orlikoff, R., & Kahane, J. (1996). Structure and function of the larynx. In N. Lass (Ed.), *Principles of experimental phonetics* (pp. 112–181). St. Louis, MO: Mosby.

Pontes, P., Yamasaki, R., & Behlau, M. (2006). Morphological and functional aspects of the senile larynx. *Folia Phoniatrica et Logopaedica, 58,* 151–158.

Pressman, J. (1942). Physiology of the vocal cords in phonation and respiration. *Archives of Otolaryngology, 35,* 355–398.

Reidenbach, M. (1998). The muscular tissue of the vestibular folds of the larynx. *European Archives of Otorhinolaryngology, 255,* 365–367.

Roscow, D. E., & Pan, D. R. (2019). Presbyphonia and minimal glottic insufficiency. *Otolaryngologic Clinics of North America, 52,* 617–625.

Rothenberg, M. (1968). *The breath-stream dynamics of simple released-plosive production* (Bibliotheca Phonetica No. 6). Basel, Switzerland: S. Karger.

Rothenberg, M. (1983). An interactive model for the voice source. In D. Bless & J. Abbs (Eds.), *Vocal fold physiology: Contemporary research and clinical issues* (pp. 155–165). San Diego, CA: College-Hill Press.

Rubin, A., Praneetvataku, V., Gherson, S., & Moyer, C. (2006). Laryngeal hyperfunction during whispering: Reality or myth? *Journal of Voice, 20,* 121–127.

Rubin, H. (1963). Experimental studies in vocal pitch and intensity in phonation. *Laryngoscope, 72,* 973–1015.

Russell, A., Penny, L., & Pemberton, C. (1995). Speaking fundamental frequency changes over time in women: A longitudinal study. *Journal of Speech and Hearing Research, 38,* 101–109.

Sampson, S., & Eyzaguirre, C. (1964). Some functional characteristics of mechanoreceptors in the larynx of the cat. *Journal of Neurophysiology, 27,* 464–480.

Sanders, I., Han, Y., Wang, J., & Biller, H. (1998). Muscle spindles are concentrated in the superior vocalis subcompartment of the human thyroarytenoid muscle. *Journal of Voice, 12,* 7–16.

Sanders, I., Wu, L., Mu, Y., & Biller, H. (1993). Innervation of the human larynx. *Archives of Otolaryngology-Head and Neck Surgery, 119,* 934–939.

Sanudo, J., Maranillo, E., Xavier, L., Mirapeix, R., Orus, C., & Quer, M. (1999). An anatomical study of anastomoses between the laryngeal nerves. *Laryngoscope, 109,* 983–987.

Sato, K., Kurita, S., Hirano, M., & Kiyokawa, K. (1990). Distribution of elastic cartilage in the arytenoids and its physiologic significance. *Annals of Otology, Rhinology, and Laryngology, 99,* 363–368.

Sawashima, M., Abramson, A., Cooper, F., & Lisker, L. (1970). Observing laryngeal adjustments during running speech by use of a fiberoptics system. *Phonetica, 22,* 193–201.

Schonharl, E. (1960). *Die stroboskopie in der praktischen laryngologie.* Stuttgart, Germany: Thieme-Verlag.

Segre, R. (1971). Senescence of the voice. *Eye, Ear, Nose, and Throat Monthly, 50,* 223–233.

Sekizawa, K., Sasaki, H., & Takishima, T. (1985). Laryngeal resistance immediately after panting in control and constricted airways. *Journal of Applied Physiology, 58,* 1164–1169.

Selbie, W., Zhang, L., Levine, W., & Ludlow, C. (1998). Using joint geometry to determine the motion of the cricoarytenoid joint. *Journal of the Acoustical Society of America, 103,* 1115–1127.

Sellars, I., & Keen, E. (1978). The anatomy and movements of the cricoarytenoid joint. *Laryngoscope, 88,* 667–674.

Shipp, T., & McGlone, R. (1971). Laryngeal dynamics associated with voice frequency change. *Journal of Speech and Hearing Research, 14,* 761–768.

Sodersten, M., & Lindestad, P. (1990). Glottal closure and perceived breathiness during phonation in normally speaking subjects. *Journal of Speech and Hearing Research, 33,* 601–611.

Solomon, N., McCall, G., Trosset, M., & Gray, W. (1989). Laryngeal configuration and constriction during two types of whispering. *Journal of Speech and Hearing Research, 32,* 161–174.

Sonesson, B. (1959). Die funktionelle anatomie des cricoarytaenoidgelenkes. *Zeitschrift fur Anatomie und Entwicklungs geschichte, 121,* 292–303.

Sonninen, A. (1968). The external frame function in the control of pitch in the human voice. *Annals of the New York Academy of Sciences, 155,* 68–90.

Stathopoulos, E., Huber, J., & Sussman, J. (2011). Changes in acoustic characteristics of the voice across the life span: Measures from individuals 4 to 93 years of age. *Journal of Speech, Language, and Hearing Research, 54,* 1011–1021.

Stevens, K. (2000). *Acoustic phonetics.* Cambridge, MA: MIT Press.

Stoicheff, M. (1981). Speaking fundamental frequency characteristics of nonsmoking female adults. *Journal of Speech and Hearing Research, 24,* 437–441.

Story, B. (2002). An overview of the physiology, physics and modeling of the sound source for vowels. *Acoustical Science and Technology, 23,* 195–206.

Story, B., & Titze, I. (1995). Voice simulation with a bodycover model of the vocal folds. *Journal of the Acoustical Society of America, 97,* 1249–1260.

Strocchi, R., De Pasquale, V., Messerotti, G., Raspanti, M., Franchi, M., & Ruggeri, A. (1992). Particular structure of the anterior third of the human true vocal cord. *Acta Anatomica, 145,* 189–194.

Takano, S., & Honda, K. (2005). Observation of the cricothyroid joint by high-resolution MRI. *Japanese Journal of Logopedics and Phoniatrics, 46,* 174–178.

Timcke, R., von Leden, H., & Moore, P. (1958). Laryngeal vibrations: Measurements of the glottic wave, I: The normal vibratory cycle. *Archives of Otolaryngology, 68,* 1–19.

Titze, I. (1989). On the relation between subglottal pressure and fundamental frequency in phonation. *Journal of the Acoustical Society of America, 85,* 901–906.

Titze, I. (1994). *Principles of voice production.* Englewood Cliffs, NJ: Prentice-Hall.

Titze, I. (2006). *The myoelastic aerodynamic theory of phonation.* Iowa City, IA: National Center for Voice and Speech.

Titze, I., Jiang, J., & Drucker, D. (1988). Preliminaries to the body-cover theory of pitch control. *Journal of Voice, 1,* 314–319.

Titze, I., Luschei, E., & Hirano, M. (1989). Role of the thyroarytenoid muscle in regulation of fundamental frequency. *Journal of Voice, 3,* 213–224.

Titze, I., & Story, B. (2002). Rules for controlling lowdimensional vocal fold models with muscle activation. *Journal of the Acoustical Society of America, 112,* 1064–1076.

Tucker, J., & Tucker, G. (1979). A clinical perspective on the development and anatomical aspects of the infant larynx and trachea. In G. Healy & T. McGill (Eds.), *Laryngotracheal problems in the pediatric patient* (pp. 3–8). Springfield, IL: Charles C Thomas.

Tucker, L. (1963). *Articulatory variations in normal speakers with changes in vocal pitch and effort* (Unpublished master's thesis). University of Iowa, Iowa City.

van den Berg, J. (1956). Direct and indirect determination of the mean subglottic pressure. *Folia Phoniatrica, 8,* 1–24.

van den Berg, J. (1957). Subglottic pressure and vibrations of the vocal folds. *Folia Phoniatrica, 9,* 64–71.

van den Berg, J. (1958). Myoelastic-aerodynamic theory of voice production. *Journal of Speech and Hearing Research, 1,* 227–244.

van den Berg, J., & Moll, J. (1955). Zur anatomie des men schlichen musculus vocalis. *Zeitschrift fur Anatomie und Entwicklungsgeschichte, 118,* 465–470.

van den Berg, J., & Tan, T. (1959). Results of experiments with human larynxes. *Practica Oto-Rhino Laryngologica, 21,* 425–450.

van den Berg, J., Vennard, W., Berger, D., & Shervanian, C. (1960). *Voice production* [Black and white 16-mm sound motion picture film]. Utrecht, Netherlands: SFW-UNFI.

van den Berg, J. W., Zantema, J., & Doornenbal, P. (1957). On the air resistance and the Bernoulli effect of the human larynx. *The Journal of the Acoustical Society of America, 29,* 626–631.

Vennard, W. (1967). *Singing: The mechanism and the technic.* New York, NY: Carl Fischer.

von Leden, H., & Moore, P. (1961). The mechanics of the cricoarytenoid joint. *Archives of Otolaryngology, 73,* 541–550.

Vorperian, H., Wang, S., Chung, M. K., Schimek, E. M., Durtschi, R. B., & Kent, R. D. (2009). Anatomic development of the oral and pharyngeal portions of the vocal tract: An imaging study. *Journal of the Acoustical Society of America, 125,* 1666–1678.

Wang, R. (1998). Three-dimensional analysis of cricoarytenoid joint motion. *Laryngoscope, 108,* 1–17.

Watson, P., Ciccia, A., & Weismer, G. (2003). The relation of lung volume initiation to selected acoustic properties of speech. *Journal of the Acoustical Society of America, 113,* 2812–2819.

Wind, J. (1970). *On the phylogeny and the ontogeny of the human larynx.* Groningen, Netherlands: Wolters-Noordhoff.

Wustrow, F. (1953). Bau und funktion des menshlichne musculus vocalis. *Zeitschrift fur Anatomie und Entwick-lungsgeschichte, 116,* 506–522.

Zemlin, W. (1998). *Speech and hearing science: Anatomy and physiology.* Boston, MA: Allyn & Bacon.

Zemlin, W., Davis, P., & Gaza, C. (1984). Fine morphology of the posterior cricoarytenoid muscle. *Folia Phoniatrica, 36,* 233–240.

Zenker, W. (1964). Questions regarding the function of external laryngeal muscles. In D. Brewer (Ed.), *Research potentials in voice physiology* (pp. 20–40). New York: State University of New York.

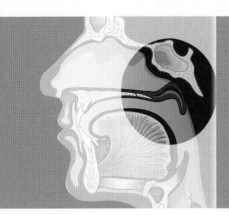

Velopharyngeal-Nasal Structure and Function

INTRODUCTION

The velopharyngeal-nasal component of the speech mechanism is located within the head and neck and comprises a system of valves and air passages that interconnects the pharynx (throat) and the atmosphere through the nose. Although most textbooks focus on the velopharyngeal part of this system, this chapter covers the complete velopharyngeal-nasal mechanism as a single functional entity. This is because the nasal part of the apparatus can have a significant influence on speech production, especially when velopharyngeal function is impaired.

This chapter covers velopharyngeal-nasal anatomy, followed by discussion of the forces and movements of the velopharyngeal and nasal parts of the mechanism, control variables and neural substrates, and velopharyngeal-nasal function for ventilation and speech production. The chapter concludes with some clinical notes. The nature of velopharyngeal-nasal function during swallowing is addressed in Chapter 7.

Duane C. Spriestersbach (1916–2011)

Spriestersbach had a distinguished career as a clinical investigator of the communication problems of children with cleft palate and craniofacial disorders. "Sprie," as he was affectionately called, served for many years as the program director of a large federally funded research grant on cleft palate at the University of Iowa. His leadership fostered much of the research done over two decades on normal velopharyngeal function for speech production and on the mechanisms involved in control of the velopharynx in individuals with velopharyngeal incompetence. Many of the names in the reference list to this chapter cut their research teeth under his guidance. Spriestersbach was an exceptional thinker. He had an enormous impact on translating the products of research into practical clinical applications for those with speech disorders caused by cleft palate. In his spare time, he took to the stage, where he performed in the Iowa City Community Theatre, and to the card table, where he played a legendary mean hand of poker.

VELOPHARYNGEAL-NASAL ANATOMY

The valves and air passages of the velopharyngeal-nasal mechanism are linked together, some arranged in series (one after another) and some arranged in parallel (side by side). The mechanism is supported by a skeletal framework and includes the pharynx, velum, nasal cavities, and outer nose, as described in this section. The velopharyngeal-nasal muscles are discussed in the next section on Forces of the Velopharyngeal-Nasal Mechanism.

Skeletal Framework

The skeletal framework of the velopharyngeal-nasal mechanism consists of the first six cervical vertebrae and various bones of the skull. The bones of the skull include cranial (braincase) bones and facial (forehead, eyes, nose, mouth, and upper throat) bones. These bones are individually intricate structures that are rigidly joined together and contribute to formation of the walls, floor, and roof of the velopharyngeal-nasal mechanism, as well as provide anchors to which many of the velopharyngeal-nasal muscles attach. The velopharyngeal-nasal and the pharyngeal-oral components of the speech mechanism share many bones of the skull. Therefore, the bones discussed in this section pertain to Chapter 5 as well.

Figure 4–1 depicts the cranial bones. Some of these bones are paired and some are not. The eight cranial bones are the temporal (two), parietal (two), occipital (one), frontal (one), sphenoid (one), and ethmoid (one) bones. Each temporal bone includes a narrow prominence called the styloid process to which muscle and ligament attach (other relevant features of the temporal bone are discussed in Chapter 6). The sphenoid bone, a double-winged structure, sits behind the eyes and forms the back wall of the nasal cavities. The ethmoid bone forms the upper side walls of the nasal cavities and the upper part of their medial wall.

Figure 4–2 depicts the facial bones, most of which are paired. These 14 bones are the maxillary (two), palatine (two), vomer (one), inferior nasal conchae (two), lacrimal (two), nasal (two), and zygomatic (two) bones and mandible (one). The bones most closely associated with structure of the velopharyngeal-nasal mechanism are the maxillary bones, which form the front of the floor of the nasal cavities; the palatine bones, which form back of the floor of the nasal cavities; the vomer bone, which forms the lower part of the medial wall of the nasal cavities; the inferior nasal conchae (plural for concha), which form the lower side walls of the nasal cavities; and the nasal bones, which form the bridge of the outer nose. The zygomatic bones form the prominences of the cheeks and are also called the cheekbones. The small and fragile lacrimal bones form part of the orbits (the cavities that contain the eyes) and articulate (connect) with the inferior nasal concha, ethmoid, frontal, and maxillary bones. The mandible is a moveable facial bone that is discussed in detail in Chapter 5.

Pharynx

Figure 4–3 depicts some of the salient features of the pharynx (throat). The pharynx is a tube of tendon and muscle that extends from the base of the skull to the cricoid cartilage in the front and to the sixth cervical vertebra in the back. The pharyngeal tube is widest at the top and narrows down its length and is oval in cross section, being larger side to side than front to back. As shown in the figure, the front wall of the pharynx is partially formed by the back surfaces of the velum (defined below), tongue, and epiglottis. Otherwise, the structure is open at the front and connects, from top to bottom, with the nasal cavities, oral cavity, and laryngeal aditus (upper entrance to the larynx).

The mix of tendon and muscle varies along the length of the pharynx. The upper part is the made up solely of connective tissue, called the pharyngeal aponeurosis, which effectively suspends the pharyngeal tube from above (the way the rim of a basketball goal suspends the net). Muscular tissue increases in proportion down the length of the pharynx until it predominates nearer the bottom. Muscle tissue encircles the pharynx, making its architecture resemble that of a sphincter. In fact, its overall arrangement is similar to that of the gut. This should come as no surprise, given that the pharynx is an active component of the digestive system and its lower part is continuous with the esophagus (gullet), where its front and back walls are in contact. This contact is broken during activities such as swallowing and regurgitation.

The pharynx comprises three cavities that are designated, from top to bottom, as the nasopharynx, oropharynx, and laryngopharynx. The boundaries of these cavities are shown in Figure 4–4. The nasopharynx lies behind the nose and above the velum. Because the velum is mobile, the lower boundary of the nasopharynx is somewhat arbitrary. Thus, a common convention is to specify this boundary by a reference line extending between the upper surface of the hard palate and the most forward point on the uppermost vertebra.

The nasopharynx always remains patent (open), a feature that distinguishes it from the other subdivisions

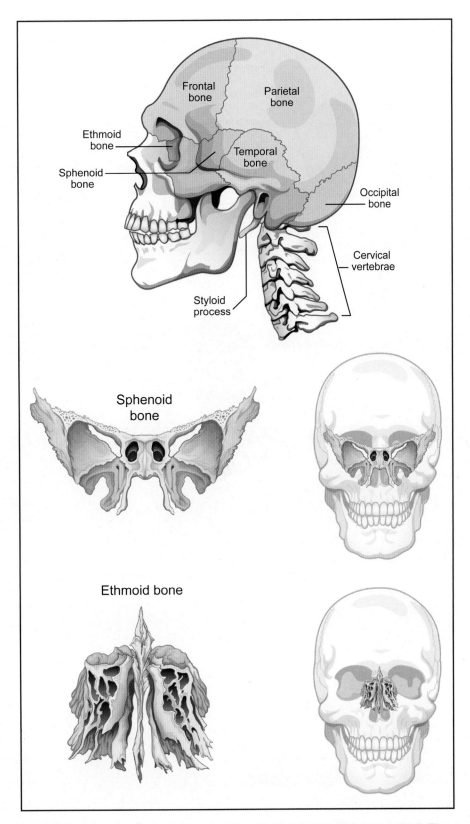

FIGURE 4-1. The cranial bones of the skull, two of which are paired. They include the temporal (two), parietal (two), occipital, frontal, sphenoid, and ethmoid bones.

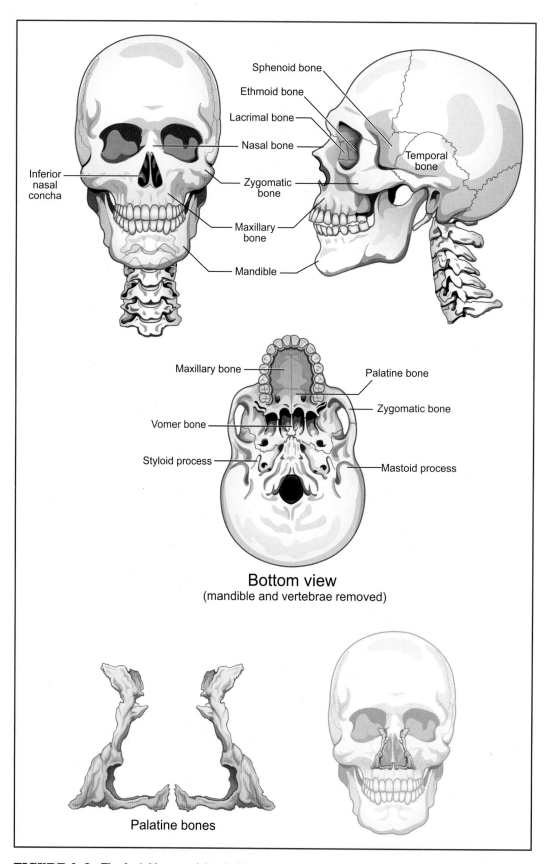

FIGURE 4-2. The facial bones of the skull, most of which are paired. They are the maxillary (two), palatine (two), vomer (one), inferior nasal conchae (two), lacrimal (two), nasal (two), and zygomatic (two) bones and mandible (one).

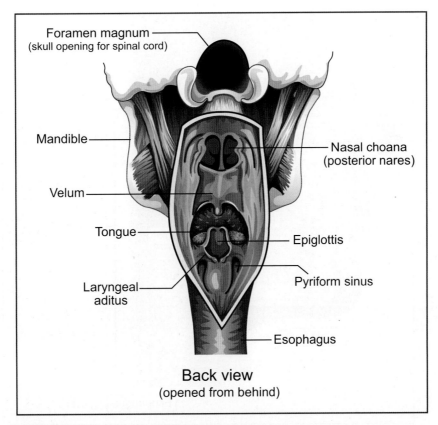

FIGURE 4–3. Salient features of the pharynx as revealed from a back view in which the posterior pharyngeal wall is opened from behind. The skull and mandible are shown for reference.

of the pharynx. The pharyngeal ends of the paired auditory tubes (also called the eustachian tubes) are located on the lateral walls of the nasopharynx. When these tubes open, they allow the pressure to equilibrate between the middle ears and atmosphere. Across the back surface of the nasopharynx, between the pharyngeal orifices of the auditory tubes, lies a large mass of lymphoid tissue called the pharyngeal tonsil. This tissue is also referred to as the nasopharyngeal tonsil and, when abnormally enlarged, is designated as adenoid tissue (or just the adenoids; see Figure 4–24 for an example). At the front, the nasopharynx connects to the nasal cavities through the nasal choanae (funnel-like openings), also called the posterior nares (nostrils) or internal nares. These are two oval-shaped apertures that are about twice as long (top to bottom) as they are wide (side to side) and are oriented in the vertical plane (see Figure 4–3).

The oropharynx forms the middle part of the pharyngeal tube. Its upper boundary is coextensive with the lower boundary of the nasopharynx, and its lower boundary is the hyoid bone. As shown in Figure 4–5, the front of the oropharynx opens into the oral cav-

ity through the faucial isthmus (the passage situated between the velum and the base of the tongue). This isthmus is bounded on the left and right sides by the anterior and posterior faucial pillars, pairs of muscular bands that resemble pairs of legs. The palatine tonsils are located between the anterior and posterior faucial pillars on each side of the isthmus. They are also often called the faucial tonsils and are "the" tonsils most often referred to colloquially. The back surface of the tongue is the site of yet another tonsil, the so-called lingual tonsil. This tonsil is a broad aggregate of lymph glands distributed across much of the posterior (root) part of the tongue. The oropharynx is the only subdivision of the pharynx that can be visualized without special equipment. The back wall of the oropharynx is best viewed when the velum is elevated, as in "open your mouth wide and say 'ah.'"

The laryngopharynx constitutes the lowermost part of the pharynx. The upper boundary of the laryngopharynx is the hyoid bone and the lower boundary is the base of the cricoid cartilage where the pharynx is continuous with the esophagus. At the front, the laryngopharynx is bounded by the back surface of the

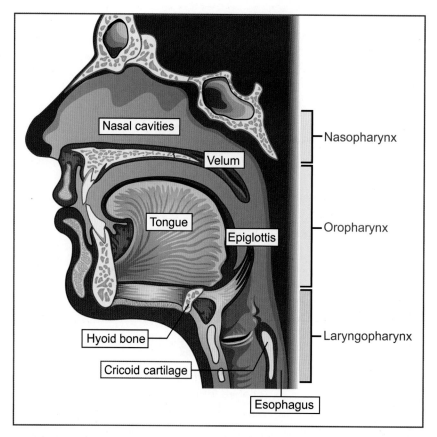

FIGURE 4–4. Boundaries of the nasopharynx, oropharynx, and laryngopharynx. The boundary between the nasopharynx and oropharynx can be arbitrary; in this figure, it is defined by an imaginary line extending backward at the level of the hard palate. The boundary between the oropharynx and laryngopharynx is the hyoid bone, and the lower boundary of the laryngopharynx is the base of the cricoid cartilage.

tongue (and the lingual tonsil), the laryngeal aditus (the opening into the larynx formed by the epiglottis and aryepiglottic folds), and the pyriform sinuses (pear-shaped cavities located to the sides of the aryepiglottic folds; see Figure 4–3).

Velum

The velum, which means *curtain*, is a pendulous flap consisting of the soft palate and uvula (meaning *little grape*). In this case, the velum is the curtain that hangs

Show Me Your Hand

They were twin girls. Each had speech that was a dead ringer for the other and was characterized by multiple misarticulations and hypernasality. What was the cause? Had they developed some sort of twin speech? Did one have a problem and the other was imitating it? Oral examinations revealed identical structural anomalies. Each girl had a short velum. Nasoendoscopic examinations further revealed that, for each girl, the velum elevated only occasionally during speech production but

never came close to the posterior pharyngeal wall. The girls' parents were with them and being interviewed by a student clinician and her supervisor. The moment the mother spoke, there were suspicions. She had a severe speech disorder characterized by multiple misarticulations, hypernasality, and pronounced nasal grimacing when speaking. She allowed an oral examination. She had a short velum. It was three of a kind.

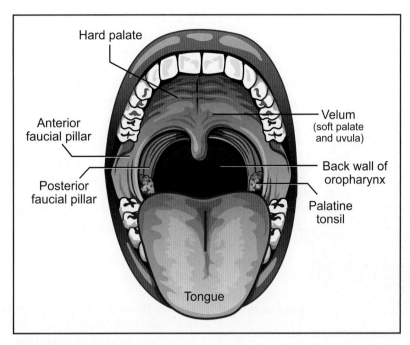

FIGURE 4–5. The oropharynx as seen from the front. The oropharynx is best viewed when instructed to "open your mouth wide and say 'ah.'" The opening between the velum and the tongue (*top to bottom*) and between the anterior and posterior faucial pillars (*side to side*) is called the faucial isthmus.

down from the back of the roof of the oral cavity, as illustrated in Figures 4–3 (back view), 4–4 (side view), and 4–5 (front view). A broad sheet of connective tissue, the palatal aponeurosis, forms a fibrous skeleton for the velum.

Patterns of muscle fiber distribution differ along the length of the velum (Kuehn & Moon, 2005). These include (a) a front portion that is void of muscle fibers, (b) a middle one-third that is rich with muscle fibers that course in various directions (including across the midline) and include insertions into the lateral margins of the structure, (c) a proportioning of muscle fibers that tapers off toward the front and back of the structure, and (d) a uvular (back) portion that is sparsely interspersed with muscle fibers. The uvula also has a richer vascular system than does the soft palate, perhaps to prevent excessive cooling of this region (Moon & Kuehn, 2004).

Nasal Cavities

The nasal cavities, also called the nasal fossae (rhymes with posse), lie behind the outer nose. They are two large chambers that run side by side and are separated from each other by the nasal septum (not often per-

fectly vertical). As shown in Figure 4–6, the nasal septum has (a) a front part composed of cartilage, (b) an upper back part that is the perpendicular plate of the ethmoid bone, and (c) a lower back part that is the vomer bone. The floor of the nasal cavities is broad and slightly concave and is formed by two sets of bones that constitute the hard palate. The palatine processes of the maxillary bones (left and right upper jaws) form the front three fourths, and the horizontal processes of the palatine bones form the back one fourth of the hard palate (this can be seen in the middle image in Figure 4–2). The roof of the nasal cavities, in contrast to the floor, is quite narrow and formed by part of the ethmoid bone called the cribriform plate. The configuration of the two cavities is similar to the roofline of an A-frame house.

By far the most complex formations within the nasal cavities are located on their lateral walls. These formations are convoluted and labyrinthine and contain many nooks and crannies. Three shell-like structures give rise to this complexity. These structures, portrayed in Figure 4–7, are the superior, middle, and inferior nasal conchae, also called the nasal turbinates. The nasal conchae extend along the length of the nasal cavities and have corresponding meatuses (passages) named for the conchae with which they are associated.

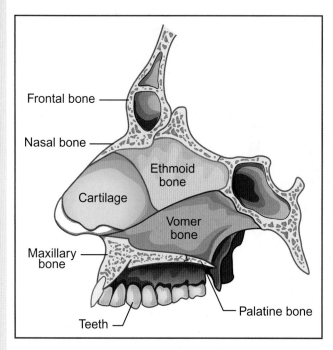

FIGURE 4–6. Components of the nasal septum (partition between the two nasal cavities). The nasal septum consists of cartilage at the front and bone (ethmoid and vomer) in the back. Selected other bones and teeth are shown for reference.

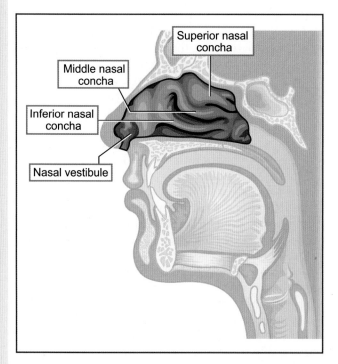

FIGURE 4–7. Superior, middle, and inferior nasal conchae (also called nasal turbinates). These conchae contain many nooks and crannies and create a large surface area to the inner nose.

The enfolding structure of the nasal cavities provides a large surface area to the inner nose and has a rich blood supply. Near the front of each nasal cavity is the nasal vestibule, a modest dilation just inside the aperture (opening) of the anterior naris.

There are four sinuses (hollows) that surround and extend from the nasal cavities. Called the paranasal sinuses, they include the maxillary, frontal, ethmoid, and sphenoid sinuses, each located within the bone of corresponding name. Three of these are shown in Figure 4–8. The sphenoid, not pictured, is located behind and above the superior nasal conchae within the sphenoid bone. They are usually air-filled but can become liquid-filled when infected.

Outer Nose

Unlike the other parts of the velopharyngeal-nasal mechanism, the outer nose is familiar to everyone. The outer nose is hard to ignore because it is in the center of the face and projects outward and downward conspicuously. The more prominent surface features of the outer nose include the root, bridge, dorsum, apex, alae, base, septum, and anterior nares, as shown in Figure 4–9.

Disposing of Things

Mucus (a slimy substance) is formed in the nose to the tune of about half a pint a day (more when you have a cold). Particles filtered by the nose are collected in a blanket of mucus and moved through the nose by the action of cilia (tiny hair cells that collectively form a fringe). Things that get trapped are moved along toward the back of the throat and then swallowed into the stomach. Some material dries before reaching the back of the throat and fractionates into pieces containing filtered particles. This happens at different spots within the nose and in residues of various consistencies. Prim and proper folks refer to these residues as nasal exudates. Most of us refer to them as "boogers." They are best gently blown into a tissue to rid them from the nose, but we all know other manual methods that are commonly practiced.

The root (point of attachment) of the outer nose is at the bottom of the forehead. Following downward along the center line are the bridge (upper bony part),

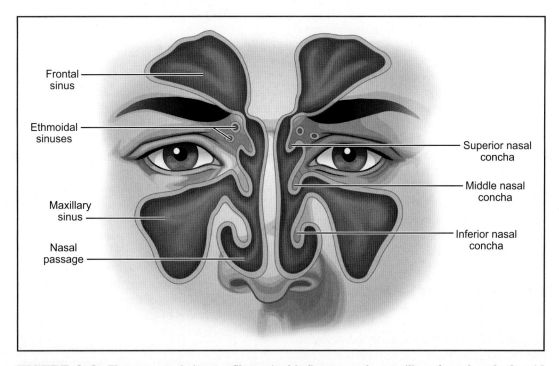

FIGURE 4-8. The paranasal sinuses. Shown in this figure are the maxillary, frontal, and ethmoid sinuses. Not shown are the paired sphenoid sinuses, which are located behind and above the superior nasal conchae.

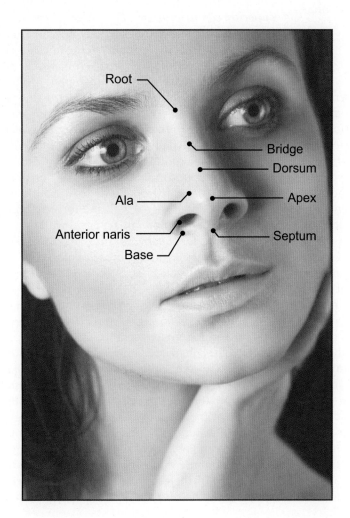

FIGURE 4-9. Surface features of the outer nose.

dorsum (prominent upper surface), and apex (tip). The alae (wings) form much of the sides of the nose and contribute significantly to its general shape. The base of the nose is partitioned down the middle (more or less) by the lowermost part of the nasal septum and includes the anterior nares (plural of naris, meaning nostrils), also called the external nares. The anterior nares are somewhat pear-shaped apertures, typically about twice as long (front to back) as they are wide (side to side). Margins of the anterior nares contain stiff hairs, called vibrissae. These hairs arrest the passage of particles riding on air currents.

FORCES OF THE VELOPHARYNGEAL-NASAL MECHANISM

Both passive and active forces operate on the velopharyngeal-nasal mechanism. Passive force is inherent and always present (although subject to change) and arises from the natural recoil of muscles, cartilages, and connective tissues, the surface tension between structures in apposition, the pull of gravity, and aeromechanical forces. Active force is applied by muscles of the pharynx, velum, and outer nose.

Muscles of the Pharynx

Figure 4–10 portrays the muscles of the pharynx and Figure 4–11 summarizes their actions. They are the *superior constrictor*, *middle constrictor*, *inferior constrictor*, *salpingopharyngeus*, *stylopharyngeus*, and *palatopharyngeus* muscles. These muscles influence the size and shape of the lumen (cavity) of the pharyngeal tube. Of course, other structures along the front side of the pharynx can also influence the lumen of the pharynx through their adjustments (velum, tongue, and epiglottis).

The *superior constrictor* muscle is located in the upper part of the pharynx. It is a complex muscle with multiple origins that arises from the front of the pharyngeal tube. Front points of attachment include the medial pterygoid plate of the sphenoid bone, the pterygomandibular ligament (a tendinous inscription between the *superior constrictor* muscle and the *buccinator* muscle, described in Chapter 5), the mylohyoid line (site of attachment of the *mylohyoid* muscle, described in Chapter 5, on the inner surface of the body of the mandible), and the side of the back part of the tongue. Fibers from the multiple origins of the *superior constrictor* muscle course backward, toward the midline, and upward to insert into the fibrous median raphe (seam) of the posterior pharyngeal wall. There, they join with fibers of the paired muscle from

the opposite side. The uppermost fibers of the *superior constrictor* muscle are horizontal and located at the level of the velum. When the *superior constrictor* muscle contracts, it reduces the regional cross section of the pharyngeal lumen by forward movement of the posterior pharyngeal wall and forward and inward movement of the lateral pharyngeal wall on the same side. The paired *superior constrictor* muscles encircle the posterior and lateral walls of the upper pharynx so that their simultaneous contraction constricts the lumen of that part of the pharyngeal tube in the manner of a sphincter.

The *middle constrictor* muscle is a fan-shaped structure located midway along the length of the pharyngeal tube. Fibers of the muscle arise from the greater and lesser horns of the hyoid bone and the stylohyoid ligament (which runs between the downward and forward projecting styloid process of the temporal bone and the lesser horn of the hyoid bone) and radiate backward and toward the midline, where they insert into the median raphe of the pharynx. The uppermost fibers of the *middle constrictor* muscle course obliquely upward and overlap the lower fibers of the *superior constrictor* muscle, whereas the lowermost fibers of the muscle run obliquely downward beneath the fibers of the *inferior constrictor* muscle. The middle fibers of the *middle constrictor* muscle run horizontally. The overlapping arrangement of the muscle fibers between the *middle constrictor* and *superior constrictor* muscles and between the *inferior constrictor* and *middle constrictor* muscles resembles the way roof shingles partially overlap. When the *middle constrictor* muscle contracts in conjunction with its paired mate on the opposite side, the cross section of the pharynx is constricted regionally by forward movement of the posterior pharyngeal wall and forward and inward movement of the lateral pharyngeal wall.

The *inferior constrictor* muscle is the most powerful of the three constrictor muscles of the pharynx. The fibers of this muscle arise from the sides of the thyroid and cricoid cartilages. The *inferior constrictor* muscle is sometimes thought of as consisting of two muscles, called the *thyropharyngeus* and *cricopharyngeus* muscles (upper and lower sections, respectively). Fibers of the *inferior constrictor* muscle diverge from their origins in a fan-like configuration and course backward and toward the midline. There, they interdigitate with fibers from the *inferior constrictor* muscle of the opposite side at the median raphe of the pharyngeal tube. The middle and upper fibers of the *inferior constrictor* muscle ascend obliquely, whereas the lowermost fibers run horizontally and downward and are continuous with those of the esophagus. When the *inferior constrictor* muscle contracts, it draws the lower part of the

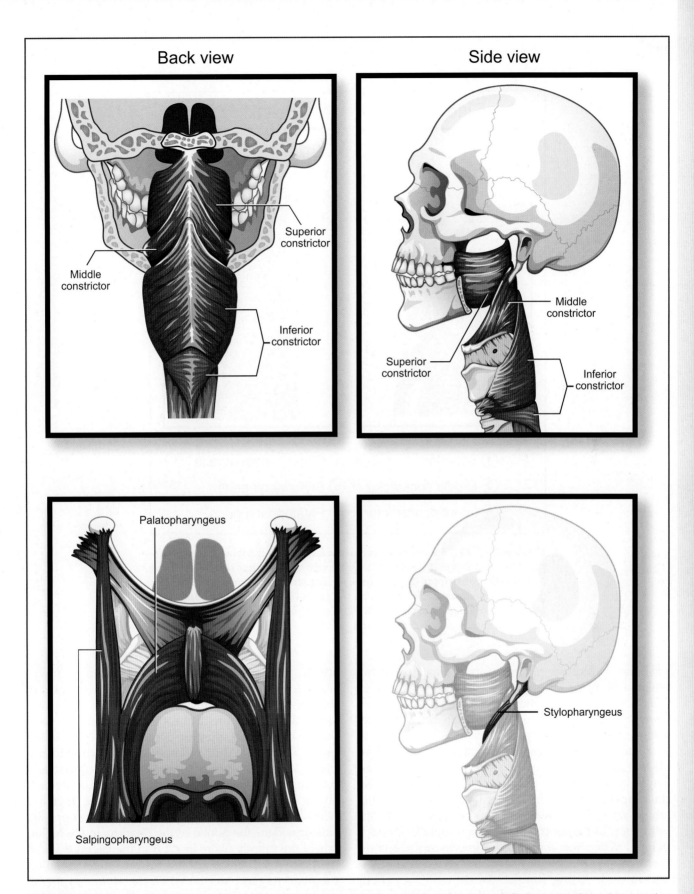

FIGURE 4–10. Muscles of the pharynx. The ***superior constrictor***, ***middle constrictor***, ***inferior constrictor*** (its superior section is called the ***thyropharyngeus*** muscle and its inferior section is called the ***cricopharyngeous*** muscle), ***salpingopharyngeus***, and ***palatopharyngeus*** muscles constrict the pharynx, whereas the ***stylopharyngeus*** muscle dilates the pharynx. Some of these muscles can also move the pharynx in other ways (see Figure 4–11).

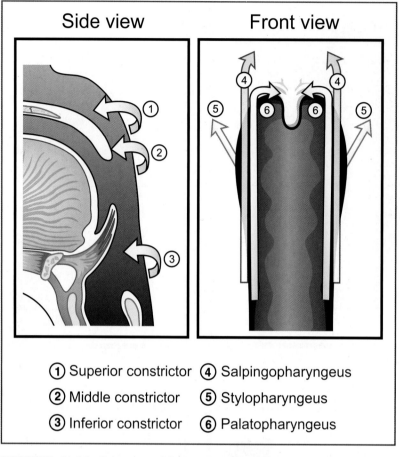

FIGURE 4–11. Summary of force vectors of the muscles of the pharynx. The muscles that constrict the pharynx are the **superior constrictor** (1), **middle constrictor** (2), and **inferior constrictor** (3) muscles. Muscles that pull both upward and inward on the pharynx are the **salpingopharyngeus** (4) and **palatopharyngeus** (6). The **stylopharyngeus** muscle (5) pulls upward and outward on the pharynx.

posterior wall of the pharynx forward and pulls the lateral walls of the lower pharynx forward and inward. This action, in conjunction with that of the *inferior constrictor* muscle on the opposite side, constricts the lumen of the lower pharynx.

The *salpingopharyngeus* muscle is a narrow muscle that arises from near the lower border of the pharyngeal orifice of the auditory tube. The fibers of the muscle course downward vertically and insert into the lateral wall of the lower pharynx, where they blend with fibers of the *palatopharyngeus* muscle (discussed below). When the *salpingopharyngeus* muscle contracts, it pulls the lateral wall of the pharynx upward and inward. Acting simultaneously with its paired muscle from the opposite side, the effect achieved is one of decreasing the width of the pharynx.

The *stylopharyngeus* muscle is a slender muscle that runs a relatively long course. It originates from the styloid process of the temporal bone and runs downward, forward, and toward the midline. Most fibers of the muscle insert into the lateral wall of the pharynx at and near the juncture of the *superior constrictor* and *middle constrictor* muscles. Some fibers extend lower in the pharyngeal wall and insert into the thyroid cartilage. When the *stylopharyngeus* muscle contracts, it pulls upward on the pharyngeal tube and draws the lateral wall of the pharynx toward the side. Together with similar action of its paired mate from the opposite side, it widens the lumen of the pharynx in the region where the muscle fibers insert into the lateral walls of the pharynx. There is also an upward pull placed on the pharynx (and larynx) when the *stylopharyngeus* muscles contract.

The *palatopharyngeus* muscle runs the length of the pharynx. It is a pharyngeal muscle as well as a muscle of the soft palate (in that context, it is called the *pharyngopalatine* muscle). The muscle is considered here from the pharyngeal perspective. The *palatopharyngeus* muscle arises mainly from the soft palate. The uppermost fibers are directed horizontally and intermingle with fibers of the *superior constrictor* muscle. A major fiber course is downward and toward the side through the posterior faucial pillar. Below the pillar, the fibers continue into the lower half of the pharynx and spread to the lateral wall of the structure and the thyroid cartilage. When the velum is relatively stable, contraction of the *palatopharyngeus* muscle results in two movements. The uppermost fibers of the muscle draw the lateral pharyngeal wall inward to complement the action of the *superior constrictor* muscle of the pharynx, whereas the lowermost fibers of the muscle pull upward on the lateral pharyngeal wall and elevate the pharynx (attachments to the thyroid cartilage also effect an upward and forward pull on the larynx).

Having It Both Ways

A muscle is usually thought of as having an origin and an insertion. The origin is its anchored end and the insertion is its movable end. This is all well and good in textbooks, but in real life, things are a bit more complicated. What may be the anchored end of a muscle for one activity may be the movable end of that muscle for another activity. A lot of it has to do with what neighboring muscles are doing. Thus, a muscle's function may change from time to time because various forces cause the mobility of its two ends to change in relation to one another. The convention adopted in this book is to reflect such change by alternately labeling a muscle in accordance with its perceived primary function in a given context. Some purists may not embrace this convention, but it carries instructive power and simply points out that in the busy world of the muscle, turnabout is fair play.

Muscles of the Velum

The muscles of the velum are shown in Figure 4–12. They are the *palatal levator, palatal tensor, uvulus, glossopalatine,* and *pharyngopalatine* muscles. These muscles influence the positioning, configuration, and mechanical status of the velum. Their force vectors are illustrated in Figure 4–13.

The *palatal levator* muscle (also called the *levator veli palatini* muscle) forms much of the bulk of the velum. The *palatal levator* is a flattened cylindrical muscle that arises from the petrous (hard) portion of the temporal bone and from the cartilaginous portion of the auditory tube. From there, it courses downward, forward, and toward the midline, passing on the outside of the posterior naris. Fibers of the *palatal levator* muscle insert into the side of the velum and spread out, where they join those of the *palatal levator* muscle from the opposite side. The spread of muscle fibers in each of the *palatal levator* muscles is to the midline and beyond to the other side of the velum (Kuehn & Moon, 2005). Fibers extend from behind the hard palate to the front of the uvula, encompassing approximately the middle 40% of the velum (Boorman & Sommerlad, 1985) or more (Kuehn & Kahane, 1990). The paired *palatal levator* muscles form a muscular sling from their cranial attachments through the velum. Each *palatal levator* muscle inserts into the velum at an angle of about 45°. When the *palatal levator* muscle contracts, it draws the velum upward and backward. Simultaneous contraction of the paired *palatal levator* muscles lifts the velum toward the posterior pharyngeal wall along an angular trajectory. The velum and the posterior pharyngeal wall come into contact frequently, sometimes with significant contact force. The upper surface of the velum can withstand such forces, in part, because of the stratified squamous epithelium that covers it. Frictional forces can also result from the sliding of the velum up and down the posterior pharyngeal wall. These are mitigated by glandular secretions of the velum that lubricate the contact areas (Kuehn & Moon, 2005).

The *palatal tensor* muscle (also known as the *tensor veli palatini* muscle) lies on the outer side of the *palatal levator* muscle. It arises from the pterygoid and scapular fossae and angular spine of the sphenoid bone as well as the cartilaginous portion of the auditory tube. From there, fibers course vertically downward to terminate in a tendon and insert into the hook-shaped hamulus of the medial pterygoid plate of the sphenoid bone. The tendon of the *palatal tensor* muscle (along with a sparse number of *palatal tensor* muscle fibers) courses inward and inserts into the hard palate and the velum (Barsoumian, Kuehn, Moon, & Canady, 1998). The *palatal tensor* muscle plays an important role in dilating the auditory (eustachian) tube, possibly in conjunction with other velopharyngeal muscles (Okada et al., 2018). Earlier conceptions of the function of the *palatal tensor* muscle also suggested that its contraction would tense the velum, because it was thought that the muscle itself wrapped around the hamulus to contribute to the horizontal portion of the structure. However,

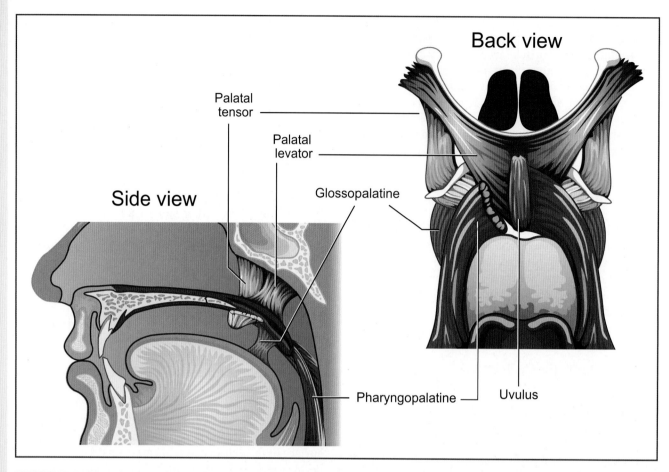

FIGURE 4–12. Muscles of the velum. They are the **palatal levator, palatal tensor, uvulus, glossopalatine,** and **pharyngopalatine** muscles. Most of these muscles act primarily to move the velum upward and backward and downward and forward. Their individual actions are shown schematically in Figure 4–13.

the fact that the *palatal tensor* muscle is now known to insert on the hamulus, with only a few fibers continuing on to insert into the velum, indicates that it does not have the mechanical means to tense the velum to any significant degree. In contrast, the tendon does seem to play an important mechanical role. The prominent size of this tendon suggests that it may relieve stress at the junction between the hard and soft palates, stress induced by frequent up-and-down movements of the velum. The stress-relief function can be thought of as analogous to a reinforced collar at the junction between an electrical plug and the wire extending from it (Kuehn, 1990).

The *uvulus* muscle is the only intrinsic muscle of the velum (both ends of its fibers are within the velum). Fibers of the *uvulus* muscle originate to the side of the posterior nasal spine formed by the palatine bones and behind the hard palate near the sling formed by the *palatal levator* muscles and about a fourth of the way along the length of the soft palate from the front. The

muscle courses downward and backward, extending through much of the length of the soft palate. Very few fibers of the *uvulus* muscle actually enter the uvula proper, from which the muscle historically derived its name (Azzam & Kuehn, 1977; Huang, Lee, & Rajendran, 1997). This has prompted some to argue (and seemingly rightfully so) that the designation of this muscle as the *uvulus* muscle is both a misnomer and anatomically misleading (Moon & Kuehn, 2004). When the *uvulus* muscle contracts, it has several effects that can be realized alone or in combination. These include that it (a) shortens the velum, (b) lifts the velum, and (c) increases the thickness (bulk) of the velum in the third quadrant of its length.

The *glossopalatine* muscle is both a muscle of the tongue (called the *palatoglossus* muscle in that context) and a muscle of the velum; it is discussed here as a muscle of the velum. Fibers of the *glossopalatine* muscle arise from the side of the tongue where they are closely blended with longitudinal fibers of the dor-

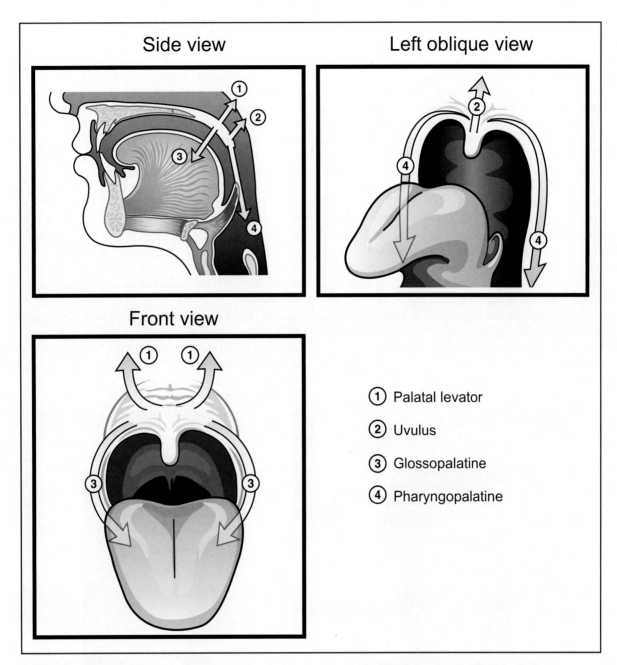

FIGURE 4–13. Summary of force vectors of the muscles of the velum. The ***palatal levator*** muscle (1) pulls the velum upward and backward. The ***uvulus*** muscle (2) shortens, lifts, and increases the thickness of the velum. The ***glossopalatine*** muscle (3) pulls the velum downward and forward and the ***pharyngopalatine*** muscle (4) pulls the velum downward and backward. The ***palatal tensor*** muscle is not included in this figure because it is not thought to have a significant effect on the velum.

sum of the tongue. They course upward and inward, forming the substance of the anterior faucial pillar, and insert into the lower surface of the palatal aponeurosis. The location of attachment to the soft palate is reported to vary across individuals, with some having insertions forward near the hard palate and others having insertions rearward near the uvula (Kuehn & Azzam, 1978). When the dorsum of the tongue is relatively fixed, contraction of the *glossopalatine* muscle places a downward and forward pull on the velum. Although the *glossopalatine* muscle has force potential on the velum, that potential is limited in comparison to the force potential of the *pharyngopalatine* muscle (Moon & Kuehn, 2004).

The *pharyngopalatine* muscle (discussed above as the *palatopharyngeus* muscle in the context of the pharynx) is considered here in the context of the velum. Its fibers arise from the lower half of the lateral wall of the pharynx and thyroid cartilage and course upward and toward the midline, where they pass through the posterior faucial pillar and insert into the soft palate (also the *superior constrictor* muscle). Its fibers do not approach or cross the midline of the soft palate but insert more laterally within the structure (Kuehn & Kahane, 1990). One notion of mechanical prominence is that there is a downward directed sling formed by the *pharyngopalatine* muscles that is antagonistic to the upward directed sling provided by the *palatal levator* muscles (Fritzell, 1969), although this has been questioned on anatomical grounds. When the pharyngeal attachment of the *pharyngopalatine* muscle is relatively fixed, contraction of its fibers (especially those that are vertically oriented) places a downward and backward pull on the velum. The action suggested here is founded on assumed muscle vector pulls inferred from anatomical observations. This approach may or may not be wholly correct.

Muscles of the Outer Nose

All of the muscles of the outer nose can be used for facial expression to convey meaning. For the purposes of this chapter, however, interest in these muscles is in their potential to influence velopharyngeal-nasal function. Five muscles of the outer nose, shown in Figure 4–14, have this potential.

The *levator labii superioris alaeque nasi* muscle (the muscle with the longest name of any muscle in animals) is a thin structure located at the side of the outer nose between the orbit of the eye and the upper lip. Its origin is from the frontal process and infraorbital margin of the maxilla. From there, the muscle courses downward and toward the side, subdividing into two muscular slips. One slip inserts into the upper lip (blending with the *orbicularis oris* muscle, described in Chapter 5) and the other slip (of more interest here) inserts into the cartilage of the nasal ala (wing at the side of the nose). Contraction of this latter muscular slip draws the ala upward on the same side of the outer nose (like lifting a side flap on a tent) and enlarges the corresponding anterior naris.

The *anterior nasal dilator* muscle is a small muscle positioned on the lower lateral surface of the

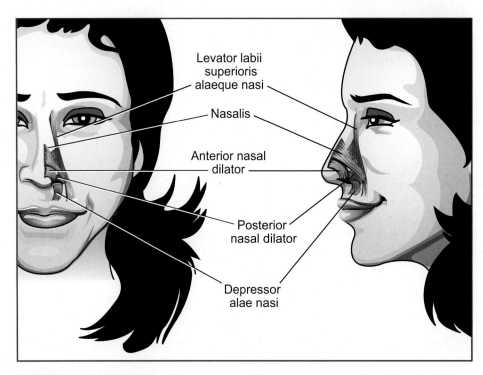

FIGURE 4–14. Muscles of the outer nose. Three muscles can dilate the nares (*levator labii superioris alaeque nasi*, *anterior nasal dilator*, and *posterior nasal dilator* muscles) and two can constrict the nares (*nasalis* and *depressor alae nasi* muscles) when activated.

outer nose. It arises from the lower edge of the lateral nasal cartilage and runs downward and outward. Following a short course, it inserts into the deep surface of the skin near the outer margin of the naris on the same side. Contraction of the *anterior nasal dilator* muscle enlarges the anterior naris on that side of the outer nose.

The *posterior nasal dilator* muscle is a small muscle located on the lower lateral surface of the outer nose. It lies behind the *anterior nasal dilator* muscle. Fibers of the *posterior nasal dilator* muscle originate from the nasal notch of the maxilla and adjacent cartilages of the outer nose. From this origin, they follow a short course and insert into the skin near the lower part of the alar cartilage along the outer margin of the naris on the same side. Contraction of the *posterior nasal dilator* muscle enlarges the corresponding anterior naris.

The *nasalis* muscle is located on the side of the outer nose. It originates from the maxilla, above and lateral to the incisive fossa (a depression in the maxilla above the incisor teeth). Fibers run upward and toward the midline and insert into an aponeurosis that is continuous with its paired muscle from the opposite side. When the *nasalis* muscle contracts, it draws down the cartilaginous part of the outer nose on the same side (like pulling down a side flap on a tent) and decreases the aperture of the corresponding anterior naris. Strong contraction of this muscle and its counterpart from the opposite side may bring the two alae of the outer nose together or compress them against one another.

The *depressor alae nasi* muscle is a short muscle that originates from the incisive fossa of the maxilla and radiates upward to insert into the back part of the ala and the cartilaginous septum of the outer nose. When the *depressor alae nasi* muscle contracts, it draws the ala of the outer nose downward on the side of action and decreases the aperture of the corresponding naris.

MOVEMENTS OF THE VELOPHARYNGEAL-NASAL MECHANISM

The velopharyngeal-nasal mechanism comprises several moveable parts. Movements of the pharynx, velum, and outer nose are considered here.

Movements of the Pharynx

The pharynx is a highly mobile tube. As illustrated in Figure 4–15, this mobility is vested in structures of the pharynx itself and in structures that comprise its lower and front boundaries. These movement capabilities are

(a) lengthening and shortening through downward and upward movements of the larynx, (b) inward and outward movements of the lateral pharyngeal walls, (c) forward and backward movements of the posterior pharyngeal wall, and (d) forward and backward movements of velum, tongue, and epiglottis. These movements, which dilate or constrict the pharynx at multiple sites, can change the size and shape of its internal cavity. In fact, one part of the pharynx may be constricted, another part dilated, and yet another part alternately constricted and dilated during the performance of a given activity. These size and shape changes can have a profound influence on the acoustic signal during speaking. They are also critical to certain phases of the swallowing process.

Sonar in a Teacup

Early study of lateral pharyngeal wall movement was problematic because x-ray techniques of the day did not provide good frontal views of the pharynx. Two speech scientists and a medical physicist from the University of Wisconsin provided the first clean data on lateral pharyngeal wall movement through the use of pulsed ultrasound. This technique sounded the depth of a point on the pharyngeal wall (like tracking a submarine). To learn the technique, they attended a short course on obstetrics where the uses of ultrasound were being taught as a pioneering means for scanning the abdomen of pregnant women. The first monitoring of lateral pharyngeal wall movement during speech production was done at that short course on an individual immersed (except for the face) in a water-filled gunner's turret of a bomber (envision an enormous teacup). Gels were only just starting to be used to transmit ultrasound into the body for medical purposes. Cheers to some of our best speech science pioneers (Kelsey, Ewanowski, Hixon, & Minifie, 1968)!

Movements of the Velum

The velum is a fleshy flap that is largely muscular. Most of the time, it hangs pendulously in the oropharyngeal space, but for many activities, it moves substantially. Movements of the velum are mainly along an upward-backward or downward-forward path, in which those in one direction closely trace those in the other. The

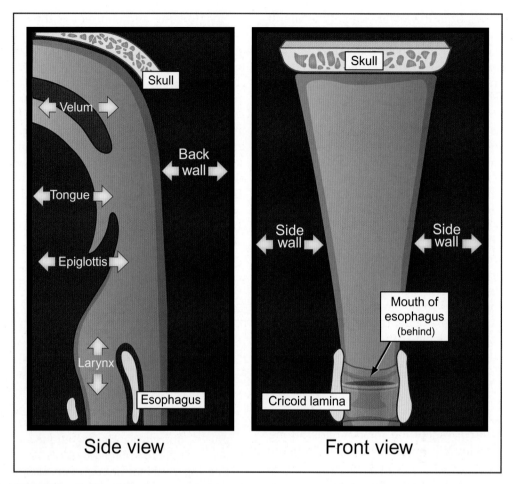

FIGURE 4–15. Movements of the pharynx. These movements can be downward and upward, inward and outward, and forward and backward and can lengthen, shorten, widen, and constrict the pharyngeal tube. Some of these movements are carried out by parts of the pharynx and others are carried out by nearby structures (velum, tongue, epiglottis, and larynx).

angular trajectory is reported to be slightly curvilinear (Kent, Carney, & Severeid, 1974) or linear (Kuehn, 1976). Maximum upward movement of the velum places its upper surface within the nasopharynx (above the boundary specified by convention to separate the oropharynx and nasopharynx).

The velum is a flap and in some ways resembles a trapdoor, but it does not move like a trapdoor (as if were swinging from a hinge). Rather, as depicted in Figure 4–16, the shape of the velum changes when it moves. The farther up and back it moves, the more hooked its appearance (as viewed from the side), and the farther down and forward it moves, the more pendulous its appearance (as viewed from the side). This is because the major lifting force that pulls the velum upward (by activation of the *palatal levator* muscles) is applied toward the middle of the velum. The hooked

appearance of the velum results in identifiable landmarks during movement. The top of the hook (on the upper surface of the velum) is referred to as the velar eminence (also called the velar knee) and the undersurface of the hook (on the lower surface of the velum) is designated as the dimple of the velum.

Movements of the Outer Nose

Movements of the outer nose result mainly from outward or inward movements of the nasal alae that may change the cross sections of the apertures of the anterior nares (nostrils). Under most circumstances, these movements are small. Exceptions occur when signaling emotions (disdain, contempt, and anger) and during certain breathing activities.

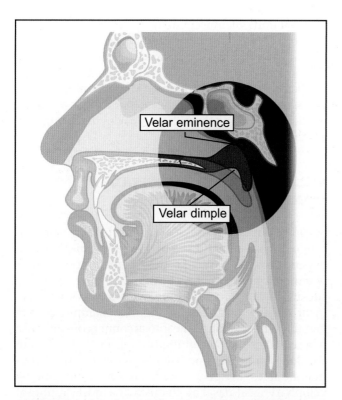

FIGURE 4-16. Elevated configuration of the velum as viewed from the side. Note its hooked appearance. The upper surface of the hook is called the velar eminence (or velar knee) and the undersurface of the hook is called the velar dimple.

The anterior nares are relatively open most of the time to accommodate nasal breathing. The nares can be dilated or constricted through the actions of muscles of the outer nose and opposed or supplemented by aeromechanical forces. For example, muscles that dilate the anterior nares may activate to resist the tendency of the nares to collapse in response to low air pressures created by high airflows moving through them. (Try this: sniff briskly while watching your outer nose in a mirror. Your nares and alae will be sucked inward by the low nasal air pressure, unless you resist with your nasal muscles.)

Although not a typical pattern, there are times when the anterior nares constrict during expiration as a means of slowing airflow through the nose. An exaggerated version of such constriction is often observed in individuals with velopharyngeal incompetence (those whose velopharynx cannot close) during speech production. Referred to clinically as "nares constriction," this is often taken as a cardinal sign of velopharyngeal dysfunction and is thought to represent an attempt to valve the airstream to compensate for an inability to valve it at the velopharynx (Warren, Hairfield, & Hinton, 1985).

Movements That Change the Size of the Velopharyngeal Port

The size of the velopharyngeal port changes when performing different activities, thereby changing the degree of coupling between the oral and nasal cavities. The port can range from wide open, such as during nasal breathing, to fully closed, such as during swallowing. Velopharyngeal closure is accomplished primarily through actions of the velum, often with participation of the pharynx. This closure pattern can be described as a flap-sphincter action, the flap being upward and backward movement of the velum and the sphincter being inward movement of the pharynx.

There is no universal pattern for achieving velopharyngeal closure. On the contrary, several movement strategies for achieving closure of the velopharyngeal port have been identified and involve actions or combinations of actions of the velum, lateral pharyngeal walls, and posterior pharyngeal wall (Croft, Shprintzen, & Rakoff, 1981; Finkelstein et al., 1995; Poppelreuter, Engelke, & Bruns, 2000; Shprintzen, 1992; Skolnik, McCall, & Barnes, 1973). These movement strategies include (a) elevation of the velum alone, (b) inward movement of the lateral pharyngeal walls with little to no participation of the velum, (c) elevation of the velum combined with inward movement of the lateral pharyngeal walls, and (d) elevation of the velum combined with inward movement of the lateral pharyngeal walls and forward movement of the posterior pharyngeal wall. The prevailing wisdom is that different movement strategies for achieving velopharyngeal closure are rooted in differences in anatomy (Finkelstein et al., 1995; Schleif et al., 2020). For example, individuals with smaller front-to-back than side-to-side dimensions of the resting velopharyngeal port may be more likely to use elevation of the velum alone as the strategy for achieving closure. In contrast, those with more equal front-to-back and side-to-side dimensions to the velopharyngeal port may be more likely to incorporate inward movement of the lateral walls of the pharynx in their closure pattern. It should be noted that velopharyngeal closure patterns are not necessarily fixed within an individual but can change over time, such as during development. Figure 4–17 illustrates a typical pattern of velopharyngeal closure in a normal individual (Croft et al., 1981). For a demonstration of various closure patterns, see Video 4–1 (Velopharyngeal Closure).

The positioning of the velum for velopharyngeal closure is most often attributed to action of the *palatal levator* muscles (Dickson, 1972). Thought typically has been that lifting of the velum follows from the contractile force provided by the *palatal levator* muscles and

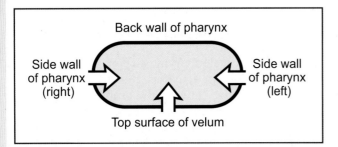

FIGURE 4-17. A typical pattern of velopharyngeal closure as seen from above. In this pattern, the velum elevates and the lateral pharyngeal walls move inward. Several other closure patterns are possible.

accounts for the fact that the midportion of the velum usually attains the highest elevation during closure of the velopharyngeal port (see Figure 4–16) (Bell-Berti, 1976; Fritzell, 1963; Lubker, 1968; Seaver & Kuehn, 1980). Although action of the *palatal levator* muscles seems to be clearly associated with the flap component of the flap-sphincter closure adjustment, correlations between *palatal levator* muscle activity and the elevation of the velum are weaker (albeit positive) than would be expected were the *palatal levator* muscles alone responsible for positioning the velum (Fritzell, 1979; Lubker, 1968). This suggests that other muscles must also be active in positioning the velum. Research, in fact, supports this inference. For example, different

Where's the Rest?

Many studies have examined the correlation between velopharyngeal incompetence and articulation skill in children with repaired cleft palates. The highest correlation found in these studies is 0.5. Square that number and you find that velopharyngeal incompetence predicts only 25% of the variance in articulation skill. Where's the rest? Some have suggested it's to be found in "learning." We believe 75% is far too much to be attributed to such a notion. Rather, we suspect that the rest is confounded by the fact that the children studied were never categorized with regard to the magnitude of their nasal airway resistance. Not knowing or controlling for this factor would have an important influence on the strength of the correlation obtained between velopharyngeal incompetence and articulation skill. Where's the rest of the variance of interest? We think it's probably in the nose and has been overlooked.

combinations of muscle activity among the *palatal levator*, *glossopalatine*, and *pharyngopalatine* muscles have been found to be associated with the same positioning of the velum (Kuehn, Folkins, & Cutting, 1982). This and other evidence (Moon, Smith, Folkins, Lemke, & Gartlan, 1994) suggest that there is a trading relationship among these three muscles that contribute to movements of the velum.

VELOPHARYNGEAL-NASAL CONTROL VARIABLES

Several control variables are important in velopharyngeal-nasal function. Their relative significance depends on the particular activity being performed, whether it is breathing, speaking, singing, blowing, sucking, swallowing, gagging, whistling, wind instrument playing, or glass blowing. For example, control variables for speaking take into account acoustic goals, whereas those for breathing do not. In contrast, both speaking and breathing involve aeromechanical control variables. For people with a normally functioning velopharyngeal-nasal mechanism, the most significant features of control pertain to its velopharyngeal component. There are times, however, when control of the nasal portion can become important.

Attention is devoted to three control variables that influence aeromechanical and acoustic aspects of velopharyngeal-nasal function. These are (a) the magnitude of the airway resistance offered by the velopharyngeal-nasal mechanism, (b) the magnitude of the muscular pressure exerted by the velopharyngeal sphincter to accomplish and maintain velopharyngeal closure, and (c) the magnitude of the acoustic impedance offered by the velopharyngeal-nasal mechanism.

Velopharyngeal-Nasal Airway Resistance

Resistance is defined, in a mechanical sense, as opposition to movement that results in a loss of energy through friction (similar to that of direct current in an electrical circuit). Velopharyngeal-nasal airway resistance is the opposition to the mass flow of air (the breath) through structures of the velopharyngeal-nasal airway. This is analogous to the resistance to airflow through the larynx discussed in Chapter 3.

Adjustments of the velopharyngeal port, nasal cavities, and/or outer nose can change airway resistance between the oral cavity and atmosphere through the nasal route, as portrayed in Figure 4–18. Specifically, an increase in velopharyngeal-nasal airway resis-

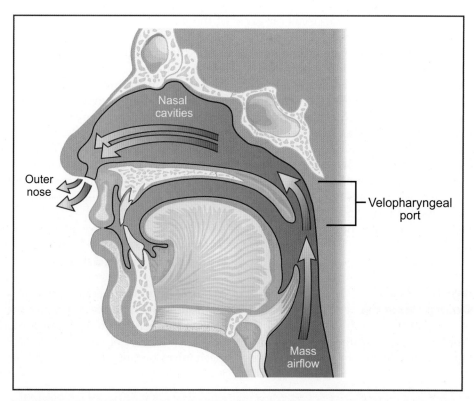

FIGURE 4–18. Velopharyngeal-nasal airway resistance. The resistance of the velopharyngeal-nasal apparatus to air flowing through it can be altered by adjustments of the velopharyngeal port, the nasal cavities, and the outer nose. Changes in the rate at which air flows through the airways can also alter the resistance.

tance may occur with a decrease in cross-sectional area and/or an increase in length of the velopharyngeal port, engorgement of the nasal cavities, or a decrease in cross-sectional area of the anterior nares. Airflow also alters the resistance because resistance is airflow dependent. That is, resistance increases with increases in airflow, even when the physical dimensions of the velopharyngeal-nasal airway remain unchanged.

The Flap Flap

Pharyngeal flaps are secondary surgical procedures usually performed on persons with repaired cleft palates who persist with velopharyngeal incompetence or insufficiency following primary surgery. Flaps are constructed using tissue from the posterior pharyngeal wall (peeled away like the skin on a banana) and attaching it to the velum to form a bridge. Flaps have also been used in children with cerebral palsy who have paresis (weakness) of the velum. They have been found to improve speech in such children, but they also have been found to have a major negative side effect. They may raise the resistance to breathing through the nose and cause some children to switch from nose breathing to mouth breathing. Mouth breathing opens the door (pun intended) to drooling. The negative social consequences of drooling are often judged to outweigh the positive social consequences of improved speech. Thus, flaps have sometimes had to be removed.

Velopharyngeal-nasal airway resistance can range from very low, such as during resting tidal breathing with patent nasal cavities (following administration of a nasal decongestant), to infinite (completely obstructed). Infinite airway resistance is usually caused by airtight closure of the velopharyngeal port. Once airtight velopharyngeal closure is attained, adjustments of the nasal cavities and outer nose have no further influence on the resistance value. Infinite velopharyngeal-nasal airway resistance can also be achieved in the case of an open velopharynx under circumstances where there is complete nasal blockage. This is an example of why it is critical to include the nasal component in this subsystem rather than focus exclusively on the velopharyngeal component.

Velopharyngeal-Nasal Sphincter Compression

Once airtight velopharyngeal closure is attained, the force of that closure can be adjusted to meet the needs of the situation. This force, depicted in Figure 4–19, is represented by the compressive muscular pressure exerted to keep the velopharyngeal sphincter closed. The muscular pressure exerted at any moment must exceed the magnitude of the air pressure difference across the velopharyngeal sphincter (whether it be positive or negative) to prevent the velopharynx from being forced (blown or sucked) open. Thus, only a low compressive force is required to maintain airtight velopharyngeal closure for an activity involving low oral air pressure, whereas a high compressive force is required for an activity involving high positive oral air pressure.

Velopharyngeal-Nasal Acoustic Impedance

Acoustic (sound) impedance, like airway resistance, is opposition to flow. However, it is opposition to the flow of sound rather than to mass airflow. Thus, the acoustic impedance offered by the velopharyngeal-nasal mechanism pertains to the rapid to-and-fro bumping

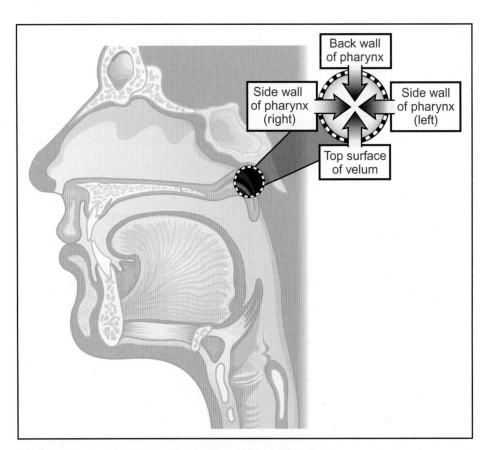

FIGURE 4–19. Compressive muscular pressure during velopharyngeal closure. The greater the air pressure difference across the velopharynx, the higher the compressive pressure needed to maintain velopharyngeal closure.

Some Things Are Not Quite What They Seem

There seems to be a relatively large number of musicians who complain of "air leaks out the nose" during wind instrument playing. Such complaints are red flags for what might be stress-induced velopharyngeal incompetence, a condition that may require medical intervention such as augmentation of the posterior pharyngeal wall. Sometimes physical measurements confirm that, in fact, the velopharynx is open during sound production. But sometimes physical measurements show that, surprisingly, the velopharynx is closed during sound production, despite what the musician is feeling. Why the mismatch? A study of trombonists may have found the answer. By sensing changes in air pressure at the anterior nares, a graduate student and her mentor (Bennett & Hoit, 2013) discovered that some trombonists open the velopharynx at the beginning of expiration before the sound begins and then close the velopharynx right as the sound starts. What they felt was correct—the velopharynx was open. But it was not open while they were actually playing. Sometimes the senses play tricks on us.

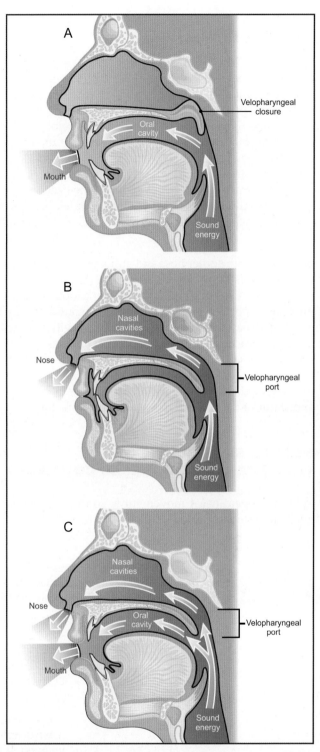

FIGURE 4–20. Oral-nasal sound wave propagation through the velopharyngeal-nasal pathway (velopharynx, nasal cavities, and outer nose) and/or oral pathway (oral cavity and mouth). The conditions shown are (A) the velopharynx closed with sound routed through the oral pathway, (B) the oral pathway closed with sound routed through the velopharyngeal-nasal pathway, and (C) both pathways open so that sound is routed through both simultaneously.

of air molecules in which each molecule stays in a very restricted region and passes energy on to its neighbors. The opposition to acoustic flow is frequency dependent (similar to that of an alternating current in an electrical circuit). Acoustic impedance influences flow propagation of sound waves (not breath).

As portrayed in Figure 4–20, the velopharyngeal port can be adjusted to influence the degree of coupling between the oral and nasal cavities and thereby change the velopharyngeal-nasal acoustic impedance. The greater proportion of sound energy will be directed through the airway (oral or nasal) having the lower acoustic impedance. When the port is closed (see Figure 4–20A), the oral and nasal airways are separated and nearly all of the sound energy passes through the oral airway and mouth. In this case, the acoustic impedance looking into the nasal cavities from their velopharyngeal end is nearly infinite, although a small amount of sound energy may be transmitted through the closed velopharynx via sympathetic vibration (with the velum acting like a drumhead). When the velopharyngeal port is open (see Figures 4–20B and 4–20C), the oral and nasal cavities are free to exchange sound energy and interact with one another acoustically, and sound energy may

Which Hunt

It is often stated that velopharyngeal incompetence or insufficiency allows air to pass into the nasal cavities, thereby causing hypernasality. This is a misconception. Significant quantities of air can pass into the nasal cavities through the velopharynx during utterance production without there being a perception of hypernasality. Also, hypernasality may be heard when no air is passing into the nasal cavities, such as when the tissue covering a submucous cleft palate vibrates and excites the nasal cavities into sympathetic vibration. Flow of air into the nose does not cause hypernasality. In fact, hypernasality may be present when speech is produced on inspiration and airflow is passing through the nasal cavities in the opposite direction from usual. It's instructive to go through written discussions about velopharyngeal dysfunction and see which authors get it right and which authors get it wrong. Think of it as sort of a "which" hunt.

pass between the outer nose and atmosphere. A demonstration of this is provided in Video 4–2 (VP-N Acoustic Impedance). Changes in the size of the velopharyngeal port are important to determining how sound energy is divided between the oral and nasal cavities. Also important are configurations of the oral and nasal cavities themselves and the extent to which each impedes the flow of sound energy. In the case of the nasal part of the system, degree of engorgement of the nasal cavities and status of the anterior nares are relevant factors.

NEURAL SUBSTRATES OF VELOPHARYNGEAL-NASAL CONTROL

Velopharyngeal-nasal movement is controlled by the nervous system. Although different parts of the central nervous system are responsible for that control, depending on the nature of the activity, all control commands are sent to velopharyngeal-nasal muscles through the same set of cranial nerves. These nerves originate in the brainstem and course outward to provide motor innervation to the pharynx, velum, and outer nose.

As shown in Table 4–1, motor innervation of the pharynx and velum comes from the pharyngeal plexus, a network that includes fibers from cranial nerves IX (glossopharyngeal), X (vagus), and possibly XI (accessory). An exception is found in the case of the *palatal tensor* muscle, whose motor innervation is provided by cranial nerve V (trigeminal). There may also be additional motor innervation to the pharynx and velum through cranial nerve VII (facial), especially related to the *palatal levator* and *uvulus* muscles. Motor innervation to the outer nose is provided by cranial nerve VII.

TABLE 4–1. Summary of the Motor and Sensory Nerve Supply to the Pharynx, Velum, and Outer Nose Components of the Velopharyngeal-Nasal Mechanism

	INNERVATION	
COMPONENT	**MOTOR**	**SENSORY**
Pharynx[a]	IX, X, (XI)[b]	V, VII, IX, X
Velum[a]	IX, X, (XI) (except **palatal tensor** muscle, which is innervated by V)	V, VII, IX, X
Outer Nose	VII	V

Note. Cranial nerves include V (trigeminal), VII (facial), IX (glossopharyngeal), X (vagus), and possibly XI (accessory).

[a]There may be additional motor innervation from cranial nerve VII to certain muscles of the pharynx and velum, especially the **palatal levator** muscle and **uvulus** muscle (Shimokawa, Yi, & Tanaka, 2005).

[b]The branches of cranial nerves IX and X (and possibly XI) that innervate parts of the velopharynx are sometimes called the pharyngeal plexus.

One might think that information about the motor nerve supply to different parts of the velopharyngeal-nasal apparatus would be straightforward and agreed upon. This is, indeed, the case for motor innervation to the outer nose but not for motor innervation to the pharynx and velum. This is because the linkage between specific cranial nerves and the motor supply to specific muscles is equivocal in some cases (Cassell & Ekaldi, 1995; Dickson, 1972; Moon & Kuehn, 2004) and because conducting research on motor nerve function in the velopharyngeal-nasal region of human beings is extremely difficult (Perry, 2011).

Sensory innervation to the pharynx and velum comes from cranial nerves V, VII, IX, and X, and sensory innervation to the outer nose is provided by cranial nerve V. Neural information traveling along the sensory nerve supply from the pharynx, velum, and outer nose comes from receptors that respond to various types of stimuli, including mechanical stimuli. For example, receptors located in the mucosa of the velum and pharynx respond to light touch, and receptors located in and near the velopharyngeal-nasal muscles relay information about muscle length and tension.

Much of the incoming information from the velopharyngeal portion of the velopharyngeal-nasal apparatus is not sensed or perceived. The potential for sensing the position of the velum in space (proprioception) and its movement (kinesthesia) is believed to be rudimentary or nonexistent. Empirical evidence for this can be found in studies in which normal speakers have been shown to have difficulty controlling velopharyngeal movements voluntarily (Ruscello, 1982; Shelton, Beaumont, Trier, & Furr, 1978). Thus, it seems likely that control of the velopharyngeal apparatus relies more heavily on other types of information, such as that associated with the sensing of air pressure and airflow (Liss, Kuehn, & Hinkle, 1994; Warren, Dalston, & Dalston, 1990) and that associated with the sensing of the acoustic signal (Netsell, 1990) via cranial nerve VIII (auditory-vestibular).

VELOPHARYNGEAL-NASAL FUNCTION AND VENTILATION

Recall from Chapter 2 that ventilation is the movement of air in and out of the pulmonary system for the purpose of gas exchange. This movement of air can be routed through the nose, the mouth, or both.

Resting tidal breathing usually occurs through the nose alone. This may seem somewhat counterintuitive, given that the airway resistance through the nasal pathway is much greater than through the oral pathway. Nevertheless, the nasal route typically prevails.

This is because it provides advantages for both inspiration and expiration. Advantages of nasal inspiration are that it converts the temperature of incoming air to that of the body, increases the humidity of incoming air, and filters dust, bacteria, and other contaminants from the incoming air before they reach the lungs and lower airways. An advantage of nasal expiration is that it helps slow the flow of expired air to ensure adequate alveolar gas exchange (Hairfield, Warren, Hinton, & Seaton, 1987) by providing an additional braking mechanism (Jackson, 1976) to accompany the laryngeal braking mechanism that also serves to slow expiration (Gautier, Remmers, & Bartlett, 1973).

Although nasal breathing is the norm, there are times when it becomes necessary to switch to mouth breathing (or combined mouth and nose breathing) to maintain adequate ventilation. This occurs when the nasal pathway resistance becomes too high due to high air flow, nasal pathway constriction, or both. Interestingly, the magnitude of resistance that leads to switching from solely nasal breathing to nasal-oral breathing turns out to be slightly lower than the resistance value that leads to the sensation of breathing discomfort (Warren, Hairfield, Seaton, Morr, & Smith, 1988; Warren, Mayo, Zajac, & Rochet, 1996). This means that the switch from nasal breathing to oral-nasal breathing occurs before any awareness of breathing difficulty.

VELOPHARYNGEAL FUNCTION AND SPEECH PRODUCTION

The velopharyngeal-nasal mechanism has two important roles during speech production. One is to manage the airstream to produce certain types of oral consonant sounds (especially those that require high oral pressure). This requires that the velopharynx be closed, or nearly closed, so that aeromechanical energy be directed through the oral channel. The other role is to manage the flow of acoustic energy into the oral and nasal cavities, which is important for the production of vowels and both oral and nasal consonants. This section considers these roles in the contexts of sustained utterances and running speech activities.

Sustained Utterances

Sustained vowels and consonants are usually produced with relatively stable configurations of the velopharyngeal-nasal mechanism. Slight differences in velopharyngeal configuration have been observed across different sustained vowels, and obvious differences can be seen in sustained oral consonants when contrasted with sustained nasal consonants.

Observations of the velopharynx during sustained vowel production have shown that the velum moves upward and backward toward the posterior pharyngeal wall in anticipation of the upcoming vowel (Bzoch, 1968; Lubker, 1968; Moll, 1962). At the same time, the lateral pharyngeal walls may move inward and the posterior pharyngeal wall may move forward slightly (Iglesias, Kuehn, & Morris, 1980). The velum is usually elevated maximally in its midportion during vowel production, and contact with the posterior pharyngeal wall is typically achieved by the third quadrant of the velum (Graber, Bzoch, & Aoba, 1959). There is also a tendency for the velum to be elevated to a higher position when sustained vowels are produced at higher vocal effort levels (Tucker, 1963).

Airtight velopharyngeal closure may or may not occur during sustained vowel production. The probability of airtight closure favors high vowels (such as /i/ in peek) over low vowels (such as /ae/ in cat). For example, Moll (1962), in an x-ray motion picture study of young adults, found that some were opening the velopharyngeal port during nearly 40% of their low vowel productions but less than 15% of their high vowel productions.

Whether or not airtight velopharyngeal closure is achieved, high vowels and low vowels contrast in still other ways. Compared to low vowel production, high vowel production is associated with (a) greater velar height, (b) greater extent of velar contact with the posterior pharyngeal wall when the two surfaces are in apposition, and (c) smaller distance between the velum and the posterior pharyngeal wall when closure is not complete (Iglesias et al., 1980; Lubker, 1968; Moll, 1962). High vowel production also involves greater velopharyngeal sphincter compression (closing force) than low vowel production when velopharyngeal closure is complete (Gotto, 1977; Kuehn & Moon, 1998; Moon, Kuehn, & Huisman, 1994; Nusbaum, Foly, & Wells, 1935). Velar height differences during sustained vowel productions are relatively strongly correlated with the electrical activity of the *palatal levator* muscles (Bell-Berti, 1976; Fritzell, 1969; Lubker, 1968). Less than perfect correlations may relate to partial influences of other nearby muscles (Fritzell, 1969; Kuehn et al., 1982).

Two possible mechanisms have been proposed to account for the differences observed in velar height between high and low vowel productions. One is that the velum elevates to different degrees because of anatomical constraints imposed through interconnections to structures below it (Harrington, 1944; Kaltenborn, 1948; Lubker, 1968; Moll, 1962). Likely candidates include the *glossopalatine* and *pharyngopalatine* muscles that have originating attachments from below the velum. The *glossopalatine* muscle is considered the more important of the two candidates. The hypothesis is that the *glossopalatine* muscle tethers the velum so that low vowels (involving low tongue positions) restrict elevation of the velum and lead to lesser degrees of closure of the velopharyngeal port. The influence of tethering is less for high vowels (involving high tongue positions) because less restriction is placed on velar elevation.

The second mechanism proposed to account for velar height differences between high and low vowel productions has an acoustic-perceptual basis. Specifically, it may be that the velum elevates to different degrees because of acoustic requirements involved in ensuring that the utterance is not perceived as nasal (Curtis, 1968; Lubker, 1968; Moll, 1962). This speculation is based on the results of electrical analog studies of the nasalization of vowels conducted by House and Stevens (1956) and more recently with a computational speech production model by Bunton and Story (2012). Both studies demonstrated that less nasal coupling (velopharyngeal opening) is required to produce the auditory-perceptual judgment of nasal quality on high vowels than on low vowels. Thus, the velar height differences observed for high and low vowels could be purposive adjustments to control the degree of nasalization in the face of different tongue adjustments that influence the flow of acoustic energy through the oral and nasal cavities. In effect, at any given moment, the particular shape of the oral and pharyngeal cavities (primarily due to position of the tongue) influences how the velopharynx must adjust to maintain the perception of nonnasal speech.

Sustained fricative and nasal consonant productions are produced with contrasting velopharyngeal configurations. Sustained fricatives, such as /s/ and /z/, are accompanied by airtight velopharyngeal closure in children as young as 3 years and adults of all ages (Hoit, Watson, Hixon, McMahon, & Johnson, 1994; Thompson & Hixon, 1979). Airtight closure of the velopharyngeal port is clearly a priority for speech sounds that rely on the management of the oral airstream for their production. Such closure has also been found to be accompanied by higher velar elevation and more forward displacement of the posterior pharyngeal wall compared to closure during vowel productions (Iglesias et al., 1980). This difference in velar elevation can be seen by comparing the vowel and fricative images in Figure 4–21.

Sustained nasal consonants, such as /m/ and /n/, are produced with large openings of the velopharyngeal port, as shown in the rightmost image in Figure 4–21. The position of the velum is the same (or slightly higher) for sustained /m/ and /n/ productions as it is for resting tidal breathing, and *palatal*

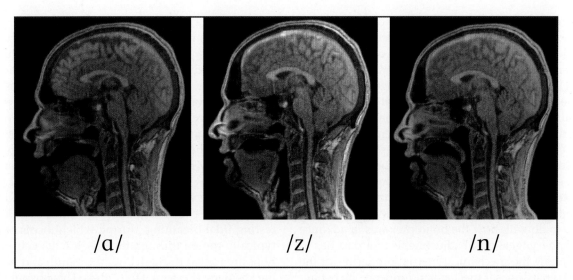

FIGURE 4-21. Sagittal magnetic resonance (MR) images showing different velar elevations associated with production of the vowel /ɑ/, the voiced fricative /z/, and the nasal consonant /n/. (Courtesy of Adam Baker)

levator muscle activity is not discernible (Iglesias et al., 1980; Lubker, 1968). Predictably, sustained nasal consonant productions are accompanied by substantial nasal airflow (Hoit et al., 1994; Thompson & Hixon, 1979).

Velopharyngeal-Nasal Function and Running Speech Activities

Running speech activities require rapid adjustments of the velopharynx. A few minutes spent watching x-ray or real-time magnetic resonance (MR) imaging recordings of running speech production reveals that velopharyngeal articulation is every bit as fast and intricate as are movements of the mandible, tongue, and lips. This can be seen in Video 4–3 (Grandfather Passage). In fact, velar elevating and lowering gestures can each occur within a time interval of about a tenth of a second (Kuehn, 1976). The precise pattern of opening and closing and the degree to which the velopharyngeal port is opened or closed relate to the nature of the speech sounds being spoken, the influence of surrounding sounds on the sound being spoken, and the rate at which they are produced (Kent et al., 1974).

When consonants and vowels are combined as they are in running speech activities, primacy of control of the velopharyngeal-nasal mechanism is vested in consonant productions. This is because the production of many consonant elements relies heavily on appropriate management of the airstream. Sacrificing the aeromechanical requirements of these consonants by opening the velopharynx may result in sacrificing

---

Playing by Her Own Rule

She was a young woman with a profound bilateral hearing loss. She had received intensive behavioral therapy for imprecise articulation, but essentially no progress was being made. A puzzled speech-language pathologist made the referral. What was preventing improvement in speech? The answer was found in a recording of nasal airflow. A large burst of airflow was found to accompany each segment of speech that included a voiceless consonant. The young woman had apparently developed a rule that said, "Only close your velopharynx for speech when your voice is on." It turned out to be a rule that could be changed by displaying nasal airflow for her to monitor on a storage oscilloscope (today, it would be displayed on a computer screen) so that she could see her rule in action and adopt a more appropriate one with some guidance. Her velopharynx cooperated and her articulation improved.

---

the intelligibility of speech. In contrast, sacrificing closure for vowel productions may increase nasalization but has only a minimal effect on speech intelligibility. The consonant elements that rely most on aeromechanical management of the airstream are often referred to as "the pressure consonants" because they are characteristically produced with high oral air pressure and a closed velopharynx. The pressure consonants include stop-plosive, fricative, and affricate speech sounds (see Chapter 5 for specific definitions). In contrast, nasal consonants are produced with a low oral air pressure and a relatively wide-open velopharyngeal port.

The control of the velopharyngeal-nasal mechanism during running speech production is not simply a sequencing of separate and independent position and movement patterns for different speech sounds. Rather, the position and movement patterns for two or more speech sounds may occur simultaneously, such that their productions actually overlap and intermingle. This is illustrated in Video 4–4 (Nasalization). Part of this has to do with how the brain prepares in advance for velopharyngeal-nasal adjustments and part has to do with how the mechanical-inertial properties of the velopharyngeal-nasal mechanism influence its behavior. More is said about these principles in Chapter 5.

Underlying the assembling of velopharyngeal-nasal positions and movements is the general principle that consonants influence the velopharyngeal-nasal adjustments of all speech sounds (consonants and vowels) within their interval of preparation. The precise influence depends on both the type of consonant and type of vowel. For example, the preparation period for oral consonants results in smaller velopharyngeal port openings (or no opening) for vowels that precede them, whereas the preparation period for nasal consonants results in larger velopharyngeal port openings for vowels that precede them (Warren & DuBois, 1964), as can be seen in Figure 4–22.

Understandably, the study of velopharyngeal-nasal function for speech production has focused on the expiratory phase of the breathing cycle, the phase of the cycle during which speech is produced. Nevertheless, the velopharyngeal-nasal mechanism also plays an important role during the inspiratory phase of the speech breathing cycle. Running speech breathing usually demands quick inspirations to minimize interruptions to the flow of speech, and quick inspirations require a low resistance pathway. The best way to create such a low resistance pathway is to abduct the lips and open the velopharynx simultaneously, and this is, in fact, what people typically do. Thus, in contrast to resting tidal breathing, during which inspirations are typically routed through the nose exclusively, inspirations are routed through both the mouth and nose during speaking (Lester & Hoit, 2014). This not only allows for quick inspirations but may also preserve some of the benefits of nasal inspirations, such as air filtration and humidification.

VARIABLES THAT INFLUENCE VELOPHARYNGEAL-NASAL STRUCTURE AND FUNCTION

There are many variables that can influence velopharyngeal-nasal function, some of which have already been mentioned. Three that are covered in this section are body position, age, and sex.

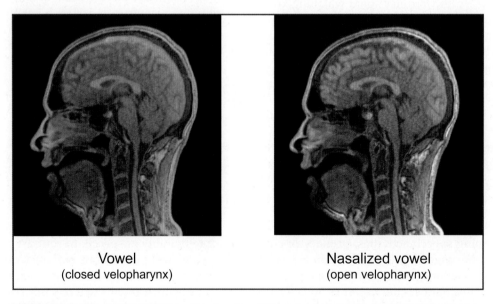

Vowel
(closed velopharynx)

Nasalized vowel
(open velopharynx)

FIGURE 4–22. Sagittal MR images showing different velar elevations for the production of a neutral vowel preceding an oral consonant (*left*) and for the same vowel preceding a nasal consonant (*right*). (Courtesy of Adam Baker)

Body Position

Velopharyngeal-nasal function changes with changes in body position, primarily because of the influence of gravity. Each time the velopharyngeal-nasal mechanism is reoriented within a gravity field, alternate mechanical solutions are required to meet the goals for adjusting the velopharyngeal port.

When in an upright position, the pull of gravity tends to lower the velum. In contrast, when in the supine body position, gravity acts to pull the velum toward the posterior pharyngeal wall (Bae, Perry, & Kuehn, 2014; Perry, 2011, Perry, Bae, & Kuehn, 2012), as shown in Figure 4–23.

Movements of the velum away from this rest position, such as those associated with speech production, require different force solutions in the two body positions. In upright, the muscle force required to elevate the velum must overcome the pull of gravity, whereas muscle force required to lower the velum is augmented by this pull. The opposite situation prevails in supine, where the muscle force to move the velum toward the posterior pharyngeal wall is augmented by the pull of gravity, and the muscle force to move the velum away from the posterior pharyngeal wall must overcome the pull of gravity. As might be expected, these different force solutions for upright and supine are accompanied by different muscle activities (Moon & Canady, 1995). Specifically, peak muscle activity for the *palatal levator* muscle (velar elevator) is lower in the supine body position compared to the upright body position, suggesting that less activation is required when the pull of gravity is in the same direction (toward the posterior pharyngeal wall). Also, the activation of the *pharyngopalatine* muscle (velar depressor) is usually greater in the supine body position where the pull of gravity is counter to movement of the velum away from the posterior pharyngeal wall.

Reorientation of the velopharyngeal-nasal apparatus in space is not restricted to changes in body position. Reorientation can also mean that the body is maintained in a fixed position and the head is moved about different axes. For example, when the head is rotated downward (toward a position where the chin would rest on the rib cage wall), gravity tends pull the velum away from the posterior pharyngeal wall. In contrast, when the head is rotated upward, gravity pulls the velum toward the posterior pharyngeal wall. Whereas head rotation may not have much effect on the velopharyngeal function in most people, it may have a profound effect on someone with weakness of the *palatal levator* muscles by enhancing movement

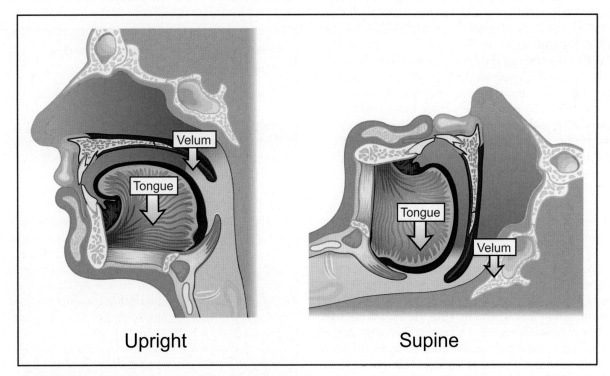

FIGURE 4–23. The velum at rest in upright and supine body positions. In upright body positions, gravity exerts a downward pull on the velum, whereas in the supine body position, gravity pulls the velum toward the posterior pharyngeal wall.

of the velum toward the posterior pharyngeal wall and, thereby, improving velopharyngeal closure for speech production.

Gravitational influences also affect the function of the nasal cavities. For example, nasal patency (openness) decreases and nasal airway resistance increases in downright as compared to upright body positions (Rudcrantz, 1969). This change in patency appears to relate to vascular changes that cause nasal congestion (Hiyama, Ono, Ishiwata, & Kuroda, 2002).

Age

The structure of the velopharyngeal-nasal mechanism changes across the life span as does its function, with the most significant changes occurring during the developmental years. Its function for speech production undergoes maturation during infancy and childhood, but once adulthood is reached, it appears that this function is maintained into senescence. Discussed here are age-related anatomical and physiological changes in the velopharyngeal-nasal mechanism; discussion of other associated upper airway structures is found in Chapter 5.

At birth, the larynx is located high within the neck and the velum and epiglottis are approximated (Kent & Murray, 1982). Around 4 to 6 months of age, the velum and epiglottis separate (Sasaki, Levine, Laitman, & Crelin, 1977) as the larynx moves from the level of the first cervical vertebra to the level of the third cervical vertebra. This downward movement is accomplished primarily by rapid growth of the pharynx in the vertical dimension from about 4 cm in the newborn pharynx (Crelin, 1973) to approximately three times that length in the adult (Sasaki et al., 1977). As children continue to grow during their first decade, so does the size of the velopharyngeal-nasal structures (Kazlin & Perry, 2016; Vorperian et al., 2009). These developmental changes affect the geometry and mechanical effectiveness of certain muscles. For example, as the palates grow, the orientation of the paired *palatal levator* muscles changes in ways that improve their mechanical advantage for elevating the velum (Fletcher, 1973).

The birth cry, the first utterance for most human newborns, is produced with an open velopharynx (Bosma, Truby, & Lind, 1965). Velopharyngeal closure for nondistress vocalizations (the vocalizations that eventually become speech) increases gradually across the first year and a half of life until it closes for such utterances around 19 months of age (Bunton & Hoit, 2018; Thom, Hoit, Hixon, & Smith, 2006). A closer look at this developmental trajectory shows that velopharyngeal closure in infants and toddlers is also condi-

tioned by the types of sounds being produced, with sounds that require high oral pressure (such as stops and fricatives) being much more likely to be produced with a closed velopharynx than those that do not require such pressure. Interestingly, other types of utterances do not seem to follow this developmental trajectory and are either closed at all ages (cries, screams, and raspberries) or open at all ages (precry windups, whimpers, and laughs). Children 3 years and older produce imitative speech with a closed velopharynx (Thompson & Hixon, 1979; Zajac, 2000), although certain temporal features of velopharyngeal function during speech production continue to be modified into the teenage years (Leeper, Tissington, & Munhall, 1998; Zajac, 2000; Zajac & Hackett, 2002).

Although speech is produced with airtight velopharyngeal closure by early childhood, the means for achieving this closure may change with development. One example relates to children who have enlarged lymphoid tissue masses in the nasopharyngeal tonsils (adenoids). These tonsils typically grow during the first decade of life and then begin to atrophy (Jaw, Sheu, Liu, & Lin, 1999; Subtelny & Koepp-Baker, 1956) until they are fully atrophied by adulthood. This is illustrated in Figure 4–24. During velopharyngeal closure, children with enlarged nasopharyngeal tonsils typically exhibit velar to adenoid contact, and those with larger adenoids show less *palatal levator* muscle con-

---

When Is a Bad Nose Good and a Good Nose Bad?

This chapter stresses the functional unity of the velopharyngeal and nasal components of the normal velopharyngeal-nasal mechanism. This unity is often even better illustrated in an abnormal mechanism. For example, not all speakers with significant velopharyngeal openings during oral consonant productions are destined to exhibit significant speech problems. With the velopharynx and nose being in mechanical series (being in line), an abnormally blocked nose may actually counteract an abnormally opened velopharynx. That is, a bad nose can be a good thing for speech, even if not for breathing. Conversely, a good nose can be a bad thing for speech when there is significant velopharyngeal impairment. The surgeon who attempts to "clean up" a bad nose and does not take into account the status of the velopharynx will sometimes figure this out after the fact when confronted with a child whose speech is worse after nasal surgery.

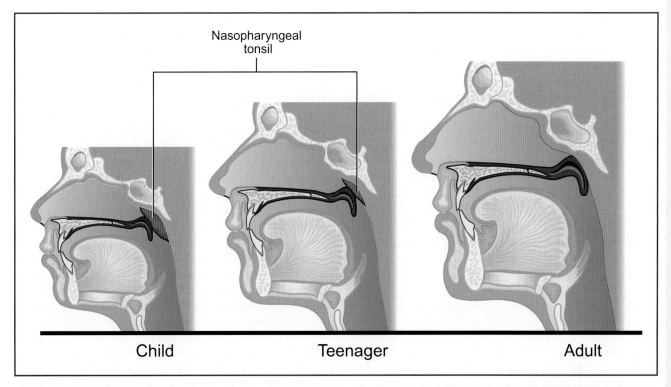

Nasopharyngeal tonsil

Child   Teenager   Adult

FIGURE 4–24. Changes in nasopharyngeal tonsil mass during development. The nasopharyngeal tonsil is large in children and atrophies with age. The velopharyngeal structures accommodate to these changes to achieve velopharyngeal closure.

traction (Perry, Kuehn, Sutton, & Fang, 2017). As the nasopharyngeal tonsil tissue recedes with age, velopharyngeal closure must go through a slow reorganization in those children who have been accomplishing closure through abutment of the velum and walls of the pharynx against the enlarged adenoidal tissue. This accommodation is obviously successful given the continuation of airtight velopharyngeal closure during the normal developmental schedule, but it may be interrupted if an adenoidectomy (removal of the adenoids) is performed in a child who is at risk for velopharyngeal problems (Andreassen, Leeper, MacRae, & Nicholson, 1994; Finkelstein, Berger, Nachmani, & Ophir, 1996; Morris, 1975; Siegel-Sadewitz, & Shprintzen, 1986).

Once adulthood is reached, changes in velopharyngeal-nasal structure and function occur slowly. Examples of age-related changes are that the pharyngeal muscles weaken and the pharyngeal lumen enlarges (Zaino & Benventano, 1977), sensory innervation declines (Aviv et al., 1994), density of palatal structures changes (Tomoda, Morii, Yamashita, & Kumazawa, 1984), and muscle bulk and bone density decrease in this region and elsewhere (Fremont & Hoyland, 2007). Although such changes seem to have the potential to alter velopharyngeal-nasal function for speech production, it appears that they do not.

He's an Old Smoothie

He was a distinguished looking white-haired grandfather. He agreed to serve as a person to be examined by graduate students learning to administer an examination for velopharyngeal-nasal function. Students had been assigned different parts of the examination and told to practice the administration of their part on at least half a dozen people so they could get "calibrated." One student, who had dutifully practiced on a group of her peers, proceeded to ask the gentleman to open his mouth while she turned on a flashlight and looked in. She methodically looked at structures and made comments to the class as she went along. When she shined the light on the gentleman's hard palate, she paused briefly and said to him, "That's the smoothest hard palate I've ever seen." He smiled and said back, "That's a denture, young lady." And so it was. He took it out and showed it to the class. The moral of this story is: Don't just practice on your classmates.

The question of whether velopharyngeal function for speech production changes with age in adults has been addressed using acoustic and aeromechanical measurements, with somewhat different outcomes. Whereas studies that used an acoustic measure called nasalance (the quotient of nasal sound pressure level to nasal + oral sound pressure level) provided ambiguous evidence (Hutchinson, Robinson, & Nerbonne, 1978; Seaver, Dalston, Leeper, & Adams, 1991), studies that used measures of air pressure and airflow (Hoit et al., 1994; Zajac, 1997) showed no influence of age. This combined evidence from these studies indicates that velopharyngeal function for speech production does not deteriorate with age, even in the very old. However, it is possible that other variables, such as age-related thinning of bone and tissue and reductions in size of mouth opening, might affect the acoustic speech product.

Sex

Sex-related differences in size and other anatomical relationships within the velopharyngeal-nasal mechanism begin to emerge after about 11 years of age and become more pronounced by the second decade of life (Perry, Kollara, Sutton, Kuehn, & Fang, 2019). By adulthood, the most obvious differences relate to size. For example, men, when compared to women, have longer pharynges (Fitch & Giedd, 1999; Jordan et al., 2017; Vorperian et al., 2009), longer *palatal levator* muscles (Bae, Kuehn, Sutton, Conway, & Perry, 2011; Ettema, Kuehn, Perlman, & Alperin, 2002), longer hard palates (Bae et al., 2011), larger and longer soft palates (Jordan et al., 2017; Kuehn & Kahane, 1990; Perry, Kuehn, Sutton, Gamage, & Fang, 2016), and longer noses (Zankl, Eberle, Molinari, & Schinzel, 2002). But do these differences influence velopharyngeal-nasal function for speech production?

There have been many studies comparing velopharyngeal function during speech production in men and women. These studies, which have used a variety of measurement techniques, have revealed some sex-related differences; however, they are small, idiosyncratic, or contradictory among studies. The only consistent finding has been that the magnitude of airflow during nasal productions is greater in men than women. This is to be expected, given that men have larger airways than women. Therefore, although men and women differ in certain details of velopharyngeal-nasal function in speech production, it is not clear that these differences make a difference functionally or in their application to clinical concerns (McWilliams, Morris, & Shelton, 1990).

CLINICAL NOTES

The focus of this chapter is on the structure and function of the healthy velopharyngeal-nasal mechanism. Nevertheless, it is also important to have some familiarity with velopharyngeal dysfunction (abnormal function) and how it can impair speech production. There are two general types of organic velopharyngeal dysfunction (those with an obvious physical basis): velopharyngeal insufficiency and velopharyngeal incompetence. Velopharyngeal insufficiency is caused by structural abnormalities that make it impossible to completely separate the oral airway from the nasal airway, usually associated with an inability to close the velopharyngeal port. This could be due to congenital anomalies (those that an infant is born with), trauma-induced injury, the presence of tumors or their surgical resection, and many other conditions. In the case of velopharyngeal incompetence, the physical structure is intact, but weakness or paralysis of the muscles makes it difficult or impossible to close the velopharyngeal port. This is usually caused by a disease or injury to the nervous system. Another type of velopharyngeal dysfunction is due to mislearning. The sidetrack called Playing by Her Own Rule is an example of velopharyngeal mislearning.

One relatively common example of velopharyngeal insufficiency is caused by a congenital anomaly called cleft (split) lip and cleft palate, a condition found in about 1 in every 1,600 infants born in the United States (https://www.cdc.gov/ncbddd/birthdefects/cleftlip.html). The photograph in Figure 4–25 shows an infant with a cleft of both the lip and palate. This is caused by a failure of the two sides of the lip, hard palate, and soft palate to fuse during development in utero. Infants such as the one pictured typically go through two or more surgeries to repair the cleft during the first 2 years of life. These surgeries are critical to the infant's quality of life because the cleft causes significant problems with speaking as well as drinking and eating. Given what has been discussed in this chapter regarding the importance of closing the velopharynx for certain speech sounds, it is easy to imagine that the speech of someone with a cleft would sound abnormal.

There are two major speech problems that can arise from velopharyngeal dysfunction. One is that it is difficult or impossible to build air pressure in the oral cavity to produce high-pressure sounds such as "p," "s," and "ch." This can have a devastating impact on speech intelligibility. The second problem is that voiced speech sounds, especially vowels and vowel-like consonants, take on a hypernasal quality. Hypernasality is a perception of how the speech sounds and is the result of the larynx-generated sound passing through

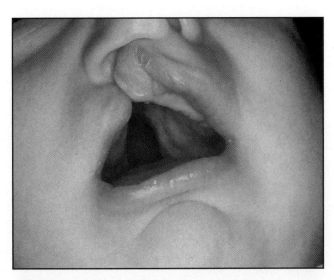

FIGURE 4–25. Photograph of an infant with a complete cleft lip and palate. From *Cleft Palate Speech* (3rd ed., p. 8), by S. Peterson-Falzone, M. Hardin-Jones, and M. Karnell, 2001, St. Louis, MO: Elsevier Mosby. Copyright 2001 by Elsevier Mosby. Reproduced with permission.

the nasal part of the velopharyngeal-nasal mechanism and being filtered differently than it would be if it were being directed through the oral pathway. The association between velopharyngeal status (fully open, partly open, closed) and hypernasality is demonstrated in Video 4–5 (Hypernasality).

REVIEW

The velopharyngeal-nasal mechanism is located within the head and neck and comprises a system of valves and air passages that interconnects the throat and atmosphere through the nose.

The velopharyngeal-nasal mechanism includes the pharynx, velum, nasal cavities, and outer nose.

Forces of the velopharyngeal-nasal mechanism are of two types—passive and active, the former arising from several sources and the latter arising from muscles distributed within different parts of the velopharyngeal-nasal mechanism.

Muscles of the pharynx include the *superior constrictor*, *middle constrictor*, *inferior constrictor*, *salpingopharyngeus*, *stylopharyngeus*, and *palatopharyngeus*.

Muscles of the velum include the *palatal levator*, *palatal tensor*, *uvulus*, *glossopalatine*, and *pharyngopalatine*.

Muscles of the outer nose include the *levator labii superioris alaeque nasi*, *anterior nasal dilator*, *posterior nasal dilator*, *nasalis*, and *depressor alae nasi*.

Movements of the pharynx enable its lumen (tubular cavity) to be changed along its length, either by constriction or dilation at different sites.

Movements of the velum involve shape changes of the structure and are mainly along an upward-backward or downward-forward path.

Movements of the outer nose are produced by muscle activities and aeromechanical events and influence the cross sections of the anterior nares, which allow airflow to pass more easily (decrease the nasal pathway resistance) or less easily (increase the nasal pathway resistance).

Closure of the velopharyngeal port can be achieved through a variety of movement strategies that involve different actions or combinations of actions of the velum, lateral pharyngeal walls, and posterior pharyngeal wall, strategies that may be conditioned by velopharyngeal anatomy.

The control variables of velopharyngeal-nasal function include airway resistance offered by the velopharyngeal-nasal mechanism, muscular pressure exerted by the velopharyngeal sphincter to maintain closure, and acoustic impedance in opposition to the flow of sound energy.

Different parts of the central nervous system are responsible for the control of the velopharyngeal-nasal mechanism, but all motor commands and sensory information travel through cranial nerves.

The warming, moistening, and filtering aspects of nasal function are important to health, and nasal breathing prevails until airway resistance becomes excessive, whereupon a switch is made to oral-nasal breathing.

During sustained utterance production, high vowels (as compared to low vowels) are produced with a higher velar position, more extensive contact between the velum and the posterior pharyngeal wall, and greater velopharyngeal compressive force.

Sustained fricatives are more likely to be produced with airtight velopharyngeal closure than sustained vowels, and nasal consonants are produced with an open velopharyngeal port.

Running speech activities involve the combining of consonants and vowels with primacy of velopharyngeal control being vested in consonant productions, especially those that are associated with high oral pressure that require closure (or near closure) of the velopharyngeal port.

Position and movement patterns of the velopharynx may reflect the occurrence of two or more speech sounds simultaneously, such that their productions overlap and intermingle and show evidence of how the brain prepares in advance for velopharyngeal adjustment and how the mechanical properties of the velopharyngeal-nasal mechanism influence its behavior.

Body position has effects on the velopharyngeal-nasal mechanism due to the influence of gravity.

Velopharyngeal closure for speech production develops gradually during infancy and appears to be relatively stable by 19 months of age with continuing modifications of temporal events during childhood and essentially no change in function throughout adulthood.

The sex of the speaker does not have a clear influence on velopharyngeal-nasal function for speech production.

Velopharyngeal dysfunction can be classified as velopharyngeal insufficiency (which includes disorders such as clefts of the lip and palate), incompetence (which results from muscle weakness or paralysis), or mislearning, all of which can result in problems with speech intelligibility and hypernasality.

REFERENCES

Andreassen, M., Leeper, H., MacRae, D., & Nicholson, I. (1994). Aerodynamic, acoustic, and perceptual changes following adenoidectomy. *Cleft Palate–Craniofacial Journal*, *31*, 264–270.

Azzam, N., & Kuehn, D. (1977). The morphology of musculus uvulae. *Cleft Palate Journal*, *14*, 78–87.

Bae, Y., Kuehn, D., Sutton, B., Conway, C., & Perry, J. (2011). Three-dimensional magnetic resonance imaging of velopharyngeal structures. *Journal of Speech, Language, and Hearing Research*, *54*, 1538–1545.

Bae, Y., Perry, J., & Kuehn, D. (2014). Videofluoroscopic investigation of body position on articulatory positioning. *Journal of Speech, Language, and Hearing Research*, *57*, 1135–1147.

Barsoumian, R., Kuehn, D., Moon, J., & Canady, J. (1998). An anatomic study of the tensor veli palatini and dilatator tubae muscles in relation to eustachian tube and velar function. *Cleft Palate–Craniofacial Journal*, *35*, 101–110.

Bell-Berti, F. (1976). An electromyographic study of velopharyngeal function in speech. *Journal of Speech and Hearing Research*, *19*, 225–240.

Bennett, K., & Hoit, J. (2013). Stress velopharyngeal incompetence (SVPI) in collegiate trombone players. *Cleft Palate–Craniofacial Journal*, *50*, 388–393.

Boorman, J., & Sommerlad, B. (1985). Levator palati and palatal dimples: Their anatomy, relationship and clinical significance. *British Journal of Plastic Surgery*, *38*, 326–332.

Bosma, J., Truby, H., & Lind, J. (1965). Cry motions of the newborn infant. *Acta Paediatrica Scandinavica*, *163*, 63–91.

Bunton, K., & Hoit, J. (2018). Development of velopharyngeal closure for vocalization during the first two years of life. *Journal of Speech, Language, and Hearing Research*, *61*, 549–560.

Bunton, K., & Story, B. (2012). The relation of nasality and nasalance to nasal port area based on a computational model. *Cleft Palate–Craniofacial Journal*, *49*, 741–749.

Bzoch, K. (1968). Variations in velar valving: The factor of vowel changes. *Cleft Palate Journal*, *5*, 211–218.

Cassell, M., & Ekaldi, H. (1995). Anatomy and physiology of the palate and velopharyngeal apertures. In R. Shprintzen & J. Bardach (Eds.), *Cleft palate speech management: A multi-disciplinary approach* (pp. 45–61). St. Louis, MO: Mosby.

Crelin, E. (1973). *Functional anatomy of the newborn*. New Haven, CT: Yale University Press.

Croft, C., Shprintzen, R., & Rakoff, S. (1981). Patterns of velopharyngeal valving in normal and cleft palate subjects: A multiview videofluoroscopic and nasendoscopic study. *Laryngoscope*, *91*, 265–271.

Curtis, J. (1968). Acoustics of speech production and nasalization. In D. Spriestersbach & D. Sherman (Eds.), *Cleft palate and communication* (pp. 27–60). New York, NY: Academic Press.

Dickson, D. (1972). Normal and cleft palate anatomy. *Cleft Palate Journal*, *9*, 280–293.

Ettema, S., Kuehn, D., Perlman, A., & Alperin, N. (2002). Magnetic resonance imaging of the levator veli palatini muscle during speech. *Cleft Palate–Craniofacial Journal*, *39*, 130–144.

Finkelstein, Y., Berger, G., Nachmani, A., & Ophir, D. (1996). The functional role of the adenoids in speech. *International Journal of Pediatric Otorhinolaryngology*, *34*, 61–74.

Finkelstein, Y., Shapiro-Feinberg, M., Talmi, Y., Nachmani, A., DeRowe, A., & Ophir, D. (1995). Axial configuration of the velopharyngeal valve and its valving mechanism. *Cleft Palate–Craniofacial Journal*, *32*, 299–305.

Fitch, W., & Giedd, J. (1999). Morphology and development of the human vocal tract: A study using magnetic resonance imaging. *Journal of the Acoustical Society of America*, *106*, 1511–1522.

Fletcher, S. (1973). Maturation of the speech mechanism. *Folia Phoniatrica*, *25*, 161–172.

Fremont, A., & Hoyland, J. (2007). Morphology, mechanisms and pathology of musculoskeletal ageing. *Journal of Pathology*, *211*, 252–259.

Fritzell, B. (1963). An electromyographic study of the movements of the soft palate in speech. *Folia Phoniatrica*, *15*, 307–311.

Fritzell, B. (1969). The velopharyngeal muscles in speech. *Acta Otolaryngologica*, *Supplement 250*, 1–81.

Fritzell, B. (1979). Electromyography in the study of the velopharyngeal function—A review. *Folia Phoniatrica*, *31*, 93–102.

Gautier, H., Remmers, J., & Bartlett, D. (1973). Control of the duration of expiration. *Respiration Physiology*, *18*, 205–221.

Gotto, T. (1977). Tightness in velopharyngeal closure and its regulatory mechanism. *Journal of the Osaka University Dental Society*, *22*, 1–19.

Graber, T., Bzoch, K., & Aoba, T. (1959). A functional study of the palatal and pharyngeal structures. *Angle Orthodontist*, *29*, 30–40.

Hairfield, W., Warren, D., Hinton, V., & Seaton, D. (1987). Inspiratory and expiratory effects of nasal breathing. *Cleft Palate Journal*, *24*, 183–189.

Harrington, R. (1944). A study of the mechanism of velopharyngeal closure. *Journal of Speech Disorders*, *9*, 325–345.

Hiyama, S., Ono, T., Ishiwata, Y., & Kuroda, T. (2002). Effects of mandibular position and body posture on nasal patency in normal awake subjects. *Angle Orthodontist, 72*, 547–553.

Hoit, J., Watson, P., Hixon, K., McMahon, P., & Johnson, C. (1994). Age and velopharyngeal function during speech production. *Journal of Speech and Hearing Research, 37*, 295–302.

House, A., & Stevens, K. (1956). Analog studies of the nasalization of vowels. *Journal of Speech and Hearing Disorders, 21*, 218–232.

Huang, Z., Lee, S., & Rajendran, K. (1997). Structure of the musculus uvulae: Functional and surgical implications of an anatomic study. *Cleft Palate–Craniofacial Journal, 34*, 466–474.

Hutchinson, J., Robinson, K., & Nerbonne, M. (1978). Patterns of nasalance in a sample of normal gerontologic subjects. *Journal of Communication Disorders, 11*, 469–481.

Iglesias, A., Kuehn, D., & Morris, H. (1980). Simultaneous assessment of pharyngeal wall and velar displacement for selected speech sounds. *Journal of Speech and Hearing Research, 23*, 429–446.

Jackson, R. (1976). Nasal-cardiopulmonary reflexes: A role of the larynx. *Annals of Otology, Rhinology, and Laryngology, 85*, 65–70.

Jaw, T., Sheu, R., Liu, G., & Lin, W. (1999). Development of adenoids: A study by measurement with MR images. *Kaohsiung Journal of Medical Sciences, 15*, 12–18.

Jordan, H., Schenck, G., Ellis, C., Rangarathnam, B., Fang, X., & Perry, J. (2017). Examining velopharyngeal closure patterns based on anatomic variables. *Journal of Craniofacial Surgery, 28*, 270–274.

Kaltenborn, A. (1948). *An x-ray study of velopharyngeal closure in nasal and non-nasal speakers* (Unpublished master's thesis). Northwestern University, Evanston, IL.

Kazlin, M., & Perry, J. (2016). Relationship between age and diagnosis on volumetric and linear velopharyngeal measures in the cleft and noncleft populations. *Journal of Craniofacial Surgery, 27*, 1340–1345.

Kelsey, C., Ewanowski, S., Hixon, T., & Minifie, F. (1968, September). Determination of lateral pharyngeal wall motion during connected speech by use of a pulsed ultrasound. *Science*, pp. 1259–1260.

Kent, R., Carney, P., & Severeid, L. (1974). Velar movement and timing: Evaluation of a model for binary control. *Journal of Speech and Hearing Research, 17*, 470–488.

Kent, R., & Murray, A. (1982). Acoustic features of infant vocalic utterances at 3, 6, and 9 months. *Journal of the Acoustical Society of America, 72*, 353–365.

Kuehn, D. (1976). A cineradiographic investigation of velar movement variables in two normals. *Cleft Palate Journal, 13*, 88–103.

Kuehn, D. (1990). Commentary on Doyle, Casselbrandt, Swarts, and Bluestone (1990): Observations on a role for the tensor veli palatini in intrinsic palatal function. *Cleft Palate Journal, 27*, 318–319.

Kuehn, D., & Azzam, N. (1978). Anatomical characteristics of palatoglossus and the anterior faucial pillar. *Cleft Palate Journal, 15*, 349–359.

Kuehn, D., Folkins, J., & Cutting, C. (1982). Relationships between muscle activity and velar position. *Cleft Palate Journal, 19*, 25–35.

Kuehn, D., & Kahane, J. (1990). Histologic study of the normal human adult soft palate. *Cleft Palate Journal, 27*, 26–34.

Kuehn, D., & Moon, J. (1998). Velopharyngeal closure force and levator veli palatini activation levels in varying phonetic contexts. *Journal of Speech, Language, and Hearing Research, 41*, 51–62.

Kuehn, D., & Moon, J. (2005). Histologic study of intravelar structures in normal human adult specimens. *Cleft Palate–Craniofacial Journal, 42*, 481–489.

Leeper, H., Tissington, M., & Munhall, K. (1998). Temporal aspects of velopharyngeal function in children. *Cleft Palate–Craniofacial Journal, 35*, 215–221.

Lester, R., & Hoit, J. (2014). Nasal and oral inspiration during natural speech breathing. *Journal of Speech, Language, and Hearing Research, 57*, 734–742.

Liss, J., Kuehn, D., & Hinkle, K. (1994). Direct training of velopharyngeal musculature. *Journal of Medical Speech-Language Pathology, 2*, 243–249.

Lubker, J. (1968). An electromyographic-cinefluorographic investigation of velar function during normal speech production. *Cleft Palate Journal, 5*, 1–18.

McWilliams, B., Morris, H., & Shelton, R. (1990). *Cleft palate speech* (2nd ed.). Philadelphia, PA: B. C. Decker.

Moll, K. (1962). Velopharyngeal closure on vowels. *Journal of Speech and Hearing Research, 5*, 30–37.

Moon, J., & Canady, J. (1995). Effects of gravity on velopharyngeal muscle activity during speech. *Cleft Palate–Craniofacial Journal, 32*, 371–375.

Moon, J., & Kuehn, D. (2004). Anatomy and physiology of normal and disordered velopharyngeal function for speech. In K. Bzoch (Ed.), *Communicative disorders related to cleft lip and palate* (5th ed., pp. 67–98). Austin, TX: Pro-Ed.

Moon, J., Kuehn, D., & Huisman, J. (1994). Measurement of velopharyngeal closure force during vowel production. *Cleft Palate–Craniofacial Journal, 31*, 356–363.

Moon, J., Smith, A., Folkins, J., Lemke, J., & Gartlan, M. (1994). Coordination of velopharyngeal muscle activity during positioning of the soft palate. *Cleft Palate–Craniofacial Journal, 31*, 45–55.

Morris, H. (1975). The speech pathologist looks at the tonsils and the adenoids. *Annals of Otology, Rhinology, and Laryngology, 84*, 63–66.

Netsell, R. (1990). Commentary. *Cleft Palate Journal, 27*, 58–60.

Nusbaum, E., Foly, L., & Wells, C. (1935). Experimental studies of the firmness of the velar-pharyngeal occlusion during the production of the English vowels. *Speech Monographs, 2*, 71–80.

Okada, R., Muro, S., Eguchi, K., Yagi, K., Nasu, H., Yamaguchi, K., Miwa, K., & Akita, K. (2018). The extended bundle of the tensor veli palatini: Anatomic consideration of the dilating mechanism of the Eustachian tube. *Auris Nasus Larynx, 45*, 265–272.

Perry, J. (2011). Variations in velopharyngeal structures between upright and supine positions using upright magnetic resonance imaging. *Cleft Palate–Craniofacial Journal, 48*, 123–133.

Perry, J., Bae, Y., & Kuehn, D. (2012). Effect of posture on deglutitive biomechanics in healthy individuals. *Dysphagia, 27,* 70–80.

Perry, J., Kollara, L., Sutton, B., Kuehn, D., & Fang, X. (2019). Growth effects on velopharyngeal anatomy from childhood to adulthood. *Journal of Speech, Language, and Hearing Research, 62,* 682–692.

Perry, J., Kuehn, D., Sutton, B., Gamage, J., & Fang, X. (2016). Anthropometric analysis of the velopharynx and related craniometrics dimensions in three adult populations using MRI. *Cleft Palate–Craniofacial Journal, 53,* e1–e13.

Perry, J., Kuehn, D., Sutton, B., & Fang, X. (2017). Velopharyngeal structural and functional assessment of speech in young children using dynamic magnetic resonance imaging. *Cleft Palate–Craniofacial Journal, 54,* 408–422.

Poppelreuter, S., Engelke, W., & Bruns, T. (2000). Quantitative analysis of the velopharyngeal sphincter function during speech. *Cleft Palate–Craniofacial Journal, 37,* 157–165.

Rudcrantz, H. (1969). Postural variations of nasal patency. *Acta Otolaryngologica, 68,* 435–443.

Ruscello, D. (1982). A selected review of palatal training procedures. *Cleft Palate Journal, 19,* 181–193.

Sasaki, C., Levine, P., Laitman, J., & Crelin, E. (1977). Postnatal descent of the epiglottis in man. *Archives of Otolaryngology, 103,* 169–171.

Schleif, E. P., Pelland, C. M., Ellis, C., Fang, X., Leierer, S. J., Sutton, B. P., . . . Perry, J. L. (2020). Identifying predictors of levator veli palatini muscle contraction during speech using dynamic magnetic resonance imaging. *Journal of Speech, Language, and Hearing Research, 63,* 1726–1735.

Seaver, E., Dalston, R., Leeper, H., & Adams, L. (1991). A study of nasometric values for normal nasal resonance. *Journal of Speech and Hearing Research, 34,* 715–721.

Seaver, E., & Kuehn, D. (1980). A cineradiographic and electromyographic investigation of velar positioning in nonnasal speech. *Cleft Palate Journal, 17,* 216–226.

Shelton, R., Beaumont, K., Trier, W., & Furr, M. (1978). Videopanendoscopic feedback in training velopharyngeal closure. *Cleft Palate Journal, 15,* 6–12.

Shimokawa, T., Yi, S., & Tanaka, S. (2005). Nerve supply to the soft palate muscles with special reference to the distribution of the lesser palatine nerves. *Cleft Palate-Craniofacial Journal, 42,* 495–500.

Shprintzen, R. (1992). Assessment of velopharyngeal function: Nasopharyngoscopy and multiview videofluoroscopy. In L. Brodsky, L. Holt, & D. Ritter-Schmidt (Eds.), *Craniofacial anomalies: An interdisciplinary approach* (pp. 196–207). St. Louis, MO: Mosby.

Siegel-Sadewitz, V., & Shprintzen, R. (1986). Changes in velopharyngeal valving with age. *International Journal of Pediatric Otorhinolaryngology, 11,* 171–182.

Skolnick, M. (1970). Videofluoroscopic examination of the velopharyngeal portal during phonation in lateral and base projections—A new technique for studying the mechanics of closure. *Cleft Palate Journal, 7,* 803–816.

Skolnick, M., McCall, G., & Barnes, M. (1973). The sphincteric mechanism of velopharyngeal closure. *Cleft Palate Journal, 10,* 286–305.

Subtelny, J., & Koepp-Baker, H. (1956). The significance of adenoid tissue in velopharyngeal function. *Plastic and Reconstructive Surgery, 12,* 235–250.

Thom, S., Hoit, J., Hixon, T., & Smith, A. (2006). Velopharyngeal function during vocalization in infants. *Cleft Palate–Craniofacial Journal, 43,* 539–546.

Thompson, A., & Hixon, T. (1979). Nasal air flow during normal speech production. *Cleft Palate Journal, 16,* 412–420.

Tomoda, T., Morii, S., Yamashita, T., & Kumazawa, T. (1984). Histology of human eustachian tube muscles: Effect of aging. *Annals of Otology, Rhinology, and Laryngology, 93,* 17–24.

Tucker, L. (1963). *Articulatory variations in normal speakers with changes in vocal pitch and effort* (Unpublished master's thesis). University of Iowa, Iowa City.

Vorperian, H., Wang, S., Chung, M., Schimek, E. M., Durtschi, R., Kent, R., . . . Gentry, L., (2009). Anatomic development of the oral and pharygneal portions of the vocal tract: An imaging study. *Journal of the Acoustical Society of America, 125,* 1666–1678.

Warren, D., Dalston, R., & Dalston, E. (1990). Maintaining speech pressures in the presence of velopharyngeal impairment. *Cleft Palate Journal, 27,* 53–58.

Warren, D., & DuBois, A. (1964). A pressure-flow technique for measuring velopharyngeal orifice area during continuous speech. *Cleft Palate Journal, 1,* 52–71.

Warren, D., Hairfield, W., & Hinton, V. (1985). The respiratory significance of the nasal grimace. *ASHA, 27,* 82.

Warren, D., Hairfield, W., Seaton, D., Morr, K., & Smith, L. (1988). The relationship between nasal airway size and nasal-oral breathing. *American Journal of Orthodontics and Dentofacial Orthopedics, 93,* 289–293.

Warren, D., Mayo, R., Zajac, D., & Rochet, A. (1996). Dyspnea following experimentally induced increased nasal airway resistance. *Cleft Palate–Craniofacial Journal, 33,* 231–235.

Zaino, C., & Benventano, T. (1977). Functional, involutional, and degenerative disorders. In C. Zaino & T. Benventano (Eds.), *Radiologic examination of the oropharynx and esophagus* (pp. 141–170). New York, NY: Springer-Verlag.

Zajac, D. (1997). Velopharyngeal function in young and older adult speakers: Evidence from aerodynamic studies. *Journal of the Acoustical Society of America, 102,* 1846–1852.

Zajac, D. (2000). Pressure-flow characteristics of /m/ and /p/ production in speakers without cleft palate: Developmental findings. *Cleft Palate–Craniofacial Journal, 37,* 468–477.

Zajac, D., & Hackett, A. (2002). Temporal characteristics of aerodynamic segments in the speech of children and adults. *Cleft Palate–Craniofacial Journal, 39,* 432–438.

Zankl, A., Eberle, L., Molinari, L., & Schinzel, A. (2002). Growth charts for nose length, nasal protrusion, and philtrum length from birth to 97 years. *American Journal of Medical Genetic, 111,* 388–391.

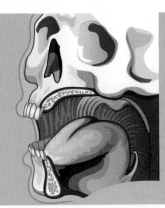

Pharyngeal-Oral Structure and Function

INTRODUCTION

The pharyngeal-oral mechanism, together with the velopharyngeal-nasal mechanism (discussed in Chapter 4), forms what is called the upper airway. In this book, the term *upper airway* is used in the context of the anatomy and physiology of this region so as to be consistent with terms such as *lower airways, laryngeal airway, velopharyngeal-nasal airway,* and *oral airway.* When referring to the acoustic properties of these regions, different terms are used: The term *vocal tract* is used for the pharyngeal-oral air spaces and the term *nasal tract* is used for the nasal air spaces.

Although most textbooks consider only the oral component (or the combined oral and velopharyngeal components), this chapter includes the pharynx in its consideration of pharyngeal-oral function. This is because the middle and lower regions of the pharynx function like articulators and acoustic filters in much the same way as do oral structures.

This chapter begins with the anatomy, forces (including muscles), and movements of the pharyngeal-oral mechanism and then discusses control variables and neural control. The final sections are dedicated to speech production, specifically, sound generation and filtering, articulatory descriptions and processes, age- and sex-related influences on structure and function, and clinical notes. Its role in swallowing is discussed in Chapter 7.

PHARYNGEAL-ORAL ANATOMY

The pharyngeal-oral mechanism is a flexible tube that extends from the larynx to the lips and undergoes an approximate 90-degree bend (like a plumber's elbow joint) at the level of the oropharynx. There, the shorter and vertical pharyngeal portion communicates through the oropharyngeal (faucial) isthmus with the longer and horizontal oral portion. The pharyngeal-oral mechanism is supported by a skeletal structure that provides the framework around which its internal topography is organized.

Skeletal Framework

The full skeletal framework that supports both the velopharyngeal-nasal and the pharyngeal-oral parts of the speech mechanism is presented and illustrated in Chapter 4. This framework consists of the cervical vertebrae, bones of the skull (see Figure 4–1), and the bones of the face (see Figure 4–2). The cervical (neck) segments of the vertebral column lie behind the three subdivisions of the pharynx—laryngopharynx, oropharynx, and nasopharynx—and form part of the substance of their back walls. The skull, made up of several irregularly shaped bones, forms the framework of the head. The facial bones contribute to the formation of the roof, floor, and sides of the oral cavity. The maxilla, mandible, and the temporomandibular joints are particularly prominent pharyngeal-oral structures and are discussed in more detail here.

Maxilla

Figure 5–1 depicts the maxilla. The maxilla forms the upper jaw and most of the hard palate. It consists of two complex bones (one on the left and one on the right) that meet at the midline. The maxilla lends strength to the roof of the oral cavity (as well as to the floor of the nasal cavities) and provides a buttress for the facial skeleton. Each bone of the maxilla has a palatine process that extends horizontally to the midline and joins with the palatine process from the opposite side to form the front three-fourths of the hard palate. The back one-fourth of the hard palate is formed by the much smaller palatine bones, which have horizontal processes that extend to the midline from each side to complete that part of the hard palate.

The alveolar process of the maxilla (sometimes called the alveolar arch) is a thick spongy projection that extends downward and houses the upper teeth. This process accommodates 16 permanent teeth (8 on each side). As shown in Figure 5–2, they are the central incisors, lateral incisors, canines (or cuspids), first and second premolars (or bicuspids), first and second molars, and third molars (or wisdom teeth). Infants and young children have only 10 teeth, called deciduous teeth (or baby teeth or milk teeth), which are later replaced by the permanent teeth.

Mandible

Figure 5–3 shows the salient features of the mandible. The mandible (lower jaw) is a large horseshoe-shaped structure when viewed from above or below. Its open end faces toward the back. The front and sides of the mandible together form what is termed the body of the structure. The left and right halves of the mandible join at the front through a fibrous symphysis (line of union)

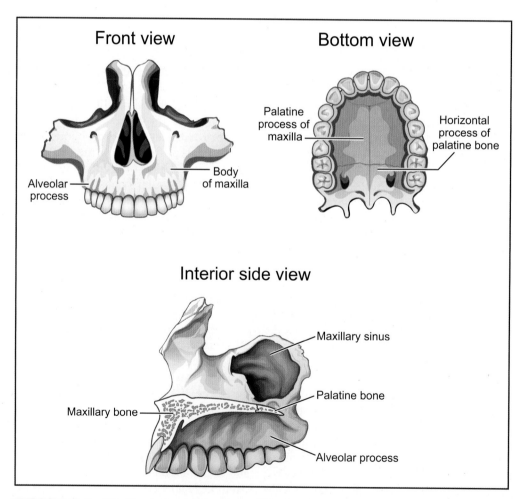

FIGURE 5–1. Maxilla as shown from three different views.

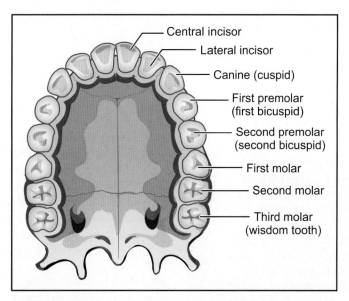

FIGURE 5-2. The upper teeth. The alveolar process of the maxilla contains 16 permanent teeth (8 on each side) that include incisors, canines, premolars, and molars. Infants and young children have fewer deciduous teeth.

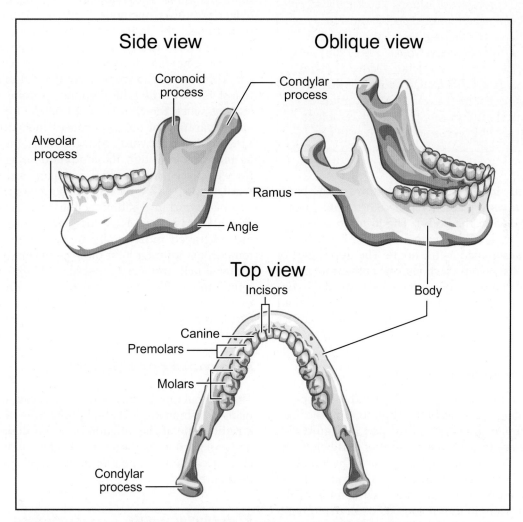

FIGURE 5-3. Mandible as seen from three different views. The mandibular alveolar process contains 16 teeth that have the same names as their maxillary counterparts.

that ossifies (turns to bone) during the first year of life. Like the maxilla, the mandible also has an alveolar process that accommodates 16 permanent teeth. These teeth bear the same names as the maxillary teeth.

Grant Fairbanks (1910–1964)

Fairbanks was a giant in speech science. He also trained others who became distinguished scientists. Fairbanks was a key figure in the development of speech science as a discipline and had a major influence in bringing it to the fore as an integrated science. One of his best-known works was the development of the notion that speech production was controlled in the manner of a servomechanism that relied on sensory feedback. His book, titled *Voice and Articulation Drillbook* (Fairbanks, 1960), is a classic and contains the famous *Rainbow Passage* that has been used in more speech research studies than any other reading. Fairbanks died while on a flight between Chicago and San Francisco. The flight was diverted to Denver, where the coroner ruled that he had choked to death while eating. Fairbanks was greatly admired as a scientist. Your authors are honored to be able to directly trace our professional lineages to him.

On each side of the mandible toward the back, there is an upward projection called the ramus (meaning a branch from the body). The location along the bottom of the mandible where each ramus diverges upward is designated as the angle. The upper part of each ramus has two projections, one at the front called the coronoid process and one at the back called the condylar process (also called the condyle). The coronoid process is somewhat rounded, whereas the condylar process has a neck and a prominent head.

Temporomandibular Joints

The mandible articulates with the left and right temporal bones along the sides of the skull to form the temporomandibular joints. As illustrated in Figure 5–4, these joints are located just in front of and below the external auditory meatuses (ear canals). The temporomandibular joints are enclosed by a fibrous capsule and lubricated by synovial fluid. Each joint is of the condyloid variety in that it consists of an ovoid (egg-shaped) process (the head of the condyle) that fits into an elliptical-shaped cavity within the temporal bone on the corresponding side (Dickson & Maue-Dickson,

1982). The condyle of the mandible (the more rearward of its two processes) is separated from its receiving cavity by a cartilaginous meniscus (crescent) called the articular disk. The surfaces of the condyle and the temporal bone are themselves covered with fibrocartilage (cartilage that contains fibrous bundles of collagen) that is devoid of vascular tissue (Sicher & DuBrul, 1975).

Three ligaments influence the function of each temporomandibular joint (see bottom image in Figure 5–4): the temporomandibular ligament, the sphenomandibular ligament, and the stylomandibular ligament. The temporomandibular ligament, which extends between the outer surface of the zygomatic arch and the outer and back surfaces of the neck of the condyle, limits the degree to which the condyle can be displaced downward and backward. The sphenomandibular ligament, which extends between the angular spine of the sphenoid bone and the inner surface of the ramus below the condyle, limits downward and backward displacement of the mandible. The stylomandibular ligament, which extends between the styloid process of the temporal bone to near the angle of the mandible, limits downward and forward displacement of the mandible.

Movements at the temporomandibular joints are conceptualized as movements of the mandible relative to a stabilized skull (although the opposite is possible, such as when the chin is rested on the top of a table and separation of the jaws causes the skull to rotate upward and backward). Movements of the mandible, as mediated through its condyloid processes, have three displacement possibilities: (a) upward and downward, made possible by a hinge-like action; (b) forward and backward in a gliding action; and (c) side to side in a gliding action. These displacement possibilities are portrayed individually in Figure 5–5; however, temporomandibular joint movements are often multidimensional and very complex. Movements of the temporomandibular joint can be felt by pressing your fingers gently against the skin near the bottom of your ears and moving your mandible in different directions.

Internal Topography

The internal topography of the pharyngeal-oral mechanism is fashioned around a hollow tube that bends at a right angle at the junction between the pharyngeal and oral portions of the structure. The pharyngeal, oral, and buccal cavities and their mucous lining are considered here.

Pharyngeal Cavity

Recall from Chapter 4 that the pharynx (throat) is a tube of tendon and muscle that extends from the base

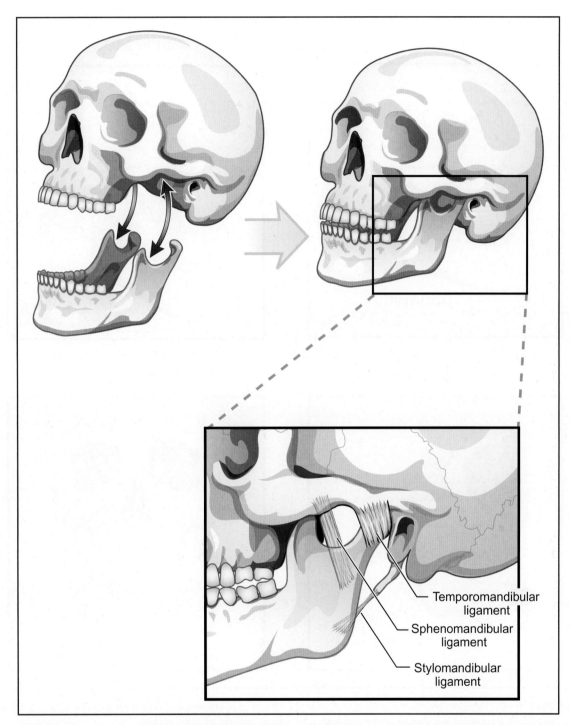

FIGURE 5–4. Temporomandibular joints and ligaments. The temporomandibular, sphenomandibular, and stylomandibular ligaments limit the motions of the joints in downward, backward, and forward directions.

of the skull to the larynx. This tube is widest at the top and narrows down its length and is larger side to side than front to back (oval shaped). The lower and middle parts of the pharyngeal tube are designated as the laryngopharynx and oropharynx, respectively, and are the parts of greatest interest in this chapter (see Figure 4–4). Pharyngeal muscles ring the back and sides of the laryngopharynx and oropharynx (see Figure 4–10). The lower part of the oropharynx is bounded by the tongue and epiglottis, and the upper part of the oropharynx opens into the oral cavity at the front through the anterior faucial pillars (palatoglossal arch). The

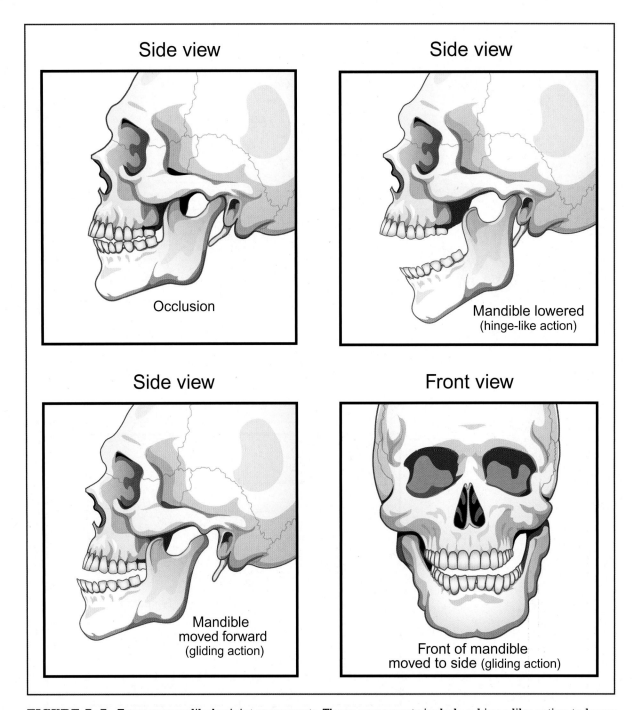

FIGURE 5–5. Temporomandibular joint movements. These movements include a hinge-like action to lower the mandible, a forward-backward gliding action, and a side-to-side gliding action.

back wall of the upper part of the oropharynx can be seen when looking back through the faucial isthmus (see Figure 4–5).

Oral Cavity

Figure 5–6 depicts the oral cavity (mouth cavity). The front entryway to the oral cavity is designated as the oral vestibule and is defined to include the lips, cheeks, front teeth, and forward-most segments of the alveolar processes of the maxilla and mandible. The oral cavity is bounded at the back by the anterior faucial pillars (palatoglossal arch), above by the hard palate and velum, and below by its floor comprising mainly the tongue.

The tongue is a prominent feature of the oral cavity, and its importance in activities such as speaking

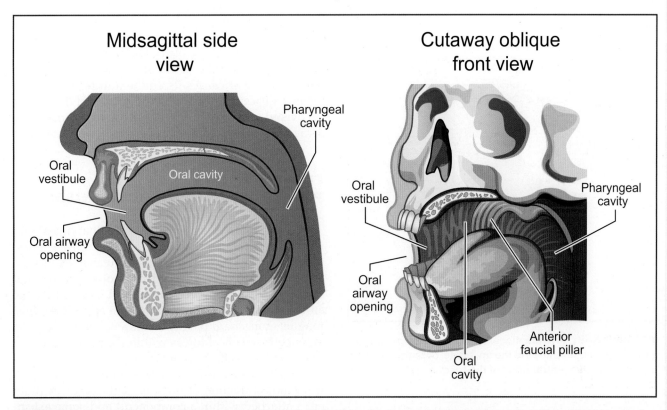

FIGURE 5–6. Oral cavity from two views. The oral vestibule is the front entryway to the oral cavity and is bounded at the front by the lips and at the back by the front parts of the alveolar processes. The back of the oral cavity is bounded by the anterior faucial pillars.

and singing has long been recognized (Figure 5–7). Although unitary in nature, the tongue is sometimes subdivided into different regions. The subdivisions can be based on anatomical schemes (e.g., Zemlin, 1998) or functional schemes (e.g., Kent, 1997). Functional schemes usually recognize regions of the tongue that are considered important to the behavior of the structure.

Figure 5–8 shows the tongue as consisting of five functional components: tip, blade, dorsum, root, and body. The tip of the tongue is the part of its surface nearest the front teeth at rest. The blade is the part of its surface that lies behind the tip and below the alveolar ridge of the maxilla and the front part of the hard palate. The dorsum of the tongue constitutes the surface that lies behind the blade and below the back part of the hard palate and the velum. The root of the tongue is the part of the tongue's surface that faces the back of the pharynx and the front of the epiglottis. The body of the tongue comprises its central mass and underlies the other four surface parts.

Buccal Cavity

The buccal cavity lies to the sides of the oral cavity. This cavity constitutes the small space between the

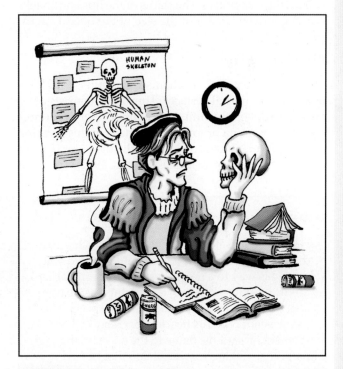

FIGURE 5–7. "That skull had a tongue in it and could sing once." (Hamlet in *Hamlet*, Act 5, Scene 1, William Shakespeare)

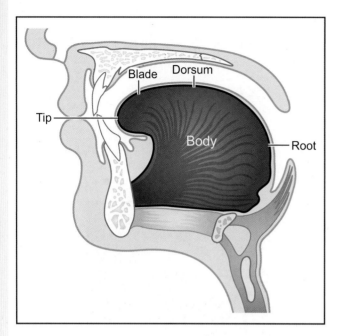

FIGURE 5–8. Five functional components of the tongue. From front to back, they are the tip, blade, dorsum, and root. The body is the central mass of the tongue that lies below the other four.

gums (gingivae) and teeth internally and the lips and cheeks (buccae) externally. The buccal cavity connects to the oral cavity through spaces between the teeth and behind the last molars. The status of the lips and cheeks is a major determinant of the size of the buccal cavity.

Mucous Lining

The pharyngeal-oral mechanism contains a mucous lining on its internal surfaces. This lining consists of an outer layer of epithelium and an inner layer of connective tissue (lamina propria). The details of this layering differ at different locations, especially the outer layer of epithelium (Dickson & Maue-Dickson, 1982). The most

prominent mucosa lining has a shiny appearance and covers all of the soft tissues except the gums, hard palate, and tongue. A so-called masticatory mucosa covers the gums and the hard palate and has a collagen subflooring that causes its epithelium to hold firmly against adjacent bone. The upper surface of the tongue is covered with a specialized mucosa that contains an array of small pockets and crypts that house taste buds.

FORCES OF THE PHARYNGEAL-ORAL MECHANISM

Two types of forces are applied to the pharyngeal-oral mechanism: passive and active. Passive force is inherent and always present but subject to change. Passive force arises from the natural recoil of structures that line the walls of the pharyngeal-oral mechanism, the surface tension between structures in apposition (lips, tongue, gums, hard palate, velum), the pull of gravity, and aeromechanical forces within the pharyngeal and oral portions of the mechanism.

The active force of pharyngeal-oral function comes from the contraction of muscles, some intrinsic (both ends attached within a component) and some extrinsic (one end attached within the component and one end attached outside the component). The function described here for individual muscles assumes that the muscle of interest is engaged in a shortening (concentric) contraction, unless otherwise specified. The tongue presents a somewhat more complex situation because of its special status as a muscular hydrostat (explained below). Discussed here are muscles of the pharynx, mandible, tongue, and lips.

Muscles of the Pharynx

The muscles of the pharynx are located within the laryngopharynx, oropharynx, and nasopharynx and

Dancing in the Moonlight

He was a pleasant young man who was honorably discharged after serving in the military. He had made his way to a large Veterans Administration Medical Center. His only complaint was hearing loss, but the audiologist thought his speech was inconsistent with his hearing test results. The moment he said his name to the speech-language pathologist, there was suspicion that he had impairment of one or both cranial nerves serving the tongue. When asked to open his mouth, the

beam of a flashlight revealed a shrunken and wrinkled tongue that seemed to dance around under the surface like a bagful of jumping beans. The signs were classic of lower motor neuron disease, and a neurologist reported presumptive bilateral congenital agenesis (failure to develop) of the hypoglossal nerves (motor nerves to the tongue). How had this escaped detection during his physical examination for the military? Perhaps he was only asked to say "ah."

are discussed in detail in Chapter 4. For the purposes of this chapter, those within the laryngopharynx and oropharynx are of primary interest and are reviewed here briefly.

Muscles of the laryngopharynx and oropharynx can influence the lumen (cavity) of the pharynx (the cross section along its length) in the region that lies behind the tongue, epiglottis, and oral cavity (the back wall of which is easily visualized through the faucial isthmus). The lumen of the pharynx in this region can also be influenced by adjustments of the tongue and epiglottis (see Figure 4–15). Muscles that attach to the laryngopharynx and oropharynx fabric proper (within the posterior and lateral pharyngeal walls) are revisited here. These include the *inferior constrictor* muscle, *middle constrictor* muscle, and *stylopharyngeus* muscle (see Figure 4–10).

The *inferior constrictor* muscle of the pharynx is located toward the bottom of the structure and is sometimes conceptualized as two muscles, the *thyropharyngeus* and *cricopharyngeus* muscles. Its fibers arise from the sides of the thyroid and cricoid cartilages and diverge in a fan-like configuration as they course backward and toward the midline. There they interdigitate with fibers of the paired mate from the opposite side. The middle and upper fibers of the muscle ascend obliquely, whereas the lowermost fibers run horizontally and downward and are continuous with those of the esophagus. When the *inferior constrictor* muscle contracts, it pulls the lower part of the back wall of the pharynx forward and draws the sidewalls of the lower pharynx forward and inward. These actions cause the lumen of the lower pharynx to constrict.

The *middle constrictor* muscle of the pharynx is located midway along the length of the pharyngeal tube. Its fibers arise from the greater and lesser horns of the hyoid bone and the stylohyoid ligament and course backward and toward the midline, where they insert into the median raphe (seam) of the pharynx. The uppermost fibers of the *middle constrictor* muscle course obliquely upward and overlap the lower fibers of the *superior constrictor* muscle, whereas the lowermost fibers of the muscle run obliquely downward beneath the fibers of the *inferior constrictor* muscle. Recall that this fiber arrangement is akin to the way in which roof shingles partially overlap. When the *middle constrictor* muscle contracts, it decreases the cross-sectional area of the oropharynx by pulling forward on the posterior pharyngeal wall and forward and inward on the lateral pharyngeal wall. Simultaneous contraction of the left and right *middle constrictor* muscles causes the pharyngeal lumen to constrict regionally in the manner of a sphincter.

The *stylopharyngeus* muscle extends between the styloid process of the temporal bone and the lateral wall of the pharynx near the juncture of the *superior constrictor* and *middle constrictor* muscles. Its fibers run downward, forward, and toward the midline. When the *stylopharyngeus* muscle contracts, it pulls the pharyngeal tube upward and draws the lateral wall of the pharynx toward the side. Together with similar action of its paired mate from the opposite side, it widens the lumen of the pharynx, especially in the region of the oropharynx, but also elsewhere along the length of the pharyngeal tube.

Muscles of the Mandible

Seven muscles provide active forces that operate on the mandible. These muscles are depicted in Figure 5–9 and are responsible for positioning the mandible in accordance with the movements allowed by the temporomandibular joints. Included among these muscles are the *masseter, temporalis, internal pterygoid, external pterygoid, digastric, mylohyoid,* and *geniohyoid.* Their general force vectors are depicted in Figure 5–10.

The *masseter* muscle is a flat, quadrilateral structure that covers much of the outer surface of the ramus of the mandible. Fibers of this muscle are in two layers. An outer layer forms the bulk of the muscle and courses from an aponeurosis along the front two-thirds of the zygomatic arch downward and backward to insert on the angle and nearby outer surface of the ramus of the mandible. An inner layer of fibers courses from the entire length of the zygomatic arch downward and forward to insert into the outer surface of the upper half of the ramus and its coronoid process. Contraction of the outer layer of the *masseter* muscle results in elevation of the mandible and approximation of the mandible and maxilla. The elevation is along a path that is at a right angle to the plane of occlusion of the molars. If the elevation is sufficient, pressure is brought to bear on the molars. Contraction of the inner layer of the muscle also results in elevation of the mandible and additionally exerts a force on the mandible that pulls it backward and aids in approximating the jaws.

The *temporalis* muscle is a broad, fan-shaped muscle that covers much of the side of the cranium. Its fibers originate from the inferior temporal line of the parietal bone and the greater wing of the sphenoid bone. These converge as they course downward under the zygomatic arch and insert on the inner surface and front border of the coronoid process and the front surface of the ramus of the mandible. Fibers toward the front and middle of the muscle course vertically, whereas those toward the back of the muscle have a more horizontal orientation. Contraction of the *temporalis* muscle results in an upward and backward pull on the mandible, with vertically oriented fibers

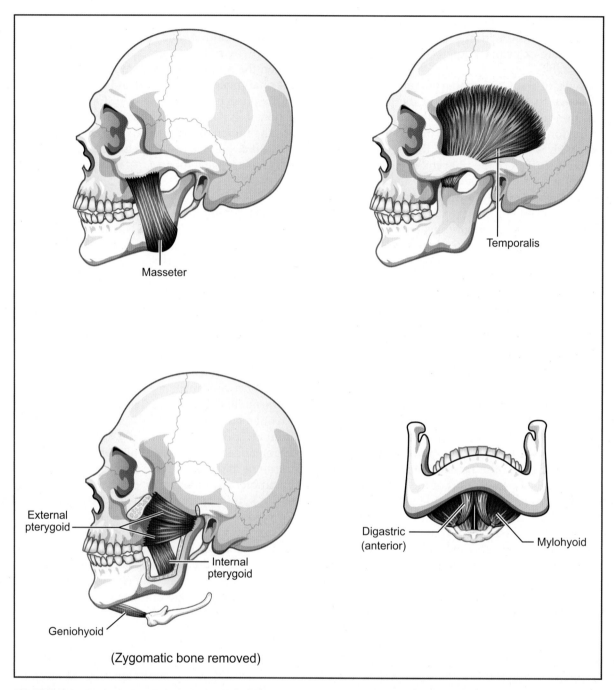

Masseter

Temporalis

External pterygoid

Internal pterygoid

Geniohyoid

Digastric (anterior)

Mylohyoid

(Zygomatic bone removed)

FIGURE 5–9. Muscles of the mandible. These muscles can raise the mandible (*masseter, temporalis, internal pterygoid*), lower the mandible (*external pterygoid, digastric* [*anterior* belly], *mylohyoid, geniohyoid*), move the mandible laterally (*masseter, temporalis, internal pterygoid, external pterygoid*), move the mandible forward (*external pterygoid*), and move the mandible backward (*masseter, temporalis*).

contributing to the upward component and horizontally oriented fibers contributing to the backward component. Activation of the *temporalis* muscle on only one side may result in retraction of the mandible on that side and movement of the front of the mandible toward the activated side.

The *internal pterygoid* muscle is a quadrilateral structure that follows an orientation that generally parallels that of the *masseter* muscle. Fibers of the *internal pterygoid* muscle originate from the lateral pterygoid plate and the perpendicular plate of the palatine bone. From there, they course downward, backward, and

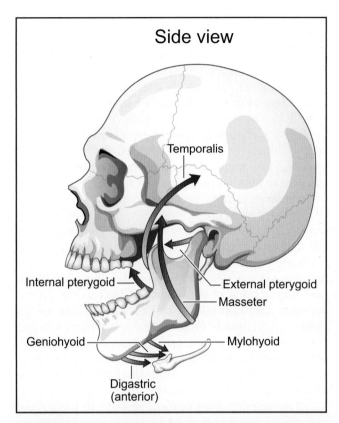

Side view

Temporalis

Internal pterygoid

External pterygoid

Masseter

Geniohyoid

Mylohyoid

Digastric (anterior)

FIGURE 5–10. Actions of muscles of the mandible. The *masseter* and *temporalis* muscles raise the mandible and pull it backward, the *external pterygoid* muscle slides the mandible downward and forward, and the *internal pterygoid*, *digastric* (*anterior* belly), *mylohyoid*, and *geniohyoid* muscles lower the mandible.

outward to insert on the inner surface of the angle and ramus of the mandible. Contraction of the *internal pterygoid* muscle results in elevation of the mandible. Sufficient elevation causes pressure to be placed on the opposing teeth of the mandible and maxilla. Activation of the muscle on only one side may result in slight movement of the corresponding condyle toward the opposite side.

The *internal pterygoid* muscle has a special relationship with the *masseter* muscle. Together these two muscles form a muscular sling that surrounds the angle of the mandible. This anatomical sling holds the angle from above and effectively straps the ramus to the skull. The result is a functional articulation between the mandible and the maxilla, with the temporomandibular joint acting as an enabling guide for movements of the mandible (Zemlin, 1998).

The *external pterygoid* muscle is one of the smaller muscles of the mandible. Its fibers have two origins toward the front, one from the greater wing of the sphenoid bone and one from the lateral pterygoid plate.

Fibers from these two points of origin tend to converge as they run generally horizontally backward to insert into the neck of the condyle of the mandible. Contraction of the *external pterygoid* muscle causes the condyle to slide downward and forward. Contraction of the *external pterygoid* muscle on only one side tends to move the front of the mandible toward the opposite side.

Three other muscles have a role in actions of the mandible. These are the *digastric* (*anterior* belly), *mylohyoid*, and *geniohyoid* muscles, all supplementary muscles of the larynx. The structure and function of these muscles are presented in detail in Chapter 3 (and illustrated in Figure 3–24) and are reviewed here only briefly.

The *digastric* muscle is a two-bellied muscle arranged such that it can pull upward on the hyoid bone and/or downward on the mandible. Its action is dependent on the degree to which either or both of these structures are fixed in position by other muscles. With greater relative fixation of the hyoid bone, contraction of the *anterior* belly of the *digastric* muscle lowers the mandible.

The *mylohyoid* muscle is positioned along the floor of the oral cavity. It is oriented such that its fibers can exert an upward and forward pull on the hyoid bone or a downward pull on the mandible. With greater relative fixation of the hyoid bone, contraction of the *mylohyoid* muscle lowers the mandible.

The *geniohyoid* muscle is a cylindrical muscle that lies above the *mylohyoid* muscle. The course of its muscle fibers is essentially parallel to the fiber course of the *anterior digastric* muscle. The *geniohyoid* muscle is oriented so that it can pull upward and forward on the hyoid bone or downward on the mandible. With greater relative fixation of the hyoid bone, contraction of the *geniohyoid* muscle lowers the mandible.

Muscles of the Tongue

Skeletal support for the overall pharyngeal-oral mechanism comes from vertebrae and bones of the skull and face, but the tongue is endowed with its own soft skeleton. This personal skeleton is largely connective tissue that surrounds and separates different parts of the tongue, including its left and right halves (Dickson & Maue-Dickson, 1982). This skeleton also includes a dense felt-like network of fibrous elastic tissue that lies below the epidermis (surface of the epithelium) and encapsulates the tongue like a bag (Zemlin, 1998). It is through this special soft skeleton that the eight muscles of the tongue (four intrinsic and four extrinsic) are able to bring about the wide variety of tongue movements that are possible.

Gone But Not Forgotten

Arm and leg amputations occurred in large numbers during the Civil War. Amputees from this era reported that pain or other sensations continued to arise from where their missing limbs had been. Some described them as sensory ghosts and many doctors of the time thought that those who reported them had mental problems. Not so. Phantom limb pain or other sensations are now recognized to be common following amputation of any body part, and scientists have embraced a number of theories about their origins. Those who have had their tongues amputated (usually surgically and because of cancer) also report tongue pain or other sensations that are analogous to those associated with their better-known phantom-limb counterpart. Ghost tongues are most prominent right after surgery and tend to fade away with time, although they are known to abruptly reappear on occasion. All of this is really quite haunting when you think about it.

The intrinsic muscles of the tongue are the *superior longitudinal*, *inferior longitudinal*, *vertical*, and *transverse* muscles. They are depicted in Figure 5–11.

The *superior longitudinal* muscle is a broad, flat muscle that lies just beneath the expansive upper surface (dorsum) of the tongue. Fibers originate within the root of the tongue from the hyoid bone and course forward in an imbricated pattern (like overlapping fish scales) along the long axis of the tongue. Forward attachments of the muscle are in the region of the front edges of the tongue and the upper surface of the tongue tip. Fibers near the midline course downward to their attachments, whereas fibers toward the side course obliquely toward the lateral boundary of the tongue. Contraction of the entire *superior longitudinal* muscle can shorten the tongue and increase its convexity from front to back. Because the muscle is composed of a series of short imbricated fibers, it can also activate in patterns that differentially affect different regions of the tongue. For example, contraction of fibers toward the front of the tongue can pull the tongue tip upward and toward the side of muscle activation. Simultaneous contractions of comparable fibers in the paired *superior longitudinal* muscles elevate the tongue tip without deviation to either side. For another example, contraction of fibers that insert obliquely into the edges of the tongue can pull the lateral margins of the structure upward to create a longitudinal trough down the center of the tongue toward the front.

The *inferior longitudinal* muscle is positioned near the undersurface of the tongue somewhat toward the side. It arises from the body of the hyoid bone at the root of the tongue and courses forward through the body of the tongue to insert near the lower surface of the tongue tip. Fibers of the *inferior longitudinal* muscle blend with the fibers of different extrinsic muscles

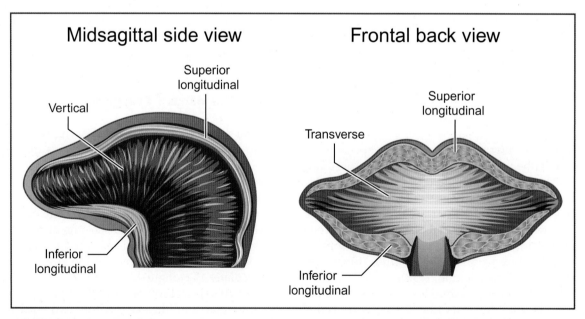

FIGURE 5–11. Intrinsic muscles of the tongue. These are the ***superior longitudinal***, ***inferior longitudinal***, ***vertical***, and ***transverse*** muscles.

of the tongue (discussed below) within the body of the tongue. Contraction of the *inferior longitudinal* muscle shortens the tongue and pulls its tip downward and toward the same side. Simultaneous contraction of comparable fibers in the paired *inferior longitudinal* muscles pulls the tongue tip downward symmetrically.

The *vertical* muscle originates from just beneath the dorsum of the tongue and courses downward vertically and toward the side through the body of the tongue. Fibers of the *vertical* muscle terminate near the sides of the tongue along its lower surface. Contraction of the *vertical* muscle results in a flattening of the tongue on the side of action, especially toward its lateral margins. This muscle can also lower the more midline parts of the upper tongue surface.

The *transverse* muscle, as its name implies, courses side to side within the tongue. Fibers of the muscle arise mainly from the median fibrous skeleton of the tongue and course laterally, where they terminate in fibrous tissue along the side of the tongue. Upper fibers fan out in an upward direction, whereas lower fibers fan out in a downward direction. The intermingling of *transverse* muscle fibers with those of other intrinsic and extrinsic tongue muscles is extensive and makes it hard to determine their precise course and location within different parts of the tongue. The *transverse* muscle is a major constituent in the mass of interwoven muscle fibers that comprise the bulk of the tongue. Contraction of the *transverse* muscle results in narrowing the tongue from side to side and elongating it.

The extrinsic muscles of the tongue include the *styloglossus, palatoglossus, hyoglossus,* and *genioglossus* muscles. These are depicted in Figure 5–12.

The *styloglossus* muscle originates from the front and side of the styloid process of the temporal bone and the stylomandibular ligament. Fibers of the muscle course forward, downward, and toward the midline to insert into the sides of the root of the tongue. From there, they run in various directions but primarily toward the midline and forward within the body of the tongue. Some fibers of the *styloglossus* muscle interdigitate with fibers of the *inferior longitudinal* muscle, whereas others interdigitate with fibers of the *hyoglossus* muscle. Ultimate blending of different fibers makes it difficult to distinguish those of one muscle from another. Contraction of the *styloglossus* muscle can have multiple consequences, including that it can (a) draw the body of the tongue upward and backward, (b) pull the side of the tongue upward to influence the tongue's concavity, (c) shorten the tongue, and (d) pull the tongue tip toward the side.

The *palatoglossus* muscle is discussed in Chapter 4 (and illustrated in Figure 4–12) as a part of the velopharyngeal-nasal mechanism. There it is referred

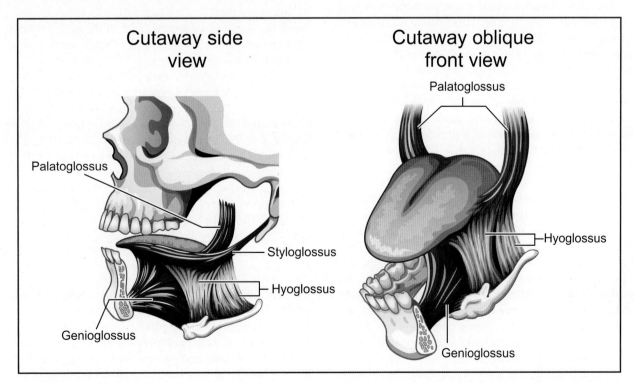

FIGURE 5-12. Extrinsic muscles of the tongue. These are the *styloglossus*, *palatoglossus*, *hyoglossus*, and *genioglossus* muscles.

to as the *glossopalatine* muscle (its origin and insertion being reversed in that context). For present purposes, the *palatoglossus* muscle can be thought of as originating from the lower surface of the palatal aponeurosis with its fibers coursing downward, forward, and toward the side (forming the anterior faucial pillar) and inserting into the side of the root of the tongue. There the fibers of the *palatoglossus* muscle blend with those of the *transverse*, *styloglossus*, and *hyoglossus* muscles of the tongue. When the *palatoglossus* muscle contracts, it pulls upward, backward, and inward on the root of the tongue. Through its action, the muscle can displace the tongue mass backward in the oral cavity and increase the concavity of its upper surface. When the left and right *palatoglossus* muscles contract simultaneously, the result is a lengthwise grooving of the upper surface of the tongue.

The *hyoglossus* muscle (see also Chapter 3 and Figure 3–24) is a quadrilateral structure that originates from the upper border of the body and greater cornua of the hyoid bone and extends upward and forward to insert into the side of the tongue toward the rear. Fibers of the *hyoglossus* muscle intermingle with those of the *styloglossus* and *palatoglossus* muscles. Contraction of the *hyoglossus* muscle lowers the body of the tongue and moves it backward. The lowering effect is most pronounced along the sides of the tongue (Dickson & Maue-Dickson, 1982).

The *genioglossus* muscle is complex and makes up a large portion of the tongue. This muscle is fan shaped and originates as three groups of fibers from the inner surface of the body of the mandible near the midline. The lower fibers course backward to insert into the root of the tongue. The middle fibers course backward and extend upward into the tongue in the region of the juncture between the dorsum and blade of the structure. The upper fibers run vertically and forward to insert near or within the tip of the tongue. Collectively, fibers of the *genioglossus* muscle travel through the body of the tongue between layers of muscle fibers formed by the *vertical, transverse*, and *superior longitudinal* muscles. Contraction of the *genioglossus* muscle can have a diverse set of consequences, depending on which particular fibers of the muscle are activated and in what patterns. Possible outcomes are that (a) the root of the tongue can be moved forward so as to force the tip of the tongue against the teeth or out of the mouth, (b) the front of the tongue can be pulled backward, and (c) the center line of the tongue can be pulled downward so as to form a trough-like depression along the upper surface of its length.

Figure 5–13 depicts the general force vectors associated with actions of the eight muscles of the tongue. Although discussion of the individual capabilities of the tongue muscles is instructive, it does not do justice to the intricate and interacting forces that can operate on and within the tongue to move it in different ways. Much of this has to do with special properties of the tongue that qualify it as a muscular hydrostat (discussed below under Movements of the Tongue).

Muscles of the Lips

The muscles of the lips are a subset of the muscles of the face. These muscles are more than a dozen in number and are portrayed in Figure 5–14 from different perspectives. The muscles of the lips include one intrinsic (contained within) and many extrinsic (one attachment within) muscles. They are the *orbicularis oris, buccinator, risorius, levator labii superioris, levator labii superioris alaeque nasi, zygomatic major, zygomatic minor, depressor labii inferioris, mentalis, levator anguli oris, depressor anguli oris, incisivus labii superioris, incisivus labii inferioris*, and *platysma*.

Street Talk About Talking

The folk language is filled with indications that the person on the street knows something about pharyngeal-oral function in speech production. Below are some expressions that we generated off the tops of our heads. Look at these and then try to add to the list from your own knowledge of the folk language. Our favorite from the list below is the last one, used during World War II to mean be careful to whom you are talking. Here goes. "That's a real tongue twister." "We were just jawing it." "He's bumping his gums." "They were flapping their cheeks." "She's lying through her teeth." "Don't give me any of your lip." "I don't chew my cabbage twice." "He's running off at the mouth again." "Hold your tongue, young man." "She's a big loudmouth." "His father told him to cork it." And our favorite, "Loose lips sink ships."

The *orbicularis oris* muscle is a ring of muscle within the lips that forms a sphincter at the oral end (mouth opening) of the pharyngeal-oral mechanism. This ring of muscle is complex and consists of fibers from both intrinsic and extrinsic sources that intertwine to form an airway valve and the most mobile part of the face. Fibers of the *orbicularis oris* muscle that are exclusive to the lips (intrinsic) are arranged in concentric

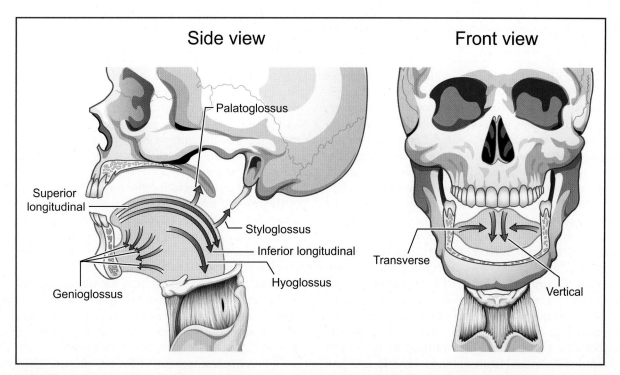

FIGURE 5-13. Actions of the eight muscles of the tongue as shown from side and front views (with parts cut away). These actions are extremely complex and not easily summarized. Shown here are major actions of each muscle, although other actions are possible.

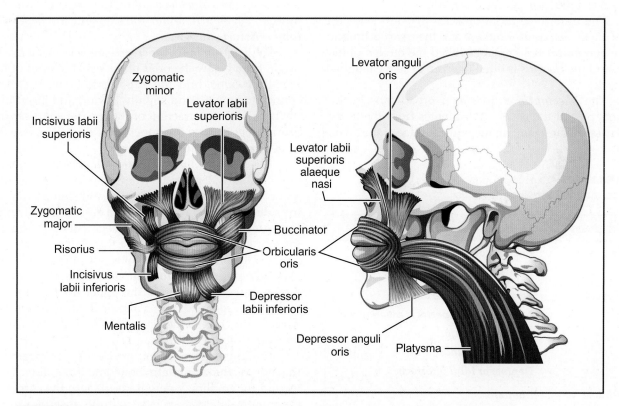

FIGURE 5-14. Muscles of the lips. All but one of these 14 muscles are extrinsic lip muscles—the exception being a subset of fibers of the *orbicularis oris* muscle. These extrinsic muscles are subgrouped into the transverse (*buccinators* and *risorius*), angular (*levator labii superioris*, *levator labii superioris alaeque nasi*, *zygomatic major*, *zygomatic minor*, *depressor labii inferioris*), vertical (*mentalis*, *levator anguli oris*, *depressor anguli oris*), and parallel (*incisivus labii superioris*, *incisivus labii inferioris*) muscles. The *platysma* muscle is a neck muscle and is included here because it has extrinsic influences on the lower lip.

rings around the border of the sphincter. These rings follow the outer contour of the upper and lower lips. The course of the intrinsic fibers of the *orbicularis oris* muscle changes with changes in the angular circumference of the mouth opening. Contraction of the *orbicularis oris* muscle can result in several positional changes of the lips. These include movements of the lips toward one another and forward, which, if extensive enough, can result in closure of the mouth and a forcing together of the lips. The corners of the mouth may also move as a result of activation of the *orbicularis oris* muscle. Such movement can be upward, downward, toward the side, or toward the midline. Action of the *orbicularis oris* muscle may also force the lips and/or corners of the mouth against the teeth.

Those lip muscles that are extrinsic are sometimes subgrouped into sets that follow fiber courses that are transverse (horizontal), angular (oblique to the corners of the mouth), vertical (from above or below), and parallel (adjacent to and alongside the lips). These subsets are considered, in turn, below, and are summarized in Table 5–1. The *platysma*, which is classified as a cervical (neck) muscle, is also discussed because it has extrinsic influences on the lower lip.

The transverse facial muscles that influence the lips are the *buccinator* muscle and the *risorius* muscle. The *buccinator* is sometimes called the bugler's muscle, and the *risorius* is often referred to as the laughter muscle.

The *buccinator* muscle is a broad muscle that forms part of the cheek. It originates from the pterygomandibular ligament, the outer surface of the alveolar process of the maxilla, and the mandible from the region of the last molars. Fibers course horizontally forward and toward the midline to insert into the upper and lower lips near the corner of the mouth. Uppermost fibers of the muscle enter the upper lip, whereas lowermost fibers enter the lower lip. Fibers of the central part of the muscle converge near the corner of the mouth and cross such that the lower fibers of that part of the muscle insert into the upper lip and the upper fibers insert into the lower lip. Contraction of the *buccinator* muscle can pull the corner of the mouth backward and toward the side. It can also force the lips and cheek against adjacent teeth.

The *risorius* muscle is a small muscle located within the cheek but closer to the surface than the *buccinator* muscle. It arises from fascia of the *masseter* muscle and courses horizontally forward and toward the midline to insert into the corner of the mouth and the lower lip. Contraction of the *risorius* muscle draws the corner of the mouth backward and toward the side; it may also force the lips against adjacent teeth.

The angular muscle group includes five muscles. These are the *levator labii superioris* muscle, *levator labii superioris alaeque nasi* muscle, *zygomatic major* muscle, *zygomatic minor* muscle, and the *depressor labii inferioris* muscle.

The *levator labii superioris* muscle has a broad origin from below the orbit of the eye, the front of the maxillary bone, and the zygomatic bone. Its fibers course downward and slightly inward and insert into the upper lip. Contraction of the *levator labii superioris* muscle elevates the upper lip; it may also cause the upper lip to turn outward (evert).

The *levator labii superioris alaeque nasi* muscle originates as a slender slip from the front of the maxilla and courses vertically downward and slightly toward the side. The muscle divides into a nasal segment and a lip segment. Fibers from the lip segment of the muscle insert into the upper lip, where they intermingle with fibers of the *orbicularis oris* muscle. Contraction of the lip segment of the *levator labii superioris alaeque nasi* muscle causes elevation of the upper lip. Contraction of the nasal segment of this muscle dilates the anterior naris on the corresponding side, as described in Chapter 4 (and shown in Figure 4–14).

The *zygomatic major* muscle has its origin on the side of the zygomatic bone and runs down and toward the midline where it inserts into the corner of the mouth. Fibers associated with its insertion intermingle with those of the *orbicularis oris* muscle. Contraction of the *zygomatic major* muscle pulls backward on the corner of the mouth. At the same time, action of this muscle lifts the corner of the mouth upward and toward the side.

TABLE 5–1. Extrinsic Tongue Muscles Organized According to Their Subgroupings

Subgroups	Muscles
Transverse	*Buccinator*
	Risorius
Angular	*Levator labii superioris*
	Levator labii superioris alaeque nasi
	Zygomatic major
	Zygomatic minor
	Depressor labii inferioris
Vertical	*Mentalis*
	Levator anguli oris
	Depressor anguli oris
Parallel	*Incisivus labii superioris*
	Incisivus labii inferioris

The *zygomatic minor* muscle originates from the inner surface of the zygomatic bone. Its fibers course downward and toward the midline, where they insert into the upper lip and interweave with fibers of the *orbicularis oris* muscle. Contraction of the *zygomatic minor* muscle elevates the upper lip and pulls the corner of the mouth upward.

The *depressor labii inferioris* muscle is a small, flat muscle located off the midline of the lower lip. Fibers of the muscle originate from the front surface of the mandible and course upward and inward to insert into the lower lip from near the midline to the corner of the mouth. Contraction of the *depressor labii inferioris* muscle pulls the lower lip downward and toward the side. It may also cause the lower lip to turn outward.

The vertical facial muscles are three in number. They include the *mentalis* muscle, *levator anguli oris* muscle, and the *depressor anguli oris* muscle.

The *mentalis* muscle lies on the front of the chin. It is a small muscle that arises from the front and side of the mandible near the midline and inserts into the *orbicularis oris* muscle and the skin overlying the chin. Contraction of the *mentalis* muscle results in upward displacement of the soft tissue of the chin, a forcing of the lower part of the lower lip against the alveolar process of the mandible, and an outward curling of the lower lip. The lower lip may also elevate somewhat during contraction of the *mentalis* muscle. These actions are consistent with the familiar signs of pouting, and indeed, the *mentalis* muscle is sometimes called the pouting muscle.

The *levator anguli oris* muscle (also referred to as the *caninus* muscle) originates from the front of the maxilla and courses downward and forward to insert into both the upper lip and the lower lip near the corner of the mouth. There, its fibers intermingle with those of the *orbicularis oris* muscle. Contraction of the *levator anguli oris* muscle draws the corner of the mouth upward and toward the side. Activation of this muscle can also elevate the lower lip against the upper lip and force the lips together.

The *depressor anguli oris* muscle is also sometimes referred to as the *triangularis* muscle. As its alternate name implies, the muscle is roughly triangular in form. This muscle has a broad origin from the outer surface of the mandible. Its fibers course upward and converge before inserting into the *orbicularis oris* muscle at the corner of the mouth and into the upper lip. Contraction of the *depressor anguli oris* muscle pulls the corner of the mouth downward. It also forces the lips together by drawing the upper lip downward against the lower lip.

There are two parallel facial muscles. These are the *incisivus labii superioris* muscle and the *incisivus labii inferioris* muscle.

The *incisivus labii superioris* muscle is a small, narrow muscle that lies beneath the *levator labii superioris* muscle. Fibers of the *incisivus labii superioris* muscle originate from the maxilla in the region of the canine tooth and course parallel to the transverse fibers of the *orbicularis oris* muscle of the upper lip. This muscle inserts near the corner of the mouth, where its fibers intermingle with the fibers of other muscles. Contraction of the *incisivus labii superioris* muscle pulls the corner of the mouth upward and toward the midline.

The *incisivus labii inferioris* muscle constitutes the lower lip counterpart of the *incisivus labii superioris* muscle. The *incisivus labii inferioris* muscle lies below the corner of the mouth and underneath the *depressor labii superioris* muscle. It originates on the mandible in the region of the lateral incisor tooth and courses parallel to the transverse fibers of the *orbicularis oris* muscle of the lower lip. The insertion of the *incisivus labii inferioris* muscle is into the region of the corner of the mouth. Contraction of the muscle results in a downward and inward pull on the corner of the mouth. The downward component of this action is antagonistic to the upward pull provided by the *incisivus labii superioris* muscle.

The *platysma* muscle is a very broad muscle that covers most of the front and side of the neck and much of the side of the face. The muscle has an extensive origin from a sheet of connective tissue within the neck above the clavicle and may even extend from as far below as the front of the chest wall and regions of the back of the torso. Fibers of the *platysma* muscle run upward and forward to attach to the lower edge of the mandible along the side and interweave with fibers of the opposite side at the front of the mandible. Its fibers have a broad distribution about the face, which includes a blending of fibers associated with different muscles of the lower lip and the corner of the mouth. Contraction of the *platysma* muscle draws the skin of the neck toward the mandible. It may also pull the lower lip and corner of the mouth to the side and downward and/or force the lower lip against the lower teeth and the alveolar process of the mandible.

Figure 5–15 portrays the general force vectors for the 14 muscles of the lips. These vectors summarize the active forces operating on the lips and their consequences on the positioning of the lips and corners of the mouth up and down and side to side, as well as compression of the lips against the teeth and/or alveolar processes of the maxilla and mandible. When the actions of these muscles are combined, they create a seeming infinite variety of lip adjustments that are intricately involved in human expression.

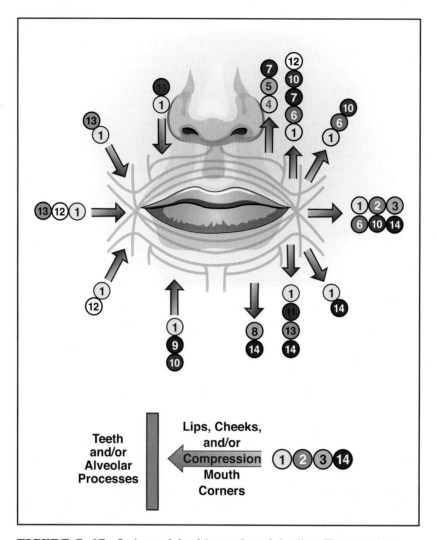

FIGURE 5–15. Actions of the 14 muscles of the lips. The muscles represented are *orbicularis oris* (1), *buccinator* (2), *risorius* (3), *levator labii superioris* (4), *levator labii superioris alaeque nasi* (5), *zygomatic major* 6) *zygomatic minor* (7), *depressor labii inferioris* (8), *mentalis* (9), *levator anguli oris* (10), *depressor anguli oris* (11), *incisivus labii superioris* (12), *incisivus labii inferioris* (13), and *platysma* (14).

MOVEMENTS OF THE PHARYNGEAL-ORAL MECHANISM

Movements of the pharyngeal-oral mechanism allow it to perform a variety of functions involved in speech production and swallowing as well as many other activities. Movements of its component parts—the pharynx, mandible, tongue, and lips—are considered individually below.

Movements of the Pharynx

The potential movements of the overall pharynx are discussed in detail in Chapter 4 and illustrated there (see Figure 4–15). Focus here is on potential movements of the laryngopharynx and oropharynx and their roles in changing the regional lumen of the pharynx and the degree of coupling between the oropharynx and the oral cavity through the palatoglossal arch (anterior faucial pillars). These portions of the pharyngeal tube are relatively mobile and present three movement capabilities: (a) inward and outward movement of their sidewalls, (b) forward and backward movement of their back wall, and (c) forward and backward movement of their front wall (tongue and/or epiglottis). These movements enable the lumen of the laryngopharynx and oropharynx to be changed in size and shape.

The pharynx can change in size from a maximally enlarged pharyngeal airway to one that is fully obstructed. In the case of complete obstruction, the walls of the pharynx may not only come in contact but also undergo forceful compression against one another. Inward movements of the sides of the pharynx are produced mainly through contractions of the *inferior* and *middle constrictor* muscles and outward movements through contractions of the *stylopharyngeus* muscle. The sides of the pharynx can also be moved inward by lowering of the mandible (thereby creating a smaller and more circular lumen) and moved outward by raising the mandible again (Minifie, Hixon, Kelsey, & Woodhouse, 1970). Inward movements of the back wall can be carried out by those same constrictor muscles, and inward movement of the front wall is usually accomplished by the tongue and epiglottis. The position of the upper front wall of the pharyngeal lumen can be changed by the velum, and the lower boundary of the lumen is changed when the height of the larynx changes.

The degree of coupling (connection) between the pharyngeal cavity and oral cavity can be changed by (a) upward and downward movements of the tongue, (b) upward and downward movements of the velum, and (c) side-to-side movements of the pillars of the palatoglossal arch (anterior faucial pillars). Maximum coupling is brought about by a combined maximum elevation of the velum and maximum depression of the tongue. Decoupling (disconnection) of the pharyngeal and oral cavities results when the undersurface of the velum and the upper surface of the tongue are placed in full apposition and the oropharyngeal airway is occluded. When contact between the tongue and the velum occurs, it is also possible to have openings on the left and right sides through which the pharynx and oral cavity are coupled.

Movements of the Mandible

The mandible is capable of a wide range of movements that derive from actions of the temporomandibular joints (see Figure 5–5). Upward and downward movements of the mandible are rotational and take place about a lateral axis that passes through the condyloid processes on the left and right sides of the skull (resembling the swinging of a two-hinged trap door about an axis that extends through the center pins of its hinges). Forward-and-backward and side-to-side movements are accomplished through gliding movements of the mandible along the articular facets of the temporomandibular joints. These three movement possibilities often combine in activities such as the crushing and grinding associated with chewing.

The mandible can be adjusted in position but not in shape. Such adjustment is usually considered in relation to the maxilla because it constitutes the opposing

Early X-Games

This isn't about sports but about x-rays. Early uses of x-rays to study structures of the upper airway during speech production were quite interesting. A few tidbits should give you an appreciation. A narrow gold chain was often placed down the midline of the tongue to make its longitudinal configuration easy to visualize on single-shot lateral head x-rays. Some of the first findings from different laboratories were not in agreement concerning tongue positions during vowel productions. Despite public arguments about linguistic bases for the differences, it turned out that the head had not been fixed in position and variation was related to its rotation from one exposure to another. Then, there were dangers. A pioneer in the use of x-rays for speech research entered old age unable to grow a beard on one side of his face, the side he had frequently bombarded with x-rays to get the view of the speech production mechanism he wanted to study.

jaw for the mandible and is critical to functions that the two structures carry out collaboratively, such as chewing and speaking. Adjustments that lower the mandible result from the action of one or more muscles that include the *external pterygoid*, *digastric* (*anterior* belly), *mylohyoid*, and *geniohyoid* muscles; adjustments that elevate the mandible result from the action of one or more muscles that include the *masseter*, *temporalis*, and *internal pterygoid* muscles. Side-to-side movements are the domain of the *masseter*, *temporalis*, *internal pterygoid*, and *external pterygoid* muscles. And forward movements are caused by actions of the *external pterygoid* muscle and backward movements by actions of the *masseter* and *temporalis* muscles.

Movements of the Tongue

The tongue is a fleshy muscular structure that is exceedingly mobile. Its mobility derives from the fact that (a) it rides with the mandible and goes as a whole where the mandible goes, (b) its position within the oral cavity can be shifted en masse as a body (akin to moving a closed fist around in space), and (c) its shape can be changed markedly and relatively independently of the first two sources of mobility. Movements of the tongue are often segmental and differ along its major (longitudinal) and minor (transverse) axes. Movements of different points on the surface of the structure can be upward and downward, forward and backward, side to side, or different combinations of these. Vertical movements can extend from the trough to the roof of the oral cavity. Front-to-back movements can range from a maximally forward displacement of the tongue out of the mouth to a maximally rearward displacement against the back wall of the pharynx. Side-to-side movements can range from the stretchable limits of one cheek to the other.

The enormous variety of possible tongue adjustments is truly amazing. The tongue can protrude, retract, lateralize, centralize, curl, point, lick, bulge, groove, flatten, rotate, and do many other things such as picking between the teeth. What seems to be a near-infinite array of adjustments relates to its special mechanical endowment that allows it to function as a muscular hydrostat (Kier & Smith, 1985; Smith & Kier, 1989). A muscular hydrostat is a pliable structure without bones that has connective tissue that allows it to change shape while maintaining its overall volume. It is a pliable structure that is incompressible and behaves somewhat like a water-filled balloon. Examples of other muscular hydrostats are octopus tentacles and elephant trunks, as depicted in Figure 5–16.

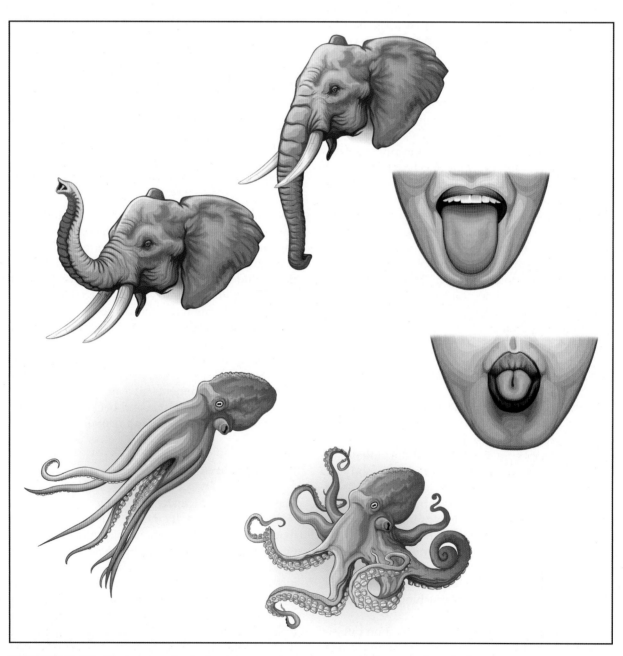

FIGURE 5–16. Three muscular hydrostats: an octopus arm, an elephant trunk, and a human tongue.

This special property of the tongue, along with its personal soft skeleton that encapsulates it, provides leverages for the eight muscles that give rise to its motive force. Because of its hydrostatic properties, inward displacement of one part of the tongue brings about outward displacement of another part (like squeezing one part of a water-filled balloon and seeing another part bulge outward). The selective contraction of different muscle fibers can change the location and shape of the tongue.

Although conceptualization of the tongue as a muscular hydrostat has been largely accepted for decades, it has been difficult to study tongue movements from this perspective until recently. New technological advances have allowed the entire tongue volume to be tracked during speaking in a four-dimensional landscape (three-dimensional space by time) (Woo, Xing, Lee, Stone, & Prince, 2016), even in disordered tongues (Woo et al., 2019).

Take It Away

The tongue rides with the mandible and goes where it goes. Thus, when trying to interpret changes in the configuration of the tongue surface, it's necessary to determine how much is attributable to adjustment of the tongue and how much is attributable to adjustment of the mandible. Suppose you had a client with a hyperkinetic disease in which both the tongue and mandible went through adventitious involuntary excursions. How could you go about parsing them in your evaluation? Not to worry! Have the client speak through clenched teeth or while biting down on a small stack of tongue depressors. Then, the abnormal movements of the tongue are on their own and not confounded by the abnormal movements of the mandible. It's called removing a degree of freedom of performance, and the principle can be applied in many ways when analyzing different structures involved in speech production.

Movements of the Lips

The mobility of the face in the region of the lips rivals that of the fine movements of the fingers. Movements of the lips can occur along vertical, side-to-side, and front-to-back dimensions. Each lip can be moved independently of the other or the two lips can be coordinated in their movements. The upper lip is fixed in spatial coordinates to the fixed position of the maxilla, whereas the lower lip rides with the mandible so that its movements are dictated, in part, by the prevailing position of the mandible. The lips can be puckered, protruded, retracted, spread, pointed, curled inward and outward, rounded, and plumped and can be associated with a host of facial expressions, such as smiling, smirking, sulking, and sneering. The multitude of possible lip adjustments is created by different combinations of the more than a dozen muscles that impart forces to the lips (see Figure 5–15). Experimenting with lip movements in front of a mirror gives one an appreciation for the degrees of freedom of lip movement.

The Cold War

With prolonged exposure to very cold weather, your face tightens up and your speech slows down. Certain parts of your speech production mechanism actually get stiffer as you chill down. You can live with this because your body, although coping with change at the periphery, is still winning the cold war. Should things get worse, however, such that hypothermia sets in, you'll be in trouble. Hypothermia occurs when your body can't replace heat lost to its surroundings and your core temperature begins to drop. From the usual 98.6°F down to 95°F, your speech will continue to sound normal. Below 95°F down to 90°F, your speech will become slurred and progressively more so as temperature decreases. Once your core temperature passes below 90°F, your speech will be unintelligible. The cooling of the body is simply too much for the nervous system to handle, and all remaining resources are devoted to preserving the organism.

Adjustments of the lips can be viewed from a variety of perspectives, such as (a) the position and shape of each lip, (b) the position and shape of the corners of the mouth, (c) the compression between the lips and/or between one or both lips and the teeth and gums, and (d) the configuration (cross section and length) of the channel that forms the airway opening. The first two of these are often considered significant contributors to facial expression, whereas compression between the lips is relevant to activities such as drinking through a straw. The configuration of the channel that forms the airway opening is especially critical to the formation of the acoustic speech product. During speaking, this channel is frequently lengthened or shortened, changed in shape, and moved from side to side (consider talking out one side of the mouth, the so-called sidewinder). The lips may even be in apposition on one side and be parted on the other, as in the dying breed of the smoker who talks with a cigarette hanging from one side of the mouth.

PHARYNGEAL-ORAL MECHANISM CONTROL VARIABLES

Several control variables may be important in pharyngeal-oral function, depending on the activity being performed, whether it is breathing, speaking, singing, whistling, wind instrument playing, blowing, sucking, chewing, or swallowing. Discussion here is devoted to four control variables: (a) pharyngeal-oral lumen size and configuration, (b) pharyngeal-oral contact pressure, (c) pharyngeal-oral airway resistance, and (d) pharyngeal-oral acoustic impedance.

Pharyngeal-Oral Lumen Size and Configuration

The lumen of the pharyngeal-oral mechanism (its inner open space) can be changed in both size and shape by adjusting the positions of structures that line the pharyngeal-oral airway. These adjustments can change physical dimensions such as length, longitudinal configuration, diameter, cross-sectional area, and cross-sectional configuration.

Open Wide

Your mandible and maxilla are separated by only a small distance when you produce speech. Activities such as calling your dog, yelling at a football game, or singing often get you to open up more. Classical (opera) singing is one activity that gets people to open very wide. One form of classical singing teaches what is referred to as a four-finger jaw position. Try it. Place the four fingers of one hand together and then, with your thumb on that hand pointing upward, insert your fingers vertically at the midline between your upper and lower front teeth. Quite a stretch, isn't it? It comes close to maximum separation between your mandible and maxilla and gives you nearly as large a mouth opening as you can achieve (or tolerate). What a great way to get that beautiful singing voice to radiate outward from the singer to the audience.

The open space that constitutes the pharyngeal-oral lumen can be either increased or decreased from the resting configuration. Figure 5–17 summarizes the structures that may contribute individually or in combination to changing the lumen of the airway in the pharyngeal cavity, the oral cavity, and the oral vestibule. Length changes of the pharyngeal-oral lumen can be achieved (a) within the pharyngeal cavity, by different combinations of adjustments of the velum and larynx; (b) within the oral cavity, by different combinations of adjustments of the tongue and mandible; and (c) within the oral vestibule, by different combinations of adjustments of the lips and mandible. Cross-sectional changes can be achieved (a) within the pharynx, by different combinations of adjustments of the tongue, epiglottis, posterior pharyngeal wall, and lateral pharyngeal walls; (b) within the oral cavity, by different combinations of adjustments of the tongue and mandible; and (c) within the oral vestibule, by different combinations of adjustments of the lips, mandible, cheeks, and tongue.

Given the lengthwise and cross-sectional adjustment possibilities noted, the number of options for luminal changes in the pharyngeal-oral apparatus is exceedingly large. This underpins the fact that the acoustic products that emanate from the pharyngeal-oral mechanism (such as speech and song) can be richly variable.

Pharyngeal-Oral Structural Contact Pressure

Adjustments of the pharyngeal-oral mechanism can result in full obstruction of the pharyngeal-oral lumen at different locations. Full obstruction can be accomplished through structural contact of (a) the tongue against the pharynx, velum, hard palate, alveolar process of the maxilla, teeth, and lips and (b) the lips against the teeth and against one another. Once two structures are in apposition, the contact pressure between them can be adjusted to meet the needs of the situation. Figure 5–18 portrays structural contact and its resultant compressive force between the tongue and the alveolar process of the maxilla.

Structural contact pressure can be influenced by several factors. These include (a) muscular pressure exerted by muscular components of the contacting surfaces (tongue against alveolar ridge or two lips against one another), (b) surface tension between apposed surfaces that are moist (tongue against hard palate) and hold them together, and (c) gravity that weighs down structures and acts on them differently in different

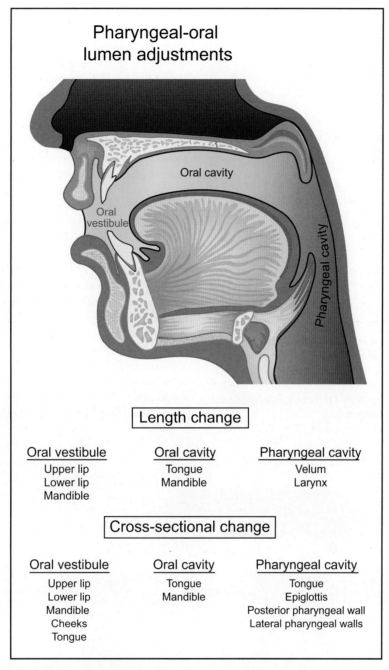

FIGURE 5–17. Regional structures contributing to adjustments of the pharyngeal-oral lumen. Length changes in the lumen can be achieved by movements of the larynx, velum, tongue, mandible, and lips. Cross-sectional changes in the lumen can be achieved by movements of the pharyngeal walls, epiglottis, tongue, mandible, lips, and cheeks.

body positions. The most significant of these three is the muscular pressure. Contact pressure for an activity may require low-level muscular exertion for soft contact between structures or it may require high contact pressure when it is necessary to fortify the contact in the face of high air pressures in the vicinity.

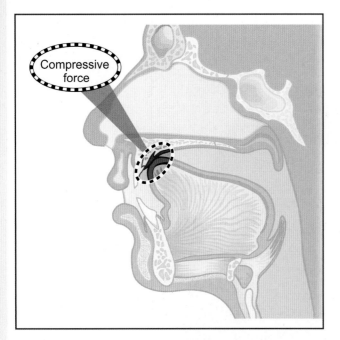

FIGURE 5–18. Structural contact pressure between the tongue and alveolar process of the maxilla. The magnitude of the contact pressure is determined by the muscular pressure exerted by the different structures, the surface tension between the surfaces, and gravity. Of these three, muscular pressure is by far the most important.

Pharyngeal-Oral Airway Resistance

Pharyngeal-oral airway resistance, portrayed in Figure 5–19, is a calculated measure of the opposition provided by the pharyngeal-oral mechanism to mass airflow through it. Airway resistance is calculated from the quotient of the pressure drop across any segment of interest and the airflow through that segment. As was the case with laryngeal airway resistance, pharyngeal-oral airway resistance is a property of the airway itself and is airflow dependent. This means that resistance increases or decreases with increases or decreases in the rate at which air moves, even without changes in the physical dimensions of the pharyngeal-oral airway. However, it is the change in the cross section of the airway that causes the greatest change in pharyngeal-oral airway resistance. By decreasing the cross-sectional area of the airway anywhere within these regions, the airway resistance will likely increase. Such change can occur anywhere along the length of the pharyngeal-oral airway, from larynx to lips, but is most prominently the result of adjustments within the oropharynx, oral cavity, and oral vestibule. The range of potential airway resistance values is from very low (associated with a wide open pharyngeal-oral airway) to infinity (associated with a completely closed pharyngeal-oral airway).

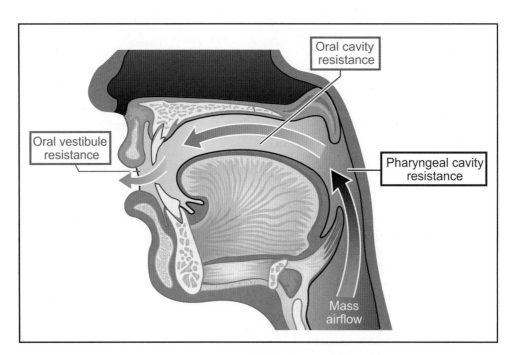

FIGURE 5–19. Pharyngeal-oral airway resistance is a calculated measure of the opposition of the pharyngeal-oral airway to mass airflow through it. The greatest changes in pharyngeal-oral airway resistance are due to changes in cross-sectional area in the oropharynx, oral cavity, and oral vestibule.

Pharyngeal-Oral Acoustic Impedance

The pharyngeal-oral mechanism plays an important role in the control of acoustic impedance, which, like airway resistance, involves opposition to flow. However, this opposition is not to mass airflow but to the movement of energy in the form of sound waves through the mechanism (Figure 5–20). These waves function like an alternating current in which adjacent air molecules collide with each other and pass energy on to their neighbors. Acoustic impedance influences how well sound waves propagate through the pharyngeal-oral airway.

Acoustic impedance is determined to a great extent by cross-sectional adjustments of the pharyngeal-oral mechanism. When the cross section of the pharyngeal-oral lumen is large, sound waves pass relatively freely through it. In contrast, when the cross section of the lumen is small, sound energy does not pass as freely. Relative decreases in the cross section of the lumen at different locations simultaneously may also influence the degree to which different segments of the pharyngeal-oral lumen interact with one another acoustically.

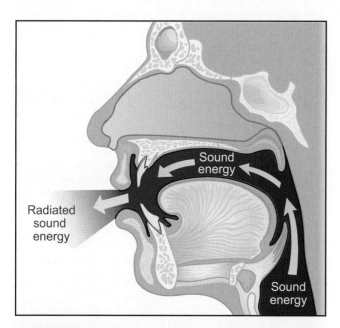

FIGURE 5–20. Pharyngeal-oral acoustic impedance. This impedance relates to the ease with which sound waves propagate through the pharyngeal-oral airway. The more open the airway, the lower the acoustic impedance. Note that, in this figure, the velopharynx is closed so that velopharyngeal-nasal impedance is near infinite (a small amount of sound energy may be transmitted through the velum via sympathetic vibration).

Low-Energy Physics

Speech is clearly an energy producing enterprise. But just how much energy is involved? One scientist has calculated that 300 to 400 ergs of energy is expended in the resultant sound wave when the sentence "Joe took father's shoe-bench out" is produced at usual loudness (Fletcher, 1953). That's not a sentence that most people run around saying, and many readers might not have an appreciation for how 300 to 400 ergs relate to their everyday lives. Perhaps we can help a bit. You and 499 of your closest friends (that's a Boeing-747 aircraft with all the seats filled or an Airbus A380 with a few empty seats) would have to say "Joe took father's shoe-bench out" together at your usual loudness continuously for a year to produce enough energy to heat a cup of coffee. Holy Starbucks! That's a lot of talking. It would undoubtedly contend for a Guinness World Record, but on nature's energy scale, it wouldn't amount to much.

NEURAL SUBSTRATES OF PHARYNGEAL-ORAL CONTROL

Pharyngeal-oral movements are controlled by different parts of the central nervous system, depending on the activity being performed. Thus, speaking and swallowing, while engaging the same pharyngeal-oral structures, are under different central nervous system control; however, all control commands are sent through the same set of peripheral nerves. Much more consideration is given to central and peripheral nervous system control for speaking and swallowing elsewhere in the book (see Chapters 7 and 8). A brief summary of the peripheral nerves that innervate the pharyngeal-oral mechanism is provided here.

As shown in Table 5–2, motor innervation of the pharynx is provided through the pharyngeal plexus, which includes fibers from cranial nerves IX (glossopharyngeal), X (vagus), and possibly XI (accessory). Motor innervation to the mandible comes from cranial nerve V (trigeminal) and the first cervical spinal nerve (C1). Motor innervation of the tongue includes cranial nerves X and XII, whereas motor innervation of the lips is through cranial nerve VII (facial).

Sensory innervation to the pharynx is carried by cranial nerves IX and X, and sensory innervation to the mandible is supplied by cranial nerve V. The tongue

Ten Four, Good Buddy

Bell's palsy is a relatively common condition that affects cranial nerve VII, the nerve that innervates the muscles of the face. Upper and lower facial muscles can become weak or paralyzed and speech production can be impaired. Most often the cause is unknown and the problem is on one side. It may involve an autoimmune inflammatory response, a herpes viral infection, or a swelling of the nerve because of allergy. Most people who get Bell's palsy make a full recovery, especially if they're young. Exposure to cold can be a factor in Bell's palsy. Truck drivers who keep the driver's-side window down may contract Bell's palsy from the cold because wind chill for a prolonged period across the side of the face near the window is believed to be a contributing factor to onset of the problem. Which side depends on the country in which you're driving.

TABLE 5–2. Summary of Motor and Sensory Nerve Supply to the Pharynx, Mandible, Tongue, and Lips

COMPONENT	INNERVATION	
	MOTOR	SENSORY
Pharynx	IX[a], X, (XI)[b]	IX, X
Mandible	V, C1[c]	V
Tongue	X[d], XII	V, VII, IX
Lips	VII	V

Note. Peripheral nerves indicated in the table and notes are cranial nerves V (trigeminal), VII (facial), IX (glossopharyngeal), X (vagus), XI (accessory), and XII (hypoglossal) and cervical spinal nerve 1 (C1).

[a]The only pharyngeal muscle innervated by cranial nerve IX is the **stylopharyngeus** muscle.

[b]The branches of cranial nerves IX and X (and possibly XI) that innervate parts of the pharynx are sometimes called the *pharyngeal plexus*.

[c]The only mandibular muscle innervated by C1 is the **geniohyoid** muscle.

[d]The only tongue muscle innervated by cranial nerve X is the **palatoglossus** muscle.

receives sensory supply from cranial nerves V, VII, and IX, whereas supply to the lips is from cranial nerve V. Neural information traveling along the sensory nerves supplying the pharynx, mandible, tongue, and lips results from the activation of receptors of various types within those structures. These receptors include an array of mechanoreceptors that are differentially distributed (some occurring in certain locations more than others) throughout the tissues of the pharyngeal-oral mechanism. When sound results from pharyngeal-oral activity, mechanoreceptors formed by hair cells within the cochlea (end organ of the auditory system) may be activated. Sensory information from the auditory system travels via cranial nerve VIII (auditory-vestibular nerve; see Chapter 6).

The mechanoreceptors within the pharyngeal-oral mechanism are sensitive to a variety of stimuli and are capable of providing the nervous system with many types of information, including information about (a) muscle length, (b) rate of change in muscle length, (c) muscle tension, (d) joint position, (e) joint movement, (f) touch, (g) surface pressure, (h) deep pressure, (i) surface deformation, (j) temperature, and (k) vibration, among others. Mechanoreceptors within the pharyngeal-oral mechanism (and within the auditory system during speech production) provide the central nervous system with information that is used to keep track of the recent status of the mechanism and to guide anticipated actions.

Myth Conceptions

The history of speech-language pathology is rich with clinical theories and methods that don't actually involve speech production directly. These have taken many forms. One early one took the point of view that language had its beginnings in chewing and that chewing exercises had a prominent role in the treatment of speech and voice disorders. The originator of this idea said that he conceived the notion when confronted with two Egyptian hieroglyphic scripts that showed a similar sign for eating and speaking. Despite using some of the same pharyngeal-oral structures, chewing and speaking are controlled differently by the nervous system, and one is not a precursor or analog of the other. Other forms of nonspeech activities and devices continue to be used even today as if they were somehow beneficial to speech production. We don't subscribe to any of these misconceptions. You shouldn't either.

SPEECH PRODUCTION: SOUND GENERATION AND FILTERING

The pharyngeal-oral mechanism performs many functions. Of particular relevance to this book are those related to speaking and swallowing. This section provides a brief description of the role of the pharyngeal-oral mechanism in sound generation and filtering, and the next two sections cover articulatory descriptions and processes. Its role in swallowing (including chewing) is covered in Chapter 7.

Sound generation refers to the creation of a sound (acoustic) source, and filtering refers to the shaping of a sound. The pharyngeal-oral mechanism does both: It generates and filters sound. The concepts of source (sound generation) and filtering were introduced in Chapter 3 and explained in reference to the larynx in Video 3–7. These concepts are revisited in this section as they pertain to the pharyngeal-oral mechanism.

A speaker of general American English produces two types of sound sources (for consonants) using the pharyngeal-oral mechanism: (a) transient (popping) sounds, in which the oral airstream is momentarily interrupted and then released, and (b) turbulence (hissing) sounds, in which air is forced through a narrow constriction. Speakers can produce other types of pharyngeal-oral sounds, such as trills and raspberries, but

discussion here is restricted to sounds used by adults speaking general American English.

Transient sounds are produced by obstructing the airflow somewhere along the pharyngeal-oral airway and then releasing it quickly. This is analogous to the transient sound produced by the larynx (glottal stop; see Chapter 3, Figure 3–36). Figure 5–21 provides an illustration of the production of the transient sound "t." On the left is shown a sagittal view of the pharyngeal-oral airway with the tongue in full contact with the maxillary alveolar ridge and air pressure building behind the obstruction. On the right is shown the sudden decoupling of the tongue from the hard palate and release of air through the constriction. A "t" sound is classified as a stop-plosive: "stop" for the obstruction phase of the production (when no sound is heard) and "plosive" for the release phase (when the "pop" is heard). The classification of stop-plosives and other speech sounds is discussed in more detail in the next section on articulatory descriptions.

Turbulence sounds are also produced in the pharyngeal-oral airway in much the same way as they are in the larynx (during whispering or "h" productions; Chapter 3, Figure 3–37): by forcing air through a small constriction. One example is an "s," depicted in Figure 5–22. This figure illustrates the forcing of air through a small constriction formed between the

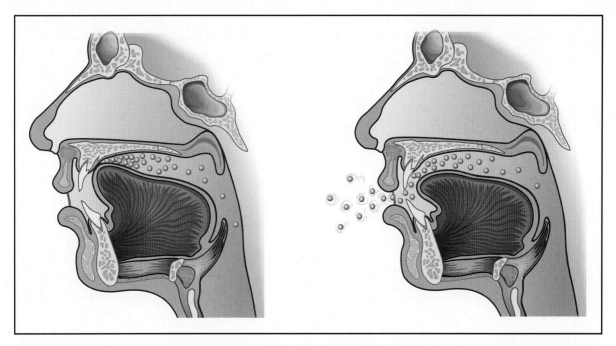

FIGURE 5–21. Sagittal view of the production of a "t," including the obstruction phase (*left*) and plosive phase (*right*). Air molecules are depicted as blue spheres. Air pressure builds behind the obstruction created by the tongue against the maxillary alveolar ridge (shown as a clustering of molecules), and then the air is released quickly when the tongue rapidly decouples from the palate.

tongue tip and the alveolar ridge. The resulting turbulence creates the noise we hear as an "s."

The pharyngeal-oral mechanism not only generates sounds but also filters the sounds it generates. For example, the "sh" sound is produced by placing the tongue in a somewhat flattened configuration, positioning it near (but not touching) the alveolar ridge and pushing air through the relatively small constriction. What we hear is the "sh" sound, whether produced in isolation or in the context of a word like "sheet" or "shoe." To be more explicit, what we actually hear is not only the sound created by the air moving through the constriction (the sound source) but the sound source *plus* how the sound source is filtered by the cavity in front of the constriction. This can be illustrated by "looking" at the "sh" under two conditions: when it is produced with spread lips and with rounded lips. The sound produced under these two conditions is shown in the form of a spectrogram (time on the horizontal axis and frequency on the vertical axis) in Figure 5–23. Even without knowledge of how the spectrogram is made or what it means, it is clear that the two "sh" sounds—that produced with spread lips ("spread" in the figure) and that produced with rounded lips ("rounded" in the figure)—look different. For example, the sh-spread production created a dark band in the region of 3000 to 4000 Hz, whereas the sh-rounded production did not but instead created a dark band in the 4000- to 5000-Hz region. These two "sh" productions look different because the filter through which the sound source passed was different: One filter was wide and open (spread lips), and the other was long and constricted (rounded lips). What is particularly

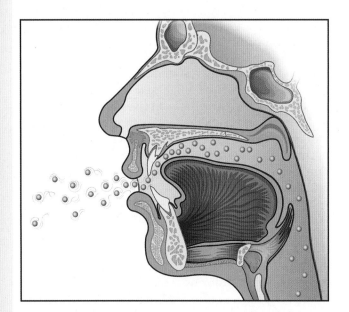

FIGURE 5–22. Sagittal view of the production of an "s" as air is forced through the narrow constriction created between the tongue tip and the alveolar ridge. Notice the turbulence in the airflow (swirling molecules) as it exits the lips, causing the noisy sound that we recognize as "s."

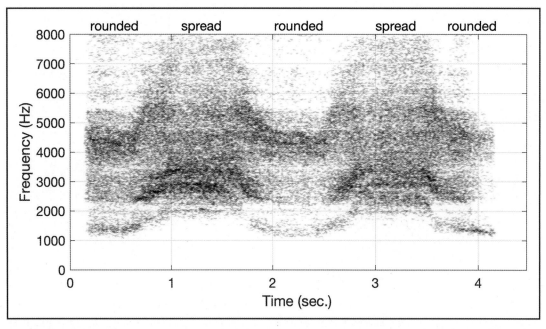

FIGURE 5–23. Spectrogram of "sh" produced (alternately) with spread lips and rounded lips. Frequency is on the *y*-axis and time on the *x*-axis. The darker areas indicate the frequency regions that contain the most energy.

interesting about this example is that these two "sh" sounds, although they appear acoustically quite different, are both perceived as "sh." The explanation for this is beyond the scope of this book; motivated readers are encouraged to read further on the fascinating topic of speech perception (e.g., Hixon, Weismer, & Hoit, 2020, Chap. 12).

The pharyngeal-oral mechanism not only filters its own sounds but also filters sounds that are generated by the larynx. Any sound generated by the larynx—via vocal fold vibration, sustained turbulence (such as whisper), or glottal stop production—must pass through the pharyngeal-oral airway (and sometimes the velopharyngeal-nasal airway). Thus, the sound that emerges from the lips is different from the sound that was generated at the larynx. This has been discussed briefly in Chapter 3 and illustrated in Video 3–6 (Source-Filter) for a voiced sentence and a whispered sentence. Another example is provided here in Figure 5–24. This figure is a spectrogram that reflects the frequency distributions of two vowels, "ee" and "oo," produced in an alternating pattern. Without concern for the details of what the spectrogram reveals about the acoustic content of these two sounds, it is clear that these two sounds are very different; in fact, we hear them as two different vowels. However, if we were to listen to the sound coming from the larynx (without the pharyngeal-oral mechanism attached), they would sound the same. This is a dramatic illustration of how much the pharyngeal-oral part of the speech mechanism influences the sound that emerges from the lips.

Duck and Cover

Aeromechanical and acoustic energies come out of your mouth during speech production. Other things also make their way out. One of these is saliva. Today your salivary glands might produce up to a quart of liquid. Tiny drops of saliva spew from your mouth when you speak. These are usually invisible and emerge as wet clouds that can hang around an hour or more and settle on nearby listeners. Each word spoken sends about 2.5 droplets of saliva into the atmosphere (Bodanis, 1995). Read this sidetrack aloud and you'll expel about 400 droplets of saliva. Do the same with the Gettysburg Address and the number will reach 700. The U.S. Constitution would get you about 11,000 droplets. And what would an assembly of 500 people reciting the Pledge of Allegiance get you? Forty thousand droplets dispersed in 500 wet clouds. This heretofore rarely noticed phenomenon suddenly became an international topic of discussion as we came to recognize the serious risk posed by speaking in the era of COVID-19 (Stadnytskyi, Bax, Bax, & Anfinrud, 2020).

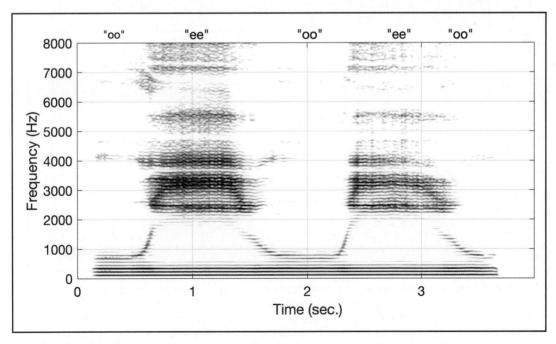

FIGURE 5–24. Spectrogram of alternating productions of "ee" and "oo." Frequency is on the *y*-axis and time on the *x*-axis, and the darker areas indicate the frequency regions that contain the most energy.

SPEECH PRODUCTION: ARTICULATORY DESCRIPTIONS

The pharyngeal-oral mechanism is often referred to as the articulatory part of the speech mechanism (in this context, an articulator is defined as a movable structure that contributes to the production of speech sounds). This section focuses on how speech sounds are described and categorized; the next section covers articulatory processes and how they play out in real time.

Articulatory descriptions of speech sounds are often separated into different types. For each type of speech sound (e.g., vowels), a finer description is made to characterize articulatory differences within the type. These descriptions for the sounds of American English are considered here. For an excellent introduction to articulatory descriptions for virtually all sounds in languages of the world, see https://en.wikipedia.org/wiki/International_Phonetic_Alphabet

The articulatory description presented here is simplified from more detailed schemes (https://www.internationalphoneticassociation.org/IPAcharts/inter_chart_2018/IPA_2018.html). This description uses the International Phonetic Alphabet (IPA) and considers the broad categories of sonorants and obstruents. Sonorants are sounds produced with a relatively open pharyngeal-oral airway (vocal tract) or nasal airway (nasal tract), which allows air and sound to flow freely from the glottis and through the lips or nose. The sonorants include vowels, diphthongs, and two types of consonants: semivowels and nasals. In American English, all sonorants are produced with vocal fold vibration. Obstruents are sounds produced with a constriction or obstruction and include three types of consonants: stops, fricatives, and affricates. In Figures 5–25 and 5–26, sonorants are shown in blue and obstruents are shown in orange.

Vowels

Vowels are usually produced with voicing by the larynx and with velopharyngeal closure (although they can be nasalized and are even intentionally nasalized in many languages). All vowels are sonorants; thus, all of Figure 5–25 is colored blue. Vowels can be described using the three dimensions of *place of major constriction* within the pharyngeal-oral mechanism, *degree of major constriction*, and *degree of lip rounding*.

Degree of major oral constriction	Place of major oral constriction				
	Front	**Central**		**Back**	
High	i beat ɪ bit			u tooth ʊ hook	Increasing lip-rounding
Mid	e bait ɛ bet	ɝ word ʌ bug	ɚ onward ə above	o boast ɔ taught	
Low	æ bat			ɑ cot	

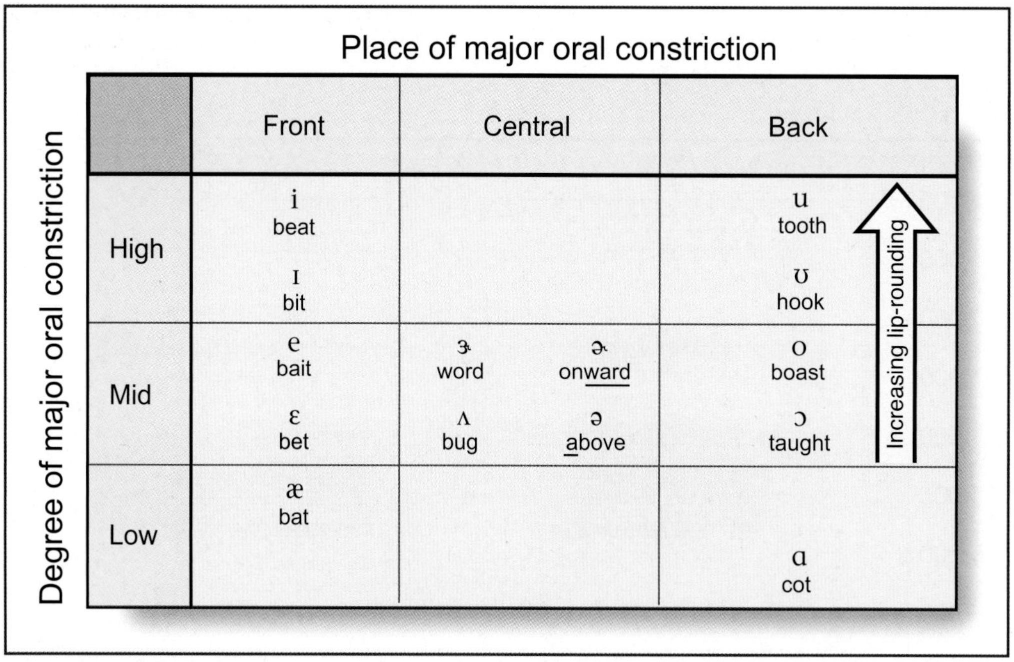

FIGURE 5–25. Vowel description. Vowels are sonorants and are categorized for American English in terms of place of major constriction, degree of major constriction, and degree of lip rounding. Vowel symbols are from the International Phonetic Alphabet. Note that for the words "onward" and "above," the target part of the word is underlined. Most word exemplars are from Fairbanks (1960).

Place of Major Constriction

Place of major constriction specifies the location at which the pharyngeal-oral airway is maximally constricted during vowel production. Three locations are specified: *front*, *central*, and *back*. The term *front* is used to designate constrictions formed between the tongue blade and the alveolar process of the maxilla. The term *central* is used to indicate constrictions formed between the tongue and the hard palate or when no obvious constriction exists. And the term *back* designates constrictions formed between the tongue and the velum, or between the tongue and the posterior pharyngeal wall. Five vowels fall under the rubric *front* vowels, four are classified as *central* vowels, and five are considered *back* vowels. Changes across the *place of major constriction* dimension can be viewed as shifts in the position of the tongue along the length coordinate of the pharyngeal-oral mechanism.

Degree of Major Constriction

Degree of major constriction designates the cross-sectional size of the constricted region of the airway.

This dimension typically specifies a *high*, *mid*, or *low* degree of major constriction and corresponds, in most circumstances, to the location of the highest point of the tongue surface in relation to the roof of the oral cavity. Exceptions occur when the major constriction is formed between the back of the tongue and the posterior pharyngeal wall. *High* degrees of constriction correspond to small cross-sectional areas at the major constriction, *mid* degrees of constriction are associated with intermediate size cross sections, and *low* degrees of constriction involve large cross-sectional areas. The size of the constricted area of the airway is influenced by the position of the mandible, which influences the height of the tongue. For example, low vowels typically have lower mandible positions as compared to high vowels.

Lip Rounding

Lip rounding designates the degree to which the lips are protruded and the area between them is reduced. Protrusion often correlates directly with the size of the airway opening at the lips. Thus, an increase in lip

		Place of production						
Manner of production		Bilabial (lips)	Labiodental (lip-teeth)	Dental (tongue-teeth)	Alveolar (tongue-gum)	Palatal (tongue-hard palate)	Velar (tongue-velum)	Glottal (vocal folds)
	Stop-plosive −	p (pole)			t (toll)		k (coal)	
	+	b (bowl)			d (dole)		g (goal)	
	Fricative −		f (fat)	θ (thigh)	s (seal)	ʃ (ash)		h (hot)
	+		v (vat)	ð (thy)	z (zeal)	ʒ (azure)		
	Affricate −					tʃ (choke)		
	+					dʒ (joke)		
	Nasal −							
	+	m (sum)			n (sun)		ŋ (sung)	
	Semivowel −							
	+	w (watt)			l (lot)	j,r (yacht, rot)		

FIGURE 5–26. Consonant description. Consonants can be obstruents (*orange*) or sonorants (*blue*). Consonants for American English are categorized in terms of manner of production, place of production, and voicing. Voiceless and voiced elements are designated by − and + signs, respectively. Consonant symbols are from the International Phonetic Alphabet. Word exemplars are from Fairbanks (1960).

rounding corresponds to a simultaneous lengthening and narrowing of the lip channel along the oral vestibule, whereas a decrease in lip rounding corresponds to a simultaneous shortening and opening up of the lip channel. This relationship between lip protrusion and decrease of the channel size is not an anatomical necessity as demonstrated by the fact that some languages have vowels sounds with substantial narrowing of the lip channel without protrusion of the lips. In American English, lip rounding occurs only on *mid*-constriction and *high*-constriction *back* vowels.

Real-Life Vowels

One way to bring this classification system to life is to see what vowels actually look like when produced by a person. The images in Figure 5–27 show mid-sagittal magnetic resonance (MR) images of an adult male producing seven vowels that correspond to the place and degree of major constriction represented in the vowel chart (see Figure 5–25). Video 5–1 (Vowel Articulation) shows how vowel production plays out in real time.

Diphthongs

Diphthongs are sonorant sounds that are vowel-like in nature. The classic phonetic view is that they are transitional hybrids of vowels that are formed by rapidly changing from one vowel position to another. Thus, they are transcribed as pairs of vowels, there being five such pairs in American English—/ɑɪ/ (as in bide), /ɔɪ/ (as in boy), /ɑʊ/ (as in bough), /eɪ/ (as in bait), and /oʊ/ (as in boat)—although diphthongs vary sub-stantially across American dialects. The fact that the "ai" in the word "bait" is included here as a diphthong and above as a vowel (in Figure 5–25) is a perfect example of this. In some parts of the country, the "ai" in the word "bait" is produced as a vowel, and in other parts of the country, it is pronounced as a diphthong. Each of these diphthongs is formed by a vowel pair in which the first vowel is characterized by a lesser degree of major constriction than the second vowel. Diphthongs may comprise vowel pairs that transition (a) within the same place of major constriction, (b) from back to front places of constriction, and (c) from mid to high degrees of constriction that include increases in lip rounding. Given that diphthongs are viewed as transitional hybrids of vowel pairs in the classic phonetic view, their production description may be conceptualized in terms of their vowel beginning and ending points and nearly continuous adjustments in between. Nevertheless, this usual phonetic conceptualization of diphthongs is not without controversy. Acoustic studies of diphthong formation have suggested that they have unique features that are different from pure vowels and that their transitional components contain defining features that show them to be a different sound class than vowels.

Consonants

Consonants can be classified as obstruents or sonorants, as represented in the color scheme in Figure 5–26. Consonants are described along three dimensions: *manner of production* (five categories), *place of production* (seven categories), and *voicing* (two categories). These three

---

More on Real-Life Vowels

The IPA vowel chart in Figure 5–25 is a general guide to the vowel categories of American English. It does not show the vowels of other languages, which can differ substantially from the vowels of English. For example, Swedish has a vowel that is very much like a lip-rounded version of American English /i/ (as in "beat"). A vowel chart that shows all vowel categories currently known in languages of the world is available at https://www.internationalphoneticassociation.org/IPAcharts/inter_chart_2018/IPA_2018.html. The phonetic symbols in the IPA vowel chart are idealized representations of vowel categories. This is different from the way speakers produce vowels in "real life." Dialect variation provides examples of the difference between IPA symbols and the actual sound of vowels in spoken language. For example, the IPA vowel chart shows /ɔ/ and /ɑ/ as different vowel categories, and in many American English dialects, this indeed is the case. In parts of the eastern United States, the vowel in "cot" (/ɑ/) is different from the vowel in "caught" (/ɔ/). In contrast, in other parts of the western United States, words like "cot" and "caught" are spoken with very similar vowel quality—they both sound like /ɔ/. In yet other parts of the country, vowels in these words (and others like them) also sound the same, but in this case like /ɑ/! The examples of /ɔ/ and /ɑ/ are good demonstrations of the potential distance between the IPA vowel symbols and vowels in real life.

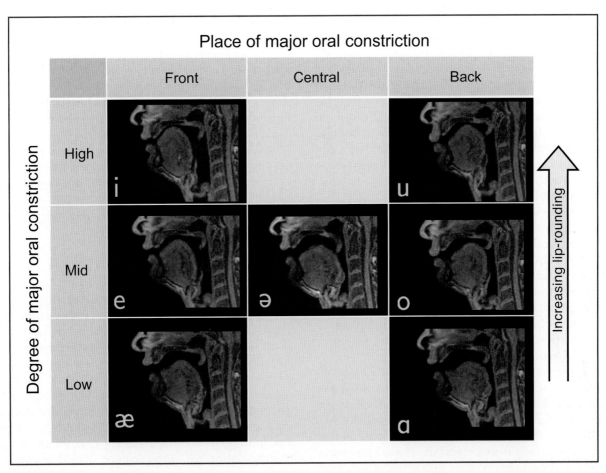

FIGURE 5–27. Mid-sagittal magnetic resonance (MR) images of a man producing seven different vowels (MR images courtesy of Adam Baker).

dimensions yield 70 (5 × 7 × 2) unique consonant possibilities. About one-third of these are used in American English.

Manner of Production

Manner of production specifies the way in which structures of the larynx, velopharynx, and pharyngeal-oral mechanism constrict or obstruct the airway to produce a consonant. The manner of production dimension includes the five categories referred to as *stop-plosive*, *fricative*, *affricate*, *nasal*, and *semivowel*. Both semivowels and nasals are sonorants but are often described as consonants.

Stop-plosive consonants begin with occlusion of the oral airway and a buildup of oral air pressure behind the occlusion followed by an abrupt opening of the airway and burst of airflow (recall the "t" production in Figure 5–21). Such actions are usually generated with airtight closure of the velopharynx. Sometimes stop consonants do not include a burst of airflow following occlusion; rather, the pent-up air is released through a lowered velum to escape inaudibly through

Raspberries

Raspberries are sounds that resemble sustained flatulence (farting). Raspberries are made by blowing air between a protruded tongue and the lips. Adults use raspberries to indicate derision, sarcasm, or silliness. All cultures seem to have a fondness for them. Infants especially like them and use them in their early sound play. Raspberries aren't used as sounds in human languages. Thus, they fade from the repertoire of experimental noises as the infant figures out that they're not an important part of the linguistic code. Nevertheless, the skill acquired is not wasted. They return later on as full-blown Bronx cheers to be used to put someone down, sarcastically cheer a poor sports performance, or be the final gesture after a lost argument. Blow a raspberry the next time you see a primate at a zoo. Most primates make raspberries. You'll either get one back or get a weird look from a resident.

the nose. Stop consonants produced in this fashion are referred to as imploded stop consonants. This type of stop consonant occurs in American English but is not phonemically distinctive (that is, does not constitute a different sound category). Recall that it is also possible to produce a stop-plosive with the larynx and that this is called a glottal stop (see Chapter 3). Glottal stops are not typically phonemic in American English, although they are in some other languages. It is, however, not uncommon for some talkers to substitute a glottal stop for a "t" sound, for example, to replace the "t" in "button" with a glottal stop.

Fricative consonants are generated when air is forced at high velocity through a narrowly constricted pharyngeal-oral or laryngeal airway (such as the "sh" in Figure 5–22). Such sounds derive their acoustic energy from turbulence airflow near their constrictions and from airflow striking nearby obstacles such as the teeth. Fricative consonants are usually produced with a closed velopharynx, although this is not obligatory if the constriction is upstream of the velopharynx, as in a fricative produced within the larynx (/h/).

Affricate consonants start out much like stop-plosive consonants with an occluded oral airway and air pressure building up behind the occlusion. The occlusion for affricate consonants is released, but less abruptly than it is for stop-plosive consonants so that the burst of airflow is less vigorous. The release phase of affricate consonants is what distinguish them from stop-plosives. Affricates consonants are usually produced with a closed velopharynx.

Nasal consonants are produced with an occluded oral airway and an open velopharynx. The aeromechanical and acoustic energy associated with their production is transmitted through the nasopharynx and nasal cavities and is emitted from the external nares. They can be described as sonorants because the airway is open via the velopharyngeal airway and to the atmosphere via the nares.

Semivowel sounds are consonant sounds produced with an oral airway that is more constricted than vowels but not as constricted as obstruents. Semivowels are generated with the velopharynx closed and the aeromechanical and acoustic energy associated with their production passing through the pharyngeal-oral airway and emerging from the mouth.

Place of Production

Place of production describes the location of the consonant constriction or occlusion along the pharyngeal-oral or laryngeal airway. This dimension encompasses seven sites: *bilabial, labiodental, dental, alveolar, palatal, velar,* and *glottal*. In the order listed, these constriction or occlusion sites lie progressively farther inward along the pharyngeal-oral and laryngeal airways.

Bilabial means that only the two lips participate in the primary action having to do with place of production. An exception exists for the semivowel /w/, which is also specified as requiring a high-back tongue configuration. *Labiodental* indicates that the place of production is between the lower lip and the upper teeth. *Dental, alveolar, palatal,* and *velar* places of production designate locations where the tongue contacts or comes very close to contacting the teeth, upper gum ridge (inside the teeth), hard palate, and velum (soft palate and uvula), respectively. The *glottal* place of production occurs between the two vocal folds.

Voicing

The *voicing* dimension for stop-plosives, fricatives, and affricates is binary. That is, voice is either on or off for consonant productions, so consonants are categorized as either *voiced* or *voiceless*. Many of the consonants of American English form cognate pairs that differ only on the voicing dimension. Thus, two consonants in a cognate pair match one another in their manner of production and place of production but differ from one another because one is *voiced* and the other is *voiceless*. In English, cognate pairs exist for the three places of articulation for stop-plosives, the four places for fricatives, and for the single place of articulation for affricates. The nasal and semivowel consonants are all *voiced*.

Real-Life Consonants

Figure 5–28 presents real-life images of 13 different consonant productions. By comparing across the images, it is possible to detect differences in positions of the tongue, lips, and velum. It is not possible to determine if the consonant is voiceless or voiced in images such as these. To see how productions of consonants play out in real time, see Video 5–2 (Consonant Articulation).

SPEECH PRODUCTION: ARTICULATORY PROCESSES

The previous section provides articulatory descriptions related to place-constriction-lip rounding for vowels and place-manner-voicing for consonants. A serious limitation of these descriptions is that they are timeless. The speech production process is not a linear assemblage of a series of idealized sounds, nor is it a series of invariant positions and movement sequences

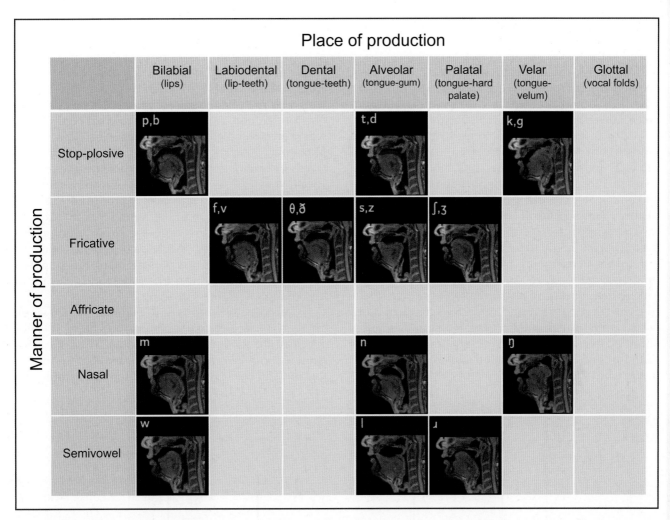

FIGURE 5–28. Mid-sagittal MR images of a man producing 13 consonants. For seven of these (p/b, t/d, k/g, θ/ð, s/z, f/v, and tʃ/dʒ), both the voiceless and voiced cognates are listed because it is not possible to determine whether or not they are voiced from MR images (MR images courtesy of Adam Baker).

strung together like beads on a string (MacNeilage, 1970). In fact, it is no exaggeration to say that the continuous and changeable movements of the articulators correspond poorly with discrete symbols of phonetic transcription, such as those presented in Figures 5–25 and 5–26. To truly understand articulatory processes in speech production, it is important to take into account the displacements and speeds of articulatory movements, coordination among articulators, and the way in which the articulatory movements of one sound influence other sounds. An important concept that has helped explain certain departures from the idealized descriptive scheme is that of coarticulation.

Coarticulation

Coarticulation is the influence of the articulatory movements of one sound on another sound (Daniloff & Hammarberg, 1973; Farnetani & Recasens, 2010). The examination of images of articulatory movements during speech production clearly shows the mutual influence between adjacent sounds and, in certain contexts, even nonadjacent sounds. One example of coarticulation is found in the production of the word "sue" [su] in which the lip rounding that is a part of the phonetic description for /u/ is observed during the [s] part of the articulatory sequence.[1] The same thing happens

---

[1]This discussion identifies speech sounds with symbols between virgules (i.e., forward slashes) or brackets. Virgules are used when the sound category is a phoneme that presumably reflects an abstract sound component; for example, the first sound category of a word such as "sue" would be written as /s/. The representation in the brain of all sound categories (not letters!) in this word includes two phoneme categories: /s/ and /u/. When a sound symbol is shown in brackets as in [su], the word and its component sounds are actually produced to be heard by

when the sequence is reversed, as in "toots" [tuts] (the sound made by a horn): Lip rounding for the /u/ may extend to the second lingua-alveolar stop-plosive [t] and the fricative [s]. These influences of immediately adjacent and nonadjacent sounds on one another explain, in part, why it is so hard to identify clear phonetic category boundaries from records of articulatory movement.

Speech scientists usually agree that there are two kinds of coarticulation. These are illustrated in Figure 5–29 for the words "sue" and "toots." Forward coarticulation (also called right-to-left coarticulation and anticipatory coarticulation) occurs when the articulatory characteristics of an upcoming sound influence the characteristics of a currently produced sound. The production of lip rounding during the [s] in "sue" is an example of an upcoming articulatory requirement (the lip rounding for /u/) occurring during the current /s/ articulation. Backward coarticulation (also called left-to-right coarticulation and carryover coarticulation) occurs when a currently articulated sound is influenced by the articulatory characteristics of a previous sound in the speech production stream. For example, in the word "toots," the articulatory characteristics of

the /t/ and /s/ include some lip rounding because of the previously articulated [u].

The traditional theory of coarticulation (Daniloff & Hammarberg, 1973) is based on the idea that each speech sound consists of a bundle of features, consistent with the phonetic descriptions discussed in the previous section. An example is shown in Figure 5–30, where an incomplete list of features is included for the phonemes (speech sound categories) that form two words: *tune* and *newt*. Each of the three features can be specified as "+," "–," or left blank. A feature specified as "+" means that the phoneme is produced with that feature, a specification of "–" represents the explicit absence of that feature from the production, and a blank means that the phoneme is not specified one way or the other for the feature. It is the blank (unspecified) features that are the most interesting and relevant to the concept of feature spreading.

Consider the word *tune* in Figure 5–30 (left side). The /t/ is specified as –sonorant and –nasal; it is not specified for the lip rounding feature. Thus, the phoneme /t/ can be produced with or without lip rounding and still be classified as a /t/. In this example, the

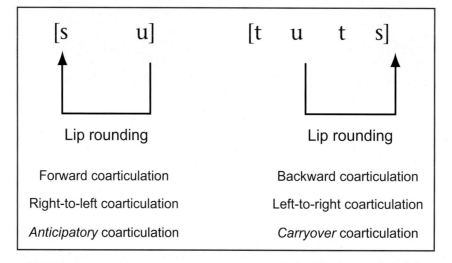

FIGURE 5–29. Schematic illustration of forward and backward coarticulation. Forward coarticulation (also called right-to-left and anticipatory coarticulation) means that a sound later in a sequence influences the production of an earlier sound in the sequence. Backward coarticulation (also called left-to-right and carryover coarticulation) means that an earlier sound in a sequence influences the production of a later sound. The symbols represent the words *sue* and *toots*.

a listener. Following the example in the text, the /s/ in /su/ has no specification for lip rounding, but when produced as [su], it is likely to have some lip rounding due to the influence of the vowel [u]. In contrast, the production of the word "see" [si] (where /i/ is the symbol for the sound "ee") does not have lip rounding for the produced [s] because /i/ does not have an abstract phonemic specification of lip rounding. Thus, the [s] in [su] and [si] is produced somewhat differently, but both are members of the abstract phoneme category /s/. Sounds that are produced differently but belong to the same phoneme category are called *allophones* of the phoneme category. The difference between phonemes and their allophones is especially important in clinical phonetics, an example of which is a child who produces a "slushy" [s] that may be corrected by a speech-language pathologist if the child is too old to be producing this kind of error. The slushy [s] is an allophone of /s/ but not an acceptable one (i.e., it is heard as a speech sound error).

	/t	u	n/	/n	u	t/
Sonorant	–	+	+	+	+	–
Lip rounding		+			+	
Nasal	–		+	+		–

FIGURE 5–30. Articulatory sequences conceptualized as strings of phonemes composed of bundles of features, with only selected features represented. Sonorant means that a sound is made with a relatively open pharyngeal-oral airway or free passage through the nasal cavities, lip rounding refers to vowels or consonants in which rounding of the lips is an integral feature, and nasal means that the sound is made with an open velopharyngeal port. These features are shown as specified (+), absent (–), or not specified (left blank). The symbols represent the words *tune* and *newt* (a semiaquatic salamander).

actual real-life [t] is produced with lip rounding in anticipation of the upcoming /u/ phoneme. This is an example of feature spreading that reflects forward (anticipatory) coarticulation. The /u/ is +sonorant and +lip rounding, but it is not specified for the nasal feature. This means that it can be nasalized or not and still be recognized as a /u/. If it is nasalized (which it almost certainly would be in this context), this would also demonstrate forward coarticulation. Finally, the /n/ is specified for +sonorant and +nasal, but not for lip rounding; therefore, a lip-rounded [n] and an [n] pro-

duced without lip rounding are both classified as /n/. The lip-rounded [n] would be considered an example of backward (carryover) coarticulation because it is carried over from the [u] production. The second example, shown on the right side of Figure 5–30, consists of the same set of limited features as applied to the word *newt*. We recommend that the reader go through the same exercise as was just described for the word *tune* as a way to understand the concept of feature spreading.

A real-life example of coarticulation is shown in Figure 5–31. This figure shows sagittal MR images of

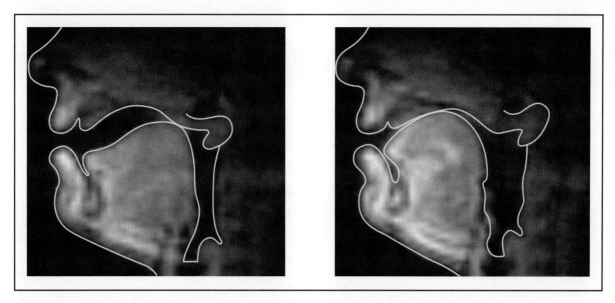

FIGURE 5–31. Two MR images of /k/ productions, one in the context of a low back vowel (/aka/, *left*) and one on the context of a high front vowel (/iki/, *right*). Note the much more forward placement of the /k/ production in the context of the front vowel compared to the back vowel (MR images courtesy of Signal Analysis and Interpretation Laboratory, University of Southern California, Shrikanth Narayanan).

someone producing a [k] in two phonetic contexts: /ɑkɑ/ and /iki/. Note that the location where the tongue makes contact with the palate for the [ɑkɑ] production is about where one would expect it from the standard description of the /k/ as a velar stop-plosive (consonant chart in Figure 5–26). In contrast, the tongue placement for the [iki] production is much farther forward along the palate and, therefore, does not fit our standard description. Why is the /k/ in [iki] different from that in [ɑkɑ]? Viewed from the perspective of coarticulation, this can be explained by the idea that the tongue has just produced a high front vowel and is getting ready to produce another high front vowel immediately after the [k]. Thus, the forward [k] placement can be explained by both backward and forward coarticulation.

Explanations and mechanisms have been proposed to account for anticipatory coarticulation (Farnetani & Recasens, 2010; Kent, 1976). One explanation is that this type of coarticulation constitutes the ability to anticipate an articulatory feature before it is needed (i.e., for a phoneme that is "+" for that feature) and is one of the ways in which speech production movements are smoothed out and made continuous across a sequence of sounds. Thus, the continuous movements of the articulators are an expression of speech motor (movement) efficiency. A proposed mechanism for anticipatory coarticulation is one in which the plan for articulatory behavior is in the form of a sequence of phonemes and their respective feature specifications, such as depicted in Figure 5–30. Quite literally, the phoneme sequence and component features are believed to be represented in the brain. A programming operation, often referred to as a look-ahead operator (Daniloff & Hammarberg, 1973; Henke, 1966), scans the phoneme sequence from left to right—the intended output order—and finds features that can be anticipated without compromising the articulatory identity of a sound.

Explanations and mechanisms have also been proposed for carryover (left-to-right or backward) coarticulation. In the traditional view, carryover coarticulation is believed to be the result of articulators being unable to move immediately from one position to the next because they have mass and demonstrate inertia. Anticipatory and carryover coarticulation are regarded as very different phenomena, even though they both involve feature spreading. Anticipatory coarticulation is thought of as a planning or programming phenomenon that occurs in the brain, whereas carryover coarticulation is thought to be the result of the physical characteristics of the speech production mechanism.

The traditional theory of coarticulation has fallen into disfavor over the past 20 years. In fact, soon after the theory was developed and publicized in the late 1960s and early 1970s, some of its problems became apparent. Several criticisms have been voiced over the years, but perhaps the most serious is the requirement of an input representation (phonemes) that may have no reality in the speech production process. Further, it seems awkward and unnecessary to imagine a speech production process in which a digital representation of speech (discrete phonemes) must be translated to an analog form (the smooth and continuous movements of the articulators). In other words, the traditional theory lacks a representation of the time element of articulatory behavior. The alternative proposed by these critics is an input to the speech production process that represents articulatory behavior as it unfolds over time.

Raymond D. Kent

Kent has been one of the leading speech scientists in the world for over three decades. He has written extensively on a variety of topics, including speech development, normal speech acoustics, and the acoustics of speech associated with neuromotor speech disorders. His work, along with colleagues, has elucidated much of what is known about speech acoustics and inferred articulatory dynamics in speakers with dysarthria. A distinguishing feature of Kent's work is its multidisciplinary nature. Those who read his articles and books come away with an appreciation for his ability to integrate diverse literatures and bring them to bear on issues in his own discipline. Few can match him, and those who know him well affectionately refer to him as "Clark Kent," the character of Superman fame, because of their awe for his powerful influence in speech science. He is retired and lives in Madison, Wisconsin.

Articulatory Phonology or Gesture Theory

Theories that reject the ideas of phonemes and their translation to speech motor behavior are variously called articulatory phonology (Browman & Goldstein, 1992) or gesture theories (Byrd, 1996; Saltzman & Munhall, 1989). The details of these different approaches to the production of articulatory behavior are less important than is a broad understanding of how these theories differ from the traditional theory of coarticulation. Figure 5–32 presents a model of the speech production process in which the focus is entirely on articulatory gestures (movements). The identity and timing of selected gestures are shown for production of the word *sinew* [sinju]. Five gestures are idealized, including those of the tongue tip, tongue body, velopharyngeal port, lips, and larynx. These gestures unfold in time, from left to right, just as the sounds for the word *sinew* occur in sequence. The time course of each gesture is indicated by the length of its associated rectangle. The onset and offset of the lip rounding gesture are shown to illustrate how the timing of each rectangle should be interpreted.

The primary impression from this display is of the different articulatory gestures occurring at different onset and offset times throughout the utterance, and of gestures overlapping in time. For example, in addition to the overlap between the open velopharyngeal port gesture and the tongue tip-raising gesture for [n], the open port gesture also overlaps with the tongue body gestures for both the preceding [i] and the following [ju]. Thus, the sounds preceding and following the nasal sound are produced with a somewhat open velopharyngeal port. In the traditional theory, the partial nasalization of [i] is an example of antici-patory coarticulation, and the partial nasalization of [ju] is an example of carryover coarticulation, both the result of feature spreading. In articulatory phonology or gesture theory, the term *coproduction* has been used (rather than coarticulation) to indicate that the over-lap of the open velopharyngeal port gesture with the tongue body gestures for the two flanking vowels is just that—overlap—and does not reflect the operation of an extra programming process (anticipatory coartic-ulation) or the physical limitation of articulatory move-ment (carryover coarticulation).

The foregoing discussion emphasizes the dynamic process of speech production. Although it seems con-venient to categorize speech sounds according to cer-tain features, such as those shown in the vowel and consonant charts provided above (Figures 5–25 and 5–26), they do not tell the true story. Far from it. Some time spent watching the movements of multiple artic-ulators producing a complex string of syllables will convince you of the elaborate coordination involved in speaking (see Video 5–3 [Microbeam "Abracadabra"]). With the temporal precision required, it is also easy to appreciate how even a slight offset in the timing of one or more articulatory movements could be devas-tating to the acoustic (speech) output (see Video 5–4 [Sliding Gestures]).

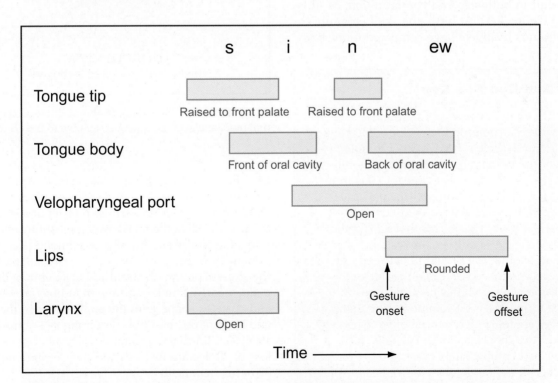

FIGURE 5–32. Model of speech production in which the focus is on articulatory gestures (move-ments). Rectangles delimit the time course of individual gestures of selected articulators. This rep-resents the production of the word *sinew*.

VARIABLES THAT INFLUENCE PHARYNGEAL-ORAL STRUCTURE AND FUNCTION

One need only look at a group of men, women, and children and listen to them speak to know that age and sex have an influence on the structure and function of the pharyngeal-oral mechanism. The effects of age are most apparent during the first couple of decades of life, although they continue on a more gradual time scale throughout the remainder of the life span. The influence of sex emerges early in life and is maintained through senescence.

Age

Age brings change, and these changes affect the anatomical and physiological substrates that support speaking and swallowing. The pharyngeal-oral mechanism at birth is a far cry from that in adulthood, and the senescent apparatus shows the wear and tear of the aging process when held up against its younger counterpart. Some of the more salient structural and functional age-related changes are described here.

The skeletal framework of the pharyngeal-oral mechanism of the newborn infant differs from that of the adult in both size and configuration, as illustrated in Figure 5–33. At birth, the skull (cranium) of the newborn is relatively large compared to the body,

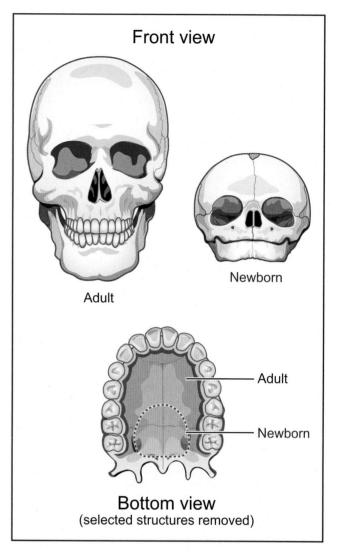

FIGURE 5–33. The skeletal framework of the pharyngeal-oral mechanism of the newborn infant and the adult.

and the facial part of the skull is small. Although the cranium approximates adult size relatively early in childhood, perhaps as early as 6 years of age (Melsen & Melsen, 1982), the facial skeleton continues to grow into adolescence and possibly adulthood (Kent & Vorperian, 1995; Richtsmeier & Cheverud, 1986). During this growth period, the front-to-back depth of the bony palate nearly doubles and the mandible grows in size and changes shape with the angle between the ramus and body of the mandible becoming less obtuse (Scott, 1976; Zemlin, 1998). Dental development involves the loss of 20 deciduous teeth and their replacement with 32 permanent teeth.

Soft structures of the pharyngeal-oral mechanism also undergo nonlinear developmental change during infancy and childhood (Vorperian et al., 2009). In the

Eye Eye Eye Eye Eye

This title should catch your eye (pun intended). As a clinician, you need to develop a good eye for eyes. Eyes can be an eye opener for identifying syndromes that include pharyngeal-oral problems. We can bear eyewitness to this from our own experiences. Consider the physical spacing of the eyes. Most faces are five eyes wide at eye level. This means that a space the width of one eye should fit between the two eyes and another eye should fit between the outside corner of each eye and the side of the face. Departures from this pattern come in several forms, the most common being that the two eyes are too widely spaced or too narrowly spaced. Any abnormal pattern should catch your eye and immediately cause you to eye the pharyngeal-oral mechanism for frank and subtle abnormalities. Hopefully, we see eye to eye on this. Work on developing your eye for eyes.

newborn infant, the pharyngeal cavity is about 4 cm in length and appreciably shorter than the oral cavity (Crelin, 1973). The contour of the junction between the pharyngeal and oral parts of the pharyngeal-oral mechanism is rounded in the newborn infant, assumes an oblique angle at about 5 years of age, and approximates the right-angle configuration of the adult around the time of puberty (Kent & Vorperian, 1995). The predominant feature of pharyngeal development is its vertical enlargement (Vorperian et al., 2005, 2009). The tongue of the newborn infant essentially fills the oral cavity (Crelin, 1976), and then, during the first year of life, it begins to descend within the neck and continues to do so until about 5 years of age (Laitman & Crelin, 1976). The lips undergo significant developmental change between birth and adulthood: They form a near-circular sphincter in the newborn infant, whereas they form a transverse, elliptical sphincter in the adult. Major reconfiguration of the lips occurs during the first 2 years of life (Burke, 1980), and rapid growth of the lips is reported to occur between 10 and 17 years of age (Vig & Cohen, 1979).

Along with the anatomical changes described above, various aspects of the nervous system also undergo development well into adolescence. This development reflects change in cognition, memory, motor control, and other nervous system functions that are relevant to pharyngeal-oral movements. Characteristic of the development of pharyngeal-oral movement control are sensitive periods in which skill acquisition is continuous but nonlinear and during which incremental increases in performance take what appear to be jumps forward (Netsell, 1986).

Studies of speech production have revealed differences in pharyngeal-oral control in children when compared to adults. For example, whereas lip movements during speech production are primarily vertical in adults, they begin as more horizontal (spreading) in infants and develop a more vertical movement com-

ponent over the first few years of life (Iuzzini-Seigel, Hogen, Rong, & Green, 2015). Nevertheless, the most prominent speech production difference between children and adults is that children speak more slowly and with greater variability in amplitude, velocity, timing, and general patterning of pharyngeal-oral movements (Goffman & Smith, 1999; Green, Moore, Higashikawa, & Steeve, 2000; Green, Moore, & Reilly, 2002; Grigos, 2009; Kent & Forner, 1980; Maner, Smith, & Grayson, 2000; Nittrouer, 1993; Sharkey & Folkins, 1985; Smith & Goffman, 1998; Smith & McLean-Muse, 1986; Smith, Sugarman, & Long, 1983; Steeve, Moore, Green, Reilly, & McMurtrey, 2008; Sturm & Seery, 2007; Watkin & Fromm, 1984). Adult-like speech production movements are not acquired until near the end of the teenage years (Smith & Zelaznik, 2004; Walsh & Smith, 2002).

Speech production is a motor skill that is functional throughout much of life and is preserved even in the oldest of the old. Once this skill is fully mature, it gives the appearance of involving little effort, proceeding automatically, and being highly ingrained. Most senescent people use this practiced motor skill exceedingly well and produce fully intelligible speech. This does not mean, however, that their speech production is unchanged from what it was decades earlier, with the majority of age-related changes manifest after the fifth decade of life (Kahane, 1990).

The pharyngeal part of the pharyngeal-oral mechanism changes during adulthood. Overall, it gets larger, lengthening as the larynx lowers and widening as the muscles of the pharynx tend to weaken and atrophy (Linville & Fisher, 1985; Wind, 1970; Zaino & Benventano, 1977). The oral part of the mechanism (oral cavity and oral vestibule) also undergoes a gradual increase in size with age (Israel, 1968, 1973). Salivary production declines and saliva thickens and alters in composition (Baum, 1981; Chauncey, Borkan, Wayler, Feller, & Kapur, 1981), possibly accounting for why the elderly have more oral infections, more oral lesions (sores),

---

Coming and Going

He could feel when it was coming. It would come on slowly, be there for a while, and then go away slowly. When it was gone, the speech sounded normal. But, when it was there, his speech sounded as if he were drunk. We studied him, using him as his own control. What could be better? He perfectly matched himself. The psychiatrist thought the problem was all in his mind. But it turned out otherwise. What made his speech alternately normal and abnormal was a condition called paroxysmal ataxia, an uncontrollable physiological change in the ability to transmit neural signals within the cerebellum. The neurologist who diagnosed the problem was concerned. Paroxysmal ataxia can be a harbinger of another diagnosis to come: multiple sclerosis. The unwanted coming and going of speech signs can mean the ultimate coming of something else unwanted. And so it turned out that this was the fate for this middle-aged man.

and more loose teeth than their younger counterparts (Sonies, 1991). Sensory and motor capabilities of the pharyngeal-oral mechanism also decrease with age and are manifest in loss of muscle strength, reduced sensitivity, and less vigorous reflexes.

Slowing is a hallmark of aging and is viewed as the most pervasive motor characteristic of getting older. Slowing of speech production has two bases, one being that articulatory rate slows and the other being that older speakers pause more often (Bilodeau-Mercure & Tremblay, 2016; Bona, 2014; Gollan & Goldrick, 2019; Hartman & Danhauer, 1976; Hoit & Hixon, 1987; Liss, Weismer, & Rosenbek, 1990; Ryan, 1972; Smith, Wasowicz, & Preston, 1987; Wohlert & Smith, 1998). There is also an increase in movement variability with advanced age (Liss et al., 1990; Smith et al., 1987; Weismer, 1984; Weismer & Fromm, 1983). Speech accuracy has also been shown to decline in older individuals, particularly during the production of complex movement and sound sequences (Bilodeau-Mercure et al., 2015).

Sex

Everyone knows that speech usually sounds different when produced by men and women. From discussion in previous chapters, it is clear that sex-related differences in speech production are strongly associated with sex-related differences in laryngeal structure and function, but that structure and function of the respiratory system and velopharyngeal-nasal mechanism are only minimally different between the sexes (see Chapters 2, 3, and 4). Here, attention turns to the potential contribution of pharyngeal-oral structure and function to sex-related differences in speech production.

Perhaps the most obvious structural difference between men and women is size. Men tend to be larger than women overall, and this size difference is also reflected in the pharyngeal-oral mechanism. Although sex-related size differences emerge strongly at puberty, there are sex-related size differences in selected regions of the pharyngeal-oral apparatus even prior to puberty (Vorperian et al., 2011). Pharyngeal-oral size differences in adults are reflected in speech (acoustic product) in the form of lower resonant (formant) frequencies in men than women across adulthood (Eichhorn, Kent, Austin, & Vorperian, 2017). One of the most important sex-related differences is that the pharynx is longer in men compared to women at rest (Fitch & Giedd, 1999) and during vowel production (Story, Hoffman, & Titze, 1997).

Pharyngeal-oral function during speech production has also been shown to differ somewhat between the sexes. For example, men speak faster and exhibit faster articulatory movements than women (Nicholson & Kimura, 1996; Simpson, 2001, 2002; Smith et al., 1987). This difference in speed may or may not be related to the observation that female talkers are more generally more intelligible than male talkers (Yoho, Borrie, Barrett, & Whittaker, 2018).

Faster Than a Herd of Turtles

When you watch someone reading aloud, things are moving all over the place. The mandible, tongue, and lips can all be seen to move from here to there and back and then off again to somewhere else. The coordination among these structures is exquisite, and the speech sounds come so fast that they blend together into a beautiful constant stream that flows quickly after the thoughts of the speaker. Running speech production is a truly a marvelous thing to watch. The speed of articulatory movements is what impresses many observers. Look at those structures go. But just how fast are they moving? What would you guess? Put it in miles per hour. 500? 250? 125? Or would you guess 65 like a car traveling along a freeway? Well, things aren't always what they seem. The actual speed is less than 1 mile per hour. That's not much faster than a thundering herd of turtles and probably considerably less than your usual walking speed.

CLINICAL NOTES

If one had to select a "favorite articulator" in the pharyngeal-oral part of the speech mechanism, it would likely be the tongue. The tongue is a key player in almost all of the speech sounds discussed in this chapter, and a viewing of the pharyngeal-oral articulators in action (for example, in the real-time MR images of a reading passage in Video 4–3 and the microbeam tracings of "abracadabra" in Video 5–3) shows the tongue to be in continuous motion during speech production. We couldn't do without it. Or could we?

There are times when a life-threatening cancer makes it necessary to resect (cut out) all or part of the tongue. This surgery is called glossectomy (or partial glossectomy), and the person who undergoes the surgery is sometimes referred to as a glossectomee (however, those who advocate the use of person-first language would reject this term). The National Cancer Institute estimates the number of new tongue cancer cases in 2020 to be over 17,000, with cases generally on the rise (https://seer.cancer.gov/statfacts/html/tongue.html). When cancer is found in the tongue, the approach to treatment must take into account the potential trade-off between saving a life and harming its quality. Quality of life is a significant consideration in this form of cancer because loss of tongue tissue can impair speaking, chewing, and swallowing, all of which are core to well-being. As surgical techniques have evolved and supportive treatments (e.g., radiation, chemotherapy) have improved, surgeons have been able to be more conservative in how much tongue tissue they remove. This, along with advances in surgical reconstruction and prosthetics, has helped to improve functional outcomes. Nevertheless, there are still people who must undergo total glossectomy and learn to live without a tongue.

With the tongue being such an important articulator, how is it possible to produce speech without one? The answer is quite amazing and illustrates how skillful our nervous systems are in their ability to "reorganize" movements so as to achieve the desired goal. In the case of speech production, the goal is to produce sounds that can be understood and carry the message we want to convey; in brief, the goal is to produce intelligible speech. Although the previous four chapters have offered a relatively accurate description of how speech is typically produced by healthy people, it is not the only way. Discussion of speech produced by someone without a tongue (and reinforced with a video example) will illustrate this.

We suggest that you take a short break from your reading to look at an x-ray image and watch an old x-ray film (circa early 1960s) of a man with a total glossectomy. Figure 5–34 contains a lateral x-ray image of most of his head and neck. Although the image is somewhat blurry, it should be apparent that much is missing from the image: Where there should be a tongue and teeth, there is nothing. Now take a moment to watch Video 5–5 (Glossectomee). This is the x-ray film of the same man reading part of the first paragraph of the *Rainbow Passage* (Fairbanks, 1960). For those of you who know this passage by heart (as do your authors), the speech should be quite intelligible. For those of you who are not familiar with this famous passage, the speech will not be as understandable. (This is an excellent example of one of the many variables that influences speech intelligibility—a topic for another day.) But even for those listeners who have difficulty understanding his speech, you will likely understand at least some sounds, words, and phrases. How is this possible when he was speaking without a tongue? The answer is that he was using other articulatory movements to produce (or approximate) the acoustic targets.

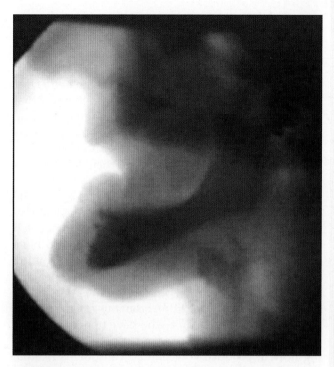

FIGURE 5–34. Lateral x-ray image of man who has undergone total glossectomy. He is also edentulous.

Although it is not possible to know with certainty how this man was producing relatively understandable speech without the benefit of a tongue, it is possible to conjecture based on what can be seen in the film and what can be reasoned from knowledge of anatomy and physiology. The first thing to notice is that this man is edentulous (without teeth). Under normal circumstances, missing teeth would be considered a disadvantage (and certainly must have limited the food he could eat); however, this may have actually been advantageous for his speech production. Without teeth, he was able to move his mandible a greater distance (toward his maxilla) and thereby change the size of the oral cavity to a greater degree than he could have if he still had his teeth. By using this expanded range of oral cavity sizes, he would be able to change the "filter" in ways that might help compensate for what he could no longer do with his tongue. Another thing to notice about this man's speech production is that he uses somewhat exaggerated lip protrusion and retraction gestures. These, too, would alter the filter in ways that might help approximate certain vowel-like sounds that are normally produced with the tongue. There are other ways that the pharyngeal-oral mechanism can be manipulated with intact structures that may have helped this man hit (or approximate) his acoustic targets. Examples are that he could make larger-than-usual vertical movements of the larynx (thereby changing the length of his pharyngeal cavity extensively); he could exaggerate the lateral movements of his pharyngeal walls; he could use his two lips to produce consonants that he would normally produce with his tongue, teeth, and lips (e.g., an approximated /f/ or /s/); and he could "trick" the listener into thinking that a /t/ was produced by using his two lips and changing subtle timing features of, for example, voicing onsets and offsets. Perhaps you can think of additional ways he might have used his remaining articulators to produce reasonably understandable speech.

Over the past few decades, there has been some research on how people who undergo glossectomy recover speech production skills. More sophisticated instrumentation and measurement approaches have allowed for more fine-grained observations of the types of movement adaptations made by speakers who have lost all or part of their tongues (Ha, Sung, Son, Stone, Ord, & Cho, 2016). From this research, it has become clearer that people who have undergone glossectomy (partial or total) are more successful in relearning how to produce vowels than consonants (Kaipa, Robb, O'Beirne, & Allison, 2012). There is also some evidence that behavioral speech intervention (speech therapy) may help improve intelligibility (Furia et al., 2001), although the evidence is far from adequate (Blyth, McCabe, Madill, & Ballard, 2015).

This topic is interesting, not just from the perspective of understanding speech problems associated with glossectomy but also from the perspective of recognizing how well the nervous system can reorganize movements to accomplish a goal. Our case example should provide hope that, even in the face of severe physical impairment, it may still be possible to continue to communicate using our most efficient and usually most effective modality: speech.

REVIEW

The pharyngeal-oral mechanism (along with the velopharyngeal-nasal mechanism) forms the upper airway, also called the vocal tract, when referring to its acoustic properties.

The pharyngeal-oral mechanism is a flexible tube that extends from the larynx to the lips and undergoes an approximate 90-degree forward bend within the oropharynx.

The skeleton of the pharyngeal-oral mechanism consists of the cervical vertebrae and various bones of the skull and especially those of the face.

The maxilla comprises two complexly shaped bones that combine at the midline to form the upper jaw, most of the hard palate, and the alveolar process that houses the upper teeth.

The mandible is a large horseshoe-shaped bone that forms the lower jaw and holds the lower teeth.

The mandible articulates with the left and right temporal bones along the sides of skull to form the temporomandibular joints, the only freely movable joints of the skull.

Movements of the mandible are conditioned by the mechanical arrangements of the temporomandibular joints, which allow a hinge action of the mandible in relation to the temporal bone, a front-to-back gliding action, and a side-to-side gliding action.

The oropharynx is located midway along the pharyngeal cavity and is the part of the pharynx that moves the most during speech production.

The oral cavity is formed by the teeth, alveolar processes of the maxilla and mandible, hard palate, velum, floor of the mouth (mainly the tongue), and the anterior faucial pillars, as well as a forward vestibule (entryway) that is formed by the lips, cheeks, teeth, and alveolar processes of the maxilla and mandible.

The buccal (cheek) cavity constitutes the small space between the gums and teeth internally and the lips and cheeks externally and connects to the oral cavity through spaces between the teeth and behind the last molars.

The pharyngeal-oral mechanism contains a mucous lining that consists of epithelium and connective tissues that are different at different locations within the mechanism and includes a general lining mucosa, a masticatory mucosa, and a specialized mucosa.

Passive and active forces act on the pharyngeal-oral mechanism, with active force coming from the contraction of muscles of the pharynx, mandible, tongue, and lips.

Muscles of the pharynx include the *middle constrictor*, *inferior constrictor*, and *stylopharyngeus*.

Muscles of the mandible include the *masseter*, *temporalis*, *internal pterygoid*, *external pterygoid*, *digastric*, *mylohyoid*, and *geniohyoid*.

Muscles of the tongue include the *superior longitudinal*, *inferior longitudinal*, *vertical*, *transverse*, *styloglossus*, *palatoglossus*, *hyoglossus*, and *genioglossus*.

Muscles of the lips include the *orbicularis oris*, *buccinator*, *risorius*, *levator labii superioris*, *levator labii superioris alaeque nasi*, *zygomatic major*, *zygomatic minor*, *depressor labii inferioris*, *mentalis*, *levator anguli oris*, *depressor anguli oris*, *incisivus labii superioris*, *incisivus labii inferioris*, and *platysma*.

Movements of the pharynx are vested in its sidewalls, back wall, and front wall and enable the lumen of the pharynx to be adjusted in size and shape, as well as the degree of coupling between the oropharynx and the oral cavity (through the palatoglossal arch) to be modified.

Movements of the mandible are conditioned by the physical arrangements of the temporomandibular joints and can involve both rotation and translation that combine to provide for vertical, front-to-back, and side-to-side adjustments of the structure.

Movements of the tongue derive from movements of the mandible, shifting of the tongue mass within the oral cavity, and changing of the shape of the tongue in various dimensions, all of which are facilitated by the biomechanical property of the tongue that enables it to function like a liquid-filled, incompressible, and pliable structure (a muscular hydrostat).

Movements of the lips are exceptionally versatile, with each lip being able to move independently or with the two lips coordinated in their movements, and with the range of possible adjustments including puckering, protruding, retracting, spreading, pointing, curling, groping, rounding, and plumping, among others.

The control variables of pharyngeal-oral function include pharyngeal-oral lumen size and configuration, pharyngeal-oral structural contact pressure, pharyngeal-oral airway resistance, and pharyngeal-oral acoustic impedance.

Pharyngeal-oral movements are controlled by the nervous system, with the final forms of control commands sent through cranial nerves to muscles, and with sensory innervation provided through cranial nerves to guide anticipated actions of the pharyngeal-oral mechanism and to keep track of its recent status.

The pharyngeal-oral mechanism can generate sound and also filter that sound, as well as filter sound coming from the larynx.

The pharyngeal-oral mechanism, well known for its articulatory role in speech production, contributes significantly to the formation of different speech sounds and those sounds that can be described and categorized as sonorants and obstruents and vowels and consonants.

Vowel and diphthongs are sonorants and are produced with voicing by the larynx, exclusion of nasal participation by velopharyngeal closure, and using combinations of structural positions and movements that result in relatively unconstricted configurations of the pharyngeal-oral airway that are classified according to place of major constriction, degree of major constriction, and degree of lip rounding.

Consonant sounds include both obstruents and sonorants and are usually produced with a relatively constricted or obstructed airway, with or without voicing by the larynx, and/or with or without velopharyngeal closure, and using combinations of structural positions and movements that are classified accord-

ing to the manner of production, place of production, and voicing.

The speech production stream is fluid and ongoing, and structures of the pharyngeal-oral apparatus move smoothly and nearly continuously from one position to another.

Traditional theory of coarticulation proposes that sounds in the speech production stream influence their neighbors through processes that are anticipatory and scan ahead and processes that are a reflection of the inertial properties of the speech production apparatus.

Traditional theory of coarticulation has been criticized for certain weaknesses and has been replaced by more recent articulatory phonology or gesture theories that propose that sounds in the speech production stream are assembled by the phasing of overlapping movement gestures of different structures and do not require schemes of phoneme representation to account for speech production behavior.

The development of pharyngeal-oral function in speech production involves a transition to faster speech production rates and more stable speech production movements across childhood, along with the development of muscle synergies and movement routines, whereas aging is manifested in changes in the resonances of the pharyngeal-oral airway, a slowing of speech production, and greater variability of performance.

Sex has certain influences on pharyngeal-oral function in speech production and speech that are related to faster utterance rates and movements in men than women and a longer pharyngeal airway in men than women that results in nonuniform differences in formants (resonances) between the sexes.

It is possible to produce reasonably understandable speech, even when missing an articulator as critical as the tongue, by reorganizing the movements of the other intact articulators to achieve or approximate the acoustic (speech) targets.

REFERENCES

Baum, B. (1981). Evaluation of stimulated parotid saliva flow rate in different age groups. *Journal of Dental Research, 60,* 1292–1296.

Bilodeau-Mercure, M., Kirouac, V., Langlois, N., Ouellet, C., Gasse, I., & Tremblay, P. (2015). Movement sequencing in normal aging: speech, oro-facial, and finger movements. *Age, 37,* 1–13.

Bilodeau-Mercure, M., & Tremblay, P. (2016). Age differences in sequential speech production: Articulatory and physiological factors. *Journal of the American Geriatrics Society, 64,* e177–e182.

Blyth, K., McCabe, P., Madill, C., & Ballard, K. (2015). Speech and swallow rehabilitation following partial glossectomy:

A systematic review. *International Journal of Speech-Language Pathology, 17,* 401–410.

Bodanis, D. (1995). It's in the air: Skin, stardust, radio waves, vitamins, spider legs. *Smithsonian, 26,* 76–81.

Bona, J. (2014). Temporal characteristics of speech: The effect of age and speech style. *Journal of the Acoustical Society of America, 136,* EL116–EL121.

Browman, C., & Goldstein, L. (1992). Articulatory phonology: An overview. *Phonetica, 49,* 155–180.

Burke, P. (1980). Serial growth changes in the lips. *British Journal of Orthodontics, 7,* 17–30.

Byrd, D. (1996). A phase window framework for articulatory timing. *Phonology, 13,* 139–169.

Chauncey, H., Borkan, G., Wayler, A., Feller, R., & Kapur, K. (1981). Parotid fluid composition in healthy young males. *Advances in Physiological Sciences, 28,* 323–328.

Crelin, E. (1973). *Functional anatomy of the newborn.* New Haven, CT: Yale University Press.

Crelin, E. (1976). Development of the upper respiratory system. *Clinical Symposia, 28,* 1–30.

Daniloff, R., & Hammarberg, R. (1973). On defining coarticulation. *Journal of Phonetics, 1,* 239–248.

Dickson, D., & Maue-Dickson, W. (1982). *Anatomical and physiological bases of speech.* Boston, MA: Little, Brown.

Eichhorn, J., Kent, R., Austin, D., & Vorperian, H. (2017). Effects of aging on vocal fundamental frequency and vowel formants in men and women. *Journal of Voice, 32,* 644.e1–644.e9.

Fairbanks, G. (1960). *Voice and articulation drillbook.* New York, NY: Harper & Row.

Farnetani, E., & Recasens, D. (2010). Coarticulation and connected speech processes. In W. J. Hardcastle, F. E. Gibbon, and J. Laver (Eds.), *Handbook of phonetic sciences* (2nd ed., pp. 316–352). West Sussex, UK: John Wiley.

Fitch, W., & Giedd, J. (1999). Morphology and development of the human vocal tract: A study using magnetic resonance imaging. *Journal of the Acoustical Society of America, 106,* 1511–1522.

Fletcher, H. (1953). *Speech and hearing in communication.* New York, NY: Van Nostrand.

Furia, C., Kowalski, L., Latorre, M., Angelis, E., Martins, N., Barros, A., & Ribeiro, K. (2001). Speech intelligibility after glossectomy and speech rehabilitation. *Archives of Otolaryngology-Head & Neck Surgery, 127,* 877–883.

Goffman, L., & Smith, A. (1999). Development and differentiation of speech movement patterns. *Human Perception and Performance, 25,* 1–12.

Gollan, T., & Goldrick, M. (2019). Aging deficits in naturalistic speech production and monitoring revealed through reading aloud. *Psychology and Aging, 34,* 25–42.

Green, J., Moore, C., Higashikawa, M., & Steeve, R. (2000). The physiological development of speech motor control: Lip and jaw coordination. *Journal of Speech, Language, and Hearing Research, 43,* 239–255.

Green, J., Moore, C., & Reilly, K. (2002). The sequential development of jaw and lip control for speech. *Journal of Speech, Language, and Hearing Research, 45,* 66–79.

Grigos, M. (2009). Changes in articulator movement variability during phonemic development: A longitudinal study. *Journal of Speech, Language, and Hearing Research, 52,* 164–177.

Ha, J.. Sung, I-y., Son, J-h., Stone, M., Ord, R., & Cho, Y-c. (2016). Analysis of speech and tongue motion in normal and post-glossectomy speaker using cine MRI. *Journal of Applied Oral Science, 24,* 472–480.

Hartman, D., & Danhauer, J. (1976). Perceptual features of speech for males in four perceived age categories. *Journal of the Acoustical Society of America, 59,* 713–715.

Henke, W. (1966). *Dynamic articulatory model of speech production using computer simulation* (Unpublished doctoral dissertation). Massachusetts Institute of Technology, Cambridge, MA.

Hixon, T., Weismer, G., & Hoit, J. (2020). *Preclinical speech science: Anatomy, physiology, acoustics, perception* (3rd ed.). San Diego, CA: Plural Publishing.

Hoit, J., & Hixon, T. (1987). Age and speech breathing. *Journal of Speech and Hearing Research, 30,* 351–366.

Iuzzini-Seigel, J., Hogan, T., Rong, P., & Green, J. (2015). Longitudinal development of speech motor control: Motor and linguistic factors. *Journal of Motor Learning and Development, 3,* 53–68.

Israel, H. (1968). Continuing growth in the human cranial skeleton. *Archives of Oral Biology, 13,* 133–137.

Israel, H. (1973). Age factor and the pattern of change in craniofacial structures. *American Journal of Physical Anthropology, 39,* 111–128.

Kahane, J. (1990). Age-related changes in the peripheral speech mechanism: Structural and physiological changes. *ASHA Reports, 19,* 75–87.

Kaipa, R., Robb, M., O'Beirne, G., & Allison, R. (2012). Recovery of speech following total glossectomy: An acoustic and perceptual appraisal. *International Journal of Speech-Language Pathology, 14,* 24–34.

Kent, R. (1976). Models of speech production. In N. Lass (Ed.), *Contemporary issues in experimental phonetics* (pp. 79–104). New York, NY: Academic Press.

Kent, R. (1997). *The speech sciences.* San Diego, CA: Singular Publishing.

Kent, R., & Forner, L. (1980). Speech segment durations in sentence recitations by children and adults. *Journal of Phonetics, 8,* 157–168.

Kent, R., & Vorperian, H. (1995). Development of the craniofacial-oral-laryngeal anatomy: A review. *Journal of Medical Speech-Language Pathology, 3,* 149–190.

Kier, W., & Smith, K. (1985). Tongues, tentacles, and trunks: The biomechanics of movement in muscular hydrostats. *Zoological Journal of the Linnean Society, 83,* 307–324.

Laitman, J., & Crelin, E. (1976). Postnatal development of the basicranium and vocal tract region in man. In J. Bosma (Ed.), *Symposium on the development of the basicranium* (pp. 206–220). Bethesda, MD: National Institutes of Health.

Linville, S., & Fisher, H. (1985). Acoustic characteristics of women's voices with advanced age. *Journal of Gerontology, 3,* 324–330.

Liss, J., Weismer, G., & Rosenbek, J. (1990). Selected acoustic characteristics of speech production in very old males. *Journal of Gerontology, 45,* 35–45.

MacNeilage, P. (1970). Motor control of serial ordering of speech. *Psychological Review, 77,* 182–196.

Maner, K., Smith, A., & Grayson, L. (2000). Influences of utterance length and complexity on speech motor performance in children and adults. *Journal of Speech, Language, and Hearing Research, 43,* 560–573.

Melsen, B., & Melsen, F. (1982). The postnatal development of the palatomaxillary region studied on human autopsy material. *American Journal of Orthodontics, 82,* 329–342.

Minifie, F., Hixon, T., Kelsey, C., & Woodhouse, R. (1970). Lateral pharyngeal wall movement during speech production. *Journal of Speech and Hearing Research, 13,* 584–594.

Netsell, R. (1986). *A neurobiologic view of speech production and the dysarthrias.* San Diego, CA: College-Hill Press.

Nicholson, K., & Kimura, D. (1996). Sex differences for speech and manual skill. *Perceptual and Motor Skills, 82,* 3–13.

Nittrouer, S. (1993). The emergence of mature gestural patterns is not uniform: Evidence from an acoustic study. *Journal of Speech and Hearing Research, 36,* 959–972.

Richtsmeier, J., & Cheverud, J. (1986). Finite element scaling analysis of human craniofacial growth. *Journal of Craniofacial Genetics and Developmental Biology, 6,* 289–323.

Ryan, W. (1972). Acoustic aspects of the aging voice. *Journal of Gerontology, 27,* 265–268.

Saltzman, E., & Munhall, K. (1989). A dynamical approach to gestural patterning in speech production. *Ecological Psychology, 1,* 333–382.

Scott, J. (1976). *Dentofacial development and growth.* Oxford, UK: Pergamon Press.

Sharkey, S., & Folkins, J. (1985). Variability of lip and jaw movements in children and adults: Implications for the development of speech motor control. *Journal of Speech and Hearing Research, 28,* 8–15.

Sicher, H., & DuBrul, E. (1975). *Oral anatomy* (2nd ed.). St. Louis, MO: C. V. Mosby.

Simpson, A. (2001). Dynamic consequences of differences in male and female vocal tract dimensions. *Journal of the Acoustical Society of America, 109,* 2153–2164.

Simpson, A. (2002). Gender-specific articulatory-acoustic relations in vowel sequences. *Journal of Phonetics, 30,* 417–435.

Smith, A., & Goffman, L. (1998). Stability and patterning of speech movement sequences in children and adults. *Journal of Speech, Language, and Hearing Research, 41,* 18–30.

Smith, A., & Zelaznik, H. (2004). Development of functional synergies for speech motor coordination in childhood and adolescence. *Developmental Psychobiology, 45,* 22–33.

Smith, B., & McLean-Muse, A. (1986). Articulatory movement characteristics of labial consonant productions by children. *Journal of the Acoustical Society of America, 80,* 1321–1327.

Smith, B., Sugarman, M., & Long, S. (1983). Experimental manipulation of speaking rate for studying temporal variability in children's speech. *Journal of the Acoustical Society of America, 74,* 744–748.

Smith, B., Wasowicz, J., & Preston, J. (1987). Temporal characteristics of the speech of normal elderly adults. *Journal of Speech and Hearing Research, 30,* 522–529.

Smith, K., & Kier, W. (1989). Trunks, tongues, and tentacles: Moving with skeletons of muscle. *American Scientist, 77,* 28–35.

Sonies, B. (1991). The aging oropharyngeal system. In D. Ripich (Ed.), *Handbook of geriatric communication disorders* (pp. 187–203). Austin, TX: Pro-Ed.

Stadnytskyi, V., Bax, C., Bax, A., & Anfinrud, P. (2020). The airborne lifetime of small droplets and their potential importance in SARS-CoV-2 transmission. *Proceedings of the National Academy of Sciences of the United States of America (PNAS), 117,* 11875–11877.

Steeve, R., Moore, C., Green, J., Reilly, K., & McMurtrey, J. (2008). Babbling, chewing, and sucking: Oromandibular coordination at 9 months. *Journal of Speech, Language, and Hearing Research, 51,* 1390–1404.

Story, B., Hoffman, E., & Titze, I. (1997). Volumetric image-based comparison of male and female vocal tract shapes. In E. Hoffman (Ed), *Proceedings of the International Society of Optical Engineering* (pp. 25–37). Bellingham, WA: International Society of Optical Engineering.

Sturm, J., & Seery, C. (2007). Speech and articulatory rates of school-age children in conversation and narrative contexts. *Language, Speech, and Hearing Services in Schools, 38,* 47–59.

Vig, P., & Cohen, A. (1979). Vertical growth of the lips: A serial cephalometric study. *American Journal of Orthodontics, 75,* 405–415.

Vorperian, H., Kent, R., Lindstrom, M., Kalina, C., Gentry, L., & Yandell, B. (2005). Development of vocal tract length during early childhood: A magnetic resonance imaging study. *Journal of the Acoustical Society of America, 117,* 338–350.

Vorperian, H., Wang, S., Chung, M., Schimek, E., Durtschi, R., Kent, R., Ziegert, A., & Gentry, L. (2009). Anatomic development of the oral and pharyngeal portions of the vocal tract: An imaging study. *Journal of the Acoustical Society of America, 125,* 1666–1678.

Vorperian, H., Wang, S., Schimek, E., Durtschi, R., Kent, R., Gentry, L., & Chung, M. (2011). Developmental sexual dimorphism of the oral and pharyngeal portions of the vocal tract: An imaging study. *Journal of Speech, Language, and Hearing Research, 54,* 995–1010.

Walsh, B., & Smith, A. (2002). Articulatory movements in adolescents: Evidence for protracted development of speech motor control processes. *Journal of Speech, Language, and Hearing Research, 45,* 1119–1133.

Watkin, K., & Fromm, D. (1984). Labial coordination in children: Preliminary considerations. *Journal of the Acoustical Society of America, 75,* 629–632.

Weismer, G. (1984). Articulatory characteristics of parkinsonian dysarthria: Segmental and phrase-level timing, spirantization, and glottal-supraglottal coordination. In M. McNeil, J. Rosenbek, & A. Aronson (Eds.), *The dysarthrias: Physiology, acoustics, perception, management* (pp. 101–130). San Diego, CA: College-Hill Press.

Weismer, G., & Fromm, D. (1983). Acoustic analysis of geriatric utterances: Segmental and nonsegmental characteristics that relate to laryngeal function. In D. Bless & J. Abbs (Eds.), *Vocal fold physiology: Contemporary research and clinical issues* (pp. 317–322). San Diego, CA: College-Hill Press.

Wind, J. (1970). *On the phylogeny and ontogeny of the human larynx.* Groningen, Netherlands: Wolters-Noordhoff.

Wohlert, A., & Smith, A. (1998). Spatiotemporal stability of lip movements in older adult speakers. *Journal of Speech, Language, and Hearing Research, 41,* 41–50.

Woo, J., Xing, F., Lee, J., Stone, M., & Prince, J. (2016). A spatio-temporal atlas and statistical model of the tongue during speech from cine-MRI. *Computer Methods in Biomechanics and Biomedical Engineering: Imaging and Visualization, 6,* 520–531. https://doi.org/10.1080/21681163.2016.1169220.

Woo, J., Xing, F., Prince, J. L., Stone, M., Green, J. R., Goldsmith, T., . . . El Fakhri, G. (2019). Differentiating post-cancer from healthy tongue muscle coordination patterns during speech using deep learning. *Journal of the Acoustical Society of America, 145,* EL423–EL429.

Yoho, S., Borrie, S., Barrett, T., & Whittaker, D. (2018). Are there sex effects for speech intelligibility in American English? Examining the influence of talker, listener, and methodology. *Attention, Perception, & Psychophysics, 81,* 558–570.

Zaino, C., & Benventano, T. (1977). Functional, involutional, and degenerative disorders. In C. Zaino & T. Benventano (Eds.), *Radiologic examination of the oropharynx and esophagus* (pp. 141–170). New York, NY: Springer-Verlag.

Zemlin, W. (1998). *Speech and hearing science: Anatomy and physiology* (4th ed.). Boston, MA: Allyn & Bacon.

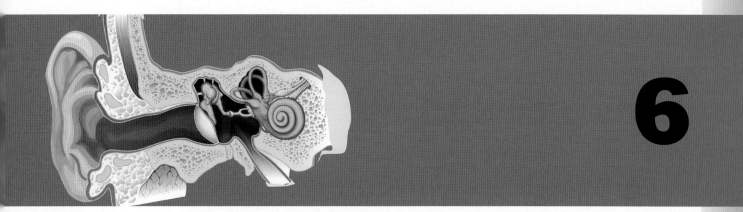

Auditory System Structure and Function

INTRODUCTION

This chapter provides an integrated description of the anatomy and physiology of the auditory mechanism. The information presented here can be found in more detailed form in textbooks and hundreds of journal publications. Here, information from Abele and Wiggins (2015); Barin (2009); Goutman, Elgoyhen, and Gomez-Casati (2015); Hudpseth (2014); Kramer and Brown (2019); Lemmerling, Stambuk, Mancuso, Antonelli, and Kubilis (1997); Luers and Hüttenbrink (2016); Mansour, Magnan, Haidar, Nicolas, and Louryan (2019); Musiek and Baran (2018); and Olsen, Duifhuis, and Steele (2012) has been used to organize a contemporary description of the relevant structures and functions of the auditory system.

A solid understanding of the auditory mechanism is critical to anyone interested in pursuing a career in audiology, speech-language pathology, hearing or speech science, or any other career related to communication. There are several reasons for this, the first of which is so obvious as to be trivial: Most children learn speech and language primarily through their auditory mechanism. Second, an understanding of the normal structures and functions of the auditory mechanism allows an appreciation of the way in which various diseases and conditions affect hearing. Finally, knowledge

of the anatomy and physiology of the auditory mechanism is essential to understanding the design and purpose of formal tests of hearing—the types of tests an audiologist performs to identify and diagnose a hearing problem. Even the simplest evaluation of hearing —when a single-frequency tone is presented through headphones and the person tested is asked to raise a hand each time it is heard—is designed with knowledge of the anatomy and physiology of the cochlea, the end organ of hearing. Other more advanced evaluations of the hearing mechanism estimate the status of different parts of the auditory system by observing behavioral, mechanical, and physiological responses to various types of sound energy. Structure and function are intimately linked in the auditory mechanism and are essential to understanding both normal hearing and disorders of hearing.

The hearing mechanism includes a peripheral component, one part of which is easily visible, and a central component comprised of pathways in the brain that are dedicated to auditory function. Discussions of *peripheral* auditory anatomy—auditory structures that are outside the central nervous system (CNS)—typically classify structures as belonging to one of three major divisions: the outer ear, the middle ear, and the inner ear. Much of the peripheral auditory mechanism is encased in the temporal bone of the skull.

TEMPORAL BONE

Figure 6–1 shows the complex shape and notable landmarks of the temporal bone. Figure 6–1A provides a view of the lateral (side) surface of the temporal bone (boundary suture highlighted). The lateral temporal bone shares boundaries with the occipital bone in back, the parietal bone above, and the sphenoid bone in front. The mastoid process of the temporal bone is behind and slightly below the bony external auditory meatus. The external auditory meatus is the bony part of the canal leading from the external ear to the tympanic membrane (eardrum). Inside the mastoid process, within the mastoid bone, are air-filled cells that communicate with the air-filled, middle ear cavity.

Figure 6–1B shows the interior base of the skull as if the top half has been removed, with the view from above. Note the position of the temporal bone relative to the sphenoid (in front) and occipital bone (behind). The temporal bone is seen to project toward the middle, forming part of the base of the skull. The temporal bone has a broad lateral base and narrows to a blunt tip at its middle termination point. The more medial part is called the petrous part of the temporal bone and is not visible from the lateral surface of the temporal

bone. The petrous part of the temporal bone encases the structures of the inner ear. Note the opening of the internal auditory meatus, a narrow canal roughly 10 mm in length through which nerve fibers run from the cochlea (inner ear structure of hearing) on their way to the brainstem, the part of the CNS that sits on top of the spinal cord (see Chapter 8). Nerve fibers running in the opposite direction, from the brainstem to the cochlea, also travel through the internal auditory meatus. All these fibers run through the inner (medial) opening of the internal meatus.

The complexity of the temporal bone is especially apparent in Figure 6–1C, where it is shown disarticulated from the other bones of the skull. The lateral surface of the bone is shown on the left, the middle surface on the right. The right-hand image shows the petrous part of the temporal bone, the wedge-like projection into the middle part of the skull base.

PERIPHERAL ANATOMY OF THE EAR

Figure 6–2 shows an artist's rendition of the peripheral anatomy of the ear (auditory structures that are outside the CNS). The structures are shown as if the

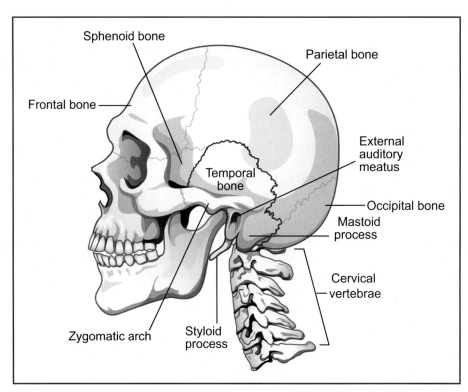

A

FIGURE 6–1. A. Sagittal view of skull showing a perimeter (*in red*) marking the boundaries of the temporal bone. *continues*

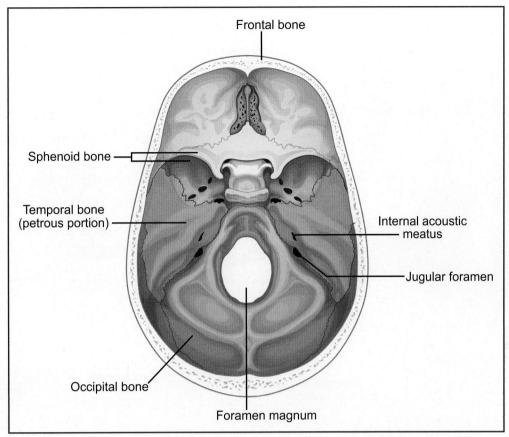

Frontal bone

Sphenoid bone

Temporal bone
(petrous portion)

Internal acoustic
meatus

Jugular foramen

Occipital bone

Foramen magnum

B

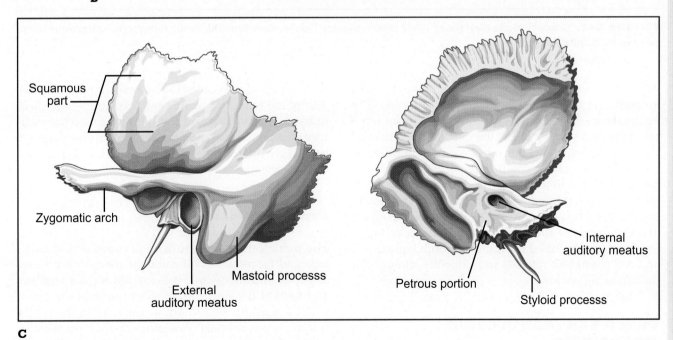

Squamous
part

Zygomatic arch

External
auditory meatus

Mastoid processs

Petrous portion

Internal
auditory meatus

Styloid processs

C

FIGURE 6–1. *continued* **B.** Interior of the base of the skull, viewed from above with top half of skull removed. **C.** Lateral (*left*) and medial (*right*) surfaces of the complexly shaped temporal bone.

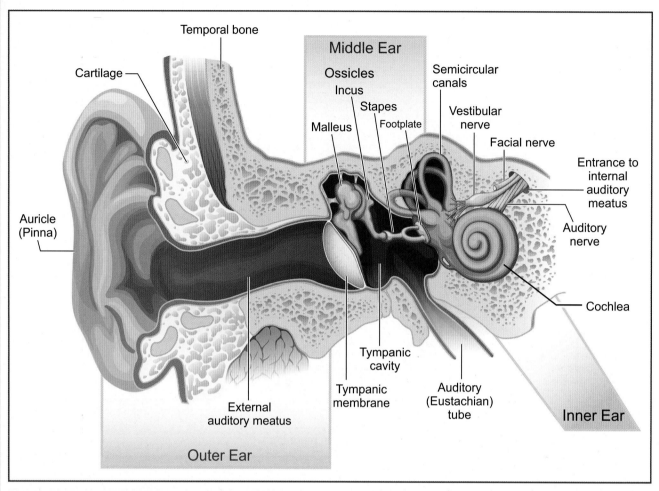

Temporal bone

Cartilage

Auricle
(Pinna)

Middle Ear

Ossicles

Incus

Stapes

Malleus

Footplate

Semicircular
canals

Vestibular
nerve

Facial nerve

Entrance to
internal
auditory
meatus

Auditory
nerve

Cochlea

Tympanic
cavity

External
auditory meatus

Tympanic
membrane

Auditory
(Eustachian)
tube

Inner Ear

Outer Ear

FIGURE 6–2. Coronal-plane view (head cut in front and back halves, view from the front) showing the structures of the peripheral auditory system.

head has been cut into front and back halves (that is, a coronal section), with the front half removed. The image shows the peripheral auditory mechanism separated into three major parts: the outer ear, the middle ear, and the inner ear. The outer ear plus middle ear are components of the conductive part of the auditory mechanism; the inner ear is the sensorineural part of the mechanism. Most of these structures are encased by the temporal bone. Figure 6–3 is a schematic diagram of the divisions of auditory anatomy, corresponding to the divisions identified in Figure 6–2. Both Figures 6–2 and 6–3 should be referred to frequently throughout the following sections.

OUTER EAR (CONDUCTIVE MECHANISM)

The outer ear includes the pinna or auricle (the structure people often refer to as "the ear") and the external

auditory canal, also called the external auditory meatus. Part of the tympanic membrane (eardrum)—the sheet of tissue that is located at the end of the external auditory meatus—is also considered a structure of the outer ear. The tympanic membrane as a whole is the boundary between the outer and middle ear.

Pinna (Auricle)

The pinna (also called auricle) is composed of cartilage and fat tissue. In humans, the pinna collects and directs sound energy into the external auditory meatus and toward the eardrum. In most humans, the pinna is not a movable body part, at least not to the extent it is in certain animals (like your cat) that use muscles to aim their pinnae, with great flexibility, at interesting sounds. Careful examination of a human's pinna shows many creases, folds, and cavities. Anatomists have names for all these features; your authors found a

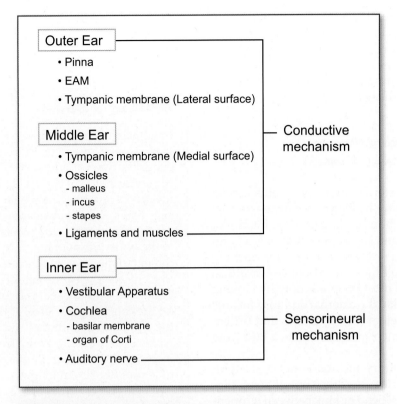

FIGURE 6–3. Schematic diagram summarizing anatomical components of the outer, middle, and inner ear, and their relationship to the functional distinction between conductive versus sensorineural auditory components.

diagram with 15 anatomical landmarks on and within the pinna! Figure 6–4 shows a human pinna with six labeled landmarks.

In humans, the shape of the pinna plays some role in the ability to locate sound sources that are elevated or lowered relative to a horizontal plane running through the head. What is known is that the pinna, by virtue of its shape, modifies the amplitudes of frequency components of sound waves striking the head. These subtle modifications provide cues to the location of a sound source in the up-down dimension.

The concha is the shallow depression of the outer ear, a sort of foyer to the ear canal. As shown in Figure 6–4, the concha may be separated into two chambers by a raised bar of cartilage that appears as a continuation of the crus of the helix, the helix being the folded edge of the pinna. The concha collects sound waves, directing them into the external auditory meatus.

The triangular fossa is the small cavity within the top and front fold of the helix. This fossa serves primarily as an anatomical landmark, and its form may be a clue in the identification of genetic syndromes in which parts of the external ear are malformed.

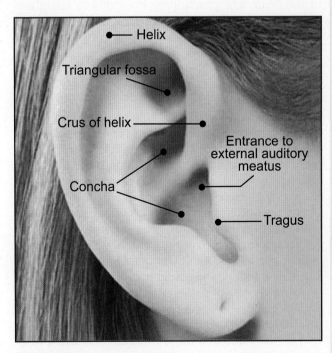

FIGURE 6–4. Photograph of human pinna (right ear) with labeled landmarks.

The tragus is a small, rounded projection from the front of the external ear, directed toward the rear of the head. Apart from the obvious value as a prominent anatomical landmark, there is some evidence for the tragus' role in locating sound along the front-rear dimension relative to the head.

External Auditory Meatus (External Auditory Canal)

The entrance of the external auditory meatus can be seen as a small opening in Figure 6–4. The external auditory meatus is a tube extending from the interior of the pinna to the tympanic membrane; *meatus* is a Latin term meaning opening or canal. This external opening into the ear, where you fit your earphones or earplugs, is fairly easy to see in most people simply by looking into the pinna. In adults, the external auditory meatus is roughly 2.5 centimeters (cm) in length and 0.7 cm in diameter. These dimensions vary quite a bit across individuals.

The external auditory meatus is not a straight, level tube; rather, it runs slightly "uphill" (see Figure 6–2) and has a small bend or kink between its opening and the tympanic membrane, where it ends. You may have noticed that your medical practitioner, when inserting an otoscope (ear scope) into your ear canal to examine the canal and view your tympanic membrane, gently pulls the pinna upward and toward the back of the head. The practitioner does this to straighten out the natural kink in the tube for a more direct view of the tympanic membrane. The kink is a backward bend in the tube that occurs in many people at the location where the canal's surrounding tissue changes from cartilage to bone.

As shown in Figure 6–2, the part of the external auditory meatus close to the concha is surrounded by cartilage; this is a continuation of the cartilaginous tissue that makes up much of the pinna. Near the bend in the external auditory meatus, the surrounding walls change from cartilage to bone; the remaining length of the ear canal, from bend to eardrum, is encased by part of the temporal bone. The external auditory meatus ends as a closed tube at the tympanic membrane.

The primary role of the external auditory meatus is to conduct sound energy from the concha to the tympanic membrane. The sound energy is in the form of pressure waves consisting of air molecules that move and vary in density over time and space (Hixon, Weismer, & Hoit, 2020, pp. 247–255). As it conducts sound energy, the external auditory meatus acts like a resonator, causing energy at certain frequencies to vibrate with greater amplitude as compared to energy at other frequencies. Specifically, the external auditory meatus of an adult amplifies energy at frequencies around 3300 Hz.

Getting a Boost

Imagine an experiment in which a pressure wave (sound) made up of frequencies of equal energy between 1 and 10000 Hz is introduced at the entrance to the ear canal (external auditory meatus). Now imagine placing a very small, sensitive microphone deep in the ear canal, precisely at the location where the ear canal ends at the tympanic membrane. You might think that the microphone would pick up the same sound that entered the ear canal. But think again. We know that the ear canal is a tube open at one end (at the concha) and closed at the other end (at the tympanic membrane) and that tubes like this have very specific resonant frequencies, depending on their length. In the case of the ear canal, a tube roughly 2.5 cm long, we can use a formula (see Hixon et al., 2020, p. 276) that identifies the primary resonant frequency as roughly 3300 Hz. Thus, the pressure wave arrives at the microphone with an energy boost around 3300 Hz. What goes in must come out, but not necessarily in the same form.

Slippery Slope of the Canal

The dead tissue that is removed through the external auditory meatus comes from the tympanic membrane. The tympanic membrane is composed of three layers of tissue. The layer on the outside is a continuation of the skin that lines the ear canal (external auditory meatus). The top layer of this skin is called keratinizing epithelium. The cells that form this epithelium lack a nucleus or other small organs that are typical of other tissue cells in the body. They are called "keratinized" because they protect the outermost layer by continuously "shedding." The shed cells do not pile up in front of the tympanic membrane like a pile of trash but rather are carried down the incline of the external auditory meatus and dispersed as they approach the concha. Something like sliding down a slippery slope.

The external auditory meatus also protects the tympanic membrane and functions as a conduit for the removal of dead tissue away from the tympanic membrane (see Slippery Slope of the Canal sidetrack on previous page). Protection of the tympanic membrane is facilitated by the production of cerumen (earwax) that is secreted by glands in the cartilaginous walls of the external auditory meatus. Cerumen presents a barrier to larger foreign objects (insects, for example) and may also block the movement of bacteria or fungal agents toward the tympanic membrane. The kinked tube of the external auditory meatus is also a barrier to foreign objects that may otherwise move easily from the outer ear to the delicate tissues of the tympanic membrane. In this sense, the shape of the canal serves a protective function.

Tympanic Membrane (Eardrum)

The tympanic membrane, or eardrum, shown in Figure 6–5, is the boundary between the outer and middle ear. The foundation of that boundary is bone. The circular perimeter of the tympanic membrane is linked to the bony foundation via a cartilage-ligamentous ring called the annulus. The annulus fits into a small circular, bony depression at the outer ear–middle ear boundary and anchors the tympanic membrane in place.

Figure 6–5 depicts the right tympanic membrane as seen through an otoscope. The otoscope has a viewing lens and a light source to illuminate the ear canal and the tympanic membrane. As a result of the shallow conical shape of the tympanic membrane and its tilt with the lower half further from the scope than the upper half, light reflects off the normal tympanic membrane in a specific way. In Figure 6–5, the reflection has the form of a narrow cone that is oriented forward, downward, and to the right. This reflection is called the "light reflex" (or "cone of light"). When the left tympanic membrane is viewed with an otoscope, the light reflex has the same form but with the downward orientation to the left. Also apparent in this otoscopic view is the circular annulus, which has a whitish appearance compared to the skin of the ear canal and is opaque in contrast to the translucent tympanic membrane. Parts of the middle ear bones (ossicles) can be seen through the membrane.

In the otoscopic view, the tympanic membrane looks more or less flat—not conical, not tilted along its top-to-bottom axis relative to the observer. The cone shape and the tilt are seen in the artist's cross-sectional rendition of the tympanic membrane (Figure 6–2). The tympanic membrane has the shape of a flattened bowl with a conical base that points into the middle ear cavity.

The tympanic membrane is composed of a three-layer sheet of tissue (see sidetrack titled Slippery Slope of the Canal). The layer at the termination of the external auditory meatus is composed of epithelial tissue that is a thinned continuation of the skin lining the canal. The layer of tissue facing the middle ear cavity is also very thin epithelium, but with a different cell structure than the layer facing the external auditory meatus. The middle layer is the primary vibratory component of the tympanic membrane and consists of fibrous tissue interlaced with collagen fibers. This middle layer is highly sensitive to very small pressures exerted by vibrating air molecules but is also capable of resisting extremely high static (nonvibratory) pressures such as those encountered in a poorly pressurized airplane cabin. The three-layer tissue structure is called the pars tensa and makes up nearly the entire surface area of the tympanic membrane. The exception is a small region in the upper part of the membrane called the pars flaccida (upper right in Figure 6–5) that lacks the middle, fibrous layer present in the rest of the tympanic membrane.

The overall thickness of the three layers of the tympanic membrane is little more than one tenth of a millimeter (0.0001 meters). The membrane has a diameter of roughly 8 to 10 mm and a surface area of about 55 mm^2. As discussed later, the surface area of the tympanic membrane plays an important role in how the middle ear mechanism transforms sound energy from the medium of air (in the external auditory meatus) to the medium of fluid (in the cochlea).

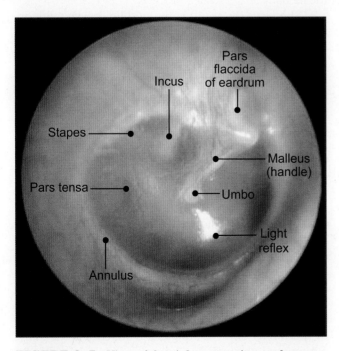

FIGURE 6–5. View of the right tympanic membrane as seen through an otoscope.

MIDDLE EAR (CONDUCTIVE MECHANISM)

The middle ear is an air-filled cavity surrounded by bone. It is a complexly shaped volume that contains tiny, movable bones (ossicles), ligaments, two muscles, nerves, and the proximal end of a tube that leads to the nasopharynx, where it terminates.

The middle ear cavity can be thought of as having six surfaces—medial, lateral, superior, inferior, posterior, and anterior—much like a cube can be described with its six surfaces. The coronal view of the middle ear cavity (see Figure 6–2) illustrates the lateral boundary of the cavity (the medial surface of the tympanic membrane plus the bone above it), the medial boundary (the bony covering of the inner ear best defined by the region around and below the attachment of the footplate of the stapes into the oval-shaped "window" of the bony labyrinth—the bony encasement of the inner ear structures), and the bony floor and roof of the cavity. This coronal section does not provide a good sense of the posterior wall of the cavity (the surface that would be seen as the back of the cavity image, if the image showed depth) or the front of the cavity, which has been cut away for this view. These different surfaces, or cavity walls, are referred to throughout the discussion of middle ear anatomy.

Chambers of the Middle Ear

The middle ear cavity is often partitioned into an upper chamber, called the epitympanum; a middle chamber, the mesotympanum; and a lower chamber, the hypotympanum. There are no clear-cut boundaries between these chambers. Nevertheless, the epitympanum is typically regarded as the chamber above the tympanic membrane and contains the head of the malleus and the body of the incus (note in Figure 6–2 their location in the small, upper cavity of the middle ear). The epitympanum also includes an airspace in its back portion called the antrum, which provides communication with air-filled cells in the mastoid process, the part of the temporal bone behind the pinna. The antrum connects the air-filled cells in the mastoid bone with the epitympanic recess (this recess can be seen in Figure 6–8, later in this chapter).

The mesotympanum is defined by the space between the top and bottom edge of the tympanic membrane. The mesotympanum contains the long processes of the malleus and incus, as well as the stapes and the oval and round windows (openings into the inner ear, described below).

The hypotympanum, or lowest space of the cavity, does not contain functional components of the middle ear but is located directly above a large vein that is separated from the floor of the middle ear cavity by a thin bony plate. Knowledge of the hypotympanum's relationship to this venous structure is critical to patient safety during middle ear surgery.

Ossicles and Associated Structures

The ossicles are the three smallest bones in the human body. They extend across the middle ear cavity from the tympanic membrane to the oval window of the cochlea. The individual ossicles plus their articulated configuration are shown in Figure 6–6. To appreciate the miniaturized size (see length calibration in Figure 6–6) of these bones, consider that all three fit (at the same time) quite easily on the lower half of the surface of a penny.

The *malleus* (also called the hammer) has a handle-like part called the manubrium, which is attached at its lower end to the tympanic membrane. The lowest attachment point of the manubrium to the tympanic membrane is called the umbo and can be seen through the translucent tissue of the tympanic membrane when viewed through an otoscope (see Figure 6–5). From this point of attachment, the handle projects upward to a thickened part, called the head of the malleus. One side of the curved edge of the malleus head articulates with the incus.

The *incus* (or anvil) is the middle ossicle, with an articular facet for the connection between it and the malleus. The upper part of the incus is made up of this facet plus a short, stubby limb that gives way to a long limb that descends to make a connection with the stapes. The hook-like end of the long limb of the incus is called the lenticular process, a subtle modification of the bone that forms the joint with the stapes.

The *stapes* (or stirrup) is the innermost (most medial) ossicle. It is the smallest of the ossicles and has an instantly recognizable shape. The very short head of the stapes is attached to the lenticular process of the incus to form the incudostapedial joint. Two arches, the anterior and posterior crura, extend from the neck and attach to an oval-shaped base, called the footplate of the stapes. The stapes fits into an oval window cut into the bony casing of the inner ear. The footplate is held in that window by a fibrous ligament (like the one securing the tympanic membrane to its circular, bony frame), the annular ligament, which adheres to the perimeter of the footplate and attaches to the bony perimeter of the oval window.

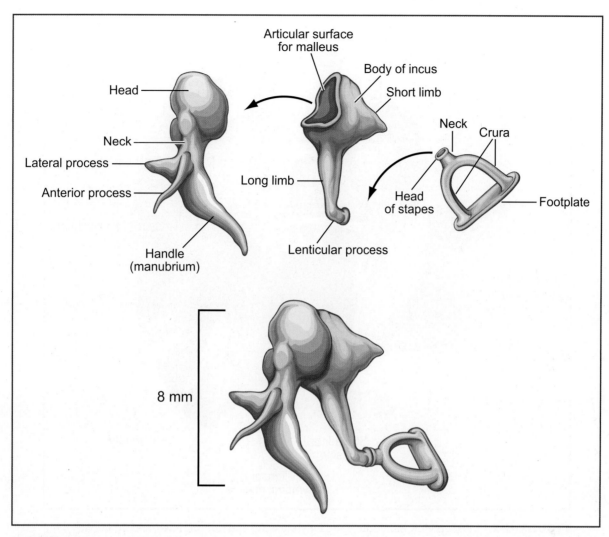

FIGURE 6–6. Artist rendition of ossicles, in their fully articulated configuration (*bottom*) and as individual, disarticulated bones (*top*). The length scale can be used to estimate the actual length or width of any of the three ossicles and its parts.

Ligaments and Muscles of the Middle Ear

The ossicles are anchored to the walls of the middle ear cavity by several ligaments and two muscles. Figure 6–7, a closeup image of the middle ear cavity, shows three ligaments attached to the ossicles (the unlabeled, pinkish-white strips extending from the ossicles in three directions to the walls of the middle ear cavity). One ligament extends from a bony point just above the tympanic membrane to the head of the malleus (lateral malleolar ligament), another is from a bony point on the "roof" of the tympanic cavity to the head of the malleus (superior malleolar ligament), and one is attached to the short process of the incus from

a point on the bony posterior wall (incudal ligament). There are two other middle ear ligaments not shown in this figure: One anchors the malleus to the front wall of the tympanic cavity (anterior malleolar ligament), and another is the annular ligament that secures the footplate of the stapes within the oval window of the bony labyrinth. All five middle ear ligaments both allow and restrict movement at the two ossicular joints—the malleolar-incudal joint (between the malleus and incus) and the incudostapedial joint (between the incus and the stapes)—as well as the movement of the footplate of the stapes into and out of the oval window.

The two muscles of the middle ear cavity are the *tensor tympani* muscle and the *stapedius* muscle (see Figure 6–7). The *tensor tympani* muscle originates

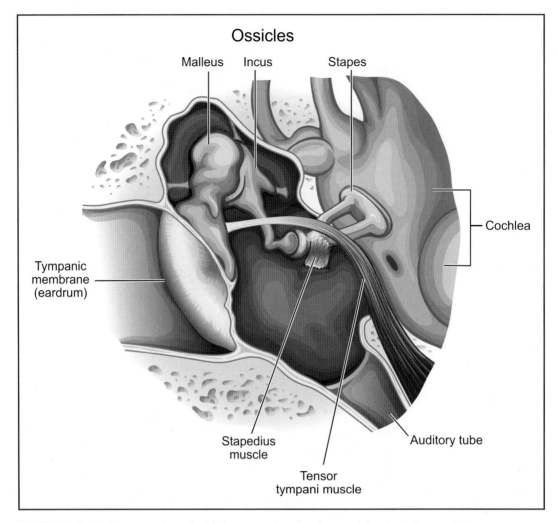

FIGURE 6–7. Closeup view of middle ear cavity, showing ossicles, muscles, and ligaments.

(Re)Flexing Your Ears

Boom! "Ouch! That hurt my ears!" It would hurt even more if you didn't have what is called an acoustic reflex. This reflex is a very quick contraction of the *stapedius* muscle in response to very loud sounds. It stiffens the ossicular chain to reduce its vibrations and protect the basilar membrane from very large displacements of cochlear fluid. Excessively strong displacement of the footplate of the stapes and the subsequent large fluid displacement has the potential to damage the cochlea's hair cells, which are the end organs of hearing. Damaged hair cells result in hearing loss. When excessive sound energy enters the ear and causes overly strong fluid displacement in the cochlea, the auditory part of cranial nerve VIII sends a signal of "too much energy" to auditory cells in the brainstem. These cells send a signal to cells that control the facial nerve (cranial nerve VII), which is the nerve that controls contraction of the *stapedius* muscle. In response, the *stapedius* muscles in both middle ear cavities contract, thus preventing the footplate of the stapes from pushing too forcefully into the cochlear fluid. The travel time around this reflex loop, from the introduction of excessive sound energy into the middle ear to the contraction of the *stapedius* muscles, is very fast, about 12 ms. But the time to the actual pull on the neck of the stapes is at least 100 ms (Gelfand, 2002). Still, a tenth of a second is pretty fast! And even better, it happens without you having to think about it.

within a bony canal in the front wall of the middle ear cavity, just next to the auditory tube (the tube that connects the middle ear cavity to the nasopharynx, also called the eustachian tube). The muscle fibers run backward to the location where the tube opens into the middle ear cavity, where they send a tiny tendon to insert into the handle of the malleus near its neck. Contraction of the *tensor tympani* muscle pulls the handle of the malleus medially, retracting the tympanic membrane into the middle ear cavity and thereby stiffening the membrane and reducing the vibratory efficiency of the conductive mechanism. The muscle is thought to provide a protective function for excessive movement of the entire conductive mechanism, which may cause damage to structures of the inner ear. Contraction of the *tensor tympani* muscle can occur in response to very high sound intensities or even during chewing.

The *stapedius* muscle originates as a tendon from a tiny hole in the back wall of the middle ear cavity, becomes a small bundle of muscle fibers, and ends in a tiny tendon at the neck of the stapes. When the muscle contracts, it pulls the stapes away from its fit into the oval window. The precise nature of the pull is to tilt the footplate out of the oval window, with the front part of the footplate most affected by this tilt. Contraction of the *stapedius* muscle stiffens the entire ossicular chain and, in so doing, protects the inner ear from excessive displacement of the footplate into the fluid of the inner ear. The *stapedius* muscle is a key component of the acoustic reflex.

Auditory (Eustachian) Tube

The auditory tube (known also as the eustachian tube, after the 16th-century Italian anatomist Bartolomeo Eustachi) is shown in Figure 6–2 as a bone-encased, open tube in the lower part of the middle ear cavity. The tube extends downward and medially from this bony part, becomes cartilaginous along its path, and terminates in a closed but flexible end in the nasopharynx at roughly the same level as the nostrils. The total length of this tube in an adult human is about 3.8 cm (1.5 inches). When the tube opens, it connects air in the middle ear cavity to air in the nasopharynx.

The nasopharynx end of the auditory tube is usually closed but can be opened by swallowing, yawning, or chewing. Immediately after the tube opens, it springs back to the closed position as a result of tissue elasticity. Intermittent opening of the auditory tube is important to expose air in the middle ear to atmospheric pressure, which is typically the pressure in the pharynx as long as the mouth or velopharynx is open. Under normal circumstances, pressure at the

lateral surface of the tympanic membrane, which is at the closed end of the external auditory meatus, is also atmospheric. This is because at its other end within the concha, the meatus is open to atmosphere. Therefore, in the absence of unusual circumstances (such as a middle ear infection), pressure on both sides of the tympanic membrane (the external ear canal side and the middle ear side) is atmospheric. This pressure balance is maintained by intermittent opening of the auditory tube.

Equal pressure across the tympanic membrane means the membrane remains in a resting position and is not pushed outward or inward by a pressure difference between the middle ear and external auditory meatus. If the auditory tube did not open intermittently, pressure in the middle ear could decrease relative to pressure in the external auditory meatus. The higher pressure in the external auditory meatus would push the tympanic membrane inward, toward the middle ear cavity. When the tympanic membrane is pulled or pushed away from its resting position, it becomes a stiffer and less efficient vibrator.

Medial and Lateral Wall View of Middle Ear: A Summary

Figures 6–8 and 6–9 offer summary views of the middle ear structures discussed above. Figure 6–8 shows middle ear structures as if they were viewed from the inner ear, looking out to the eardrum; this view looks toward the lateral wall of the tympanic cavity and associated structures. Anterior is to the left and superior to the top. The stapes has been removed so a direct view is provided of the lenticular process of the incus as well as the attachment of the handle of the malleus to the tympanic membrane. Note the *tensor tympani* muscle within the bony canal next to the auditory tube and its tendinous attachment to the handle of the malleus. The carotid artery, the main supply of blood to the cerebral hemispheres of the brain, is seen just in front and below the tympanic membrane. Cranial nerve VII (the facial nerve) is posterior to the tympanic membrane and runs in a bony canal in the back wall of the middle ear cavity. It gives off a branch called the chorda tympani that snakes between the malleus and incus before exiting the skull. The chorda tympani carries taste sensation from the anterior two thirds of the tongue to the brainstem, via cranial nerve VII.

Figure 6–9 shows middle ear structures as viewed from the vantage point of the tympanic membrane; it looks toward the medial wall of the tympanic cavity. In this view, anterior is to the right, and the incus and malleus have been removed. The crura of the stapes are shown clearly. The promontory is the bony casing of

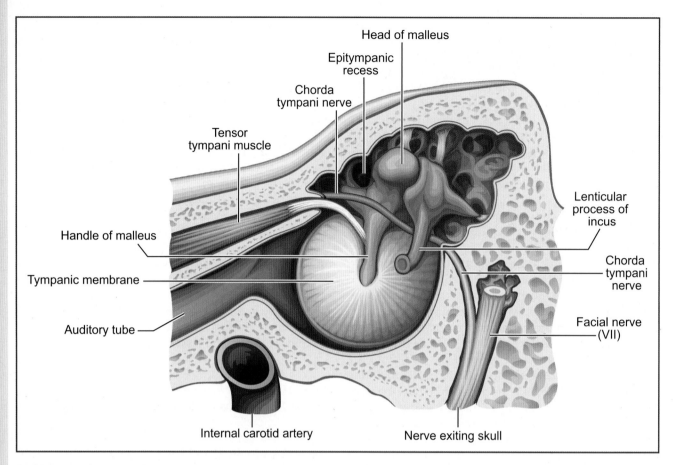

FIGURE 6–8. View of middle ear cavity as if looking at the structures from the inner ear, toward the tympanic membrane. In this view, the stapes has been removed.

the basal turn of the cochlea. Note the attachment of the *stapedius* muscle to the posterior wall of the tympanic cavity at one end and its tendon to the neck of the stapes at the other end. The bony casing (prominence) of one of the semicircular canals is also shown.

Transmission of Sound Energy by the Conductive Mechanism

The ossicles transmit vibratory energy from the tympanic membrane to the cochlea in the inner ear. This is possible because the ossicles are physically connected to the tympanic membrane on one end (where the malleus is attached) and the cochlea on the other end (where the footplate of the stapes fits into the oval window).

Although details of the cochlea have not yet been discussed, an understanding of the role of the ossicles in hearing requires the knowledge that the cochlea is composed of chambers that are filled with fluid (liquid). Displacement of this fluid is required to make auditory

nerve fibers "fire" and send impulses to the brain, where they are processed and interpreted as auditory events. The footplate of the stapes, which fits into the bony labyrinth that houses the cochlea, displaces the fluid when vibrations are transmitted through the ossicular chain (the three articulated ossicles).

The ossicular chain has special properties that help to solve the impedance mismatch between the air within the external auditory meatus and the fluid (liquid) inside the cochlea. The term *impedance mismatch* refers to the difference in displacement (movement) of two media (substances such as air and liquid) given the same applied force. Fluid such as that within the inner ear has much greater impedance (opposition to displacement) than air. Thus, a force applied to such fluid results in much less displacement than the same force applied to air. The ossicles function to match the impedance of airborne sound energy to the fluid mechanism in the cochlea. They do this by increasing the overall sound energy applied to the tympanic membrane so that it is much greater when it reaches the footplate of the stapes. This increase is done in two ways.

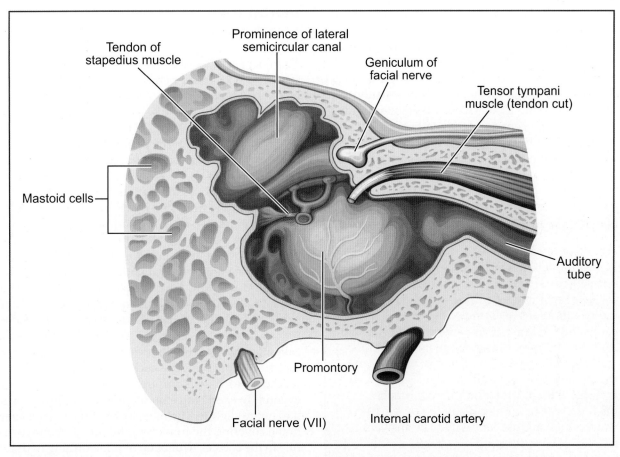

FIGURE 6-9. View of middle ear cavity as if looking at the structures from the tympanic membrane, toward the inner ear. In this view, the malleus and incus have been removed.

The first way that sound energy is increased is by augmenting the sound pressure as it travels from the tympanic membrane to the footplate of the stapes. Pressure, defined as force per unit area, is an important aspect of the strength of a sound wave. A sound wave traveling in the external auditory meatus applies force to the tympanic membrane, which has an area of roughly 55 mm^2. That force is transmitted across the ossicles and applied to the footplate of the stapes, which has an area of about 3 mm^2, nearly 20 times smaller than the area of the tympanic membrane. Thus, the force applied to the tympanic membrane by the sound wave travels across the ossicles to be applied to a much smaller area at the footplate of the stapes. As a result, the pressure (force/area) at the footplate of the stapes is much greater than it was at the tympanic membrane. In fact, the gain in pressure due to the area difference between the tympanic membrane and stapes produces an increase in sound energy of approximately 20 to 25 decibels (dB). This corresponds to a pressure gain of roughly 15:1 to 18:1. The pressure gain from tympanic membrane to stapes footplate helps to make up

for the impedance mismatch between air and the fluid within the cochlea.

The second way that sound is increased by the middle ear is that the ossicles apply a lever force to the footplate of the stapes. During tympanic membrane vibration, a very small force applied to the malleus is "levered" to the incus (the long part of the malleus is much longer than the long arm of the incus), which in turn is transmitted to the stapes. This levering action increases energy across the ossicles and contributes to matching the impedance of airborne sound waves to the fluid waves created by displacement of the footplate of the stapes into the cochlea. The lever action of the ossicular chain increases energy from the tympanic membrane to the footplate of the stapes by 1 to 3 dB.

In addition to its impedance matching function, the ossicular chain serves to emphasize certain frequencies. Specifically, the ossicular chain has a resonant frequency around 1000 to 1500 Hz, which means that it vibrates best at these frequencies. Energy between 1000 and 1500 Hz is therefore "boosted" relative to energy at other frequencies as the vibration travels across the ossicular chain. Together with the energy "boost" provided by the resonance of the external auditory meatus (around 3300 Hz), the range of frequencies between 1000 and 3500 Hz is amplified relative to other frequencies that travel through the outer and middle ear. This greater auditory sensitivity to sound energy in the 1000- to 3500-Hz frequency range is beneficial to perception of speech because much of the important energy in the speech signal—energy that serves as cues to phonetic identity—occurs within this frequency range.

No Ossicles??

What would happen if we didn't have ossicles? We wouldn't be able to hear as well. Your ossicle-less ear would have an eardrum and a cochlea, separated by an air-filled middle ear cavity. Vibrations of air molecules in your outer ear would be transmitted to the air in the middle ear cavity by the vibrating tympanic membrane, and these middle ear sound waves would strike the membrane of the oval window, behind which is cochlear fluid. Under these circumstances, is the fluid in your cochlea displaced by sound waves in the middle ear cavity? The answer is "yes," but very ineffectively because of the huge impedance mismatch between the air and fluid. If you have ever ducked your head under water in a swimming pool and listened to people talking outside the pool, you have experienced this effect. To your underwater ear, their speech sounds muffled and indistinct. This is because the sound waves traveling through the air strike the surface of the water and are mostly reflected away, with only small amount of the original energy making it to your cochlea. We should thank our lucky stars that we have ossicles!

These facts concerning the transmission of sound energy across the conductive mechanism provide examples of the interdependent nature of structure and function. Anatomical characteristics such as the relative areas of the tympanic membrane and footplate of the stapes, the relative length of "arms" of two ossicles, and the mass and stiffness which determine the resonant frequency of the linked ossicular chain determine amplitude and frequency transmission as the acoustic signal is transferred from the external auditory meatus to the cochlea. A summary of the transfer of sound energy from the external ear canal to the cochlear fluid is provided in Table 6–1.

INNER EAR (SENSORINEURAL MECHANISM)

The inner ear is housed in a complex, hollowed-out bony structure within the petrous portion of the temporal bone. The hollowed-out structure is called the bony labyrinth, or otic capsule. The bony labyrinth of the right ear is depicted in Figure 6–10. When the bony labyrinth is viewed from the perspective of the tympanic membrane (looking toward the center of the head), the semicircular canals are at the back (the left part of the Figure 6–10), the vestibule is in the middle, and the cochlea is at the front (the right part of Figure 6–10).

There are two openings into the bony labyrinth. The upper opening is called the oval window where the footplate of the stapes is attached and held in place by the annular ligament. The lower opening is the round window, which is covered by a membrane similar in structure (although not identical) to the tympanic membrane. When the footplate of the stapes moves inward, it displaces fluid within the cochlea called *perilymph.* This fluid is contained within ducts that run throughout the cochlea (see below). The displaced fluid travels through two of these ducts and eventually exerts force on the round window, causing it to bulge slightly. The movement of the flexible membrane covering the round window plays an important role in the cochlea's function of transforming hydraulic energy (energy associated with displacement of fluid) into neurochemical and electrical energy that code the frequency and intensity content of sound waves.

The Fluidity of Language

This chapter has used the term *fluid* several times to describe the contents of the bony and membranous labyrinth. The text made this terminology a bit more precise by indicating that, in the case of cochlear contents, the fluid is a liquid. Technically, any gas (like air) is a fluid; thus, the claim that the cochlea is a fluid-filled structure could mean it is filled with air, which, as you know by now, is not the case. We use the term *fluid* in the lay sense, but the distinction between the fluid air and the fluid water is an important one: As noted in the text, air has much lower impedance compared to liquid. Thus, if you wanted to be absolutely precise in your use of language, you would use the term liquid to describe the cochlear contents. However, the scientific literature always uses the term "fluid" for the contents of thr cochlear ducts, and we do as well.

TABLE 6-1. Summary of Transfer of Energy From Air in External Auditory Meatus to Cochlear Fluid

Impedance mismatch between air and fluid

- Given a constant force applied to air molecules and the fluid molecules in the cochlea, air molecules are displaced more easily compared with fluid molecules; stated otherwise, fluid in the cochlea has greater impedance compared with air.
- Sound energy applied to the tympanic membrane would be relatively ineffective in displacing the fluid in the cochlea if a solution to the impedance mismatch was not "built into" the conductive component of the auditory periphery.

The conductive component "corrects" the impedance mismatch

- Area of the tympanic membrane is much greater than area of the footplate of the stapes.
- Sound pressure (force/area) applied to the tympanic membrane is greatly increased at the footplate of the stapes because the area of the footplate is much smaller than the area of the tympanic membrane (primary mechanism of correcting the impedance mismatch).
- Lever action of the ossicles increases the movement of the stapes into the cochlear fluid.

Certain frequencies are conducted with greater amplitude than other frequencies due to the resonance characteristics of the external auditory meatus and of the ossicular chain.

- Resonance of the external auditory meatus is approximately 3300 Hz for an external auditory meatus with a length of 2.5 cm.
- Resonance of the ossicular chain is between 1000 and 1500 Hz.
- Due to these resonance effects, the frequency region between ~1000 and 3500 Hz is conducted with great amplitude compared to other frequencies.

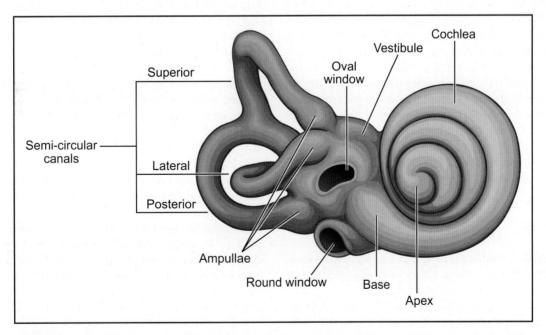

FIGURE 6-10. The bony labyrinth (otic capsule), as if viewed from the middle ear cavity of the right ear. The semicircular canals are to the left, the vestibule is in the middle, and the cochlea is to the right.

The bony labyrinth includes three major structures. These are the semicircular canals, the vestibule, and the cochlea.

Semicircular Canals

Three semicircular canals comprise the back part of the bony labyrinth. Although it cannot be seen in the two-dimensional image of Figure 6–10, a view from above the head, looking straight down to the bony labyrinth, shows the semicircular canals to be posterior and lateral to the cochlea. One semicircular canal is oriented in the superior-inferior dimension, one extends posteriorly, and one extends laterally. Note in Figure 6–10 how any one of the canals is oriented at right angles to the other two. Each of the bony canals contains perilymph, and within the perilymph is a membranous duct that follows the contour of the bony canals. These membranous ducts contain a fluid called *endolymph*. The endolymph is displaced when the head moves; this displacement causes bending of hair cells, small sensory organs (the ampullae) that include hair-like structures located at the base of the canals. The bending causes the cells to send signals to the brain that the head has been rotated from side to side (as in shaking the head "no": horizontal semicircular canal), forward and backward (as in nodding the head: superior semicircular canal), or toward and away from the shoulders (as in "wagging" the head in time with music: posterior semicircular canal). Movements of the head are typically complex combinations of these three simple dimensions.

Movements of the head are translated into motion perception by the relative displacement of endolymph and the bending of hair cells within the three canals. Bending of the hair cells results in complex patterns of neural activity that "code" head movements. The neural activity travels in nerve fibers that arise from the hair cells and gather together to form the vestibular part of cranial nerve VIII (the auditory-vestibular nerve). This nerve bundle runs through the internal auditory meatus on its way to the brainstem.

Vestibule

The vestibule contains the oval window where the footplate of the stapes is fixed. Other critical structures of the vestibule are the utricle and saccule.

The utricle, a swelling at the base of the three semicircular canals, contains hair cells. These hair cells send signals to the brain concerning the position of the head relative to the position of the body, as well as the degree of acceleration of the head (and the rest of the body). The signals sent from the utricle to the brain are integrated with signals from the eyes and other body structures to create a sense of body position and motion in space. The utricle primarily provides information on positions and motions in the horizontal plane. The saccule is another pouch-like swelling below and in front of the utricle. It performs essentially the same function as the utricle, but for motion in the vertical plane. The combined activity generated by the utricle and saccule provides information about complex positions and motions of the head.

Cochlea

The cochlea (meaning snail) is made up many smaller structures. Among the most important of these are the scalae (plural for scala), the basilar membrane, and the organ of Corti, which includes hair cells. These structures transform sound energy into neural signals via traveling waves within the cochlear fluid.

Scalae

The cochlea consists of three membranous, fluid-filled ducts that are coiled in a snail shell–shaped spiral. The membranous spiral, encased in the similarly coiled bony labyrinth, includes two and one-half turns from its base to its tip. The three ducts of the cochlea are called the *scala vestibuli, scala media* (or cochlear duct), and *scala tympani*. Figure 6–11 shows the coiled cochlea cut in several cross sections; the three ducts are visible at each cut. The tip of the cochlear spiral is called the heliocotrema (not shown in the figure), where the scala vestibuli and scala tympani are connected to allow fluid flow between these two ducts. This connection explains why the fluid displacement at the oval window (pushing into the scala vestibuli) is transmitted to the scala tympani. After a *very* brief delay (on the order of microseconds), the fluid displacement caused by movement of the oval window results in bulging of the round window (the termination of the scala tympani).

The scala media is separated from the scala tympani by a membrane called the basilar membrane, and from the scala vestibuli by Reissner's membrane. Nerve fibers emerge from the base of the middle duct (scala media) and gather in the center of the snail shell to form the auditory part of cranial nerve VIII.

The fluid in the scala vestibuli and scala tympani is perilymph, the same fluid that fills the bony semicircular canals. When the footplate of the stapes pushes

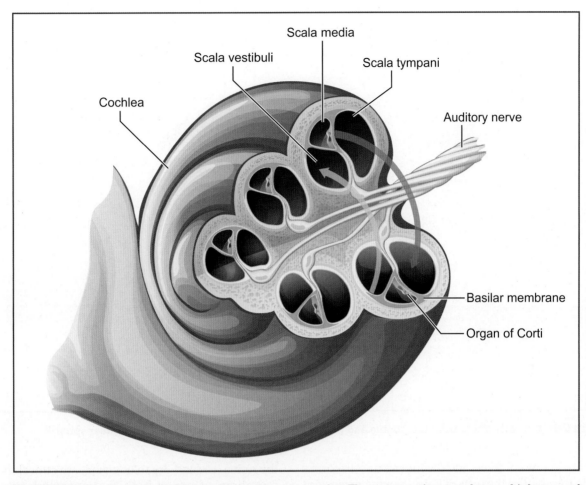

FIGURE 6–11. The spirals of the cochlea cut in cross section. The cross-section cuts show multiple turns of the cochlea. Each section of the cochlea contains three scalae: the scala vestibuli, the scala media (cochlear duct), and scala tympani.

into the scala vestibuli, perilymph is displaced toward the heliocotrema (apex of the spiral), which causes displacement of the perilymph of the scala tympani. The force exerted by the moving perilymph causes the round window to bulge. The scala media, the smaller duct that sits between the scala vestibuli and scala tympani, contains a different fluid called endolymph. Endolymph has special chemical properties that are important to the "firing" of hair cells within the cochlea.

The displacement of the perilymph not only causes the round window to bulge but also displaces fluid within the scala media, which results in movement of the membrane that forms the wall between the scala media and the scala tympani. This membrane, the basilar membrane, runs the length of the cochlea from its base near the oval window up to the heliocotrema. Sitting on top of the basilar membrane, throughout its

entire length, is the organ of Corti, which contains the sensory organs for hearing.

Basilar Membrane and Organ of Corti

An artist's rendition of the basilar membrane and organ of Corti is shown in Figure 6–12. To get an idea of how much this image has been magnified relative to the size of the actual organs, consider that the nearly vertical structures labeled "inner hair cells" and "outer hair cells" are roughly 30 micrometers (0.000030 meters, around 1/1,000th of an inch) in length and 10 micrometers in diameter. Artist renditions of the organ of Corti and hair cells depend on photographs of the scala media that use high-magnification microscopes. Figure 6–12 shows several different cell types sitting atop the basilar membrane, the most important of which (for this discussion) are the hair cells. The outer hair

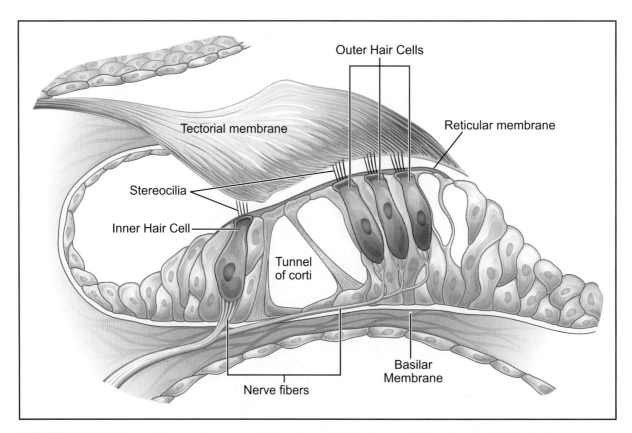

FIGURE 6–12. The basilar membrane and the organ of Corti, at one cut along the cochlear spiral.

cells are in rows of three, and the inner hair cells form a single row. Notice the tufts of hairy-looking extensions at the top of each hair cell, many of the tips of which are embedded in the tectorial membrane above. The basilar membrane, the organ of Corti and its hair cells, and the tectorial membrane form the end organ of hearing.

The image in Figure 6–12 is a cross section at a single "slice" along the scala media. If the cochlea were stretched out—uncoiled—as it is in Figure 6–13, the image in Figure 6–12 would be from a single cross-sectional slice somewhere along the length of the scala media. The view in Figure 6–12 is as if we are looking directly into the contents of the scala media (cochlear duct) at the location of the cut. The vestibular and tympanic cuts, although not included in this magnified image, are at the top and bottom, respectively, of the scala media shown in Figure 6–12.

Hair Cells

The hair cells within the organ of Corti are critical to auditory sensation, much like the rods and cones of the retina, the end organ of vision, are critical to visual sensation. Although both the inner and outer hair cells contribute to hearing sensitivity, they do so in different ways.

The inner hair cells are deformed by fluid motion within the scala media, which transforms hydraulic motion (movement of the fluid within the cochlea) into electrical impulses in nerve fibers connecting the cochlea to the brain. Note in Figure 6–12 how the inner hair cells have nerve fibers (shown in yellow) extending from their base. When all these nerve fibers are gathered together from all inner hair cells along the length of the organ of Corti, they form a major part of the auditory (or cochlear) nerve (which is part of cranial nerve VIII, the auditory-vestibular nerve). This part of the auditory nerve conducts electrical impulses to specialized auditory structures in the CNS. Because the nerve fibers from the inner hair cells send impulses from the peripheral end organ of hearing to the CNS, they are referred to as the afferent component of the auditory nerve.[1] The inner hair cells and the nerves to which they are connected perform a frequency analysis

[1]As used here, "afferent" means running from a peripheral structure such as the cochlea, in the direction of the central nervous system (CNS). The term *efferent* means the opposite—running from the CNS to a peripheral structure. See Chapter 8 for a broader definition of the terms afferent and efferent.

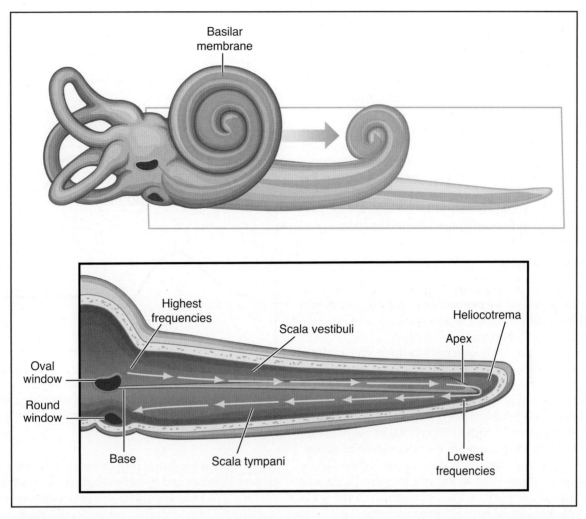

FIGURE 6–13. The cochlea as if theoretically rolled out (*top*) to form a straight tube (*bottom*). In the bottom image, the scala vestibuli is the top duct, the scala tympani is the bottom duct, and the basilar membrane is shown as the pink partition in the middle. The membrane is narrow and stiff at the base and wide and floppy at the apex.

of the acoustic signal that enters the central auditory system. In humans, this frequency analysis (pitch analysis, in perceptual terms) is exquisitely precise.

The outer hair cells are also connected to the CNS by nerve fibers, specifically by efferent fibers (see Footnote 1). These nerve fibers exit the brainstem, run in the auditory nerve, and terminate at the base of the outer hair cells. The outer hair cells, stimulated by impulses from cells in the brainstem, vibrate and in so doing amplify the response of the inner hair cells to the deformation by fluid displacement described above. This is why the outer hair cells are often referred to as the *cochlear amplifier*. This amplification is particularly effective for sounds with very little energy. A cochlea without outer hair cells would be a cochlea with very poor sensitivity to the wide range of sound energies

in the environment, including speech and music. Stimulation of the outer hair cells also increases the precision of the frequency analysis performed by the inner hair cells.

The location of the inner and outer hair cells along the basilar membrane is critical to understanding frequency analysis within the cochlea. The unrolled cochlea at the bottom of Figure 6–13 illustrates the basilar membrane, shown in pink, as narrow at its base (the left end of the membrane in the figure) and becoming increasingly wider as it extends to the apex of the cochlea. The narrow base of the basilar membrane is very stiff and the wide tip end of the membrane is relatively floppy. Sitting atop the basilar membrane all along its length are the single row of inner hair cells and three rows of outer hair cells. The hair cells at the base (narrow part) of the membrane are sensitive to the *highest* frequencies humans can hear (about 20000 Hz). Moving away from the base toward the tip of the basilar membrane, the hair cells are sensitive to increasingly lower frequencies until at the tip they are sensitive to the *lowest* frequencies humans are capable of hearing (about 20 Hz). Frequency, therefore, is represented "tonotopically" along the basilar membrane such that the location of a hair cell along the membrane determines its specific frequency sensitivity.[2] The tonotopic organization of frequency sensitivity along the basilar membrane (demonstrated in Video 6–1 [Tonotopic Organization]) is critical to the concept of fluid displacement in the cochlea as a traveling wave.

Traveling Waves

The tonotopic arrangement of the hair cells running from base to apex of the basilar membrane raises the question of how different locations along the membrane are stimulated when vibratory motions of the conductive mechanism are transferred to the cochlear fluid. The explanation of the cochlear response to vibration leads to an understanding of how nerve fibers associated with different frequencies are made to fire.

Georg von Békésy (1899–1972), a Hungarian physicist and engineer, studied the cochlea's response to sound energy in many mammals (including humans). Békésy observed that when the footplate of the stapes vibrated in response to sound energy introduced into the external auditory meatus, perilymph in the scala vestibuli was displaced and a fluid wave traveled from the base of the cochlea to the apex. Most important, he observed that the amplitude of the wave varied from base to apex. He found that the location of the highest amplitude of the wave depended directly on the frequency of the sound energy. When the frequency was low, the wave amplitude built up gradually and reached its peak near the apex of the basilar membrane, some distance from the oval window. In contrast, high-frequency sound energy produced a fluid wave that built to a peak (crested) at a short distance from the oval window (that is, near the base), with a quickly decreasing amplitude as the wave moved from its crest toward the apex of the membrane. In his world-famous 1928 paper, Békésy described this as a traveling wave.

Figure 6–14 shows a schematic view of two different traveling waves in an uncoiled representation of the cochlea. The top, unrolled cochlea shows a straight line (no wave) from base (where the stapes fits into the oval window) to tip. This is the hypothetical case

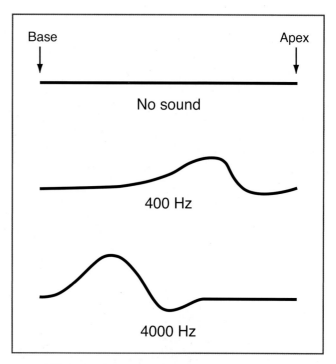

FIGURE 6–14. Schematic representation of the traveling wave in response to a 400-Hz tone (*middle*) and a 4000-Hz tone (*bottom*). The top line shows the reference pattern of no sound (and therefore no traveling wave).

when there is no sound transmitted across the conductive mechanism and therefore no traveling wave in the cochlea. The middle pattern shows what is expected for a relatively low-frequency sound, in this case, a 400-Hz tone (a sinusoid—see below). In this illustration, the wave is shown at a single instant in time. Note that the greatest amplitude of this traveling wave is relatively close to the apex of the cochlea. The bottom pattern in the figure shows a large-amplitude wave closer to the base, with rapidly decreasing amplitudes as the wave moves toward the apex. This is like the traveling wave pattern seen for a 4000-Hz sinusoid. It is relevant to note that the tendency for the basilar membrane to be maximally deformed at a particular location is due, in part, to mechanical differences in the tissue along the membrane: The stiff base of the membrane moves more easily at higher frequencies, and the floppy apex moves more easily at lower frequencies.

Békésy called these cochlear displacement patterns traveling waves because they literally traveled through the perilymph of the cochlea; that is, it took some time for fluid to move from the base to apex of the cochlea. Of course, the time delay between displacement of

---

[2]The concept of tonotopic organization of the hair cells along the basilar membrane is conceptually similar to the somatotopic organization of the primary motor and sensory cortex, as discussed in Chapter 8 and illustrated in Figure 8–5.

the stapes and arrival of the wave at the apex of the cochlea is extremely brief (on average, about 0.000090 seconds [90 microseconds, or 90 μs]). The fact that there is any delay of fluid motion between the base and apex supports the idea of a fluid wave moving over time from the point of origin (the oval window) to the apex of the cochlea.

The nature of the cochlear traveling wave also suggests that, for a given frequency, wave patterns such as those in Figure 6–14 are snapshots in time. Even for the same, single frequency—a sinusoid—the wave appears differently depending on the instant in time when the traveling wave pattern is captured. The waves "build up" over time, even if the relevant time intervals are extremely brief. For example, the 4000-Hz wave may look somewhat different if the snapshot is taken very close to the onset of the signal or at a later time when the signal has been stimulating the peripheral auditory system continuously. This buildup of the traveling wave for a 400-Hz and 4000-Hz tone can be seen in Video 6–2 (Traveling Wave).

The traveling waves shown in the middle and bottom of Figure 6–14 can be thought of as displacements of the basilar membrane and the organ of Corti riding atop it. These displacements are caused by time-dependent pressure differences between perilymph in the scala tympani versus the scala vestibuli (the scalae that surround the scala media where the basilar membrane and organ of Corti reside). The initial displacement of fluid in the scala vestibuli creates a higher pressure in its perilymph as compared to pressure in the perilymph of the scala tympani. That pressure difference causes the basilar membrane to move away from the region of higher pressure (scala vestibuli) and toward the region of lower pressure (scala tympani). The wave patterns in Figure 6–14 can be thought of as pressure differences across the basilar membrane, with greater wave amplitudes corresponding to greater pressure differences. For example, a high-frequency sinusoid results in a large pressure difference toward the base of the cochlea and much smaller pressure differences as the wave moves in the direction of the apex. The large amplitude displacement toward the base of the cochlea causes greater deformation of the hair cells in this region, which results in the firing of high-frequency nerve fibers.

The hair cells in the organ of Corti are prominently featured in the closeup cross-sectional view of the cochlea in Figure 6–12. The hairy "tufts" sticking out of the top of the single inner hair cell and each of the three outer hair cells give them their name. These tufts consist of multiple, tiny projections called *stereocilia*. Each of the stereocilia is roughly 0.025 millimeters in length (some a bit shorter, some longer). As many as 300 stereocilia may project from the tip of each hair cell.

Directly above the hair cells is the tectorial membrane. This membrane is very close to the tips of the inner hair cells and actually in contact with the tips of the stereocilia of many outer hair cells.

The inner hair cells are mechanoelectrical transducers. When the traveling wave deforms the basilar membrane at a particular location along the spirals of the cochlea, the hair cells at that location are bent by the fluid displacement and may even be pushed into the gel-like tectorial membrane directly above them. This is the "mechano" part of mechanoelectrical transduction. Sufficient bending of the hair cells causes molecule-sized pores, or channels, to open in the hair-cell membrane, allowing potassium ions (positively charged molecules) in the endolymph to rush inside the hair cell, which at rest—when the hair cells are not bent—has a negative charge relative to the tissue outside the cell. The influx of positive ions causes a quick reversal of the charge: Suddenly, the inside of the hair cell is charged positively relative to the charge outside the cell. This process is called depolarization of the cell. Depolarization of a hair cell releases a chemical, called a neurotransmitter, that causes the nerve fiber attached to the hair cell to "fire." This depolarization is the "electrical" part of the mechanoelectrical transduction. The nerve fiber exiting the base of an inner hair cell (see Figure 6–12) makes a connection (synapse) within a cluster of nerve cell bodies (called a ganglion) a short distance from the hair cell, which causes a fiber in the auditory nerve to fire and conduct an impulse to the brainstem, where the next synapse is located. These nerve fibers, from inner hair cell to ganglion and then to the brainstem, are typically referred to as afferent (inward directed, toward the CNS) fibers. As noted above, afferent fibers in the peripheral nervous system deliver input from the periphery to the CNS.

AUDITORY NERVE AND AUDITORY PATHWAYS (NEURAL MECHANISM)

The auditory nerve, a peripheral part of the auditory mechanism, and the auditory pathways within the CNS comprise the neural component of the hearing mechanism. The cochlea and the auditory nerve (the auditory part of cranial nerve VIII) are often combined to designate the "sensorineural component" of the auditory mechanism (see Figure 6–3), even though the cochlea and auditory nerve are separate structures. Audiologists—specialists in the identification of hearing loss and the structures causing the loss—use basic tests to determine how much of a hearing loss is due to sensorineural factors versus conductive factors. Within the sensorineural component, advance tests are available to separate the hearing functions of the cochlea from those of the auditory nerve; tests are also available to evaluate the role of the central auditory pathways in hearing. Musiek and Baran (2018) and Kramer and Brown (2019) are excellent sources of information for how different audiological tests are used to identify the amount of hearing loss associated with damage to conductive, sensorineural (cochlear plus auditory nerve), and central auditory structures.

Auditory Nerve

Figure 6–12 shows afferent nerve fibers attached to the base of the inner hair cells and efferent nerve fibers attached to the base of the outer hair cells. The afferent nerve fibers have a first synapse (connection) in the spiral ganglion. From there, they are gathered together to form a significant part of the auditory nerve (which is part of cranial nerve VIII). The efferent fibers, from brainstem to outer hair cells, make up another part of the auditory nerve. Both afferent and efferent fibers of the auditory nerve run through the internal auditory meatus on their way between the cochlea and brainstem (afferent) or brainstem and cochlea (efferent). The internal auditory meatus also contains the fibers of the vestibular part of cranial nerve VIII (the vestibular nerve) as well as fibers of cranial nerve VII (the facial nerve). Refer back to Figure 6–2, which shows the cochlear and vestibular components of cranial nerve VIII and the fibers of cranial nerve VII entering the distal opening of the internal auditory meatus. The close proximity of the facial nerve to the auditory nerve is significant because the former may be affected by disease of the latter, as in the case of a tumor on the auditory nerve that presses on the facial nerve. The combination of auditory problems and facial weakness may have diagnostic significance due to the proximity of the two nerves within the internal auditory meatus.

Like hair cells on the basilar membrane, the auditory nerve is arranged tonotopically. The outer or surface fibers in the nerve bundle are from the base of the cochlea and therefore carry impulses resulting from high-frequency stimulation. From the surface of the nerve bundle to its core, the fibers carry information from higher to lower frequencies. Fibers at the core of the auditory nerve carry information on very low frequencies, originating in hair cells from the apex of the basilar membrane.

Central Auditory Pathways

The term *central auditory pathways* designates structures in the nervous system that carry afferent auditory impulses from the point at which the auditory nerve enters the brainstem up to the cortex, the highest level of the CNS. It also refers to efferent pathways—nerve fibers descending in the CNS that leave the brainstem and continue in the auditory nerve to the outer hair cells on the basilar membrane. The focus in this section is on the afferent auditory pathways.

When electrical impulses are transmitted in the nervous system, they travel along nerves (or tracts, as they are called in the CNS) and make connections (synapses) in clusters of cell bodies, which issue another tract aimed at a different cluster of cell bodies. In the case of the auditory system, particular pathways are more or less dedicated to transmitting information from the auditory nerve all the way to the auditory cortex.

Figure 6–15 illustrates a broad-stroke view of the auditory pathways in the human brain. The bottom

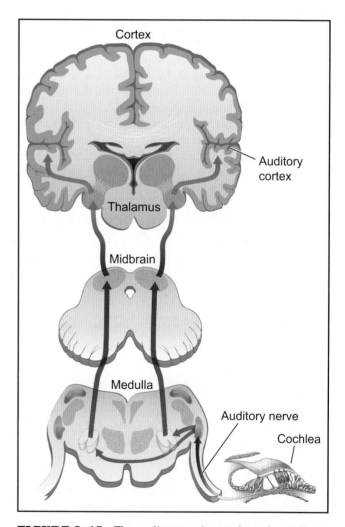

FIGURE 6–15. The auditory pathways from the auditory nerve to the primary auditory cortex in the temporal lobe. The pathways include several nuclei (clusters of cells) and fiber bundles (tracts). These pathways are "dedicated" to auditory function and for the most part maintain tonotopic arrangement.

right of Figure 6–15 shows the auditory nerve emerging from the cochlea and entering the brainstem, where the central auditory pathways begin. After the auditory nerve on one side (in this case, the left ear, as if the head is facing the viewer) enters the lowest level of the brainstem, the medulla, its fibers make synapses with specific cell groups, indicated in Figure 6–15 by brown shapes. These cell groups give off axons (projections extending from the body of a nerve cell) that cross the midline of the brainstem in a fiber bundle, shown in Figure 6–15 by a red arrow that turns purple when it reaches the opposite side. The fiber tract ascends to the midbrain, the highest level of the brainstem, where synapses are made with another cell group; these midbrain cells send fibers to a cell group in the thalamus, which send fibers to cells of the primary auditory cortex in the temporal lobe of the cerebral hemispheres. These central auditory pathways, including all cell groups (nuclei) and axon bundles (fiber tracts), typically maintain tonotopic arrangement from the brainstem to the cortex. Primary analysis in the auditory cortex, located in the temporal lobe, is sent to auditory association cortex for complex analysis of events such as speech and music.

Most (but not all) of the auditory nerve fibers that enter the brainstem on one side cross over in the medulla to the other side before ascending on their way to the cortex. This means that the auditory information that comes into the left ear is largely represented in the primary auditory cortex of the right hemisphere and vice versa for auditory information entering the right ear. Still, a large number of fibers (perhaps 25% of all the ascending fibers) stay on the same side as the side of entry of the auditory nerve. Thus, auditory information from one ear has representation on both sides of the auditory cortex.

This presentation of the central auditory pathways is purposely "stripped down." The names of the fiber tracts and the cell groups with which they make contact have not been included, nor have the more complex connections between cell groups and fiber tracts. A summary of the important information presented in this section is (1) the afferent component of the central auditory pathways consists of neural cell groups and fiber tracts that are dedicated to auditory analysis, (2) the pathways begin in cell groups within the medulla, and as they ascend make contact with cell groups in the midbrain, the thalamus, and finally the auditory cortex of the temporal lobe, (3) about 75% of the fibers that enter the brainstem via the auditory nerve on one side of the brainstem cross over within the medulla to the other side of the brainstem before ascending through the levels named in point (2), and (4) like the hair cells within the cochlea and the fibers of the auditory nerve, the cell groups and fiber tracts

of the central auditory pathways have a tonotopic arrangement.

The efferent auditory pathways are not shown in Figure 6–15, in part because the anatomy of the efferent auditory system is less well understood than that of the afferent system. The efferent fibers originate in the auditory cortex and have a complicated pathway down through the thalamus and brainstem on their way to the cochlea. There is a good evidence, as presented above, that the innervation of the outer hair cells serves to amplify and even "tune" the response of the inner hair cells to motions of the basilar membranes. The efferent pathways also play an important role in contraction of the two middle ear muscles, the *stapedius* muscle and the *tensor tympani* muscle. The efferent auditory fibers do not innervate those muscles directly, but they form reflex-type loops with other cranial nerves to control the contraction of these muscles. The central auditory pathways are described more fully in Hixon et al. (2020), as well as Musiek and Baran (2018).

It is sometimes difficult to envision how a sound enters the ear and is transduced from mechanical energy into neural signals. The reader is encouraged to take advantage of available animations that offer a dynamic look at how the auditory system processes sound; see, for example, Video 6–3 (Sound to Brain).

Transduction in the Auditory System

Transduction refers to the conversion of one form of energy into another form of energy. And transduction plays a critical role in understanding how the auditory system conducts sound through a series of transductions so that sound waves are ultimately processed in the brain as electrical signals. Sound pressure vibrations in air are transduced into mechanical vibrations of the tympanic membrane and ossicles. These mechanical vibrations are then transduced to hydromechanical energy when the footplate of the stapes pushes into the oval window and the traveling wave results in deformation of the hair cells. The transduction into electrical energy occurs when the deformed (bent) hair cells are depolarized (see more on depolarization in Chapter 8). Depolarization causes nerve fibers attached to the hair cells to "fire" and conduct electrical impulses through the auditory nerve and to the CNS. Nature has clearly devised an interesting series of transduction events to get sound wave information from the external world of air to the brain world of electrical impulses.

CLINICAL NOTES

Clinical audiology is the discipline of diagnosis and treatment of hearing disorders. Diagnosis of a hearing disorder is based not only the amount of hearing loss but also on its underlying cause. As discussed above in this chapter, the auditory mechanism has a conductive component, a sensorineural component, and a CNS component. Hearing loss can result from damage to each or any combination of these components.

Hearing loss is a common problem in people of all ages. According to the National Institute on Deafness and other Communication Disorders (NIDCD), National Institutes of Health (NIH), 2 to 3 of every 1,000 children born have some form of hearing loss, approximately 12.5% of all people aged 12 or older have a significant hearing loss, and for people aged 65 to 74, the number with hearing loss increases to 25% and rises again to 50% for people aged 75 and older. Additional statistical information on hearing loss can be found at https://www.nidcd.nih.gov/health/statistics

Part of the long history of audiology is the design of hearing tests that are tailored to diagnose the health of specific components of the auditory mechanism. Here we discuss the anatomical and physiological basis of pure-tone audiometry, a hearing test that is often the starting point in the audiologist's test protocol.

Pure-tone audiometry is performed with tones having sound energy at only a single frequency—hence the term *pure* tone. Typically, six different frequencies are used in the test, each delivered separately to a listener via headphones. The frequencies in standard pure-tone testing are 250, 500, 1000, 2000, 4000, and 8000 Hz (Hz is the abbreviation for "cycles per second").[3] The person being tested raises her hand (or pushes a button) each time she hears the tone; the tester's goal is to find the lowest sound level (intensity) below which the person never hears the tone. That sound level is called the pure-tone *threshold*.

To understand the logic of this test, think back to the earlier discussion of tonotopic representation along the basilar membrane. Across the frequency range of human hearing, the lowest frequency of about 20 Hz is represented on the basilar membrane at the tip of the cochlea, and the highest frequency is represented on the basilar membrane at the base of the cochlea. Starting at the base and moving in the direction of the tip, the frequency sensitivity of the hair cells decreases systematically all the way to the tip, where hair cell sensitivity is greatest for the lowest frequencies heard by humans. In other words, specific locations along the basilar membrane are sensitive to specific frequencies.

When sound energy is transmitted across the ossicles and the footplate of the stapes pushes into the oval window, the result is a traveling fluid wave within the cochlea. Unlike more complicated sounds, a pure tone creates a traveling wave that has a very precise "crest" at a specific point along the basilar membrane. This precise crest bends only those hair cells in a narrow region along the basilar membrane. Thus, the use of pure tones to determine hearing thresholds allows a tester to "pinpoint" locations along the basilar membrane where the hair cells are healthy and locations where they may be damaged.

A chart called an audiogram is used to record pure-tone thresholds at each of the six test frequencies. The audiograms in Figure 6–16 show hearing level represented on the *y*-axis in 10-decibel (dB) steps, with 0 dB near the top of the chart; the six test frequencies are ordered from low to high frequency along the *x*-axis. The threshold obtained at 250 Hz reflects the health of the hair cells at a point near the tip of the basilar membrane, the threshold at 500 Hz the health of hair cells at a point some distance from the tip, and so on; the threshold at 8000 Hz reflects the health of the hair cells furthest from the tip for the six test frequencies identified above. Three sample audiometric results in Figure 6–16 are described below after a brief explanation of the 0-dB line of an audiogram.

The "0-dB" line does not mean "no sound energy." It is approximately the lowest sound level at which a large sample of people with normal hearing cannot detect the presence of a tone.[4] The 0-dB line is a norm that defines healthy-hearing thresholds for each of the test frequencies. Additional information on the meth-

---

[3]Pure-tone testing may also be done at other frequencies, especially at 125, 6000, and 10000 Hz.

[4]The reader may have noticed that the terms *sound level* and *hearing level* are used throughout this discussion. The terms are different, even though they both refer to an expression of the degree of sound energy. In brief, *sound level*, expressed in dB, is used for the level of energy relative to a reference level. The reference level may be the sound energy that is the minimal audible energy that can be detected by the average listener with normal hearing, but it also may have a different reference, well above the minimal detectable sound energy, as in the statement, "typical human conversation has a sound level that is 30 dB greater than the sound level of whispered conversation." *Hearing level* is a term specific to an audiogram, in which sound energy is based on the thresholds of listeners with normal hearing, as described in the text. In this sense, a negative threshold (e.g., –10 dB) makes sense—sound energy is present at a threshold of –10 dB but is less than the average sound energy present for the average thresholds of people with normal hearing—where the reference on the audiogram chart is 0 dB. A more detailed explanation of the technical difference between sound level and hearing level is presented in Hixon et al. (2020).

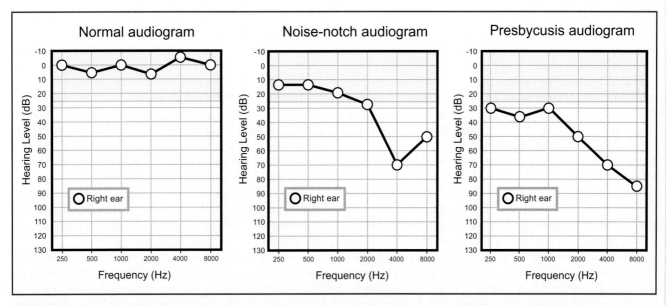

FIGURE 6–16. Audiograms showing hearing thresholds for a single ear. Pure-tone frequency is on the *x*-axis; hearing level is on the *y*-axis. *Left*, normal thresholds; *middle*, noise-notch audiogram; *right*, presbycusis audiogram.

ods used to generate audiometric norms is presented in Hixon et al. (2020).

The three audiograms in Figure 6–16 show thresholds for a single ear (for example, the right ear) as circles at each frequency–sound level coordinate (thresholds are typically determined separately for the two ears). In each audiogram, the circles are connected across the six test frequencies by straight lines. The audiogram on the left shows normal thresholds at each frequency. Note that three thresholds (250, 1000, and 8000 Hz) are on the 0-dB line; those for 500, 2000, and 4000 Hz are not. For a given frequency, normal thresholds fall within a range of hearing levels, rather than exclusively at 0 dB. This range, from −10 dB to 25 dB, is shaded light blue. The inclusion of −10 dB on the *y*-axis within the range of "normal" thresholds reflects the fact that some people can detect the presence of a pure tone at even lower sound levels than the average sound level that is designated as 0 dB on the audiogram (see Footnote 4).

The middle audiogram shows normal thresholds at the lowest three test frequencies (250, 500, 1000), the threshold at 2000 Hz just higher than the normal range, and a sudden increase (increase = worsening) in threshold for the 4000-Hz test tone. This threshold is 60 dB, which is regarded as a "moderate" hearing loss. The 8000-Hz threshold of 40 dB is better than at 4000 Hz but still reflects a hearing loss for that frequency.

Audiograms are often described by the shape of the diagram formed by the lines that connect the thresholds. This shape is referred to as the audiometric

configuration. The configuration of the middle audiogram is called a "noise-notch" because of the normal (or in some cases, near-normal) thresholds at lower frequencies, a dramatically elevated threshold at 4000 Hz, and a better threshold—though still not normal—at 8000 Hz. The dip at 4000 Hz is the "notch." The extent of the dip—the degree of the elevated threshold, in dB—may worsen over time. Noise notch audiograms are the result of chronic exposure, over many years, to high levels of environmental noise. The kind of noise levels that result in a noise notch audiogram include those generated by jet airplanes, rock-band amplifiers cranked up for arena concerts, and heavy machinery such as a jack hammer. Hair cells in the 4000-Hz region along the basilar membrane are particularly sensitive to extremely high sound levels, causing the hair cells to sustain damage and eventually die. Unfortunately, hair cells do not regenerate after damage or death.

The audiogram on the right side of Figure 6–16 shows a pattern of thresholds across frequencies that is typical in *presbycusis*, the term for hearing loss due to aging. This audiometric configuration forms when the pattern of thresholds is defined by near-normal thresholds in the lower frequencies and steadily increasing thresholds across the high frequencies. The presbycusis audiogram in Figure 6–16 shows thresholds at 250, 500, and 1000 Hz slightly greater than the range of normal thresholds, followed by thresholds of 45, 65, and 80 dB for pure tones at 2000, 4000, and 8000 Hz, respectively. Most often, the high-frequency hearing loss increases with age. A high percentage of adults over the age of 65 have hearing loss that in most cases is due to presbycusis.

Presbycusis is the result of progressive deterioration and ultimately death of hair cells. In older people, a lifetime of exposure to environmental noise may also contribute to hair cell damage and hearing loss. The audiometric pattern in presbycusis reflects a greater susceptibility to deterioration of hair cells toward the basal end of the basilar membrane, compared with hair cells toward the tip of the basilar membrane.

Pure-tone testing is based on knowledge of the anatomy and physiology of the cochlea. Specifically, the anatomical concept of tonotopic representation of frequency along the basilar membrane and the physiological concept of how the traveling wave differs according to frequency are the essential pieces of knowledge required to understand pure-tone audiometry. Fortunately, the various audiometric configurations seen in hearing loss provide guidance for treatment options. The audiometric configuration in presbycusis, for example, suggests that a hearing aid with greater amplification of high frequencies, compared to low frequencies, is likely to be effective for this kind of hearing loss. In fact, hearing aids can be precisely configured for individual hearing patterns that are revealed by pure-tone audiometry.

REVIEW

Knowledge of the structure and function of the auditory mechanism is critical to those who plan to become communication specialists, with a goal of understanding how hearing affects language learning, how diseases affect the normal mechanism, and how formal evaluations of hearing are designed and interpreted.

Most of the peripheral auditory mechanism is housed within the temporal bone, a complexly shaped bone of the skull.

The peripheral auditory mechanism can be subdivided into the conductive mechanism, comprising the outer and middle ear, and the sensorineural mechanism, comprising the inner ear and auditory nerve.

The outer ear includes the pinna, external auditory meatus, and tympanic membrane.

The pinna (or auricle) is a cartilaginous structure that is attached to the side of the head and contributes to the ability to localize a sound source.

The external auditory meatus (or external auditory canal) is a tube approximately 2.5 cm (nearly 1 inch) long and 0.7 cm in diameter that extends from the concha to the tympanic membrane, in which cerumen (ear-

wax) is produced and through which sound waves are directed to the tympanic membrane.

The external auditory meatus has a resonant frequency of roughly 3300 Hz, which explains in part the very acute sensitivity of the human auditory mechanism in this frequency region.

The tympanic membrane (or eardrum) is a small (about 55-mm^2 area) three-layered structure located at the internal end of the outer ear, the middle layer of which is sensitive to the very small pressure variations associated with sound waves.

The middle ear is an air-filled cavity, divided into three chambers, that lies between the outer ear and inner ear and contains three small ossicles (bones), several ligaments, and two muscles.

The ossicles are the malleus (which attaches to the tympanic membrane), incus, and stapes (which connects by its footplate to the oval window of the inner ear).

Connected to the ossicles are ligaments that tether the ossicles to different structures and to each other (at joints) and also tether two muscles, the *tensor tympani* muscle that attaches to the malleus and the *stapedius* muscle that attaches to the stapes, both of which serve to stiffen the ossicular chain when they contract.

The auditory tube (or eustachian tube), a 3.8-cm (1.5-inch) tube that runs from the middle ear to the nasopharynx, is bony and open to the middle ear and cartilaginous and flexible at its termination point in the nasopharynx where it is usually closed but opens occasionally to equalize middle ear air pressure with atmospheric pressure.

The structure of the ossicles minimizes the impedance mismatch between the air in the outer ear and the fluid (liquid) in the inner ear by the substantial area difference between the tympanic membrane and the oval window, as well as the lever actions of the ossicular chain.

The inner ear is housed within the bony labyrinth of the temporal bone and contains the semicircular canals, vestibule, and cochlea, all structures that communicate with the CNS via cranial nerve VIII (auditory-vestibular nerve).

Three semicircular canals, each oriented at right angles to the other two, contain hair cells that bend when the head moves and cause the vestibular part of cranial nerve VIII to fire and send information about head orientation and movements to the brain.

The vestibule includes the oval window as well as the utricle and saccule that contain hair cells, which send signals to the brain about the relative position and acceleration of the head.

The cochlea is the spiral-shaped end organ of hearing that converts hydraulic (fluid) energy into neural signals and contains many important structures, including the scalae, basilar membrane, and organ of Corti, the latter of which supports the hair cells.

Within the cochlea are three membranous, fluid-filled ducts called the scala vestibuli (containing perilymph), scala media (or cochlear duct; containing endolymph), and scala tympani (containing perilymph), the first and last of which are connected at the heliocotrema (apex), the tip of the cochlear spiral.

The scala media is separated from the scala tympani by the basilar membrane and from the scala vestibuli by Reissner's membrane.

On top of the basilar membrane sits the organ of Corti, which contains a row of inner hair cells and three rows of outer hair cells, some of the ends of which are embedded in the tectorial membrane above.

Movement of fluid in the cochlea (caused by pressure changes transmitted through the outer and middle ear) deforms inner hair cells and causes them to depolarize and fire.

The outer hair cells, referred to as the "cochlear amplifier," are stimulated by efferent neural signals originating in the CNS that cause them to vibrate and amplify the response sensitivity of the inner hair cells in the same region.

Hair cells are arranged tonotopically along the basilar membrane, ranging from those that respond best to the highest frequency at its narrow base (20000 Hz) to those that respond best to the lowest frequency at its wide apex (20 Hz).

As discovered by Georg von Békésy in the early 1900s, the hair cells are stimulated by traveling waves of cochlear fluid that are frequency dependent, with high-frequency sounds creating waves that peak near the base of the basilar membrane and low-frequency sounds creating waves that peak near the apex of the basilar membrane.

When inner hair cells are deformed by a traveling wave, they depolarize and send a signal through their associated nerve fibers, which carry the signal to a ganglion and then on to the brainstem via the auditory part of cranial nerve VIII.

The auditory nerve portion of cranial nerve VIII carries afferent fibers from inner hair cells and efferent fibers to outer hair cells, with the neural fibers arranged tonotopically just like the hair cells.

The central auditory pathways consist of tracts and clusters of cell bodies that carry auditory signals from the brainstem to the cortex, with information from both ears included in both ascending pathways and, like the hair cells and auditory nerve, are tonotopically organized.

Pure-tone audiometry is a basic test of hearing in which sound waves composed of a single frequency—pure tones—are used to determine hearing thresholds; thresholds determined for a series of pure tones ranging from low to high frequencies are used to assess the health of the hair cells at different locations along the basilar membrane.

An audiogram is a chart that displays thresholds, in decibels, for the pure-tone test frequencies, and its pattern of thresholds for different frequencies can provide insight to the basis for a hearing loss.

REFERENCES

Abele, T. A., & Wiggins, III, R. H. (2015). Imaging of the temporal bone. *Radiological Clinics of North America, 53*, 15–36.

Barin, K. (2009). Clinical neurophysiology of the vestibular system. In J. Katz, L. Medwetzky, R. Burkard, & L. Hood (Eds.), *Handbook of clinical audiology* (6th ed., pp. 431–466). Baltimore, MD: Lippincott Williams & Wilkins.

Békésy, G. (1928). ZurTheorie des Hörens; die Schwingungsform der Basilarmembran. *Physik Zeits, 29*, 793–810.

Gelfand, S. A. (2002). The acoustic reflex. In J. Katz (Ed.), *Handbook of clinical audiology* (5th ed., pp. 205–232). Philadelphia, PA: Lippincott Williams & Wilkins.

Goutman, J. D., Elgoyhen, A. B., & Gomez-Casati, M. E. (2015). Cochlear hair cells: The sound-sensing machines. *FEBS Letters, 589*, 3354–3361.

Hixon, T. J., Weismer, G., & Hoit, J. D. (2020). *Preclinical speech science: Anatomy, physiology, acoustics, perception* (3rd ed.). San Diego, CA: Plural Publishing.

Hudpseth, A. J. (2014). Integrating the active process of hair cells with cochlear function. *Nature Reviews Neuroscience, 15*, 600–614.

Kramer, S., & Brown, D. K. (2019). *Audiology: Science to practice* (3rd ed.). San Diego, CA: Plural Publishing.

Lemmerling, M. J., Stambuk, H. E., Mancuso, A. A., Antonelli, P. J., & Kubilis, P. S. (1997). CT of the normal suspensory ligaments of the ossicles in the middle ear. *AJNR American Journal of Neuroradiology, 18*, 471–477.

Luers, J. C., & Hüttenbrink, K.-B. (2016). Surgical anatomy and pathology of the middle ear. *Journal of Anatomy, 228*, 338–353.

Mansour, S., Magnan, J., Haidar, H., Nicolas, K., & Louryan, S. (2019). *Comprehensive and clinical anatomy of the middle ear* (2nd ed.). Berlin, Germany: Springer.

Musiek, F. E., & Baran, J. A. (2018). *The auditory system: Anatomy, physiology, and clinical correlates* (2nd ed.). San Diego, CA: Plural Publishing.

Olsen, E. S., Duifhuis, H., & Steele, C. R. (2012). vonBékésy and cochlear mechanics. *Hearing Research, 293*, 31–43.

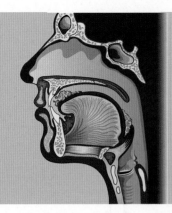

Swallowing Structure and Function

INTRODUCTION

Some of the most enjoyable activities of daily living involve eating and drinking. These include meals (where eating and drinking are the purpose of the activity), special events such as receptions (where eating and drinking enhance the celebration), and relaxation activities such as going to the movies (where eating popcorn and drinking soda are an integral part of the experience for some people). Figure 7–1 is a cartoon that depicts the anticipation of a good meal and the social context in which it is enjoyed.

The ease of eating and drinking is deceptive. These are complicated activities that require intricately coordinated actions of the lips, mandible, tongue, velum, pharynx, larynx, esophagus, and other structures. Because eating and drinking engage many of the same structures and much of the same airway as those used for speaking and breathing, it is not uncommon for there to be competition between these activities or for trade-offs to occur when trying to do them simultaneously. For example, chewing must stop to be able to speak clearly and breathing must stop to be able to swallow safely.

The entire act of placing liquid or solid substance in the oral cavity, moving it backward to the pharynx, propelling it into the esophagus, and allowing it to make its way to the stomach is called *deglutition*. Although the word *swallowing* is sometimes used as a synonym for deglutition, swallowing actually includes only certain phases of deglutition. Nevertheless, to simplify the explanations that follow, the term *swallowing* is used in place of *deglutition* and is meant to include all phases of deglutition.

ANATOMY

Figure 7–2 shows the structures that participate in swallowing. These structures extend from the lips to the stomach. Most of these same structures also participate in speech production; notable exceptions are the esophagus and stomach. The salivary glands also play a critical role in swallowing.

Respiratory, Laryngeal, Velopharyngeal-Nasal, and Pharyngeal-Oral Structures

Structures within the respiratory, laryngeal, velopharyngeal-nasal, and pharyngeal-oral subsystems participate in swallowing. These include the chest wall, vocal folds, ventricular folds, epiglottis, pharynx

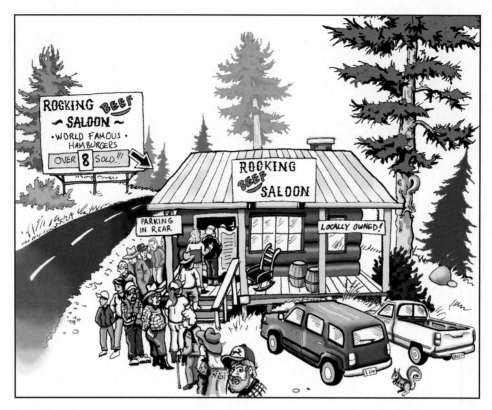

FIGURE 7–1. Cartoon depicting the anticipation of a good meal and the social context in which it is enjoyed.

(laryngopharynx, oropharynx, nasopharynx), velum, tongue, mandible, and lips. Their anatomy is described in Chapters 2, 3, 4, and 5, and their functions during swallowing are described below. The anatomy of the esophagus, stomach, and salivary glands is not covered in the other chapters and warrants attention here.

Esophagus

The esophagus is a flexible tube, about 25 cm long in adults, which extends from the lower part of the pharynx to the stomach. The esophagus begins below the base of the larynx and runs behind the trachea, pulmonary apparatus, and heart. It courses through the diaphragm (recall Figure 2–6) and enters the abdominal cavity, where it connects to the stomach. The esophagus is usually in a flattened state but can stretch to accommodate substances passing through it. The cervical (upper) esophagus consists of striated (voluntary) muscle, the thoracic (middle) region of the esophagus comprises a mixture of striated and smooth (involuntary) muscle, and the abdominal (lower) region is made up of purely smooth muscle. These regions are depicted

in Figure 7–3. The esophagus is lined with a thick layer of mucosa, beneath which lies connective tissue and glands that secrete mucus to aid in the movement of substances through it.

The esophagus is bounded at each end by sphincters. A sphincter is a muscular region that is tonically activated in its "resting" state to keep an orifice closed; when relaxed, the sphincter allows the orifice to open so that material can pass through it. It is bounded at its upper end by the upper esophageal sphincter (sometimes called the pharyngoesophageal segment, or just PE segment) and at its lower end by the lower esophageal sphincter (also called the gastroesophageal sphincter or cardiac sphincter). These sphincters mark the entrance and exit of the esophagus and are operationally defined as zones of high pressure rather than as precise anatomical entities. It is uncertain which structures are responsible for creating these high-pressure zones. Nevertheless, indirect evidence suggests that the *cricopharyngeus* muscles of the pharynx (considered by some to be part of the *inferior constrictor* muscles; see Chapter 4) are the primary contributors to the contraction-relaxation pattern of the upper esophageal sphincter (Hila, Castell, & Castell, 2001).

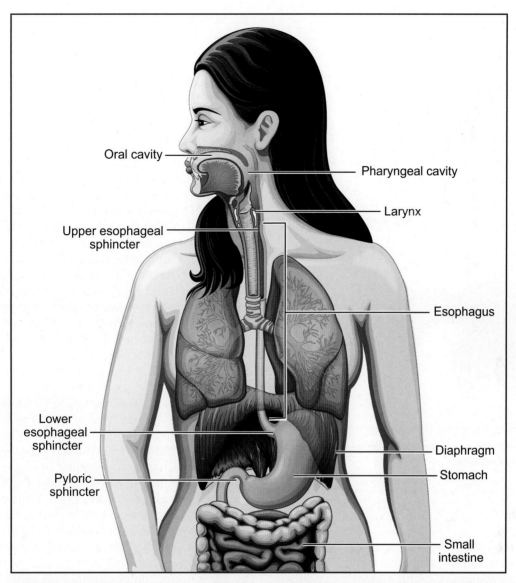

Oral cavity

Pharyngeal cavity

Larynx

Upper esophageal
sphincter

Esophagus

Lower
esophageal
sphincter

Diaphragm

Stomach

Pyloric
sphincter

Small
intestine

FIGURE 7–2. Structures of the swallowing apparatus. These include structures that participate in speech production (see Chapters 2, 3, 4, and 5 for detailed descriptions), as well as
structures that do not (esophagus, stomach, and intestines and their associated sphincters).

The upper end of the esophagus is positioned
among several of the pharyngeal and laryngeal structures discussed in Chapters 3, 4, and 5. These structures
are depicted in two different views in Figure 7–4. The
upper image depicts the laryngeal area and the top
of the esophagus (in its closed state) as viewed from
above. Of particular interest in the context of swallowing are the pyriform sinuses and the epiglottic valleculae. The pyriform sinuses are cavities that are located
near the back of the larynx and lateral to the aryepiglottic folds. The epiglottic valleculae (one vallecula on
each side) are depressions located toward the front of

the larynx on the lingual (tongue) side of the epiglottis and just behind the root of the tongue. The lower
image in Figure 7–4 shows the pharyngeal, laryngeal,
and upper esophageal areas as viewed from the back,
with the pharyngeal muscles intact (left side) and with
those muscles removed and the pharynx open at the
back (right side). The *cricopharyngeus* muscle (lower
part of the *inferior constrictor* muscle) is shown to surround the region of the upper esophagus. Also shown
in this figure is the relationship of the esophagus to one
pyriform sinus and one epiglottic vallecula, as well as
the epiglottis, tongue, and velum.

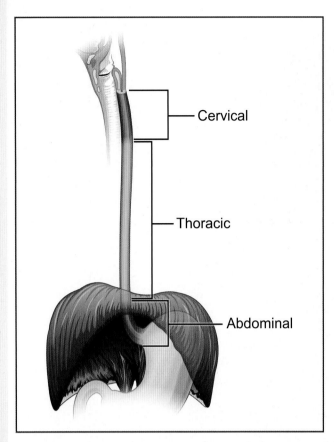

FIGURE 7–3. Three regions of the esophagus: cervical, thoracic, and abdominal.

Stomach

The stomach is a large, sac-like structure made up of smooth muscle, mucosa, and other tissue. It is on the left side of the abdominal cavity, against the undersurface of the diaphragm. The stomach connects to the esophagus via the lower esophageal sphincter and to the small intestine via the pyloric sphincter. After a typical meal, the stomach holds about a liter of solid and/or liquid substance, although it can stretch to hold much more if necessary. Gastric juices in the stomach break up ingested substances so that they can be absorbed into the body through the stomach lining.

Salivary Glands

Saliva is a liquid made up of water combined with many other elements, including enzymes that begin the process of breaking down food. There are hundreds of salivary glands that produce saliva, but about 90% of the saliva is produced by the paired parotid, submandibular, and sublingual glands. These are illustrated in Figure 7–5. The parotid glands are located in front and below the left and right ears and wrap around the corresponding ramus of the mandible. The submandibular glands lie beneath the floor of the oral cavity and above the *digastric* muscles. The sublingual glands, the smallest of the three pairs, are positioned below and to the side of the tongue and beneath the mucous membrane of the floor of the oral cavity.

The salivary glands produce saliva when stimulated by taste or when stimulated mechanically by chewing. Saliva production is controlled by parasympathetic innervation from the autonomic nervous system (see Chapter 8) traveling in cranial nerves IX (glossopharyngeal; to parotid glands) and VII (facial; to the other two glands). Saliva plays many critical roles in swallowing and digestion, including lubricating the oral cavity, protecting the health of the teeth and the oropharyngeal and esophageal mucosa, forming the bolus for swallowing, and beginning the digestive process by the introduction of enzymes (Pedersen, Sørensen, Proctor, & Carpenter, 2018). When not enough saliva is produced, the result can be xerostomia (dry mouth).

Mustard Belt Champions

Holy stomach full! Japan's Takeru Kobayashi was the six-time hot-dog-eating world champion and ate 63 hot dogs and buns (6 more than his personal best) on July 4, 2007, at Coney Island, New York. But with more than 50,000 people in attendance and in the glare of national television cameras, Kobayashi lost his crown to Joey Chestnut of San Jose, California. Sanctioned by Major League Eating, the world governing body of all stomach-centric sport, Nathan's Famous International

Fourth of July Hot Dog Eating Championship has been held each year on the 4th of July since 1916. On July 4, 2020, with 12 wins already under his belt, Joey Chestnut once again exceeded his personal best and set a new world record by ingesting 75 hot dogs and buns in just 10 minutes. And, yes, there is a women's competition too. Miki Sudo, seven-time Mustard Belt champion, set the new women's world record in 2020 by ingesting 48.5 hot dogs and buns in 10 minutes.

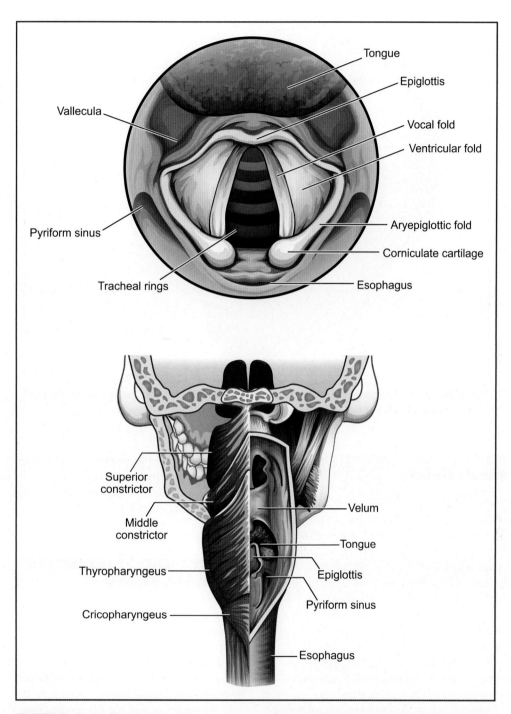

FIGURE 7-4. Two views of laryngeal and pharyngeal structures. The upper image depicts the laryngeal area viewed from above and the front of the larynx at the top. In particular, note the location of the pyriform sinuses (toward the back), esophagus (behind the larynx), and the epiglottic valleculae (toward the front, near the tongue root). The lower image is a view from the back. Its left side shows the ***superior***, ***middle***, and ***inferior*** (***thyropharyngeus*** and ***cricopharyngeus*** divisions) ***constrictor*** muscles intact. Its right side shows these muscles removed to reveal the pharyngeal and laryngeal regions (again, note the location of the pyriform sinus).

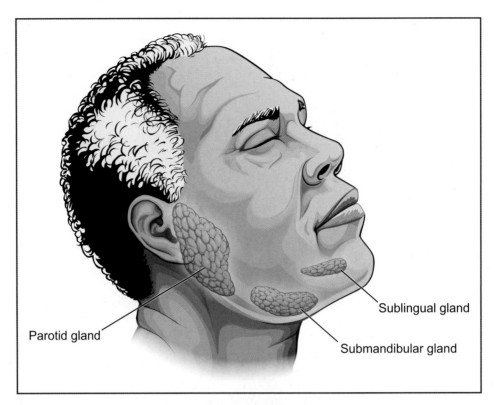

FIGURE 7–5. The main salivary glands: the parotid, submandibular, and sublingual glands. Only the salivary glands on the right side are shown.

Mmm Mmm Good!

"Mmm, mmm, good!" Does this make you think of steamy, chunky soup? Or, better yet, freshly baked cookies just out of the oven? Maybe your imagination is so good that your mouth actually starts to water, which brings us to the point of this sidetrack: saliva. Saliva is produced by salivary glands and is critical to our ability to swallow and digest. Most saliva is swallowed alone (these are called "dry swallows"). During eating, saliva mixes with the food to moisten it for easier transport through oral, pharyngeal, and esophageal parts of the digestive tract and introduces enzymes that begin the digestive process. Do you have any idea how much saliva we produce? The answer is an amazing 1 to 2 liters of saliva every 24 hours! Although saliva production is continuous, its volume and content vary rhythmically; that is, saliva production has a circadian rhythm. Much less saliva is produced during sleep than during wakefulness. That's good. Best to save that saliva for the cookie-eating waking hours.

Xerostomia can have serious consequences, including oral and pharyngeal discomfort (sore throat), halitosis (bad breath), dental erosion, gum disease, and dysphagia (difficulty swallowing).

FORCES AND MOVEMENTS OF SWALLOWING

Although many of the structures that participate in swallowing are the same as those that are used for speaking, the forces and movements for the two activities are very different. In general, the forces are greater and many of the movements are slower during swallowing than during speech production.

To set the stage for understanding the forces and movements of swallowing, it is useful to begin by considering certain pressures associated with the resting state of the swallowing mechanism. These pressures, pointed out in Figure 7–6, are shown with the swallowing mechanism at rest at the end of a tidal expiration. As expected, the pressure in the oral cavity, which is coupled to the outside via the velopharyngeal-nasal airway, is zero (equal to atmospheric pressure) at rest. The other pressures are not zero and their values as

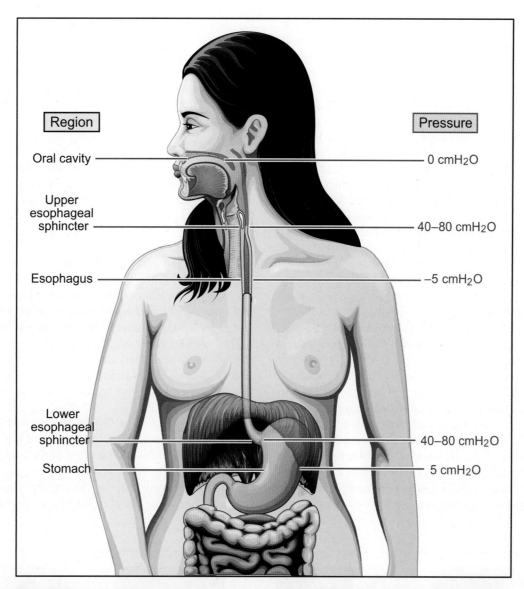

FIGURE 7–6. Relevant pressures associated with the resting state of the swallowing mechanism. Oral pressure is zero (atmospheric), esophageal pressure is slightly negative, and stomach (gastric) pressure is slightly positive. Both the upper and lower esophageal sphincters exert high pressure that can range considerably in magnitude. It is especially important that the lower esophageal sphincter pressure remain higher than the pressure within the stomach (gastric pressure) so that the contents of the stomach do not reflux.

shown in Figure 7–6 are approximations; some of them can range substantially.

At rest, the pressure within the esophagus is below atmospheric pressure (approximately –5 cmH$_2$O). To understand why, it is necessary to review the phenomenon of pleural linkage, discussed in Chapter 2. The two membranes that line the outside of the pulmonary apparatus and the inside of the chest wall, the visceral pleura and the parietal pleura, are linked together with a thin layer of liquid. In this linked state,

the pulmonary apparatus "wants" to collapse and the chest wall "wants" to expand (recall the spring analogy in Figure 2–4 representing the linked pulmonary apparatus and chest wall). This creates a negative pressure between the pleura (called pleural pressure; see Figure 2–8) and that negative pressure is transmitted across the dividing wall to the esophagus.

The pressure in the stomach (gastric pressure) is slightly above atmospheric pressure (approximately 5 cmH$_2$O). This positive pressure is, in part, the result of the muscle tone exerted by the wall of the stomach. This pressure is also attributed to the hydrostatic properties of the abdomen.

In contrast to these relatively low esophageal and gastric pressures, the pressures within the upper and lower esophageal sphincters are high. These high pressures are attributable to the high tissue forces exerted by the sphincters. Although a typical range is 40 to 80 cmH$_2$O in the resting state, their absolute magnitudes depend on the measurement approach used as well as a variety of physiological factors (Goyal & Cobb, 1981; Linden, Hogosta, & Norlander, 2007). Because the upper and lower esophageal sphincters exert such high pressures, these regions function like forcefully closed valves while at rest. In particular, it is important that the pressure in the lower esophageal sphincter be substantially higher than the pressure in the stomach. Otherwise, substances from the stomach may reflux (flow back) into the esophagus.

The act of swallowing is driven by both passive and active forces. Passive force comes from many sources, including (a) the natural recoil of connective tissues (ligaments and membranes), cartilages, and bones; (b) the surface tension between structures in apposition; (c) the pull of gravity; and (d) aeromechanical factors. Active force results from the activation of respiratory, laryngeal, velopharyngeal-nasal, and pharyngeal-oral muscles in various combinations. Their contributions to active force are described in Chapters 2, 3, 4, and 5 and are discussed here as they relate to swallowing, as are the forces exerted by the esophagus.

Forces and movements of swallowing can be described as they pertain to four phases of swallowing. These phases, depicted in Figure 7–7, are the oral preparatory phase, oral transport phase (sometimes called the oral propulsive phase or oral transit phase), pharyngeal phase, and esophageal phase. These phases are used to describe the movement of a bolus through the oral, pharyngeal, and esophageal regions of the swallowing mechanism. *Bolus* is the word used to refer to the volume of liquid or the mass of solid substance being swallowed. The physiological events associated with each of these phases are described below and summarized in Table 7–1.

Oral Preparatory Phase

The oral preparatory phase is depicted in the first panel of Figure 7–7. This phase begins as a solid or liquid substance makes contact with the structures of the anterior oral vestibule. The mandible has already lowered and the lips have abducted in anticipation of the swallow (Shune, Moon, & Goodman, 2016). What happens next largely depends on the nature of the substance to be swallowed.

If the substance is liquid, the mandible elevates and the lips adduct, forming an anterior seal to contain the bolus. The bolus is contained in the anterior region of the oral cavity by actions of the tongue and other structures and held there momentarily (usually on the order of 1 second). The anterior tongue depresses (low-

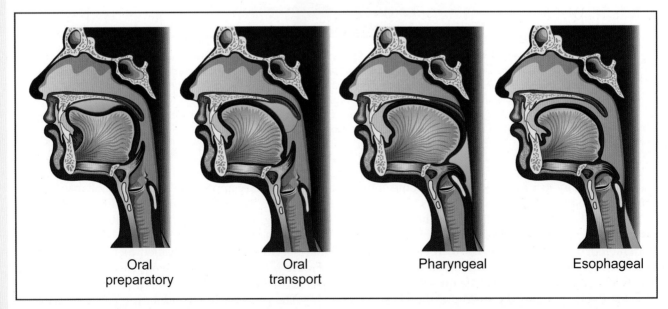

| Oral preparatory | Oral transport | Pharyngeal | Esophageal |

FIGURE 7–7. Depiction of the oral preparatory, oral transport, pharyngeal, and esophageal phases of swallowing. The actions associated with each phase are summarized in Table 7–1. The bolus is shown in green.

TABLE 7–1. Summary of the Actions Associated With the Four Phases of Swallowing

Swallowing Phase	Actions
Oral preparatory	This phase begins as the liquid or solid substance comes in contact with the oral vestibule and ends with the bolus held in the oral cavity with the back of the tongue elevated to contact the velum and create an impenetrable wall. This phase can be as short as 1 second when ingesting liquid and as long as 20 seconds when chewing (preparing) a solid food.
Oral transport	During this phase, sometimes called the oral propulsive or oral transit phase, the bolus is transported back through the oral cavity to the pharynx. To do so, the tongue elevates in progressively more posterior regions to push the bolus back toward the pharynx, the velum begins to elevate, and the upper esophageal sphincter begins to relax. This phase lasts less than 1 second.
Pharyngeal	During this phase, the bolus usually divides to run through the right and left valleculae and is transported through the pharynx to the upper esophageal sphincter. This phase is "triggered" automatically once the bolus passes the anterior faucial pillars (though the exact location can vary) and is associated with numerous and rapid events: The velopharynx closes, the tongue pushes the bolus backward, the pharynx constricts segmentally, the hyoid bone and larynx move upward and forward, the arytenoids move medially and tilt forward toward the epiglottis, the larynx closes at multiple levels (vocal folds, ventricular folds, and epiglottis), and the upper esophageal sphincter opens. This phase lasts less than 1 second.
Esophageal	This phase begins when the bolus enters the upper esophageal sphincter and ends when it enters the stomach. This phase can last from 3 to 20 seconds.

ers) and the sides of the tongue elevate to form a cup for the bolus. The bolus may be cupped in one of two ways, depending on the person. Some people hold the bolus with the tongue tip elevated and contacting the back surface of the maxillary incisors, and other people hold the bolus on the floor of the oral cavity in front of the tongue (dubbed "dipper" and "tipper" type swallows, respectively; Dodds et al., 1989). The back of the tongue elevates to make contact with the velum to form a back wall that separates the oral from the pharyngeal cavities and helps ensure that no substance can slip by and into the pulmonary airways. The velopharynx is open so that breathing can continue. Nevertheless, many people stop breathing momentarily at this point in the swallow (this is called the apneic interval) or even before the glass or straw reaches the lips (Martin, Logemann, Shaker, & Dodds, 1994; Martin-Harris, Brodsky, Price, Michel, & Walters, 2003; Martin-Harris, Michel, & Castell, 2005). This apneic interval serves to reduce the risk of aspiration (aspiration is defined as invasion of substances below the vocal folds).

These initial events are quite different when the substance to be swallowed is solid rather than liquid, primarily because solid substances need to be masticated (chewed) into smaller pieces and mixed with saliva before being transported toward the esopha-

gus. Saliva moistens the solid substance to facilitate its transport and introduces enzymes that begin to break down the substance for digestion. Actions of the mandible (and teeth), lips, tongue, and cheeks grind and manipulate the solid substance into a cohesive bolus and position it on the surface of the anterior tongue. The lips may adduct (although this is not necessary) while the mandible moves to grind the bolus. During chewing, the mandible moves up and down, forward and backward, and side to side. This is in contrast to speech production, during which the mandible moves primarily up and down. The velum makes contact with the back part of the tongue to seal off the oral from the pharyngeal cavity and prevent the bolus from moving into the pharynx and larynx. The velopharynx is open during preparation of the bolus and breathing either continues or is interrupted by apnea (McFarland & Lund, 1995; Palmer & Hiiemae, 2003). The duration of the oral preparatory phase may last from as short as 3 seconds, when chewing a soft cookie, to as long as 20 seconds, when chewing a tough piece of steak.

At the end of the oral preparatory phase, the substance in the oral cavity is ready for consumption. Usually it is immediately transported back toward the pharynx (oral transport phase). There are choices at this point, however, including that the substance can be (a) savored for a while by continued manipulation, (b) squirreled in the cheeks, or (c) expelled. The expulsion option is used when performing a sham feeding test to study the actions of the stomach in anticipation of receiving food.

Oral Transport Phase

The oral transport phase, also called the oral propulsion phase or oral transit phase, is shown in the second panel of Figure 7–7. From the ready position (either the "dipper" or "tipper" position for liquids), the bolus is transported back through the oral cavity. This is done by using the tongue tip to squeeze the bolus against the hard palate; then, progressively, more posterior regions of the tongue elevate and squeeze the bolus against the palate, moving the bolus back toward the pharynx. The tongue is an especially effective structure for moving and clearing the bolus because it behaves like a muscular hydrostat and can move and change shape in an almost infinite number of ways (see Chapter 5). The force needed to propel the bolus varies with bolus viscosity (the resistance offered by a fluid to flowing). To see how the surface of the tongue moves the bolus back during the first two oral phases, see Video 7–1 (Oral Phase Tongue Movement). The lips usually press together firmly (although this is not necessary) and the cheeks are pulled inward slightly to keep the bolus positioned over the tongue. At the same time, the velum begins to elevate while the upper esophageal sphincter relaxes. The oral transport phase is short, lasting less than a second (Cook et al., 1994; Tracy et al., 1989).

Pharyngeal Phase

The pharyngeal phase of the swallow is "triggered" once the bolus passes the anterior faucial pillars; however, the exact location of the trigger varies, depending on the bolus type and the age of the individual. During this phase, depicted in the third panel of Figure 7–7, several events occur rapidly and nearly simultaneously to move the bolus quickly through the pharynx while protecting the airway. This phase is under "automatic" neural control, so that, once triggered, it proceeds as a relatively fixed set of events that cannot be altered voluntarily (except in the magnitude and duration of the pressures generated). These events occur within about half a second (Cook et al., 1994; Tracy et al., 1989) and include velopharyngeal closure, elevation of the hyoid bone and larynx, laryngeal closure, pharyngeal constriction, and opening of the upper esophageal sphincter, as described below.

During the pharyngeal phase, the velopharynx closes like a flap-sphincter valve by elevation of the velum and constriction of the pharyngeal walls. This closure is forceful (more forceful than for speech production) so as to prohibit substances from passing through the nasopharynx into the nose.

The hyoid bone and larynx move upward and forward as a result of contraction of extrinsic tongue muscles, with major contribution from the *geniohyoid* muscles to upward movement and the *mylohyoid* muscles to forward movement (Pearson, Langmore, & Zumwalt, 2011). (Recall from Chapters 3 and 5 that several extrinsic muscles of the tongue attach to the hyoid bone.) As the hyoid bone is pulled upward and forward, the larynx is pulled along with it by its muscular and nonmuscular connections to the hyoid bone. In fact, this group of structures is often called the *hyolaryngeal complex* because of these anatomical connections and the tendency for them to move as a unit. Elevation of the larynx also causes the pharynx to shorten.

Closure of the larynx for swallowing has been described as a folding of the larynx (Fink & Demarest, 1978) that forms a seal to the entrance of the trachea to protect the pulmonary airways. Closure occurs at multiple levels, which include the vocal folds, the ventricular folds, and the aryepiglottic folds and epiglottis. The arytenoid cartilages move medially and then tilt forward to touch the epiglottis and both the vocal folds and ventricular folds adduct firmly. The epiglottis is forced down over the laryngeal aditus like a trap door and serves as a first line of defense against substances entering the larynx and pulmonary airways. Both passive and active forces appear to be responsible for downward movement of the epiglottis during swallowing (Ekberg & Sigurjonsson, 1982; Fink & Demarest, 1978; VanDaele, Perlman, & Cassell, 1995). The passive force derives from backward movement of the tongue and upward and forward movement of the hyoid bone and larynx, which mechanically deflect the epiglottis backward and downward. Upward and forward movement of the larynx simultaneously contributes to airway protection by tucking the larynx against the root of the tongue and deflecting the trachea away from the digestive pathway. The active force is somewhat less certain (Fink, Martin, & Rohrmann, 1979; Ramsey, Watson, Gramiak, & Weinberg, 1955; VanDaele et al., 1995) but is argued to derive from contraction of the *aryepiglottic* muscles (and possibly from vertically ascending lateral fibers of the *thyroarytenoid* muscles), which purportedly pull the epiglottis downward to complete the seal of the laryngeal aditus (Ekberg & Sigurjonsson, 1982).

As the tongue propels the bolus into the pharynx, the pharynx undergoes segmental contraction (from top to bottom). The tongue root moves backward and the pharyngeal walls constrict to squeeze the bolus toward the esophagus. The bolus often divides at the epiglottis as it passes through the left and right epiglottic valleculae (lateral channels between the root of the tongue and the epiglottis) and into the left and right pyriform sinuses (recesses bounded by the pharynx and larynx), or it flows down one side or through the midline of the covered laryngeal aditus (Dua, Ren, Bardan, Xie, & Shaker, 1997; Logemann, Kahrilas, Kobara, & Vakil, 1989).

As all of these events are playing out, the upper esophageal sphincter is opening to allow the bolus to pass into the esophagus. Two sets of actions appear to contribute to its opening: (a) stretching of the upper esophageal sphincter by forward and upward movement of the hyolaryngeal complex (likely accomplished by activity of the *mylohyoid*, *geniohyoid*, and *anterior* belly of the *digastric* muscles) and (b) relaxing of the *cricopharyngeus* muscles (Omari et al., 2016).

The bolus is propelled through the pharynx to the esophagus during the pharyngeal phase by a combination of mechanical (structural) forces and aeromechanical forces. The mechanical forces consist of the tongue pushing the bolus back into the pharynx and the pharynx contracting segmentally against the tongue root, as just described. The aeromechanical forces are in the form of regional pressure changes that help to move the bolus along. Specifically, backward movement of the tongue and constriction of the pharyngeal walls serve to narrow the airway and reduce the airway volume, thereby causing the pressure to rise in that region. At the same time, elevation of the larynx and dilation of the upper esophageal sphincter lower the pressure below the bolus. The pressure differential (higher pressure behind the bolus than in front of it) helps to drive the bolus toward its destination.

It is also relevant to mention that the pharyngeal phase of swallowing can be stimulated by pooling of saliva in the pharynx and can be initiated in the absence of oral preparatory and oral transport phases (Logemann, 1998). These swallows occur regularly throughout the day and night and are called nonbolus swallows, dry swallows, or saliva swallows.

Esophageal Phase

The esophageal phase, the initial part of which is illustrated in the last panel of Figure 7–7, begins when the bolus enters the upper esophageal sphincter and ends when it passes into the stomach through the lower esophageal sphincter. This phase may last anywhere from 8 to 20 seconds (Dodds, Hogan, Reid, Stewart, & Arndorfer, 1973). At the same time the upper esophageal sphincter opens to allow the bolus to pass into the esophagus, the lower esophageal sphincter relaxes. The bolus is propelled through the esophagus by peristaltic actions (alternating waves of contraction and relaxation) of the esophageal walls. Peristaltic contraction raises pressure behind the bolus and relaxation lowers pressure in front of the bolus, creating the pressure differential needed to propel it toward the stomach. The nature of the peristaltic action varies somewhat depending on the nature of the bolus (liquid or solid), body position (relation of esophagus and bolus to gravity), and other factors. When a substance is left behind following the primary peristalsis, it is cleared by subsequent peristaltic action (called secondary peristalsis). The esophagus usually transports substances toward the stomach; however, it can also transport substances or gas away from the stomach (as in the case of vomiting or burping).

Overlap of Phases

Although the phases of swallowing are described above as though they are discrete and occur one after the other, in fact, they overlap substantially. When a person is eating a solid substance, for example, preparation of part of the bolus in the oral cavity may continue while another part of the bolus moves into the pharyngeal area, as illustrated in Figure 7–8. This partial bolus may remain in the epiglottic valleculae as long as 10 seconds before it merges with the rest of the bolus and the pharyngeal transport phase of the swallow is triggered (Hiiemae & Palmer, 1999).

Overlap of phases is also apparent if swallowing is viewed in relation to the actions of individual structures, rather than in relation to the status of the bolus. Whereas the traditional description of swallowing (used in this chapter) focuses on preparation and transport of the bolus to define the phases of swallowing, there are schema that try to segment physiological events along somewhat different conceptual lines and to categorize them across different levels of observation (Martin-Harris, Michel, et al., 2005). This view of the swallowing process focuses on coordination of temporal events across structures. Figure 7–9 is an example of this type of conceptualization. Starting at the left side of the figure, the lips are abducted and the mandible and tongue tip are depressed to allow the bolus to enter the oral vestibule. Moving rightward from there, many structures (not an exhaustive list) take action to move the bolus back toward the esophagus and to protect the airways. Note that this figure presents a general representation of the sequence and relative timing of various

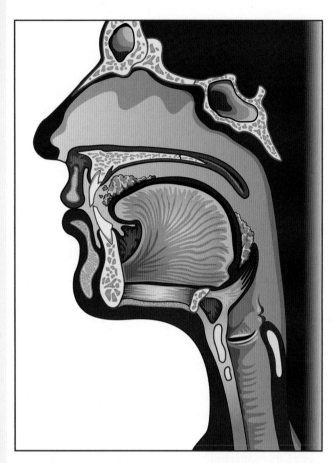

FIGURE 7–8. An illustration of eating, in which part of the bolus continues to be chewed while another part moves into the epiglottic valleculae, where it may remain for many seconds. This is an example of why the conceptualization of swallowing as comprising discrete phases can be problematic.

events; actual measures of these events reveal substantial variability within and across people (Molfenter & Steele, 2012). Schema such as these that are based on cross-structure analyses reveal the overlapping elements of swallowing behavior and interactions among its components and hold promise for developing a better understanding of the swallowing process. This approach has opened up new ways of looking at swallowing that likely will have improved clinical applications. For example, a recent proposal suggests that the mechanics of the pharyngeal phase of swallowing can be conceptualized as a set of functional modules that have clinical relevance—one that protects the airway, one that moves the bolus through the pharynx, one that shortens the pharynx and raises the larynx, and one that maintains a given head and neck posture (Hosseini, Tadavarthi, Martin-Harris, & Pearson, 2019).

BREATHING AND SWALLOWING

Protection of the pulmonary airways during swallowing depends, in large part, on the coordination of breathing and swallowing. Without such coordination, inspiration might occur at the same time a substance is being transported through the pharynx and that substance might be "sucked" through the larynx into the pulmonary airways (aspiration). This is avoided by closing the larynx (at multiple levels, as described above), an action that arrests breathing for a brief period during the swallow. This brief period of breath holding is called apnea or the apneic interval.

One Tug and Two Consequences

Breathing and swallowing cooperate in healthy individuals to prevent unwanted substances from entering the pulmonary airways. This cooperation can be more difficult with certain diseases. Chronic obstructive pulmonary disease (COPD) is one of these. When advanced, COPD expands the pulmonary apparatus and the diaphragm rides low and flat because air is trapped in the alveoli and airways. The abnormal positioning of the diaphragm has two potential consequences for swallowing. One is that a downward tug is placed on the larynx that tends to abduct the vocal folds and diminish their ability to protect the pulmonary airways. A second possible consequence is that the same downward tug lowers the laryngeal housing and tethers it from below. This means that the larynx may have difficulty moving up during a swallow because it has farther to go and because it must work against the downward pull of the diaphragm. It's no wonder that many people with advanced COPD also have problems with their swallowing.

The risk of aspiration appears to be further reduced by timing the swallow to occur during the expiratory phase of the breathing cycle. During single swallows, the most common pattern is expiration-swallow-expiration; that is, expiration begins, the swallow occurs (accompanied by apnea), and then expiration continues (Hopkins-Rossabi, Curtis, Temenak, Miller, & Martin-Harris, 2019; Martin et al., 1994; Martin-Harris, 2006; Nishino, Yonezawa, & Honda, 1985; Perlman, Ettema, & Barkmeier, 2000; Selley, Flack, Ellis, & Brooks, 1989; Smith, Wolkove, Colacone, & Kreisman, 1989). This pattern, illustrated in Figure 7–10, is the pre-

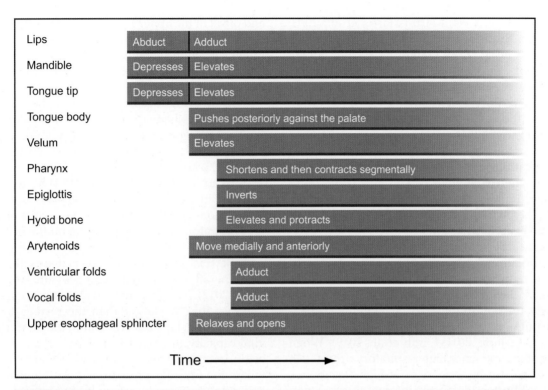

FIGURE 7–9. Schematic representation of the initiation of actions of several structures during a swallow. This is not meant to represent a fixed sequence or timing of actions (because they can differ across swallows and individuals, depending on many variables) but, rather, to illustrate that swallowing is a continuous physiological process that cannot be divided into a strict set of phases. (Figure designed in collaboration with Rosemary Lester-Smith, PhD, CCC-SLP, and based on Langmore [2001]).

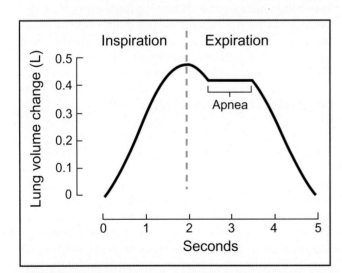

FIGURE 7–10. Typical breathing pattern during a single swallow, featuring a period of apnea (cessation of breathing). This pattern is described as expiration–swallow (accompanied by apnea)–expiration.

of serving conditions, such as presenting a liquid bolus with a syringe, drinking water from a cup or straw, or eating a solid substance (Preiksaitis & Mills, 1996; Wheeler-Hegland, Huber, Pitts, & Sapienza, 2009). This appears to be a protective mechanism for potentially "blowing" any foreign substance away from the pulmonary airways. Swallowing during expiration is associated with a reduced risk of aspiration in people with various impairments (Steele & Cichero, 2014) and is the basis for part of a training protocol used to improve breathing-swallowing coordination for clients at risk for aspiration (Martin-Harris, Garand, & McFarland, 2017). Nevertheless, it is interesting to note that, even in healthy people, not every swallow is followed by expiration; in fact, some healthy individuals occasionally inspire immediately after a swallow. This is particularly prevalent in people over age 65 years (Martin-Harris, Brodsky, et al., 2005). It is also possible for healthy individuals to swallow voluntarily during the inspiratory phase of the breathing cycle (Ulysal, Kizilay, Ünal, Güngor, & Ertekin, 2013).

Although the apneic interval during swallowing typically lasts about 1 second, it can range from less than a second to several seconds (Klaun & Perlman,

dominant one for swallowing over a broad range of bolus volumes and consistencies and under a variety

1999; Martin et al., 1994; Martin-Harris et al., 2003; Martin-Harris, Brodsky, et al., 2005; Palmer & Hiiemae, 2003; Perlman et al., 2000; Preiksaitis & Mills, 1996). In some people, the duration of the apneic interval is influenced by variables such as bolus volume (Preiksaitis, Mayrand, Robins, & Diamant, 1992). Nevertheless, most of the variability in apnea duration can be attributed to variability in the onset of apnea relative to the eating or drinking event. For example, one person may stop breathing as the food or drink is approaching the mouth, whereas another person may continue to breathe until immediately before the larynx begins to elevate for the pharyngeal transport phase of the swallow (Martin et al., 1994).

The apnea associated with swallowing can cause dyspnea (breathing discomfort) and a subsequent increase in ventilation, even in healthy people (Lederle, Hoit, & Barkmeier-Kraemer, 2012), and can be particularly uncomfortable and challenging in people with pulmonary disease (Hoit, Lansing, Dean, Yarkosky, & Lederle, 2011; Lindh et al., 2019). When healthy people experience high respiratory drive (such as might occur during exercise or at high elevations), they tend to shorten the apneic interval during swallowing (Hårdemark Cedborg et al., 2010; in this study, high respiratory drive was created by breathing gas with a greater-than-usual amount of carbon dioxide). Shortening apnea in this way likely helps to minimize dyspnea. Also observed is a tendency to shift the onset

and offset of the apnea relative to the swallow such that more time is spent breath holding after the swallow under conditions of high drive (specifically high elevation; Huff et al., 2019) possibly to increase the protective effect of the apnea.

Swallowing occurs at lung volumes that are almost always larger than the resting expiratory level (that is, the end-expiratory lung volume associated with resting tidal breathing), usually on the order of 10% to 20% larger (Lederle et al., 2012; McFarland et al., 2016; Wheeler-Hegland et al., 2009; Wheeler-Hegland, Huber, Pitts, & Davenport, 2011). This lung volume range is one in which the passive (recoil) pressure of the respiratory system is positive, on the order of 5 to 10 cmH$_2$O (see relaxation characteristic in Figure 2–16), and the tracheal pressures associated with swallowing generally fall in this recoil pressure range (Gross et al., 2012). The fact that swallowing occurs at lung volumes that are larger than the resting size of the respiratory system, but still within the midrange of the vital capacity, appears to have several advantages. To begin, because swallows are produced at lung volumes where the alveolar pressure is positive, postswallow expirations are easily driven by the respiratory recoil pressure. Also, because swallows are produced at lung volumes that are only moderately large, there is no need to exert inspiratory muscular pressure to brake excessive positive recoil pressure that prevails at large lung volumes. Finally, by avoiding larger-than-necessary lung volumes, the abductory force exerted on the vocal folds by the descent of the diaphragm is minimized (i.e., "tracheal tug," see Chapter 3). This optimal lung volume range has been incorporated as a component of a training protocol for clients with abnormal breathing-swallowing patterns who are at risk for aspiration (Martin-Harris et al., 2017).

NEURAL CONTROL OF SWALLOWING

The neural control of swallowing is complex and generally beyond the scope of this book. Here, some of the more salient features of the neural control of swallowing are discussed as they relate to the participation of the peripheral and central nervous systems. Additional details regarding the structure and functions of the nervous system are provided in Chapter 8.

Role of the Peripheral Nervous System

Nearly all the structures involved in swallowing are the same as those involved in speech production (the

---

Hungry for Air

People with chronic obstructive pulmonary disease (COPD) have other problems besides the expanded pulmonary apparatus and flattened diaphragm described in the previous sidetrack. One particularly troublesome problem is dyspnea (breathing discomfort), a condition that causes people with COPD to avoid activities that compete with their already strong drive to breathe. Perhaps surprisingly, eating is one of those activities. Most healthy people have no idea that they hold their breath when they swallow. But for people with severe COPD, it's quite a different story. They are often acutely aware of the competition that goes on between eating and breathing. The need to hold the breath during the swallow causes "air hunger" and makes eating and drinking unpleasant chores rather than pleasurable pastimes. Do everything you can to avoid COPD and your life will be happier. Have you quit smoking yet?

most notable exceptions being the esophagus and stomach). Those structures that participate in both swallowing and speech production are innervated by the spinal nerves and cranial nerves described in previous chapters and summarized in Table 7–2. As can be seen in the table, half of the cranial nerves (6 of 12) and most of the spinal nerves (22 of 31) are potential participants in swallowing (and speech production). The cranial nerves are involved in swallowing through their innervation of the lips, mandible, tongue, velum, pharynx, and larynx, whereas the spinal nerves are primarily involved in breathing and its cessation (apnea) as they relate to swallowing.

Peripheral innervation of the esophagus differs along its length. The upper (cervical) region is made up of striated muscle, the type of muscle found in other structures of the swallowing mechanism (lips, mandible, tongue, velum, pharynx, larynx, and respiratory). The cervical region, which includes the upper esophageal sphincter, is innervated by the recurrent branch of the vagus nerve (cranial nerve X), the same branch that innervates most of the intrinsic muscles of the larynx. Thus, the same peripheral nerve is responsible for the simultaneous actions of closing the larynx and opening the upper esophageal sphincter. This means that there is a strong neural link between actions that serve to protect the airway and actions that allow substances to pass into the esophagus. This strong link has obvious advantages for the coordination of the normal swallow but also has the disadvantage that damage to the recurrent branch of the vagus nerve can have serious consequences for both voice production and swallowing (Corbin-Lewis & Liss, 2015).

In lower regions of the esophagus, where smooth muscle intermingles with striated muscle (thoracic esophagus) and where smooth muscle is the only type of muscle present (abdominal esophagus), a different form of neural control operates. This control comes from the autonomic nervous system, which is generally considered to be under automatic (as opposed to voluntary) control. The autonomic nervous system has two parts, the parasympathetic and sympathetic subdivisions. The parasympathetic subdivision is important for maintaining gastrointestinal motility so that a swallowed substance moves through the esophagus easily and quickly. In contrast, the sympathetic subdivision, best known for its importance in fight-or-flight responses to stressful situations, tends to inhibit gastrointestinal motility. This is one reason why gastrointestinal problems are associated with physical and emotional stress. Many of the nerve fibers of the autonomic nervous system travel with the vagus nerve.

Role of the Central Nervous System

Although swallowing and speech production are executed using many of the same peripheral nerves, central nervous system control of these two activities is quite different. This means that a given structure, such as the tongue, is under one form of neural control during swallowing and under another form of neural control during speech production. Because of this, it is possible to have central nervous system damage that impairs the function of a structure for speech production but not swallowing and vice versa. There are two major regions

TABLE 7–2. Summary of Motor and Sensory Nerve Supply to the Respiratory System, Larynx, Velopharyngeal-Nasal Mechanism, and Pharyngeal-Oral Mechanism

SUBSYSTEM	INNERVATION	
	MOTOR	SENSORY
Respiratory	C1–C8, T1–T12, L1–L2	C1–C8, T1–T12, L1–L2
Laryngeal[a]	V, VII, X, XII, C1–C3	X[b]
Velopharyngeal-nasal	V, VII, IX, X, (XI)	V, VII, IX, X
Pharyngeal-oral	V, VII, IX, X, (XI), XII, C1	V, VII, IX, X

Note. Spinal nerves are designated by their segmental origins (C = cervical, T = thoracic, L = lumbar). Cranial nerves are V (trigeminal), VII (facial), IX (glossopharyngeal), X (vagus), XI (accessory), and XII (hypoglossal). This information is also available in Tables 2–2, 3–1, 4–1, and 5–2.

[a]Includes intrinsic, extrinsic, and supplementary laryngeal muscles

[b]Sensory innervation of extrinsic and supplementary laryngeal muscles includes other cranial nerves, such as V and VII.

within the central nervous system that are responsible for the control of swallowing. One is in the brainstem and the other is in cortical and subcortical areas.

The brainstem center is located primarily in the medulla, the part of the brainstem that is contiguous with the uppermost part of the spinal cord. Two main groups of brainstem neurons participate in swallowing: one group that appears to be primarily responsible for triggering the swallow and shaping its temporal pattern and another group that appears to allocate neural drive to the various motor nerves that participate in swallowing (Jean, 2001). This brainstem center has primary control over the more automatic phases of swallowing (pharyngeal and esophageal phases).

Many cortical and subcortical regions contribute to the generation and shaping of swallowing behaviors. The most consistent findings point to contributions of the primary motor and sensory areas of the cortex, anterior cingulate cortex, and insular cortex, with probable contributions from basal ganglia, thalamus, and cerebellum (Humbert & Robbins, 2007; also see Chapter 8 for descriptions of these structures and regions). Activity in these areas has a strong influence over the control and modulation of the more voluntary phases of swallowing (oral preparatory phase, including mastication, and oral transport phase).

Afferent input (information flowing toward the central nervous system from the periphery) is critical to the generation of a normal swallow. The sources of afferent input are many and include, but are not limited to, information related to (a) muscle length and rate of length change, (b) muscle tension, (c) joint position and movement, (d) surface and deep pressures, (e) surface deformation, (f) temperature, (g) taste, and (h) noxious stimuli. Afferent activity is generated by receptors in the swallowing mechanism and sent to the brainstem, where such activity may trigger the motor output required to elicit the pharyngeal phase

of the swallow or may modulate the motor output to accommodate, for example, a larger-than-expected bolus. Afferent activity may also be sent on to subcortical regions (such as the thalamus) or cortical regions (such as the sensorimotor cortex), where it may be consciously perceived. Often the perception is a pleasant experience, such as savoring the flavor and texture of ice cream, or it may be unpleasant (see sidetrack on Sphenopalatineganglioneuralgia).

VARIABLES THAT INFLUENCE SWALLOWING

A number of variables influence swallowing, including characteristics of the bolus, the swallowing mode, and body position. There are also developmental and aging effects on swallowing but essentially no influence of sex.

Bolus Characteristics

Although the act of swallowing occurs generally as described near the beginning of this chapter, the precise nature of the swallow is determined, in part, by what exactly is being swallowed. Bolus consistency and texture, volume, and taste are variables that have been found to influence the act of swallowing.

Consistency and Texture

One of the most important contrasts that determines swallowing behavior is the difference between liquids and solids. Whereas a liquid bolus is usually held briefly in the front of the oral cavity before being propelled to the pharynx, a solid bolus may be moved to the pharynx and left there for several seconds while

---

Sphenopalatineganglioneuralgia

Boy, that sounds like something you wouldn't want to meet in the dark. But it comes from something really good. As a child (or even as an adult), you may have said the phrase, "I scream, you scream, we all scream for ice cream." Scream has a meaning of anticipation in this context, but it can also have a meaning of hurting. You know the feeling. You take a bite of ice cream and momentarily hold it against the roof of your mouth before you swallow it. Then suddenly you get an intense, stabbing pain in your forehead. What's up? The pain is caused as your hard palate warms up after you made it cold. Cold causes vasoconstriction (reduction in blood vessel diameter) in the region, which is followed by rapid vasodilation (increase in blood vessel diameter). It's the rapid vasodilation that hurts and gets your attention. The technical term for this pain is "sphenopalatineganglioneuralgia." The common term (and the one more easily pronounced) is "brain freeze." Fortunately, the pain lasts only a few seconds. Be thankful. There's all that ice cream still waiting to be eaten.

the remainder of the bolus continues to be chewed (Hiiemae & Palmer, 1999; Palmer, Rudin, Lara, & Crompton, 1992; see Figure 7–8). Although something similar can also happen with liquids (Linden, Tippett, Johnston, Siebens, & French, 1989), it is much less common, except in cases where a combined liquid-and-solid bolus is chewed and swallowed (Saitoh et al., 2007), something that might occur during mealtime eating (Dua et al., 1997). Even when not combined, the consistency of liquids and the textures of solid food influence swallowing behavior.

Liquid substances can be characterized according to consistency, ranging from thin as water (low viscosity) to as thick as pudding (high viscosity), and differences in consistency have been shown to influence swallowing. Specifically, thick liquids or puree consistencies tend to take longer to swallow than thin liquids (Chi-Fishman & Sonies, 2002; Im, Kim, Oommen, Kim, & Ko, 2012). This slowing is due to longer oral and pharyngeal phase events and longer upper esophageal sphincter opening durations (Dantas et al., 1990; Im et al., 2012). Tongue forces are higher when swallowing thick substances compared to thin liquids (Chi-Fishman & Sonies, 2002; Miller & Watkin, 1996; Steele & van Lieshout, 2004). As might be predicted, it is more difficult to maintain a cohesive (single) bolus when swallowing thinner liquids as compared to thicker liquids. As a result, laryngeal penetration (where part of the bolus moves into the laryngeal vestibule but remains above the vocal folds; Robbins, Hamilton, Lof, & Kempster, 1992) is more common when swallowing thin liquids than when swallowing thicker substances (Daggett, Logemann, Rademaker, & Pauloski, 2006; Steele et al., 2015). The fact that vocal fold closure starts earlier and lasts longer with thinner compared to thicker liquids (Inamoto et al., 2013) is likely a mechanism to protect against this risk of aspiration.

The textures of solid substances can also influence the swallow (Steele et al., 2015). For example, the harder and drier the substance, the greater the number of chewing cycles (Engelen, Fontijn-Tekamp, & van der Bilt, 2005), the longer the duration of the initial transport of the bolus from the anterior oral cavity to the postcanine region (Mikushi, Seki, Brodsky, Matsuo, & Palmer, 2014), and the greater number of times the tongue squeezes the bolus back toward the pharynx (Hiraoka et al., 2017).

Many different terms have been used to refer to liquids of different thicknesses and substances of different textures, making it difficult to communicate clearly across clinical settings and within the research community. One proposed framework incorporates standardized terminology and rating scales for substances that are used in the evaluation and management of swallowing disorders (International Dysphagia Diet Standardization Initiative [IDDSI]; Cichero et al., 2017, 2020). In this framework, the two major categories are drinks and foods. Drinks are described as thin, slightly thick, mildly thick, moderately thick, and extremely thick, and foods are described as liquidized, pureed, minced and moist, soft and bite-sized, and regular.

Volume

It seems intuitive that the volume (size) of the bolus might affect the swallow, and most studies indicate that, in fact, it does (Chi-Fishman & Sonies, 2002; Cook et al., 1989; Kahrilas & Logemann, 1993; Logemann et al., 2000; Logemann, Pauloski, Rademaker, & Kahrilas, 2002; Perlman, Palmer, McCulloch, & VanDaele, 1999; Perlman, Schultz, & VanDaele, 1993; Tasko, Kent, & Westbury, 2002). When a person is swallowing a larger bolus compared to a smaller bolus, tongue movements are generally larger and faster, hyoid bone movements begin earlier and are more extensive, pharyngeal wall movements and laryngeal movements are larger, and the upper esophageal sphincter relaxes and opens earlier and stays open longer (Cock, Jones, Hammer, Omari, & McCulloch, 2017; Kahrilas & Logemann, 1993; Lin et al., 2014). This means that events related to tongue propulsion of the bolus, closing of the velopharynx, protection of the pulmonary airways, and opening of the upper esophageal sphincter are conditioned by bolus volume in ways that are more sustained and more vigorous for larger boluses than smaller boluses. It is unclear whether or not the duration of apnea varies with bolus volume (Krishnan, Goswami, & Rangarathnam, 2020).

Despite the success of the adjustments made to accommodate a larger bolus, there tends to be a greater frequency of laryngeal penetration as bolus size increases, at least for liquid boluses. For example, part of the bolus penetrates the laryngeal vestibule more than twice as often when swallowing a 10-mL bolus than when swallowing a 1-mL bolus (Daggett et al., 2006). Nevertheless, when laryngeal penetration occurs in healthy individuals, the substance is almost always pushed away from the larynx and transported to the esophagus without being aspirated (going below the vocal folds).

Taste

Taste contributes enormously to the enjoyment of the eating and drinking experience. Imagine, for a moment, eating a hot fudge sundae with some salty nuts on top, then think about biting into a lemon slice. Although the hot fudge sundae may be more enticing, there is evidence that the lemon elicits a more vigorous swallow response.

Gutsy Stuff

Taste receptors in the tongue get all the press and all the credit for making things taste sweet—not surprising, given that there are about 10,000 of them. Put a little sugar in your mouth and the taste receptors in your tongue will come to attention and tell your brain about it. But the taste of sweetness is not just limited to your mouth. Receptors that sense sugar have also been found in the gut. These gut receptors taste glucose in the same way that taste cells in your tongue signal sweetness to the brain. They've been found to alter the secretion of insulin and hormones that regulate blood sugar level and influence appetite. Those are two very important responsibilities. This is all very gutsy stuff and is touted by its discoverers as possibly leading to new treatment options for obesity and diabetes. Let's hope they're right.

Tastes include sweet, salty, sour, bitter, and other tastes (such as umami, meaning meaty or savory), and how something tastes can influence certain features of the swallow. For example, substances with taste (sweet, salty, sour), when compared to tasteless substances, are generally associated with higher peak tongue pressures (Pelletier & Dhanaraj, 2006; Pelletier & Steele, 2014), especially at higher taste intensities (Nagy, Steele, & Pelletier, 2014), and faster and greater activation of selected swallow-related muscle regions (Ding, Logemann, Larson, & Rademaker, 2003). Sour tastes, in particular, appear to elicit more effortful swallows (greater amplitude muscle activity) than other tastes (Leow, Huckabee, Sharma, & Tooley, 2007; Palmer, McCulloch, Jaffe, & Neel, 2005), as well as more frequent swallows (Mulheren, Kamarunas, & Ludlow, 2016). These behavioral effects are associated with taste-related differences in brain function. For example, the ingestion of tasty liquids stimulates significantly more activity in certain cortical regions when compared to ingestion of unflavored water (Babael et al., 2010; Mulheren et al., 2016). Of course, it should also be recognized that tastes are accompanied by their associated smells, so that both the gustatory (taste) and olfactory (smell) senses are usually stimulated simultaneously.

Swallowing Mode

Much of the research on swallowing has focused on single swallows that were either cued ("Swallow now") or in which the bolus was introduced directly into the oral cavity with a syringe. Clearly, this is not how swallowing usually occurs. As the research base expands, there is growing evidence that sequential swallows differ from single swallows and that spontaneously initiated swallows differ from those that are elicited with an external cue, including the cue to swallow with greater-than-usual effort.

Single Versus Sequential Swallows

During eating and drinking, there are times when a swallow occurs in isolation. There are also times when swallows occur sequentially, one immediately after the other.

A swallow is characterized by the same major events whether it is produced singly or as part of a sequence—that is, the bolus is pushed back by the tongue, the velopharynx closes, the hyoid bone and larynx rise and close off the airway, the bolus is moved through the pharynx, and the upper esophageal sphincter opens to admit the bolus into the esophagus. Nevertheless, there are some subtle, yet important, differences between single swallows and sequential swallows that involve the relative timing of certain events and the nature of certain movements.

During both single and sequential swallows, the tongue moves upward to the palate (front to back) to push the bolus backward; however, certain aspects of these movements differ under these two conditions (Chi-Fishman, Stone, & McCall, 1998). To begin, swallow time is shorter during sequential swallows compared to single swallows, something that may be accounted for by shorter contact times, faster movements, shorter movement distances, or some combination of these. Also, certain movements that usually follow one another during a single swallow, such as tongue tip lowering and tongue body elevation, may occur simultaneously during sequential swallows. During a single swallow, the hyolaryngeal complex rises and then falls back to its original (resting) position. In contrast, during sequential swallows, the hyolaryngeal complex rises for the first swallow and then falls, but only part way toward the resting position, before rising again for the next swallow (Chi-Fishman & Sonies, 2000; Daniels et al., 2004; Daniels & Foundas, 2001). The velum rises and falls in synchrony with the hyolaryngeal complex during sequential swallowing (Chi-Fishman & Sonies, 2000). The epiglottis either moves in synchrony with the hyolaryngeal complex or remains down over the laryngeal airway throughout swallow cycles with the hyolaryngeal complex maintained in a partially elevated position (Daniels et al., 2004).

During sequential swallowing, successive boluses often merge in the epiglottic valleculae before the pharyngeal phase is triggered (Dua et al., 1997; Hiiemae & Palmer, 1999). When this happens, the airway tends to stay closed for liquid substances, but not for solid substances (Chi-Fishman & Sonies, 2000). Unsurprisingly, laryngeal penetration is more common during sequential swallows than for single swallows, but in healthy individuals, the penetrated substance is almost always cleared on the next swallow. As is the case with single swallows, the swallow apnea associated with sequential swallows is usually followed by expiration (Ouahchi et al., 2019); nevertheless, it is more common for inspiration to follow the apneic interval during sequential swallows than during single swallows (Lederle et al., 2012; Preiksaitis & Mills, 1996). The average size of the bolus is larger when drinking (sequentially) from a cup than when drinking from a straw (Veiga, Fonseca, & Bianchini, 2014).

Breathing behavior also differs between single and sequential swallows. Whereas single swallows are produced within a single breathing cycle (usually during the expiratory phase), swallows within a series are usually interspersed with breathing cycles. For example, even when instructed to "drink this glass of water without stopping," people will tend to take breaths between occasional swallows (Gürgor et al., 2013; Lederle et al., 2012). This may be a strategy for minimizing dyspnea.

Esophageal behavior differs under the two swallowing conditions as well. For example, during sequential drinking of water, the pressure associated with esophageal peristalsis is lower and the frequency of peristalsis is lower than during single swallows (Meyer, Gerhardt, & Castell, 1981).

Cued Versus Uncued Swallows

The majority of swallowing studies, including those performed for both research and clinical purposes, have been conducted using external cues to swallow (Daniels, Schroeder, DeGeorge, Corey, & Rosenbek, 2007). These are usually verbal cues ("Swallow now"), but they can also be visual or tactile cues. In contrast, the swallowing associated with eating and drinking in daily life is seldom accompanied by such cuing (unless you are a child whose caregiver is saying, "Hurry up and drink your milk"). So, the question arises as to whether or not cuing alters the swallow. Studies that have addressed this question directly (Daniels

et al., 2007; Nagy et al., 2013) have shown that under a cued condition, the substance (a single liquid bolus) is loaded into the anterior oral cavity and then moved somewhat back and held between the midline of the tongue and the hard palate in preparation for the cue, whereas in the noncued condition, the bolus is moved immediately out of the anterior oral cavity as soon as loading is complete. This affects the timing measures associated with each of the phases of swallowing and has implications for how certain measures are obtained.

Sword Throats

Sword swallowing is an ancient art that continues to be practiced. There is even a Sword Swallowers Association International with both professional and amateur members from all over the world. The practice and ill effects of sword swallowing were discussed in an article in the prestigious *British Medical Journal* (Witcombe & Meyer, 2006). Major complications from sword swallowing are more likely when the swallower is distracted or when swallowing unusual swords. Sequelae can include perforation of the pharynx or esophagus, gastrointestinal bleeding, pneumothorax (collapsed lung), and chest pain. (All of this is little wonder, we think.) Novice sword swallowers must learn to desensitize the gag reflex, align the upper esophageal sphincter with the neck hyperextended, open the upper esophageal sphincter, and control retching as the blade is moved on toward the cardia. All in all, it doesn't sound like fun to us. It also makes for a very long bolus.

Another form of cuing involves having a person voluntarily change the nature of the swallow. For example, an instruction such as, "Squeeze hard when you swallow" tends to elicit higher tongue and/or pharyngeal pressures (depending, in part, on the precise wording of the instruction), greater muscle activation levels, and longer durations of several swallowing events compared to swallows produced with usual effort (Fritz et al., 2014; Fukuoka et al., 2013; Molfenter, Hsu, Lu, & Lazarus, 2018; Steele & Huckabee, 2007; Wheeler-Hegland, Rosenbek, & Sapienza, 2008; Yeates, Steele, & Pelletier, 2010). Interestingly, effortful swallow maneuvers also appear to increase amplitudes of peristaltic pressure waves in regions of the esophagus containing smooth muscle, especially the region near the lower esophageal sphincter (Lever et al., 2007; O'Rourke et al., 2014). Effortful swallow maneuvers, and other forms of conscious maneuvers, are often used as behavioral strategies to help clients with swallowing disorders (Leonard, Kendall, McKenzie, & Goodrich, 2008; Logemann, 1998) and those with weak muscles due to normal aging (Park & Kim, 2016).

Body Position

Certain details of swallowing change with body position. For example, whether a person is in an upright body position or on "all fours" (on hands and knees, facing terra firma), swallowing usually occurs during the expiratory phase of the breathing cycle (McFarland, Lund, & Gagner, 1994). Nevertheless, there can be subtle changes in the onset time of the swallow within the expiratory phase. In an upright body position, the swallow usually occurs late in the expiratory phase, whereas when a person is on "all fours," the swallow is more apt to occur earlier in the expiratory phase. It is unclear why this happens, but it may be related to the pull of gravity on the abdominal content, which, in turn, is transmitted to the larynx via its mechanical connections through the diaphragm and pulmonary apparatus (McFarland et al., 1994). In addition, a liquid bolus tends to arrive in the pharynx earlier during swallows produced in an upright body position than during swallows produced in a facedown position (Saitoh et al., 2007), although this position-related timing difference does not appear to occur when a person is swallowing a solid bolus (Palmer, 1998; Saitoh et al., 2007).

There are also differences between swallows produced in supine versus upright body positions. For example, in the supine body position (compared to an upright body position), (a) the hyoid bone moves a greater distance anteriorly, the velum moves a smaller distance posteriorly, and the pharyngeal transport phase of the swallow is longer (Perry, Bae, & Kuehn, 2012); (b) pharyngeal pressure is more positive (Dejaeger, Pelemans, Ponette, & VanTrappen, 1994; Johnson, Shaw, Gabb, Dent, & Cook, 1995); (c) the upper esophageal sphincter pressure reaches its nadir (most subatmospheric pressure) slightly earlier (Castell, Dalton, & Castell, 1990); (d) bolus flow through the upper esophageal sphincter is faster (Johnson et al., 1995); (e) peristaltic waves in the esophagus (particularly in its distal region) are slower and stronger; and (f) the pressure in the lower esophageal sphincter is higher (Sears, Castell, & Castell, 1990). In addition, pressure in the nasopharyngeal region is higher in more supine compared to more upright positions (Rosen,

Abdelhalim, Jones, & McCulloch, 2018). This is likely a compensatory neural mechanism to ensure that the velopharynx remains closed during the swallow so as to prevent nasal regurgitation. It is not clear whether or not the timing of pharyngeal events is influenced by body position (Castell et al., 1990; Ingervall & Lantz, 1973; Johnson et al., 1995; Su et al., 2015). Similarly, the timing of sensory and motor events related to vocal fold activation before, during, and after the swallow appears to be unaffected by a change from upright to supine position (Barkmeier, Bielamowicz, Takeda, & Ludlow, 2002).

Age

Infancy and childhood are times of significant anatomical and physiological development. Many of these developmental changes have been described in previous chapters (see Chapters 2, 3, 4, and 5). The focus here is on those changes that pertain to the development of feeding and swallowing.

There are many important anatomical changes that influence swallowing during the period from infancy through childhood. Some of these include the following (Arvedson & Brodsky, 2002): (a) The infant's tongue goes from nearly filling the oral cavity to filling only the floor of the oral cavity due to differential growth of oral structures; (b) the infant's oral cavity goes from being edentulous to having a full set of deciduous teeth; (c) the cheeks of the infant have fatty pads (sometimes called sucking pads) that eventually disappear, to be replaced with muscle; (d) the infant goes from having essentially no oropharynx to having a distinct one as the larynx descends; and (e) the infant's larynx goes from being one-third adult size, with relatively large arytenoid cartilages and a high position within the neck, to the adult configuration and position. It is interesting to note that although anatomical changes influence swallowing, the opposite is also true. That is, because the forces exerted during swallowing and chewing are quite large, they have a profound influence on molding the oral and pharyngeal anatomy of the infant and young child.

Swallowing (of amniotic fluid) begins well before birth, as early as 12.5 weeks' gestation (Humphrey, 1970). Interestingly, although many of the components of swallowing are in place before birth, velopharyngeal closure during swallowing is not (Miller, Sonies, & Macedonia, 2003). Perhaps this is related to the fact that the entire digestive tract is infused with amniotic fluid so that there is little consequence of having an open velopharynx; that is, the amniotic fluid would infuse the nasal passages whether the velopharynx is open or closed. Immediately after birth, the velopharynx closes for swallowing and the infant exhibits a suckling pattern characterized by forward and backward (horizontal) movements of the tongue (Bosma, 1986; Bosma, Truby, & Lind, 1965). These tongue movements are accompanied by large vertical movements of the mandible and serve to draw liquid into the oral cavity. Around the age of 6 months, this suckling pattern converts to a sucking pattern, which is characterized by raising and lowering (vertical) movements of the tongue, firm approximation of the lips, and less pronounced vertical movements of the mandible. Sucking is stronger than suckling and allows the infant to pull in thicker substances into the oral cavity and to begin the ingestion of soft food (Arvedson & Brodsky, 2002).

During the first few months of life, the infant relies on breastfeeding (or nipple feeding from a bottle) for all nutritional intake. This form of feeding consists of suck-swallow or suck-swallow-breathe sequences, typically repeated several times (8 to 12 times) and followed by a rest period (several seconds). It was once thought that infants swallow and breathe at the same time; however, they do not. Although infants can continue breathing during the suck, like adults, they stop breathing during the swallow (Wilson, Thach, Brouillette, & Abu-Osba, 1981) and their ventilation decreases as a result (Koenig, Davies, & Thach, 1990). During this period, several oral reflexes that aid in early feeding are active. These disappear around 6 months of age, with the exception of the gag reflex, which remains active throughout childhood and adulthood.

By about 6 months of age, infants are ready to begin eating solid foods and being fed by spoon. Foods such as crackers and soft fruits and vegetables are introduced during the next few months. The basic patterns for chewing are in place by 9 months and continue to develop over the next few years of life (Green et al., 1997; Steeve, Moore, Green, Reilly, & Ruark McMurtrey, 2008). By 2 to 3 years of age, the child is able to eat regular table food.

As with most physiological functions, swallowing changes with age across adulthood. The most robust age-related change is that swallowing becomes slower, particularly after age 60 years (Humbert et al., 2018; Jardine, Miles, & Allen, 2020; Leonard & McKenzie, 2006; Logemann et al., 2002; Robbins et al., 1992; Sonies, Parent, Morrish, & Baum, 1988). Certain individual components of the swallow also tend to be delayed in older compared to younger adults. For example, the trigger for the pharyngeal phase is located closer to the esophagus in older adults (Robbins et al., 1992; Tracy et al., 1989) than in younger adults (Logemann, 1998). Also, it takes longer for the bolus to move through the pharynx and for the upper esophageal sphincter to open in older adults (Logemann et al., 2002; Mendell & Logemann, 2007; Nishikubo et al., 2015; Robbins et al., 1992). The apneic interval during the swallow is generally longer in older adults than younger adults (Hirst, Ford, Gibson, & Wilson, 2002; Wang et al., 2015), and the offset of the apneic interval occurs later (Martin-Harris, Brodsky, et al., 2005). There is a greater tendency for older adults to initiate the swallow during inspiration (Yamada et al., 2017) or to inspire immediately after the swallow (Martin-Harris, Brodsky, et al., 2005). Tongue movements during swallowing are slower in older than younger adults (Steele & van Lieshout, 2009), although tongue pressures do not seem to change with age (Fei et al., 2013; Youmans, Youmans, & Stierwalt, 2009). Mastication (chewing) effectiveness remains intact, even in the very old (as long as they are healthy), although the number of chewing cycles per bolus tends to increase with age (Peyron, Woda, Bourdiol, & Hennequin, 2017).

An outcome of the age-related slowing of the swallow (combined with age-related reductions in sensory function; for example, see Malandraki, Perlman, Karampinos, & Sutton, 2011) is that the frequency of laryngeal penetration increases with age (Daniels et al., 2004; Robbins et al., 1992). Laryngeal penetration occurs in people over 50 years about twice as often as it occurs in adults under 50 years, and more frequently when swallowing liquids than when swallowing solids. Although this appears to be a dangerous situation and a possible precursor to aspiration, in healthy individuals, the substance is moved out of the vestibule to be rejoined with the rest of the bolus (Daggett et al., 2006). Despite all these age-related changes, there is no convincing evidence that aging alone is a risk for swallowing disorders (Jardine, Miles, & Allen, 2018; Namasivayam-MacDonald, Barbon, & Steele, 2018).

Sex

Several studies of swallowing have included participants of both sexes, and some of these have revealed statistically significant differences in selected measures. Nevertheless, there do not appear to be consistent findings across studies that would lead to the conclusion that swallowing is different in men and women. Sex-related differences that have been reported are likely to be attributable to chance (such as that related to participant selection or statistical chance) or to variables other than sex (such as size and strength). Thus, given the current knowledge base, it seems safe to conclude that swallowing does not differ between the sexes in any consistent or important way and does not need to be taken into account in clinical endeavors.

Chicken Dinner

Cancer had taken his tongue. He had no teeth. And signs of a stroke were on his face. His speech was remarkably good and arrangements were made to travel out of state with him to use special x-ray equipment to study his speaking and swallowing. The trip was by car and went well until a snowstorm forced an overnight stay. Dinner was instructive. To propel food toward his pharynx, he threw his head back in the way a chicken tosses its head when eating. Having no teeth helped him because he could touch his mandible to his maxilla and create a downward and backward sloping floor to his mouth. He poured liquids down this slope. When motion picture x-rays from his study were developed, they were enlightening. When he swallowed water, his epiglottis stood fully erect, as if at military attention, while liquid cascaded around it. He apparently hadn't read textbooks telling him how the epiglottis is always forced down over the larynx during swallowing.

CLINICAL NOTES

Swallowing disorders—also called dysphagia (and pronounced dis-FAY-juh)—are common, and people with dysphagia make up a large part of the caseload of speech-language pathologists who work in medical settings. Dysphagia can be caused by structural, neurogenic, and even psychogenic problems, and they can occur at any age, from infancy to senescence.

The clinical evaluation of people with dysphagia has come a long way since your authors were in college. Whereas the evaluation of swallowing used to be performed by occupational therapists without instruments, then later by speech-language pathologists without instruments, today evaluation of swallowing now includes a variety of instrumental approaches. Instrumental measurement of swallowing is especially important when considering that as many as half of the clients who aspirate do so "silently" without any signs of coughing or other signs of visible or audible struggle (Logemann, 1998). In such cases, aspiration can only be detected through instrumental examination. There are many instrumental approaches to swallowing evaluation. Our focus here is on videofluoroscopy. It is generally agreed that videofluoroscopy provides the most comprehensive evaluation of swallowing, and for many, it is considered the "gold standard" of measurement.

The videofluoroscopic swallow examination, sometimes called a modified barium swallow (MBS) study, was first described by Logemann, Boshes, Blonsky, and Fisher (1977). Barium is a contrast material that allows the bolus to be tracked visually as it travels through the oral, pharyngeal, and esophageal regions. The adjective "modified" is used to differentiate this examination from a barium swallow study, which is conducted by a gastroenterologist to evaluate esophageal structure and function. A videofluoroscopic examination is usually conducted with the client seated in a specially designed chair. The examination is performed in a radiology laboratory, with a radiologist (or radiology technician) running the x-ray equipment and a speech-language pathologist directing the swallowing protocol. The examination protocol typically consists of the swallowing of a series of liquid and solid substances (mixed with barium or accompanied by ingestion of a barium capsule to provide contrast) that vary in volume and consistency or texture. For example, the protocol might include the swallowing of thin liquid, nectar, and pudding in small and large servings and the chewing and swallowing of a cookie or cracker. The drinking of the thin liquid might be from a spoon, cup, straw, or a combination of these. The exact protocol depends on the nature of the client's swallowing complaint (in a clinical setting) or the nature of the research question (in a research setting).

Figure 7–11 shows an example of a videofluoroscopic image of the oral preparatory phase of swallowing. The bolus is the dark substance in the oral cavity; some traces of the bolus can also be seen farther down in the airway. Although this figure contains only one still frame, the actual image is a moving image that can be viewed in real time, recorded, and played back at normal speed, slow speed, or even frame by frame. Images can be obtained using a lateral view (as in this figure) and a frontal view (not shown). Each view offers different advantages for capturing certain swallowing events.

A variety of temporal and spatial measurements can be made from the videofluoroscopic images. Temporal measurements are generally in the form of objective values, for example, the time from the beginning of bolus movement from the oral cavity to its arrival at the upper esophageal sphincter. Spatial measurements may also be in the form of objective values, or they may be in the form of judgments or ratings. For example, ratings can be made of the extent of velar elevation (on a scale of none to fully elevated) or extent of hyoid bone excursion (on a scale of none to normal). One of the most popular assessment tools, the Penetration-Aspiration Scale (Rosenbek, Robbins, Roecker, Coyle, & Wood, 1996), is an 8-point categorical rating scale that provides descriptions of events that indicate laryngeal penetration or aspiration (ranging from "material does not enter

you to watch two videos. The first is a videofluoro-scopic study of a healthy adult swallowing (see Video 7–2 [Videofluoroscopy: Normal]); the second features someone with dysphagia (see Video 7–3 [Videofluoros-copy: Abnormal]).

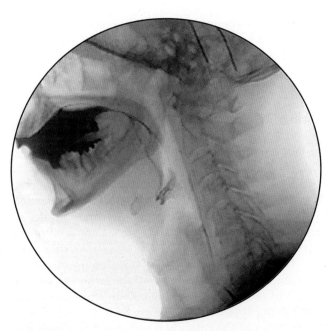

FIGURE 7–11. Videoflurosocopic image showing the oral preparatory phase of a swallow. The large, dark area in the oral region is the bolus. The thin, dark line that runs along the tongue to the epiglottal vallecula indicates that there may be some trace residue from a previous swallow or that there has been some premature spillage during the oral hold. From *Dysphagia Assessment and Treatment Planning: A Team Approach*, Second Edition (p. 273), by Rebecca Leonard and Katherine Kendall. Copyright © 2008 by Plural Publishing. All rights reserved.

the airway" to "material enters the airway, passes below the vocal folds, and no effort is made to eject").

To gain an appreciation for the movements of swallowing and how rapidly the bolus passes through the oral and pharyngeal airway to the esophagus, we invite

REVIEW

Eating and drinking involve intricately coordinated actions of the lips, mandible, tongue, velum, pharynx, larynx, esophagus, and other structures.

The act of placing liquid or solid substances in the oral cavity, moving it backward to the pharynx, propelling it into the esophagus, and allowing it to make its way to the stomach is called *deglutition*.

The term *swallowing* is ingrained as a synonym for deglutition and is used as such in this chapter, although swallowing technically involves only part of the deglutition process.

Many of the important anatomical and physiological components of the speech production apparatus, discussed in Chapters 2 through 5 of this text, are also important anatomical and physiological components of the swallowing apparatus.

The esophagus is a muscular tube that extends from the lower border of the pharynx to the stomach and is bounded at its two ends by high-pressure valves (the upper and lower esophageal sphincters) that govern the passage of liquid and solid substances into and out of the structure.

The stomach is a liter-sized sac whose upper end connects to the esophagus through the lower esophageal sphincter and whose lower end connects to the small intestine through the pyloric sphincter.

GERD and LPR

Your stomach is rich with chemicals that have about the same acidity as the battery acid in your car. That's right, that's the same battery acid that will burn a hole in your clothes if you splash some of it on you. GERD, an acronym for gastroesophageal reflux disease, is a chronic condition in which acid from the stomach backs up into the esophagus when the lower esophageal sphincter (the valve that separates the esophagus and stomach) fails to do its job properly. Although a certain amount of reflux (backflow) from the stomach into the esophagus is considered normal, too much can cause heartburn and the need to see a gastroenterologist

(GI doctor). When stomach acid travels all the way through the esophagus and spills onto the larynx, it is called laryngopharyngeal reflux, or LPR. LPR can irritate and erode laryngeal tissue. LPR can cause a hoarse voice, chronic cough, frequent throat clearing, and other problems that may lead to the need to seek help from an otolaryngologist (ENT doctor). Some helpful hints for avoiding GERD and LPR: Don't stuff yourself before you go to bed, lay off foods that make it worse, and sleep with your body inclined so that your head is higher than your feet.

The forces of swallowing are greater and the movements of swallowing are generally slower than those associated with speech production.

Passive forces of swallowing come from the natural recoil of structures, surface tension between structures in apposition, gravity, and aeromechanical factors, whereas active forces result from the activation of breathing, laryngeal, velopharyngeal-nasal, pharyngeal-oral, and esophageal muscles in various combinations.

Different pressure gradients are critical to the swallowing process and are influenced by pressures existing within the oral cavity, the upper esophageal sphincter, the esophagus, the lower esophageal sphincter, and the stomach.

The forces and movements associated with the act of swallowing can be categorized in four phases that include an oral preparatory phase, oral transport phase, pharyngeal phase, and esophageal phase.

The oral preparatory phase involves taking liquid or solid substances in through the oral vestibule and manipulating it within the oral cavity to prepare the bolus (liquid volume or lump of solid) for passage.

The oral transport phase involves moving the bolus (or a part of it) through the oral cavity toward the pharynx by rearward propulsion.

The pharyngeal phase is usually "triggered" when the bolus passes the anterior faucial pillars or beyond and consists of a combination of compressive actions that force the bolus downward toward the esophagus while at the same time protecting the lower airways.

The esophageal phase begins when the bolus enters the esophagus and continues as the bolus is moved toward the stomach by a series of peristaltic waves of muscular contraction and relaxation that progress down the muscular tube and which are followed by secondary waves that clear the esophagus.

Although it is convenient to describe swallowing as four discrete phases, the reality is that there is enormous overlap among the phases, and more physiologic schemes may offer better ways to characterize the swallowing process.

Swallowing usually occurs during expiration at lung volumes that are somewhat larger than the resting expiratory level and is associated with a brief apneic interval (cessation of breathing).

The neural control of swallowing is vested in the brainstem and in other higher brain centers that oversee automatic and voluntary aspects of the different phases of swallowing.

Characteristics of the bolus can influence the swallowing pattern, including bolus consistency and texture, volume, and taste.

The mode of swallowing has an impact on the swallowing process, with differences observed for single swallows versus sequential swallows, cued swallows versus spontaneous swallows, with dependencies on how the substance is presented and what instructions are given.

Details of the swallowing pattern may change with changes in body position, including when swallowing occurs during the breathing cycle, the timing of certain swallowing events, and the magnitudes of certain pressures.

The development of swallowing from infancy is rapid and complex and moves through different sucking and chewing patterns toward adult-like eating and drinking behaviors, carrying with it important developmental processes related to social and emotional development.

The effect of aging on the swallow is an overall slowing and a subtle deterioration in the spatial and temporal coordination among certain structures of the swallowing apparatus.

The sex of the individual makes little difference to the nature of swallowing.

There are several ways to measure and analyze swallowing, but the "gold standard" is videofluoroscopy.

REFERENCES

Arvedson, J., & Brodsky, L. (2002). *Pediatric swallowing and feeding: Assessment and management* (2nd ed.). Clifton Park, NY: Thomson Learning (Singular Publishing).

Babael, A., Kern, M., Antonik, S., Mepant, R., Ward, B., Li, S.-J., . . . Shaker, R. (2010). Enhancing effects of flavored nutritive stimuli on cortical swallowing network activity. *American Journal of Physiology: Gastrointestinal and Liver Physiology, 299,* G422–G429.

Barkmeier, J., Bielamowicz, S., Takeda, N., & Ludlow, C. (2002). Laryngeal activity during upright vs. supine swallowing. *Journal of Applied Physiology, 93,* 740–745.

Bosma, J. (1986). Development of feeding. *Clinical Nutrition, 5,* 210–218.

Bosma, J., Truby, H., & Lind, J. (1965). Cry motions of the newborn infant. *Acta Paediatrica Scandinavica, 163,* 63–91.

Castell, J., Dalton, C., & Castell, D. (1990). Effects of body position and bolus consistency on the manometric parameters and coordination of the upper esophageal sphincter and pharynx. *Dysphagia, 5,* 179–186.

Chi-Fishman, G., & Sonies, B. (2000). Motor strategy in rapid sequential swallowing: New insights. *Journal of Speech, Language, and Hearing Research, 43,* 1481–1492.

Chi-Fishman, G., & Sonies, B. (2002). Effects of systematic bolus viscosity and volume changes on hyoid movement kinematics. *Dysphagia, 17,* 278–287.

Chi-Fishman, G., Stone, M., & McCall, G. (1998). Lingual action in normal sequential swallowing. *Journal of Speech, Language, and Hearing Research, 41,* 771–785.

Cichero, J., Lam, P., Chen, J., Dantas, R., Duivestein, J., Hanson, B., . . . Vanderwegen, J. (2020). Release of updated International Dysphagia Diet Standardization Initiative Framework (IDDSI 2.0). *Journal of Texture Studies, 51,* 195–196.

Cichero, J., Lam, P., Steele, C., Hanson, B., Chen, J., Dantas, R., . . . Stanschus, S. (2017). Development of international terminology and definitions for texture-modified foods and thickened fluids used in dysphagia management: The IDDSI framework. *Dysphagia, 32,* 293–314.

Cock, C., Jones, C., Hammer, M., Omari, T., & McCulloch, T. (2017). Modulation of upper esophageal sphincter (UES) relaxation and opening during volume swallowing. *Dysphagia, 32,* 216–224.

Cook, I., Dodds, W., Dantas, R., Kern, M., Massey, B., Shaker, R., & Hogan, W. (1989). Timing of videofluoroscopic, manometric events, and bolus transit during the oral and pharyngeal phases of swallowing. *Dysphagia, 4,* 8–15.

Cook, I., Weltman, M., Wallace, K., Shaw, D., McKay, E., Smart, R., & Butler, S. (1994). Influence of aging on oral-pharyngeal bolus transit and clearance during swallowing: Scintigraphic study. *American Journal of Physiology, 266,* G972–G977.

Corbin-Lewis, K., & Liss, J. (2015). *Clinical anatomy and physiology of the swallow mechanism.* Independence, KY: Cengage Learning.

Daggett, A., Logemann, J., Rademaker, A., & Pauloski, B. (2006). Laryngeal penetration during deglutition in normal subjects of various ages. *Dysphagia, 21,* 270–274.

Daniels, S., Corey, D., Hadskey, L., Legendre, C., Priestly, D., Rosenbek, J., & Foundas, A. (2004). Mechanism of sequential swallowing during straw drinking in healthy young and older adults. *Journal of Speech, Language, and Hearing Research, 47,* 33–45.

Daniels, S., & Foundas, A. (2001). Swallowing physiology of sequential straw drinking. *Dysphagia, 16,* 176–182.

Daniels, S., Schroeder, M., DeGeorge, P., Corey, D., & Rosenbek, J. (2007). Effects of verbal cue on bolus flow during swallowing. *American Journal of Speech-Language Pathology, 16,* 140–147.

Dantas, R., Kern, M., Massey, B., Dodds, W., Kahrilas, P., Brasseur, J., . . . Lang, I. (1990). Effect of swallowed bolus variables on oral and pharyngeal phases of swallowing. *American Journal of Physiology, 258,* G675–G681.

Dejaeger, E., Pelemans, W., Ponette, E., & VanTrappen, G. (1994). Effect of body position on deglutition. *Digestive Diseases and Sciences, 39,* 762–765.

Ding, R., Logemann, J., Larson, C., & Rademaker, A. (2003). The effects of taste and consistency on swallow physiology in younger and older healthy individuals: A surface electromyographic study. *Journal of Speech, Language, and Hearing Research, 46,* 977–989.

Dodds, W., Hogan, W., Reid, D., Stewart, E., & Arndorfer, R. (1973). A comparison between primary esophageal peristalsis following wet and dry swallows. *Journal of Applied Physiology, 35,* 851–857.

Dodds, W., Taylor, A., Stewart, E., Kern, M., Logemann, J., & Cook, I. (1989). Tipper and dipper types of oral swallows. *American Journal of Roentgenology, 153,* 1197–1199.

Dua, K., Ren, J., Bardan, E., Xie, P., & Shaker, R. (1997). Coordination of deglutitive glottal function and pharyngeal bolus transit during normal eating. *Gastroenterology, 112,* 73–83.

Ekberg, O., & Sigurjonsson, S. (1982). Movement of epiglottis during deglutition: A cineradiographic study. *Gastrointestinal Radiology, 7,* 101–107.

Engelen, L., Fontijn-Tekamp, & van der Bilt, A. (2005). The influence of product and oral characteristics on swallowing. *Archives of Oral Biology, 50,* 739–746.

Fei, T., Polacco, R., Hori, S., Molfenter, S., Peladeau-Pigeon, M., Tsang, C., & Steele, C. (2013). Age-related differences in tongue-palate pressures for strength and swallowing tasks. *Dysphagia, 28,* 575–581.

Fink, B., & Demarest, R. (1978). *Laryngeal biomechanics.* Cambridge, MA: Harvard University Press.

Fink, B., Martin, R., & Rohrmann, C. (1979). Biomechanics of the human epiglottis. *Acta Otolaryngologica, 87,* 554–559.

Fritz, M., Cerrati, E., Fang, Y., Verma, A., Achiatis, S., Lazarus, C., . . . Amin, M. (2014). Magnetic resonance imaging of the effortful swallow. *Annals of Otology, Rhinology, & Laryngology, 123,* 786–790.

Fukuoka, T., Ono, T., Hori, K., Tamine, K., Nozaki, S., Shimada, K., . . . Domen, K. (2013). Effect of the effortful swallow and the Mendelsohn maneuver on tongue pressure production against the hard palate. *Dysphagia, 28,* 539–547.

Goyal, R., & Cobb, B. (1981). Motility of the pharynx, esophagus, and esophageal sphincters. In L. Johnson (Ed.), *Physiology of the gastrointestinal tract* (pp. 359–390). New York, NY: Raven Press.

Green, J., Moore, C., Ruark, J., Rodda, P., Morvee, W., & VanWitzenburg, M. (1997). Development of chewing in children from 12 to 48 months: Longitudinal study of EMG patterns. *Journal of Neurophysiology, 77,* 2704–2716.

Gross, R., Carrau, R., Slivka, W., Gisser, R., Smith, L., Zajac, D., & Sciurba, F. (2012). Deglutitive subglottic air pressure and respiratory system recoil. *Dysphagia, 27,* 452–459.

Gürgor, N., Arici, S., Incesu, T. Seçil, Y., Tokuçoglu, F., & Ertekin, C. (2013). An electrophysiological study of the sequential water swallowing. *Journal of Electromyography and Kinesiology, 23,* 619–626.

Hårdemark Cedborg, A., Bodén, K., Witt Hedström, H., Kuylenstierna, R., Ekberg, O., Eriksson, L., & Sundman, E. (2010). Breathing and swallowing in normal man: Effects of changes in body position, bolus types, and respiratory drive. *Neurogastroenterology and Motility, 22,* 1201–1208.

Hiiemae, K., & Palmer, J. (1999). Food transport and bolus formation during complete feeding sequences on foods of different initial consistency. *Dysphagia, 14,* 31–42.

Hila, A., Castell, J., & Castell, D. (2001). Pharyngeal and upper esophageal sphincter manometry in the evaluation of dysphagia. *Journal of Clinical Gastroenterology, 33,* 355–361.

Hiraoka, T., Palmer, J., Brodsky, M., Yoda, M., Inokuchi, H., & Tsubahara, A. (2017). Food transit duration is associated with the number of stage II transport cycles when eating solid food. *Archives of Oral Biology, 81,* 186–191.

Hirst, L., Ford, G., Gibson, G., & Wilson, J. (2002). Swallow-induced alterations in breathing in normal older people. *Dysphagia, 17,* 152–161.

Hoit, J., Lansing, R., Dean, K., Yarkosky, M., & Lederle, A. (2011). Nature and evaluation of dyspnea in speaking and swallowing. *Seminars in Speech and Language, 32,* 5–20.

Hopkins-Rossabi, T., Curtis, P., Temenak, M., Miller, C., & Martin-Harris, B. (2019). Respiratory phase and lung volume patters during swallowing in healthy adults: A systematic review and meta-analysis. *Journal of Speech, Language, and Hearing Research, 62,* 868–882.

Hosseini, P., Tadavarthi, Y., Martin-Harris, B., & Pearson, W. (2019). Functional modules of pharyngeal swallowing mechanics. *Laryngoscope Investigative Otolaryngology, 4,* 341–346.

Huff, A., Day, T., English, M., Reed, M., Zouboules, S., Saran, G., . . . Pitts, T. (2019). Swallow-breathing coordination during incremental ascent to altitude. *Respiratory Physiology & Neurobiology, 265,* 121–126.

Humbert, I., & Robbins, J. (2007). Normal swallowing and functional magnetic resonance imaging: A systematic review. *Dysphagia, 22,* 266–275.

Humbert, I., Sunday, K., Karagiorgos, E., Vose, A., Gould, F., Greene, L., . . . Rivet, A. (2018). Swallowing kinematic differences across frozen, mixed, and ultrathin liquid boluses in healthy adults: Age, sex, and normal variability. *Journal of Speech, Language, and Hearing Research, 61,* 1544–1559.

Humphrey, T. (1970). Reflex activity in the oral and facial area of the human fetus. In J. Bosma (Ed.), *Second symposium on oral sensation and perception* (pp. 195–233). Springfield, IL: Charles C Thomas.

Im, I., Kim, Y., Oommen, E., Kim, H., & Ko, M. (2012). The effects of bolus consistency in pharyngeal transit duration during normal swallowing. *Annals of Rehabilitation Medicine, 36,* 220–225.

Inamoto, Y., Saitoh, E., Okada, S., Kagaya, H., Shibata, S., Ota, K., . . . Palmer, J. (2013). The effect of bolus viscosity on laryngeal closure in swallowing: Kinematic analysis using 320-row area detector CT. *Dysphagia, 28,* 33–42.

Ingervall, B., & Lantz, B. (1973). Significance of gravity on the passage of bolus through the human pharynx. *Archives of Oral Biology, 18,* 351–356.

Jardine, M., Miles, A., & Allen, J. (2018). Swallowing function in advanced age. *Current Opinion in Otolaryngology & Head and Neck Surgery, 26,* 367–374.

Jardine, M., Miles, A., & Allen, J. (2020). A systematic review of physiological changes in swallowing in the oldest old. *Dysphagia, 35,* 509–532.

Jean, A. (2001). Brain stem control of swallowing: Neuronal network and cellular mechanisms. *Physiological Reviews, 81,* 929–969.

Johnson, F., Shaw, D., Gabb, M., Dent, J., & Cook, I. (1995). Influence of gravity and body position on normal oropharyngeal swallowing. *American Journal of Physiology, 269,* G653–G658.

Kahrilas, P., & Logemann, J. (1993). Volume accommodation during swallowing. *Dysphagia, 8,* 259–265.

Klaun, M., & Perlman, A. (1999). Temporal and durational patterns associating respiration and swallowing. *Dysphagia, 14,* 131–138.

Koenig, J., Davies, A., & Thach, B. (1990). Coordination of breathing, sucking, and swallowing during bottle feedings in human infants. *Journal of Applied Physiology, 69,* 1623–1629.

Krishnam, G., Goswami, S., & Rangarathnam, B. (2020). A systematic review of the influence of bolus characteristics on respiratory measures in healthy swallowing. *Dysphagia.* Advance online publication. doi.org/10.1007/s00455-020-10103-4

Langmore, S. (2001). *Endoscopic evaluation and treatment of swallowing disorders.* New York, NY: Thieme Medical Publishers, Inc.

Lederle, A., Hoit, J., & Barkmeier-Kraemer, J. (2012). Effects of sequential swallowing on drive to breathe in young, healthy adults. *Dysphagia, 27,* 221–227.

Leonard, R., Kendall, K., McKenzie, S., & Goodrich, S. (2008). The treatment plan. In R. Leonard & K. Kendall (Eds.), *Dysphagia assessment and treatment planning: A team approach* (2nd ed., pp. 295–336). San Diego, CA: Plural Publishing.

Leonard, R., & McKenzie, S. (2006). Hyoid-bolus transit latencies in normal swallow. *Dysphagia, 21,* 183–190.

Leow, L., Huckabee, M., Sharma, S., & Tooley, T. (2007). The influence of taste on swallowing apnea, oral preparation time, and duration and amplitude of submental muscle contraction. *Chemical Senses, 32,* 119–128.

Lever, T., Cox, K., Holbert, D., Shahrier, M., Hough, M., & Kelley-Salamon, K. (2007). The effect of effortful swallow on the normal adult esophagus. *Dysphagia, 22,* 312–325.

Lin, T., Xu, G., Dou, Z, Lan, Y., Yu, F., & Jiang, L. (2014). Effect of bolus volume on pharyngeal swallowing assessed by high-resolution manometry. *Physiology & Behavior, 128,* 46–51.

Linden, M., Hogosta, S., & Norlander, T. (2007). Monitoring of pharyngeal and upper esophageal sphincter activity with an arterial dilation balloon catheter. *Dysphagia, 22,* 81–88.

Linden, P., Tippett, D., Johnston, J., Siebens, A., & French, J. (1989). Bolus position at swallow onset in normal adults: Preliminary observations. *Dysphagia, 4,* 146–150.

Lindh, M., Malinovschi, A., Brandén, E., Janson, C., Ställberg, B., Bröms, K., . . . Koyi, H. (2019). Subjective swallowing symptoms and related risk factors in COPD. *European Respiratory Journal Open Research, 5,* 00081-2019.

Logemann, J. (1998). *Evaluation and treatment of swallowing disorders* (2nd ed.). Austin, TX: Pro-Ed.

Logemann, J., Boshes, B., Blonsky, E., & Fisher, H. (1977). Speech and swallowing evaluation in the differential diagnosis of neurologic disease. *Neurologia, Neurocirugia, and Psiquiatria, 18*(2–3 Suppl.), 71–78.

Logemann, J., Kahrilas, P., Kobara, M., & Vakil, N. (1989). The benefit of head rotation on pharyngo-esophageal dysphagia. *Archives of Physical Medicine and Rehabilitation, 70,* 767–771.

Logemann, J., Pauloski, B., Rademaker, A., Colangelo, L., Kahrilas, P., & Smith, C. (2000). Temporal and biomechanical characteristics of oropharyngeal swallow in younger and older men. *Journal of Speech, Language, and Hearing Research, 43,* 1264–1274.

Logemann, J., Pauloski, B., Rademaker, A., & Kahrilas, P. (2002). Oropharyngeal swallow in younger and older women: Videofluoroscopic analysis. *Journal of Speech, Language, and Hearing Research, 45,* 434–445.

Malandraki, G., Perlman, A., Karampinos, D., & Sutton, B. (2011). Reduced somatosensory activations in swallowing with age. *Human Brain Mapping, 32*, 730–743.

Martin, B., Logemann, J., Shaker, R., & Dodds, W. (1994). Coordination between respiration and swallowing: Respiratory phase relationships and temporal integration. *Journal of Applied Physiology, 76*, 714–723.

Martin-Harris, B. (2006, May 16). Coordination of respiration and swallowing. *GI Motility Online.* doi:10.1038/gimo10

Martin-Harris, B., Brodsky, M., Michel, Y., Ford, C., Walters, B., & Heffner, J. (2005). Breathing and swallowing dynamics across the adult lifespan. *Archives of Otolaryngology-Head and Neck Surgery, 131*, 762–770.

Martin-Harris, B., Brodsky, M., Price, C., Michel, Y., & Walters, B. (2003). Temporal coordination of pharyngeal and laryngeal dynamics with breathing during swallowing: Single liquid swallows. *Journal of Applied Physiology, 94*, 1735–1743.

Martin-Harris, B., Garand, K., & McFarland, D. (2017). Optimizing respiratory-swallowing coordination in patients with oropharyngeal head and neck cancer. *Perspectives of the ASHA Special Interest Groups, 2*, 103–110.

Martin-Harris, B., Michel, Y., & Castell, D. (2005). Physiologic model of oropharyngeal swallowing revisited. *Otolaryngology-Head and Neck Surgery, 133*, 234–240.

McFarland, D., & Lund, J. (1995). Modification of mastication and respiration during swallowing in the adult human. *Journal of Neurophysiology, 74*, 1509–1517.

McFarland, D., Lund, J., & Gagner, M. (1994). Effects of posture on the coordination of respiration and swallowing. *Journal of Neurophysiology, 72*, 2431–2437.

McFarland, D., Martin-Harris, B., Fortin, A., Humphries, K., Hill, E., & Armeson, K. (2016). Respiratory-swallowing coordination in normal subjects: Lung volume at swallowing initiation. *Respiratory Physiology & Neurobiology, 234*, 89–96.

Mendell, D., & Logemann, J. (2007). Temporal sequence of swallow events during the oropharyngeal swallow. *Journal of Speech, Language, and Hearing Research, 50*, 1256–1271.

Meyer, G., Gerhardt, D., & Castell, D. (1981). Human esophageal response to rapid swallowing: Muscle refractory period or neural inhibition? *American Journal of Physiology, 241*, G129–G136.

Mikushi, S., Seki, S., Brodsky, M., Matsuo, K., & Palmer, J. (2014). Stage I intraoral food transport: Effects of food consistency and initial bolus size. *Archives of Oral Biology, 59*, 379–385.

Miller, J., Sonies, B., & Macedonia, C. (2003). Emergence of oropharyngeal, laryngeal and swallowing activity in the developing fetal upper aerodigestive tract: An ultrasound evaluation. *Early Human Development, 71*, 61–87.

Miller, J., & Watkin, K. (1996). The influence of bolus volume and viscosity on anterior lingual force during the oral stage of swallowing. *Dysphagia, 11*, 117–124.

Molfenter, S., Hsu, C.-Y., Lu, Y., & Lazarus, C. (2018). Alterations in swallowing physiology as the result of effortful swallowing in healthy seniors. *Dysphagia, 33*, 380–388.

Molfenter, S., & Steele, C. (2012). Temporal variability in the deglutition literature. *Dysphagia, 27*, 162–177.

Mulheren, R., Kamarunas, E., & Ludlow, C. (2016). Sour taste increases swallowing and prolongs hemodynamic responses in the cortical swallowing network. *Journal of Neurophysiology, 116*, 203–204.

Nagy, A., Leigh, C., Hori, S., Molfenter, S., Shariff, T., & Steele, C. (2013). Timing differences between cued and noncued swallows in healthy young adults. *Dysphagia, 28*, 428–434.

Nagy, A., Steele, C., & Pelletier, C. (2014). Differences in swallowing between high and low concentration taste stimuli. *BioMed Research International.* https://doi.org/10.1155/2014/813084

Namasivayam-MacDonald, A., Barbon, C., & Steele, C. (2018). A review of swallow timing in the elderly. *Physiology & Behavior, 184*, 12–26.

Nishikubo, K., Mise, K., Ameya, M., Hirose, K., Kobayashi, T., & Hyodo, M. (2015). Quantitative evaluation of age-related alteration of swallowing function: Videofluoroscopic and manometric studies. *Auris Nasus Larynx, 42*, 134–138.

Nishino, T., Yonezawa, T., & Honda, Y. (1985). Effects of swallowing on the pattern of continuous respiration in human adults. *American Review of Respiratory Disease, 132*, 1219–1222.

Omari, T., Jones, C., Hammer, M., Cock, C., Dinning, P., Wiklendt, L., . . . McCulloch, T. (2016). Predicting the activation states of the muscles governing upper esophageal sphincter relaxation and opening. *American Journal of Physiology—Gastrointestinal and Liver Physiology, 310*, G359–G366.

O'Rourke, A., Morgan, L., Coss-Adame, E., Morrison, M., Weinberger, P., & Postma, G. (2014). The effect of voluntary pharyngeal swallowing maneuvers on esophageal swallowing physiology. *Dysphagia, 29*, 262–268.

Ouahchi, Y., Salah, N. B., Mjid, M., Hedhli, A., Abdelhedi, N., Beji, M., . . . Verin, E. (2019). Breathing pattern during sequential swallowing in heathy adult humans. *Journal of Applied Physiology, 126*, 487–493.

Palmer, J. (1998). Bolus aggregation in the oropharynx does not depend on gravity. *Archives of Physical Medicine and Rehabilitation, 79*, 691–696.

Palmer, J., & Hiiemae, K. (2003). Eating and breathing: Interactions between respiration and feeding on solid food. *Dysphagia, 18*, 169–178.

Palmer, P., McCulloch, T., Jaffe, D., & Neel, A. (2005). Effects of a sour bolus on the intramuscular electromyographic (EMG) activity of muscles in the submental region. *Dysphagia, 20*, 210–217.

Palmer, J., Rudin, N., Lara, G., & Crompton, A. (1992). Coordination of mastication and swallowing. *Dysphagia, 7*, 187–200.

Park, T., & Kim, Y. (2016). Effects of tongue pressing effortful swallow in older healthy individuals. *Archives of Gerontology and Geriatrics, 66*, 127–133.

Pearson, W., Langmore, S., & Zumwalt, A. (2011). Evaluating the structural properties of suprahyoid muscles and their potential for moving the hyoid. *Dysphagia, 26*, 345–351.

Pedersen, A., Sørensen, C., Proctor, G., & Carpenter, G. (2018). Salivary functions in mastication, taste, and textual perception, swallowing and initial digestion. *Oral Diseases, 24*, 1399–1416.

Pelletier, C., & Dhanaraj, G. (2006). The effect of taste and palatability on lingual swallowing pressure. *Dysphagia, 21,* 121–128.

Pelletier, C., & Steele, C. (2014). Influence of the perceived taste intensity of chemesthetic stimuli on swallowing parameters given age and genetic taste differences in healthy adult women. *Journal of Speech, Language, and Hearing Research, 57,* 46–56.

Perlman, A., Ettema, S., & Barkmeier, J. (2000). Respiratory and acoustic signals associated with bolus passage during swallowing. *Dysphagia, 15,* 89–94.

Perlman, A., Palmer, P., McCulloch, T., & VanDaele, D. (1999). Electromyographic activity from human laryngeal, pharyngeal, and submental muscles during swallowing. *Journal of Applied Physiology, 86,* 1663–1669.

Perlman, A., Schultz, J., & VanDaele, D. (1993). Effects of age, gender, bolus volume, and bolus viscosity on oropharyngeal pressure during swallowing. *Journal of Applied Physiology, 75,* 33–37.

Perry, J., Bae, Y., & Kuehn, D. (2012). Effect of posture on deglutitive biomechanics in healthy individuals. *Dysphagia, 27,* 70–80.

Peyron, M., Woda, A., Bourdiol, P., & Hennequin, M. (2017). Age-related changes in mastication. *Journal of Oral Rehabilitation, 44,* 299–312.

Preiksaitis, H., Mayrand, S., Robins, K., & Diamant, N. (1992). Coordination of respiration and swallowing: Effect of bolus volume in normal adults. *American Journal of Physiology, 263,* R624–R630.

Preiksaitis, H., & Mills, C. (1996). Coordination of respiration and swallowing: Effects of bolus consistency and presentation in normal adults. *Journal of Applied Physiology, 81,* 1707–1714.

Ramsey, G., Watson, J., Gramiak, R., & Weinberg, S. (1955). Cinefluorographic analysis of the mechanism of swallowing. *Radiology, 64,* 498–518.

Robbins, J., Hamilton, J., Lof, G., & Kempster, G. (1992). Oropharyngeal swallowing in normal adults of different ages. *Gastroenterology, 103,* 823–829.

Rosen, S., Abdelhalim, S., Jones, C., & McCulloch, T. (2018). Effect of body position on pharyngeal swallowing pressures using high-resolution manometry. *Dysphagia. 33,* 389–398.

Rosenbek, J., Robbins, J., Roecker, E., Coyle, J., & Wood, J. (1996) A penetration-aspiration scale. *Dysphagia, 11,* 93–98.

Saitoh, E., Shibata, S., Matsuo, K., Baba, M., Fujii, W., & Palmer, J. (2007). Chewing and food consistency: Effects on bolus transport and swallow initiation. *Dysphagia, 22,* 100–107.

Sears, V., Castell, J., & Castell, D. (1990). Comparison of effects of upright versus supine body position and liquid versus solid bolus on esophageal pressures in normal humans. *Digestive Diseases and Sciences, 35,* 857–864.

Selley, W., Flack, F., Ellis, R., & Brooks, W. (1989). Respiratory patterns associated with swallowing: Part I. The normal adult pattern and changes with age. *Age and Ageing, 18,* 168–172.

Shune, S., Moon, J., & Goodman, S. (2016). The effects of age and preoral sensorimotor cues on anticipatory mouth movement during swallowing. *Journal of Speech, Language, and Hearing Research, 59,* 195–205.

Smith, J., Wolkove, N., Colacone, A., & Kreisman, H. (1989). Coordination of eating, drinking, and breathing in adults. *Chest, 96,* 578–582.

Sonies, B., Parent, L., Morrish, K., & Baum, B. (1988). Durational aspects of the oral-pharyngeal phase of swallow in normal adults. *Dysphagia, 3,* 1–10.

Steele, C., Alsanei, W., Ayanikalath, S., Barbon, C., Chen, J., Cichero, J., . . . Wang, H. (2015). The influence of food texture and liquid consistency modification on swallowing physiology and function: A systematic review. *Dysphagia, 30,* 2–26.

Steele, C., & Cichero, J. (2014). Physiological factors related to aspiration risk: A systematic review. *Dysphagia, 29,* 295–304.

Steele, C., & Huckabee, M. (2007). The influence of orolingual pressure on the timing of pharyngeal pressure events. *Dysphagia, 22,* 30–36.

Steele, C., & van Lieshout, P. (2004). Influence of bolus consistency on lingual behaviors in sequential swallowing. *Dysphagia, 19,* 192–206.

Steele, C., & van Lieshout, P. (2009). Tongue movements during water swallowing in healthy young and older adults. *Journal of Speech, Language, and Hearing Research, 52,* 1255–1267.

Steeve, R., Moore, C., Green, J., Reilly, K., & Ruark McMurtrey, J. (2008). Babbling, chewing, and sucking: Oromandibular coordination at nine months. *Journal of Speech, Language, and Hearing Research, 51,* 1390–1404.

Su, H., Khorsandi, A., Silberzweig, J., Kobren, A., Urken, M., Amin, M., Branski, R., & Lazarus, C. (2015). Temporal and physiologic measurements of deglutition in the upright and supine position with videofluoroscopy (VFS) in healthy subjects. *Dysphagia, 30,* 438–444.

Tasko, S., Kent, R., & Westbury, J. (2002). Variability in tongue movement kinematics during normal liquid swallow. *Dysphagia, 17,* 126–138.

Tracy, J., Logemann, J., Kahrilas, P., Jacob, P., Kobara, M., & Krugler, C. (1989). Preliminary observations on the effects of age on oropharyngeal deglutition. *Dysphagia, 4,* 90–94.

Ulysal, H., Kizilay, F., Ünal, A., Güngor, H., & Ertekin, C. (2013). The interaction between breathing and swallowing in healthy individuals. *Journal of Electromyography and Kinesiology, 23,* 659–663.

VanDaele, D., Perlman, A., & Cassell, M. (1995). Intrinsic fibre architecture attachments of the human epiglottis and their contributions to the mechanism of deglutition. *Journal of Anatomy, 186,* 1–15.

Veiga, H., Fonseca, H., & Bianchini, E. (2014). Sequential swallowing of liquid in elderly adults: Cup or straw? *Dysphagia, 29,* 249–255.

Wang, C.-M., Chen, J.-Y., Chuang, C.-C., Tseng, W.-C., Wong, A., & Pei, Y.-C. (2015). Age-related changes in swallowing, and in the coordination of swallowing and respiration determined by novel non-invasive measurement techniques. *Geriatrics & Gerontology International, 15,* 736–744.

Wheeler-Hegland, K., Huber, J., Pitts, T., & Davenport, P. (2011). Lung volume measured during sequential swallowing in healthy young adults. *Journal of Speech, Language, and Hearing Research, 54,* 777–786.

Wheeler-Hegland, K., Huber, J., Pitts, T., & Sapienza, C. (2009). Lung volume during swallowing: Single bolus swallows in healthy young adults. *Journal of Speech, Language, and Hearing Research, 52,* 178–187.

Wheeler-Hegland, K., Rosenbek, J., & Sapienza, C. (2008). Submental sEMG and hyoid movement during Mendelsohn maneuver, effortful swallow, and expiratory muscle strength training. *Journal of Speech, Language, and Hearing Research, 51,* 1072–1087.

Wilson, S., Thach, B., Brouillette, R., & Abu-Osba, Y. (1981). Coordination of breathing and swallowing in human infants. *Journal of Applied Physiology, 50,* 851–858.

Witcombe, B., & Meyer, D. (2006). Sword swallowing and its side effects. *British Medical Journal, 333,* 1285–1287.

Yamada, T., Matsuo, K., Izawa, M., Yamada, S., Masuda, Y., & Ogasawara, T. (2017). Effects of age and viscosity on food transport and breathing-swallowing coordination during eating of two-phase food in nursing home residents. *Geriatrics & Gerontology International, 17,* 2171–2177.

Yeates, E., Steele, C., & Pelletier, C. (2010). Tongue pressure and submental surface electromyography measures during non-effortful and effortful saliva swallows in healthy women. *American Journal of Speech-Language Pathology, 19,* 274–281.

Youmans, S., Youmans, G., & Stierwalt, J. (2009). Differences in tongue strength across age and gender: Is there a diminished strength reserve? *Dysphagia, 24,* 57–65.

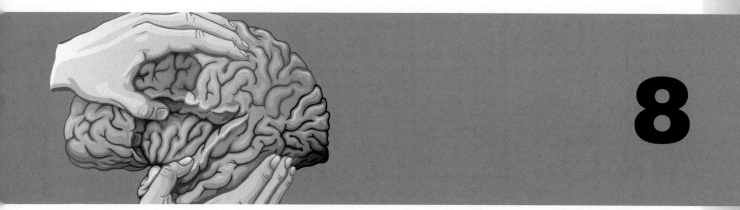

Brain Structures and Mechanisms for Speech/Language, Hearing, and Swallowing

INTRODUCTION

This chapter describes the role of the central and peripheral nervous systems in speech, language, and hearing. Although this text does not treat language function (e.g., word retrieval, sentence structure) directly, the role of the nervous system in language is central to understanding brain function for communication. Some material concerning the expressive and receptive language function of the brain is therefore included in this presentation.

The chapter begins with an overview of major concepts. Next, gross neuroanatomy is presented for the cerebral hemispheres and cerebral white matter, subcortical nuclei (e.g., basal ganglia and thalamus), cerebellum, brainstem and cranial nerves, cortical innervation patterns, and the spinal cord and its peripheral nerves. Cells within the nervous system are then discussed along with selected aspects of their function followed by description of the meninges, ventricles, and blood supply to the brain. The chapter ends with some clinical notes about Parkinson's disease. Aspects of neurophysiology are interwoven throughout the several sections of the chapter, along with selected clinical implications for the speech-language pathologist and audiologist.

THE NERVOUS SYSTEM: AN OVERVIEW AND CONCEPTS

This chapter covers both *nervous system structures* (anatomy) and *nervous system mechanisms* (physiology). Description of nervous system structures is focused primarily on gross anatomy: structures easily observable when handling and dissecting a whole brain or when viewed using modern imaging techniques. More limited information is provided on cellular and molecular anatomical levels, to provide a foundation for understanding how neurological diseases affect these fine-structure components of the nervous system and, specifically, speech, language, and hearing functions.

The term *nervous system mechanisms* refers to its physiology at the molecular, cellular, neurochemical, and system levels. *System* levels of nervous system function are the ones associated with observable *behaviors*, such as moving the articulators for speech sound production, uttering a sentence, or providing behavioral evidence for understanding spoken language (as in following an instruction).

Selected concepts are described in this section. These concepts offer a framework and set of reference terms that can be consulted throughout a reading of the chapter. They include central versus peripheral nervous system, anatomical planes and directions, white versus gray matter, tracts versus nuclei, nerves versus ganglia, efferent and afferent, and lateralization and specialization of function. Some of this information has been presented in Chapter 1 but is repeated here in the specific context of the nervous system.

Central Versus Peripheral Nervous System

The distinction between the *central nervous system* (CNS) and *peripheral nervous system* (PNS) is familiar to most readers of this textbook. The distinction is straightforward: The CNS includes the cerebral hemispheres and its contents, the brainstem, and the spinal cord; the PNS includes the nerves issued from the brainstem and spinal cord, plus clusters of sensory nerve cells, called ganglia, located in close proximity to, but outside, the brainstem and spinal cord. In Figure 8–1, the major components of the CNS are labeled, and nerves of the PNS are shown extending from the brainstem and spinal cord.

The structure of nerve cells is presented later in this chapter. For the current discussion, nerve cells (neurons) in both the CNS and PNS consist of a cell body and an axon. The axon conducts electrical impulses away from the cell body to the terminus (end) of the neuron, where the electrical energy is converted into chemical energy. Bundles of axons are abundant in both the CNS and PNS. A bundle of axons in the CNS is called a *tract*; a bundle of axons in the PNS is called a *nerve*.

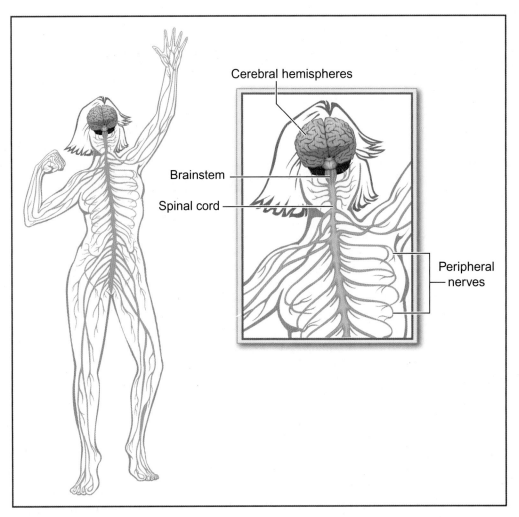

FIGURE 8–1. Major components of the nervous system, including three subdivisions of the CNS (cerebral hemispheres, brainstem, spinal cord) and the components of the PNS (peripheral nerves).

Anatomical Planes and Directions

Anatomical planes and directions have been introduced in Chapter 1. This chapter makes extensive use of the terminology of anatomical planes and directions, so the terms are reviewed and specific examples relevant to the CNS are provided.

The terminology for planes and directions differs depending on the part of the CNS under discussion. The left part of Figure 8–2 shows an artist's rendition of three anatomical planes as they are applied to the cerebral hemispheres. The *coronal plane* (also called *frontal*) cuts the cerebral hemispheres into front and back sections, the *sagittal plane* into left and right sections, and the *horizontal plane* (also called *axial* or *transverse*) into upper and lower sections. Any of the three planes can be moved along an axis perpendicular to the plane to "cut" the cerebral hemispheres at different locations. For example, the horizontal plane can be moved up and down to obtain higher or lower horizontal cuts. Similarly, the sagittal plane can be moved left or right from the midline (a midline cut is called the *midsagittal* plane) to divide the brain into left and right parts. Sagittal cuts away from the midline are referred to as *parasagittal* planes.

Several structures within the cerebral hemispheres have complex, curved shapes. Some structures are buried within the cerebral hemispheres and are difficult to visualize without multiplane views. Views of the brain in all three of the standard planes—coronal, sagittal, horizontal—are necessary to appreciate the form of these structures. A good example of the varying appearance of a single structure is the corpus callosum, shown on the right side of Figure 8–2 as magnetic

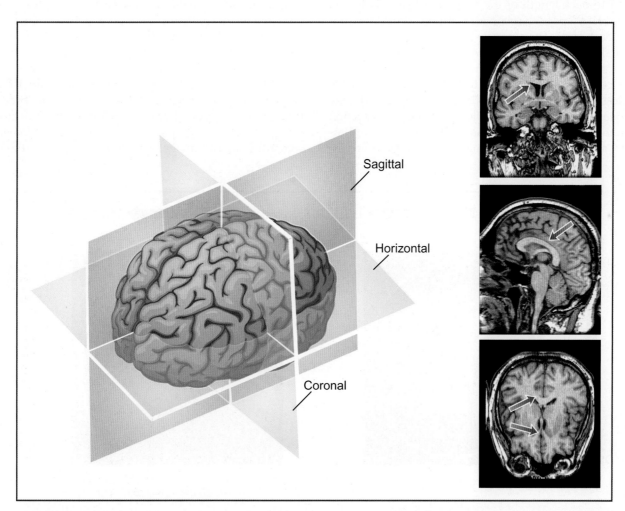

FIGURE 8–2. *Left*, major anatomical planes as seen in an anatomical drawing of the cerebral hemispheres, viewed from slightly above the hemispheres and in the sagittal plane; *right*, three MR images shown in the coronal (*top*), sagittal (*middle*), and horizontal (*bottom*) planes. In each of the MR images, the red arrows point to the corpus callosum.

resonance (MR) images. The corpus callosum is a massive bundle of fibers (a tract) linking structures in the left and right cerebral hemispheres. The top MR image is a coronal slice, roughly at the midway point between the front and back of the brain. The red arrow points to a gently concave, white band of tissue located above two black "horns." This coronal plane image intersects the corpus callosum at a single location, where the structure extends laterally from the midline into the two hemispheres. (The arrow is just off the midline, in the right hemisphere, which appears on the left from the reader's view.) The appearance of the corpus callosum in the coronal plane varies depending on where the coronal slice is located along the front-to-back extent of the brain. This is better appreciated by examining the midsagittal plane MR image (Figure 8–2, middle). The white band of callosal tissue (*callosal*, meaning *of the corpus callosum*) extends along the front-to-back length of the brain and has a flattened, arch-like shape with relatively complex form at its front and back ends. The coronal slice shown above the sagittal slice (Figure 8–2, top MR image) was taken just in front of the red arrow shown on the sagittal slice; this coronal slice intercepts the corpus callosum more or less in the middle of the flattened arch. Clearly, the appearance of the corpus callosum in a coronal section depends on where the slice is taken along the front-to-back axis of the cerebral hemispheres. The bottom MR image in Figure 8–2 shows a horizontal slice in which the white bands of corpus callosum tissue connecting the two hemispheres are indicated by two red arrows, one toward the front of the brain (lower arrow) and one toward the back (upper arrow). Between these two areas of corpus callosum tissue, other callosal fibers are not apparent. This is because the horizontal slice is placed below the highest point of the arch seen in the midsagittal slice, which means it does not intersect this part of the corpus callosum tissue.

Figure 8–3 shows a horizontal MR image on the left and a sagittal image on the right. Toward the top of the horizontal image—the front of the cerebral hemispheres—is the anterior direction, toward the bottom the posterior direction. The anterior-posterior dimension is also shown in the sagittal image on the right of Figure 8–3; here the directions are obvious because of the clarity of the facial features. This sagittal image introduces an interesting complication in the use of direction terms. Note the distinction between the dorsal-ventral and anterior-posterior dimensions: Dorsal means toward the top of the cerebral hemispheres, posterior toward the back of the cerebral hemispheres (Figure 8–3, labels to the right of the sagittal image). For neuroanatomical structures *below* the top of the brainstem, however, dorsal and posterior mean the same thing, as do ventral and anterior (Figure 8–3, labels below the sagittal image). The top of the brainstem is

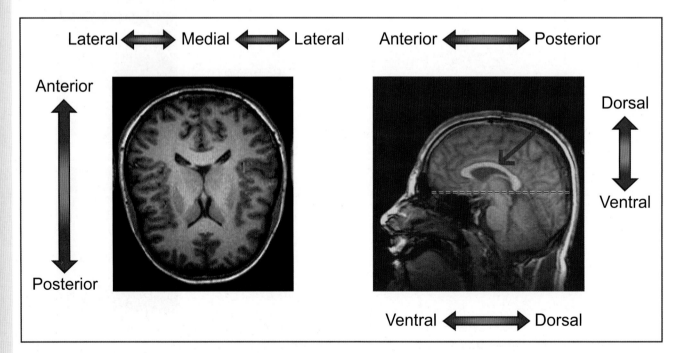

FIGURE 8–3. MR images in the horizontal (*left*) and sagittal (*right*) planes. In the right image, the dashed, red line shows approximate location for the top of the brainstem and the red arrow points to the corpus callosum. See text for discussion of direction terminology above and below the brainstem.

indicated on the sagittal image by a horizontal dashed line. The identity between the terms *dorsal/posterior* and *ventral/anterior* applies to spinal cord structures as well. (See sidetrack called Which Way Is Up? in Chapter 1 for the explanation for this apparent inconsistency.)

The terms *deep* and *superficial* are used to locate one structure relative to another. These terms are typically used to designate the relative locations of structures as a path is followed from "outside to inside" (or the reverse). The question, "What is beneath this surface?" is equivalent to asking, "What is deep to this surface?" For example, the white matter of the cerebral hemispheres is deep to the cortex (or the cortex is superficial to the white matter).

White Versus Gray Matter, Tracts Versus Nuclei, Nerves Versus Ganglia

When a brain is removed from the skull with the intention of preserving it for later study, it is "fixed" in a solution of formalin, a fluid that partially hardens biological tissue. A formalin-preserved brain shows certain regions having a grayish-brown appearance and other regions with a pale, near-white appearance. Similarly, in conventional MR images of the brain, there are regions that appear more grayish and regions that appear more whitish. Coronal and horizontal plane MR images (see Figures 8–2 and 8–3) show both *gray* and *white matter*. Gray matter consists of clusters of neuron cell bodies (*somata*, the plural of *soma*, which means cell body); white matter is formed from myelinated axons (see below) issued by those cell bodies.

Gray Matter and Nuclei

The cortex, the outermost thick covering of the cerebral hemispheres, consists of densely packed cell bodies; the cortex is a major part of the gray matter in the cerebral hemispheres. Figure 8–3 (left MR image) shows the cortical "rind" of gray matter enclosing extensive white matter. Within this white matter, near the center, are several regions of additional gray matter. A specific cluster of cell bodies inside the cerebral hemispheres, or within the brainstem or spinal cord, is referred to in the singular as a *nucleus* (as in *caudate nucleus*) or in some cases as a group of nuclei (as in *cranial nerve nuclei*, clusters of cell bodies within the brainstem). The clusters of cell bodies deep to the cortex but within the cerebral hemispheres, such as the caudate, putamen, and thalamus, are referred to as *subcortical nuclei* (described below). Some subcortical nuclei are collections of many smaller nuclei but are referred to jointly as part of a single structure (such as the *thalamus*). The term *subcortical nuclei* is reserved for clusters of cell bodies within the cerebral hemispheres and above the brainstem and does not include nuclei within the brainstem and spinal cord. Nuclei are also found in the cerebellum; these are referred to as cerebellar nuclei.[1]

Whether in the cortex, subcortical region, brainstem, cerebellum, or spinal cord, neuronal cell bodies most often cluster together for a common purpose. In a given region of cortex, for example, cell bodies related to eye movements, auditory perception, or motor control are likely to have unique areas in which they cluster together. Within a particular region of cortex, or within a subcortical or brainstem nucleus in which the cells have a common function, there is likely to be an even more fine-grained, systematic aggregation. For example, the most posterior gyrus (*gyrus* means a hill of tissue on the cortical surface, separated from other gyri by deep *fissures* or *sulci*) of the frontal lobe is the primary motor cortex, containing cells that have more or less direct control over the timing, force, and duration of muscle contractions. Within this primary motor cortex, cells associated with particular parts of the body aggregate together. Hand and finger cells, for example, are found in close proximity in the primary motor cortex. The cellular representation of the body within a specific cortical area (such as primary motor cortex) is a map-like reflection of the body plan and is called *somatotopic organization* (this is illustrated in Figure 8–5, later in the chapter, for both the motor and sensory cortices).

The concept of somatotopic representation of cells within the brain is important not only for understanding brain anatomy but also for gaining clinical perspectives on the effects of lesion location on function. For example, somatotopic organization explains (in part) how a stroke can affect the ability to walk but leave speech and language unaffected, or how a stroke can affect speech and language in the absence of other obvious problems.

White Matter and Fiber Tracts

Neurons have a cell body, an axon, and a terminal (end) structure. The primary function of a neuron is to conduct electrical impulses from the cell body along the

---

[1]The terms *nucleus* and *nuclei* are not used when referring to clusters of cell bodies in the cortex; these organizations of cell bodies are referred to as cortex, cortical region, cortical tissue, and so forth. Similarly, the term nucleus is used only sparingly when referring to gray matter in the spinal cord.

Somatotopic Representation Is Not Always "Clean"

Many studies have demonstrated somatotopic representation in primary motor and sensory cortices. These studies include correlations between highly localized lesions (damage to brain tissue) and affected body parts, electrical stimulation of discrete locations along the cortex and observation of the resulting movements or reported sensations, and functional magnetic resonance imaging (fMRI) studies in which local movements, as in raising a single finger, result in the "lighting up" of a small region of the primary motor cortex. Somatotopy, however, is not always neat and clean. For example, fMRI studies of representation of speech structures in the primary motor cortex have revealed that cells for muscles of the pharynx, tongue, and lips "share" space close to the bottom of the central fissure, where the primary motor cortex meets the Sylvian fissure (Takai, Brown, & Liotti, 2010). Takai and colleagues call the mixing of cells for these speech structures "somatotopy with overlap." Perhaps such overlap makes functional sense for the control of complex coordinated behaviors such as swallowing and speaking.

axon to the terminal structure, also called a terminal segment. As discussed in more detail below, the majority of axons in the brain are wrapped in a fatty substance called *myelin*. Myelin gives axons the whitish appearance in fixed brains and brain images. The horizontal section in Figure 8–3 shows a good deal of white matter and therefore many, many myelinated axons.

Axons connect different areas of gray matter. These connections are referred to as pathways, fiber tracts, fiber bundles, fasciculi (plural of fasciculus), and lemnisci (plural of lemniscus). Bundles of axons connect different cortical regions to one another, including cortical cells to subcortical and brainstem nuclei, spinal nuclei to brainstem and subcortical nuclei, and cerebellar nuclei to many different nuclei in the brain.

Ganglia

The term *ganglia* (plural of ganglion) is typically reserved for clusters of nerve cell bodies located *outside* the CNS, in the PNS. They receive sensory fibers coming from receptors in the limbs and trunk (such as tactile receptors) or from the cochlea or retina where a first synapse (connection with another neuron) is made prior to entry of the information into the CNS. For example, a tactile receptor in the hand is a special end organ of the PNS, embedded in skin or muscle and connected by a sensory fiber (axon) to the CNS. When the end organ is stimulated (e.g., by the compression of touch), it "fires," sending an electrical impulse to the CNS via the sensory fiber. This fiber makes a first synapse with a cell in a ganglion immediately outside the spinal cord. The ganglion cell receiving this information delivers it, via its own axon, to sensory cells in the spinal cord. Similar receptors are found in muscles of the speech mechanism, including muscles of the respiratory system, larynx, and upper airway (vocal tract).

The spinal cord is associated with a series of *dorsal root ganglia*, arranged from the top to bottom along the cord, that serve as the first synapses (connections) for much of the sensory information delivered from the limbs and trunk to the CNS. There are also ganglia immediately outside the brainstem that serve as the first synapses for sensory information from head and neck structures. For example, the hair cells of the cochlea are the specialized sensory endings for hearing, and when they are deformed by motion of the basilar membrane, they fire, sending impulses to a cluster of nerve cells outside the brainstem called the spiral ganglion, where the first synapses for hearing take place. Cell bodies in the spiral ganglion send axons into the brainstem to make synapses within the first set of nuclei along the auditory pathways (see Chapter 6). Another example is the sensory processing of touch on the face. When stimulated, tactile receptors embedded in the skin of the face send sensory fibers to a ganglion located just outside of the brainstem. The fibers make their first synapse in this ganglion, which then sends fibers into the brainstem for synapses in the CNS.

Efferent and Afferent

The terms *efferent* and *afferent* are used in two different ways to describe information flow in the nervous system. The first use of these terms concerns overall information flow for the production of muscular effort (efferent) in contrast to the information flow for the sensation of an environmental event (afferent). When motor commands are issued from cortical tissue and travel along descending pathways through one or more motor nuclei before eventually being directed by peripheral nerves to muscles, the pathways are referred to as efferent. Sometimes the term *efference* is equated with the basic components—brain-directed muscle contractions and their patterns in space and time—of motor (movement) control. In contrast, when a sensory receptor (such as a tactile receptor in a finger, or a hair cell in the cochlea) is stimulated and the resulting signal travels via peripheral nerves to the spinal cord or brainstem and through ascending pathways to a final destination in the cortex, the pathways are said to be afferent. *Afference* is often taken to mean *sensory*.

A second use of the terms *efferent* and *afferent* indicates the inputs and outputs of nuclei *within* the CNS. When a nucleus sends a fiber tract to another nucleus, the tract is said to be the output or the efferent information emerging from that nucleus. When that same nucleus receives a fiber tract from a different nucleus, the incoming information is referred to as the afferent input to the nucleus. Note that a single nucleus has both efferent projections (tracts sent to other nuclei) and afferent inputs (tracts received from other nuclei). Most nuclei, and cortical cells as well, receive and send information to multiple locations within the brain. Each cortical region or nucleus is therefore likely to have multiple efferent and afferent projections.

Lateralization and Specialization of Function

Lateralization and *specialization* may sometimes be used interchangeably, but the terms have different technical meanings. When a function is said to be *lateralized* in the brain, the technical meaning is that the function is primarily controlled by one hemisphere relative to the other. Good examples of lateralized functions include speech and language (thought to be controlled primarily by left hemisphere structures in about 95% of the right-handed population and about 85% of the left-handed population: see Papanicolaou, Rezaie, & Simos, 2019; Rasmussen & Milner, 1977; Swanson, Sabsevitz, Hammeke, & Binder, 2007), handedness (also controlled by the left hemisphere in about 95% of the population), and emotions (thought to be controlled primarily by right hemisphere structures).

How is *specialization* different from *lateralization*? Although it may seem reasonable to say that the left hemisphere is specialized for speech and language (in the same way it is lateralized for speech and language), the term *specialization* is used in a more specific sense. Specialization means that certain brain regions have evolved to serve distinct functions, whether lateralized or not. For example, specialization can be found in regions of the brain thought to be critical for the representation and programming of articulatory gestures for speech. Some scientists place these two processes in a very small portion of the posterior, ventral edge of the left frontal lobe. The actual neural tissue for the *execution* of speech sounds—where execution means transforming the represented and programmed sounds into movements—is thought to be located slightly posterior to this programming tissue but still in the frontal lobe. This is an example of specialization within lateralization: Speech is left-lateralized, and within this lateralized function, there are finer degrees of specialization for the specific functions of producing speech and language.

fMRI

Magnetic resonance images (MRI) are obtained by placing a body structure within a strong magnetic field and then, by application and withdrawal of a second magnetic field, causing cell nuclei to generate magnetic properties that are sensed by a coil. The coil detects different amounts of energy generated by the cells, depending on cell properties, cell locations, and other factors. Software processes the signals generated by all these cells and assembles them into an image of the target structure, such as those shown in Figures 8–2 (right side) and 8–3. Functional magnetic resonance imaging, or fMRI, uses the same general principles, but with a twist (a pun for those of you familiar with the magnetized behavior of brain cell nuclei). When neurons are firing, the active region attracts blood flow from arteries. This arterial blood flow is oxygen rich, and oxygen-rich blood has different magnetic properties than run-of-the-mill blood. When an area of the brain is active for a specific task, such as speaking, that area generates a different signal than an area not being used for that task. The imaging software is designed to make that active area "light up" because of increased blood flow. So, now you know that you can actually light up a room when you speak words of cheer!

CEREBRAL HEMISPHERES

The cerebral hemispheres are part of the CNS (see Figure 8–1). Each hemisphere is divided into lobes and contains gray and white matter.

Cerebral Hemispheres

Figure 8–4 shows the cerebral hemispheres in four views (the image should be viewed with the caption as the bottom of the page). The top left view is from above the brain, looking down to the dorsal surfaces of the two hemispheres. The front of the brain is toward the top of the image. This view shows the left and right cerebral hemispheres, separated by a long, front-to-back fissure called the *longitudinal fissure* (also called the *interhemispheric* or *sagittal fissure*). The visible surface tissue is *cortex*, the most complex and sophisticated part of the brain. Note the ridges or "hills" of the cortex and the "dips" between them. The ridges are called *gyri* (singular = *gyrus*) and the dips *sulci* (singular = *sulcus*) or *fissures* (the term *fissure* is typically used to mean a particularly deep sulcus, such as the longitudinal fissure). One notable difference between the human brain and the brain of animals, such as sheep, cats, and dogs, is that humans have relatively deep and numerous sulci defining the cortical surface. These deep sulci are infoldings of cortical surface, forming hidden walls of tissue that contribute to a greater volume of cortical cells in the human brain relative to other animals. This hidden cortical surface area and its corresponding thickness add to human cognitive and performance power. With the gentle separation of any sulcus on the surface of a prepared (formalin-hardened) brain, these walls of hidden cortical tissue can be revealed. Some authors have estimated that close to two-thirds of the human cortex is hidden inside sulcal walls (Zilles, Armstrong, Schleicher, & Kretschmann, 1988). This unique feature of the human brain appears to be an evolutionary solution to packing lots of cortical tissue into a container—the skull—of limited volume.

A dramatic view of "hidden" cortical tissue can be gained by putting your thumbs inside the longitudinal fissure of a prepared brain, your two hands resting on the two hemispheres, and gently separating the hemispheres without tearing the tissue. This exposes the deep inside (medial) walls of the two hemispheres. A view of the medial wall of the right cerebral hemisphere is shown in the top right view of Figure 8–4. A prominent feature of this midsagittal view of the cerebral hemispheres is the *corpus callosum*, the massive bundle of tissue that connects structures across the two hemispheres.

Figure 8–4, bottom right, shows a side view of the brain's left hemisphere. The front of the brain is toward the left of the image. This view shows the four lobes of the brain, their boundary landmarks, plus additional regions important to the discussion of the brain in speech, language, and hearing. In this figure, the four lobes are the frontal (dark and light green), parietal (orange and yellowish-brown), temporal (dark and light blue), and occipital (purple) lobes. The darker and lighter values of the color code in three of the lobes designate particularly important cortical regions for speech, language, and hearing. What follows is a more detailed consideration of each of these lobes, plus two additional cerebral regions (the insula and limbic system). The functions of these regions are discussed in broad terms, and when relevant, their assumed role in speech, language, hearing, and swallowing is noted.

Frontal Lobe

The frontal lobe (green in Figure 8–4) is bounded at the back by the *central fissure* (also called the *fissure of Rolando*) and below by the front part of the *sylvian fissure* (also called the *lateral sulcus*). The gyrus immediately in front of the central sulcus, and therefore within the frontal lobe, is the *primary motor cortex* (also called the *precentral gyrus*), shown as a lighter shade of green in Figure 8–4. The primary motor cortex contains cells, called motor neurons, that send signals to other motor neurons in the brainstem and spinal cord, which, in turn, send axons to muscles to control their contraction patterns. The pathway—primary motor cortex neurons → brainstem/spinal cord motor neurons → muscles—can be thought of as the direct route of nervous system control of the timing, strength, and speed of muscle contractions for head, neck, limb, and torso structures. As discussed later in this chapter, this direct route to muscle control is modulated and fine-tuned by activity in several different parts of the CNS, including other cortical regions (such as the supplementary motor area, primary somatosensory cortex, and Broca's area, shown in Figure 8–4, top and bottom right), the basal ganglia, and the cerebellum, to produce everyday movement and highly skilled, specialized movement.

Primary Motor Cortex

The cells (motor neurons) of the primary motor cortex are arranged along the precentral gyrus (primary motor cortex) in a *somatotopic* fashion. Imagine drawing a map of the body parts, starting at the top of the

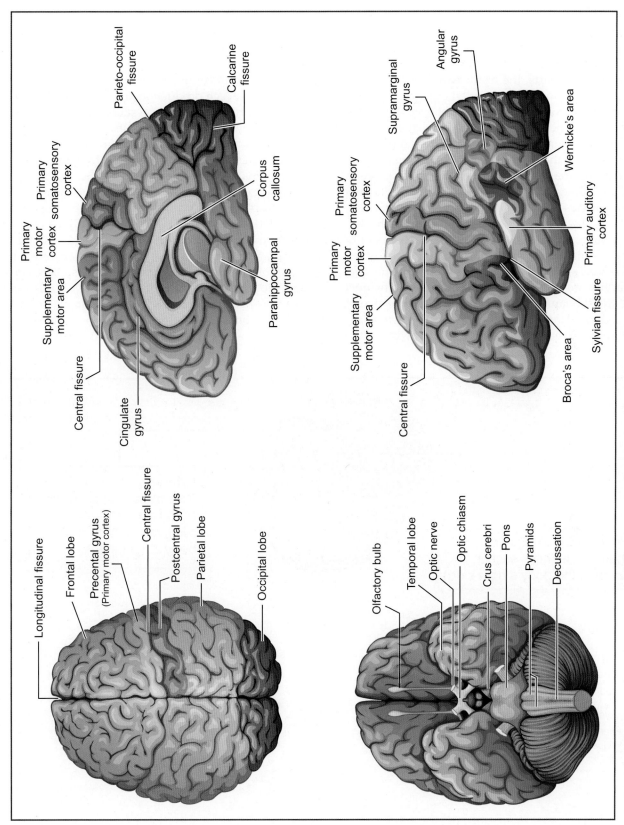

FIGURE 8–4. Four views of the cerebral hemispheres. *Top left,* dorsal surface of hemispheres; *bottom left,* ventral surface of hemispheres; *top right,* medial surface of right hemisphere, seen in midsagittal view; *bottom right,* view of lateral surface of left hemisphere.

brain (at the longitudinal fissure) and working your way down the lateral surface of the precentral gyrus of either hemisphere to the sylvian fissure. If the map reflected which body parts are represented in a specific region and the amount of cortex devoted to the control of those parts, the result would be similar to the image shown on the bottom left of Figure 8–5. The primary motor cortex (shown in light green) is a slab of tissue that, when mapped for body part representation, shows the somatotopic plan of cortical motor cells and the muscles they control. The most obvious characteristic of this map is the upside-down representation of the body along the primary motor cortex. Cells that control muscles of the lower part of the body (such as muscles of the hip and knee) are at the top of the primary motor cortex (or even along the medial wall of the cortex—note the location of cells for muscles of the toes), whereas control of muscles of the face, tongue, and larynx are toward the bottom of the gyrus, just above the sylvian fissure. In the drawing, the size of each body part represents the amount of cortical tissue devoted to that part; the larger the drawing of the

body part, the greater the number of cells devoted to its control. Note the exceptionally large size of the face and its associated structures (the tongue, lips, larynx), compared to the size of the feet or the trunk. A disproportionate number of cells in the primary motor cortex are devoted to control of the structures that play a major role in speech production and swallowing.

The disproportionate representation of cells that control movements of orofacial structures (e.g., jaw, tongue, lips) and laryngeal structures suggests the great relevance of these structures to human life. No great imagination is required to make the case for the centrality of eating and the need for sophisticated muscular control to support this behavior. The same case can be made, of course, for any mammal. But the disproportionate representation of these structures within the primary motor cortex of humans is very much a function of our unique ability to generate spoken language. Notice the phrase "spoken *language*"; it is not just the production of sounds—many animals do this for simple communicative purposes—but the extensive use of a signal system (the acoustic signal emerg-

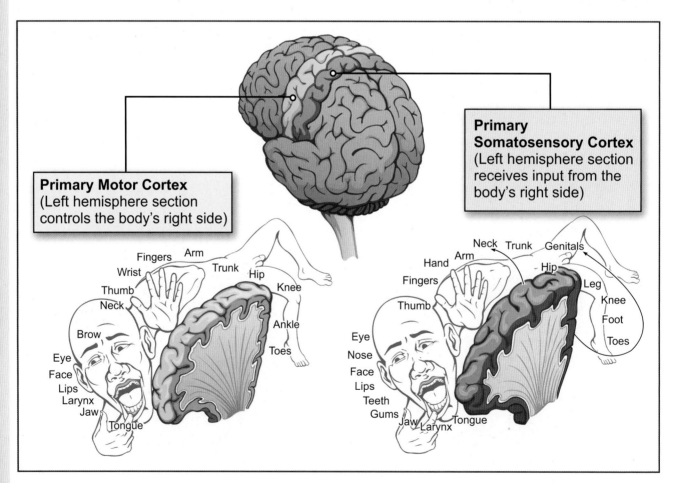

FIGURE 8–5. Somatotopic representations along the primary motor (*green*) and sensory (*orange*) cortices.

ing from the vocal tract) to give meaning to abstract, complex ideas, to convey the same idea in many different ways, and even to *create* ideas (Deacon, 1997).

Broca's Area

The inferior frontal gyrus, on the lateral surface of the left frontal lobe and immediately above the front end of the sylvian fissure, is called *Broca's area*. Broca's area is shown in Figure 8–4 (bottom right, colored dark green). Broca's area is often said to have a central role in the planning and organization of motor behavior required for speech production. In the classical (historical) understanding of brain regions and their role in speech and language performance, Broca's area was considered the site where speech expression is controlled. This conclusion was formulated by Paul Broca (1824–1880), the famous French physician who between 1861 and 1865 reported on a few patients with primarily expressive speech-language disorders resulting from neurological disease. On autopsy of the patients' whole brains (that is, brains not subjected to dissection), Broca noted lesions in and around the third frontal gyrus of the left hemisphere. If this gyrus was damaged in patients who exhibited speech-language disorders largely of an expressive nature, with minimal problems in language comprehension, the function of the gyrus in healthy individuals as the center of speech expression seemed to be a logical conclusion. The conclusion was reinforced by observations that lesions in the inferior gyrus of the right frontal lobe did not produce speech or language disorders. The emerging picture was of lateralization and specialization for expressive control of speech and language in the left hemisphere in the region of the frontal lobe where Broca had identified lesions in the brains of his patients. This view is recognized today as overly simplistic, but the general idea of speech production mechanisms having significant representation in the left frontal lobe is accepted by most scientists and clinicians.

Premotor and Supplementary Motor Area

The gyrus just forward of, and more or less parallel to, the primary motor cortex is called *premotor cortex* (often called PMA, for premotor area, not labeled in Figure 8–4; see the darker green gyrus immediately anterior to the lighter green gyrus in Figure 8–4, bottom right). Broca's area, colored dark green, is part of the premotor cortex. On the medial wall of the cortex, the tissue in front of the primary motor cortex is labeled *supplementary motor cortex* (SMA) (see Figure 8–4, top and bottom right); the SMA is also part of the PMA. There is a distinction between the presumed functions of the PMA/SMA versus the primary motor cortex: PMA/SMA *plans* movement, whereas primary motor cortex issues commands to *perform* movement. This distinction is important to speech-language pathologists, who are often asked to make a diagnostic judgment of whether a speech motor control disorder is one of execution or planning (or both). Execution disorders of speech motor control are called *dysarthrias*; planning disorders are called *apraxias*.

Prefrontal Cortex

The large mass of frontal lobe tissue anterior to the primary motor cortex and PMA/SMA is called *prefrontal cortex*. Many scientists (see, for example, Ridderinkhof, Ullsperger, Crone, & Nieuwenhuis, 2004) believe that this part of the frontal lobe performs *executive function* in the brain. Because executive function is thought to be associated with the oversight and coordination of brain functions, it is easy to understand why scientists have connected prefrontal cortex with aspects of personality. This may have direct relevance to speech-language pathologists who work with brain-injured patients exhibiting personality changes as a consequence of injury to the frontal lobes, as well as patients with dementia due (in part) to deterioration of frontal lobe tissue.

Parietal Lobe

The parietal lobe (shown in light brown in Figure 8–4, except for its most anterior gyrus, which is colored orange) is bounded at the front by the *central fissure* (or *sulcus*; also called the *fissure of Rolando*), below by the back part of the *sylvian fissure* (or *lateral sulcus*), and toward the back of the brain by the *parieto-occipital fissure*. The parieto-occipital fissure, which is the boundary between the parietal and occipital lobes, is easy to see on the medial wall of the cerebral hemisphere (see Figure 8–4, top right) but is only partially visible when viewing the external surface of the hemisphere. The boundary shown between the parietal and occipital lobes in the bottom right view of Figure 8–4 is therefore approximate. Similarly, the boundary between the lower part of the parietal lobe and the back of the temporal lobe is approximate in the bottom right view of Figure 8–4.

The gyrus immediately in back of the central (Rolandic) fissure—the most forward gyrus of the parietal lobe—is the *primary somatosensory cortex* (also called the *postcentral gyrus*, as labeled in the top left image of Figure 8–4). The primary somatosensory cortex, colored orange in Figure 8–4, runs more or less parallel to the primary motor cortex. Like the primary motor cortex, the primary somatosensory cortex is organized somatotopically, although not in precisely the same way as the motor cortex (see Figure 8–5).

Cells in the primary somatosensory cortex respond to touch and pain stimuli from all body locations. The primary somatosensory cortex is, in fact, a good deal more complicated than this broad view. There are extensive interconnections among different cell types within the somatosensory cortex. Some cortical cells receive basic touch information from lower parts of the brain (that is, subcortical and brainstem nuclei), some use this basic information to encode information on the texture or shape of touched objects, and some may respond to the magnitude and direction of a tactile stimulus (Bear, Connors, & Paradiso, 2016). Some of the cells in primary somatosensory cortex are even interconnected with cells in primary motor cortex.

The parietal cortex posterior to the primary somatosensory cortex and anterior to the occipital lobe, as well as the portion sharing a boundary with the temporal lobe, is called the *posterior parietal cortex* (PPC). The PPC contains cell groups that integrate and process different sensory stimuli to create complex sensory experiences; these cells are also involved in the planning of complex motor acts such as reaching, grasping, and tool use (Culham & Valyear, 2006). Primary analysis in auditory cortex and visual cortex is also sent to the PPC, where it is analyzed and integrated into increasingly more complex perceptions and actions. In this sense, the PPC functions as *association cortex*, literally associating different types of sensory stimuli and directing action plans on the basis of this integration.

An example of the integrative function of PPC is instructive. Object recognition by the hand requires the ability to identify size, shape, texture, hardness/softness, and other object characteristics. Activity in primary somatosensory cortex related to these simple characteristics is sent to PPC for association and integration, and ultimately recognition of the object. Recognition of an object requires an attachment of meaning to the object's properties. Individuals with damage to PPC may experience *agnosia*, which is the inability to recognize objects even though basic sensory skills (e.g., as revealed by a simple test of touch sensitivity) appear to be normal. Agnosias may also occur in the visual and auditory modalities. Although basic tests of visual and auditory sensitivity reveal apparently normal abilities, the person with damage to PPC may not be able to connect meaning to visual or auditory input.

Two other landmarks on the parietal lobe are shown in Figure 8–4. These are specific regions of parietal association cortex important to high-level language function. The *angular gyrus* is shown as the dark turquoise region immediately behind and slightly above the back end of the sylvian fissure (Figure 8–4, lower right). Note the location of the angular gyrus at the boundaries of the parietal, occipital, and temporal lobes. Clinically, lesions of the angular gyrus result in higher-order language deficits (such as difficulty understanding a metaphor) and difficulty with mathematical concepts and performance. Immediately above and slightly in front of the angular gyrus is the *supramarginal gyrus*, shown in Figure 8–4 (lower right) as a yellow region of PPC. The supramarginal gyrus is thought to be involved in word meaning, the relation of individual speech sounds to the formation of words, and the ability to connect word meanings with action patterns (i.e., to perform an action on command such as, "Show me how you whistle").

Temporal Lobe

The temporal lobe, shown in blue in Figure 8–4, is located on the lower side of each cerebral hemisphere. The sylvian fissure is the boundary between the temporal lobe and the frontal lobe above and toward the front; toward the back, the same fissure separates the temporal lobe from the parietal lobe. The upper part of the temporal lobe has a back boundary with the lower parietal lobe, and the lower parts of the temporal lobe have a boundary with the occipital lobe. These back boundaries are not always clearly defined by prominent fissures on the lateral surface of the hemispheres; thus, the color scheme for the different lobes in Figure 8–4 shows approximate temporal-parietal and temporal-occipital boundaries.

The surface of the temporal lobe when viewed from the side has three major gyri: superior, medial, and inferior. Immediately below the sylvian fissure is the prominent superior temporal gyrus. Shown in the light blue area of Figure 8–4 (lower right), the upper "lip" and some surrounding tissue of the superior temporal gyrus is called *primary auditory cortex* or *Heschl's gyrus*. This upper lip extends medially, creating a shelf of temporal lobe tissue that cannot be seen in a lateral view of either hemisphere (see below, discussion of Figure 8–6). The primary auditory cortex is the first cortical location for processing of auditory signals; more complex processing follows when this initial analysis is forwarded to other locations within the temporal lobe.

The anatomy of primary auditory cortex—Heschl's gyrus—requires additional description with the assistance of a different view of the brain. Imagine drawing an oblique line parallel to and slightly above the sylvian fissure, as shown by the "cut line" in the upper image of Figure 8–6. Think of this line as one edge of a plane cutting through the cerebral hemispheres, dividing them into upper and lower halves.

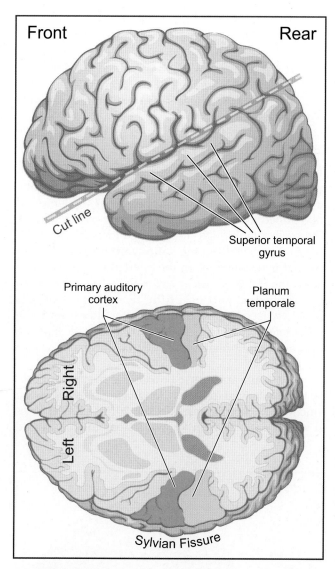

FIGURE 8–6. *Top,* lateral surface of left hemisphere, showing an oblique plane whose edge follows the upward tilt of the sylvian fissure; *bottom,* a view of the dorsal surface of the brain cut into upper and lower parts along this oblique plane. This section shows the "shelf" of auditory cortex inside the sylvian fissure, including the more anterior, primary auditory cortex (*salmon*), and the more posterior planum temporale (*blue*). Note the larger area of the planum temporale in the left, as compared to the right, hemisphere.

Specifically, this is a horizontal (axial) section angled to follow the pitch of the sylvian fissure. When this cut is made and the top half of the hemispheres removed, the top (dorsal) surface of the temporal lobes can be seen from the perspective of looking down from above (along with other structures not discussed here). This view is shown in the bottom image of Figure 8–6. Recall that the superior temporal gyrus extends medially from its upper lip, like a "shelf" of cortex. Part of this

shelf of tissue is called the *planum temporale.* The lower image in Figure 8–6 shows, for both hemispheres, primary auditory cortex (colored salmon) as well as the planum temporale (colored blue). Note the markedly larger surface area of the planum temporale in the left, as compared to right, hemisphere.

The primary auditory cortex and planum temporale have interesting features. First, the cells in the primary auditory cortex are arranged systematically (tonotopically; see Chapter 6) with respect to auditory signal frequency; this does not seem to be the case for the planum temporale (Langers, Backe, & van Dijk, 2007). Kandel, Schwartz, Jessel, Siegelbaum, and Hudspeth (2012) have described the primary auditory cortex as a core of cells surrounded by cortical tissue devoted to increasingly higher-level processing of auditory information. This surrounding cortical tissue is called secondary auditory cortex, and the planum temporale falls into this category. The basic characteristics of acoustic signals—such as frequency, intensity, and duration—are analyzed in primary auditory cortex. This basic analysis is sent to surrounding temporal

Planum Temporale

The planum temporale has a lofty-sounding name (the *temporal plane*) and a scientific history as murky as lofty ideas tend to be. This wedge of brain tissue (see Figure 8–6) tends to be larger in the left than the right hemisphere in most people, including preverbal infants (Tervaniemi & Hugdahl, 2003). Unfortunately, at least for scientists who enjoy equating size differences with functional differences, chimps also have a larger left than right planum temporale. If only chimps communicated like humans, this would not be a theoretical problem. "Oh bother," as Winnie-the-Pooh might say, if bears could actually talk. In fMRI studies, the planum temporale lights up on the left side for speech sounds and on the right side for tones. Some scientists argue that lateralization to the left hemisphere for *detection* of speech sounds can be found in the planum temporale but that the broader needs of speech processing (extracting meaning from sound sequences) are accomplished bilaterally (Hickok, 2009). Maybe if we understood more about chimp's vocal communication, we could resolve the true role of the planum temporale in human communication; according to Winnie-the-Pooh, "Some people talk to animals. Not many listen though. That's the problem."

lobe tissue (secondary auditory cortex) for higher-level analyses. One form of higher-level auditory analysis is speech and language perception and understanding. The planum temporale is thought to be important to perceptual analysis of speech and language, and the evidence of anatomical asymmetries for this part of the temporal lobe—a larger planum temporale in the left than the right hemisphere—has encouraged the view of this cortical region as important to the natural aptitude among humans to develop and use speech and language.

Just posterior to the primary auditory cortex, along the back portion of the superior temporal gyrus, is a region of the temporal lobe (perhaps including the lateroventral portion of the parietal lobe) called *Wernicke's area* (see lower right image in Figure 8–4, the dark blue area toward the back of the sylvian fissure). Wernicke's area was originally defined as the brain region associated with speech and language comprehension because postmortem examination revealed lesions in this cortical area—the superior temporal gyrus—in several patients who were known, in life, to have had difficulty comprehending spoken language. In contrast, they *produced* speech in a more or less normal way. Dr. Carl Wernicke, a Prussian physician, examined one famous patient when alive and on postmortem examination located a lesion in the brain region named for him (Figure 8–4, lower right).

Imaging research on the perisylvian (meaning surrounding the sylvian fissure) language areas, and the temporal lobe specifically, during speech perception and language comprehension tasks supports the general ideas outlined above. The primary auditory cortex, roughly in the middle of the upper lip of the superior temporal gyrus, is active when a person is required to make decisions concerning individual speech sounds, especially when these decisions do not require word, sentence, or discourse meaning. It is as if this kind of task activates the part of the auditory cortex devoted to analysis of basic acoustic signal characteristics. When a person is required to make language input decisions involving meaning, more widespread regions of the temporal lobe are activated. Single-word meaning, meaning tied to different levels of grammatical complexity, and very abstract meaning (as in metaphor) engage many different regions of the temporal lobe, including the planum temporale, as well as regions of the parietal, frontal, and occipital lobes. Price (2010) provides an excellent review of brain imaging and the perception and comprehension of speech and language.

Occipital Lobe

The occipital lobes (colored purple in Figure 8–4) comprise the posterior parts of the cerebral hemispheres;
they are the smallest of the four lobes of the brain. The occipital lobes contain the primary visual cortex, in which visual information such as light and color is analyzed. These analyses of basic visual properties are delivered to other regions of the occipital lobes that contain cells for the analysis of more abstract, elaborate visual processing.

Insula

In Figure 8–7, a lateral view of the left cerebral hemisphere is shown with the lower "lips" of the frontal and parietal lobes and the upper lip of the temporal lobe pulled away to reveal underlying gyri and sulci. These retractable "lips" are referred to as *opercula* (plural of *operculum*, from the Latin word for *lid*). The cortex that is revealed when the opercula are retracted is called the *insula* or *insular cortex*. Sometimes the insula is described as part of a fifth hemispheric lobe, the *limbic lobe* (see below). In this chapter, the terms *insula* and *insular cortex* are used to denote this cortical region without commitment to the notion of the insula as part of a fifth lobe.

The insula appears to be a critical part of the cortical tissue engaged in speech, language, and swallowing functions (Ackermann & Riecker, 2010). Clinical cases in which patients with known lesions in and around

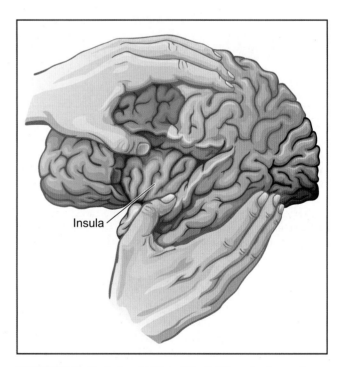

FIGURE 8–7. Lateral view of the left hemisphere, showing how the opercula (lids) of the frontal, parietal, and temporal lobes can be pulled apart to reveal the underlying insula.

the insula exhibit certain speech and language difficulties, surgical cases (brain tumors requiring resection of insular tissue), electrical stimulation of exposed brain (in patients undergoing brain resections for severe epileptic seizures), and fMRI studies of healthy individuals point to a role for the front part of the insula in speech motor control and possibly in speech perception. These speech functions of the insula appear to be lateralized to the left hemisphere, in much the same way that, in an overwhelming majority of individuals, speech and language functions are lateralized to Broca's and Wernicke's regions.

Limbic System (Limbic Lobe)

Heimer and Van Hoesen (2006) recommended the term *limbic lobe* to designate the collection of structures within the cerebral hemispheres that serve emotions, motivation, memory, and adaptive functions. Not all authors assign limbic structures the status of a lobe of the cerebral hemispheres, at least in the same sense as the frontal, parietal, temporal, and occipital lobes. Some authors refer to a limbic *system* to reflect a collection of structures within the brain, all of which play an important role, broadly speaking, in emotional and motivational aspects of behavior. Here the term *limbic system* is used.

The most easily visualized structures of the limbic system are on the medial surface of a hemisphere (see Figure 8–4, top right). The *cingulate gyrus* is one of these structures, forming an incomplete ring above and around the corpus callosum. The ring is partially completed on the lower side of the hemisphere by the upper gyrus of the medial temporal lobe, called the *parahippocampal gyrus*. The cingulate and parahippocampal gyri are part of the cortex, but their cell structure is different from (for example) cells found in the primary motor, primary somatosensory, or association cortex (Heimer & Van Hoesen, 2006). The cell structure of limbic cortical areas in humans may be described as more primitive than the cell structure in many other cortical areas.

Cerebral White Matter

The surface of the cerebral hemispheres is made up of many gyri and sulci, some of which have been identified above. This surface topography is composed of gray matter, formed by densely packed clusters of neuronal cell bodies. Cut into the cerebral hemispheres and a tremendous volume of white matter is revealed. White matter connects nearby and distant cell groups within the brain.

At any location within the white matter, there are fibers running in many different directions, to and from different cell groups. Even though fiber tracts are typically bundled together, with a given bundle running from a specific group of cell bodies to another specific group of cell bodies, white matter reflects an intermixing of several such bundles. A relatively new brain imaging technique called *diffusion tensor imaging* (DTI) allows scientists to establish the origin, course, and termination of major fiber tracts in the human brain (see sidetrack on DTI). DTI research has established a detailed map of fiber bundles within the brain. Much of the following information, including an organizational scheme for classifying fiber bundles within the cerebral hemispheres, is adapted from a review article by Schmahmann, Smith, Eichler, and Filley (2008). Table 8–1 outlines this classification system.

DTI

Because fiber tracts within the cerebral hemispheres are intermixed and so densely packed, it is difficult to establish the origins, pathways, and destinations of connections between cell groups. Techniques used in animal research, such as introducing certain chemicals into the brain that "label" specific fiber tracts, are mostly not usable in human research. Fortunately, a relatively new technique called diffusion tensor imaging (DTI) makes it possible to monitor selected pathways without posing danger to humans. Water molecules move along fiber tracts in ways that can be identified by proper computer settings of a brain scanner. In what are called region-of-interest techniques, the brain-scanning instrument is directed at the presumed target region, and computer reconstructions of the pathways show their extent, volume, and orientation. Conturo et al. (2008) provide an explanation of the DTI technique, and Saur et al. (2008) show how it can be used to understand speech and language connectivity of the brain.

Association Tracts

Association tracts connect one part of the cortex to another *within the same hemisphere (intrahemispheric)*. These *ipsilateral* (same side of the brain) connections may consist of small groups of fibers running between adjacent gyri, or between more distantly separated gyri

TABLE 8–1. An Organizational Scheme for Classifying Tracts (Central Fiber Bundles) and Their Principal Connections

Fiber Bundle Type	Connections
Association tracts	*Intra*hemispheric, both within and between lobes
Striatal tracts	From cortex to basal ganglia (principally to caudate and putamen), and from cortex to subthalamic nucleus
Commissural tracts	*Inter*hemispheric, from specific area of one hemisphere to similar area of the other hemisphere
Descending projection tracts	
Corticobulbar	Motor cortex to cell groups in brainstem
Corticospinal	Motor cortex to cell groups in spinal cord
Corticothalamic	Widespread regions of the cortex to cell groups in the thalamus
Ascending projection tracts	
Posterior column/medial lemniscus	Spinal cord to brainstem nuclei and thalamus
Anterolateral	Spinal cord to thalamus
Thalamocortical	Cell groups in the thalamus to widespread regions of the cortex

Source: Adapted and modified from Schmahmann et al. (2008).

within the same lobe. Of greater importance for the current discussion are several association tracts that are tightly organized, large bundles of axons connecting cortical areas in one lobe to cortical areas in a different lobe. Of immediate interest is the superior longitudinal fasciculus, more commonly known as the arcuate fasciculus.

Arcuate Fasciculus and Speech and Language Functions

The *superior longitudinal fasciculus*, the main part of which is the *arcuate fasciculus* (AF) (see Bernal & Ardila, 2009), connects the speech/language cortex in the parietal, frontal, and temporal lobes. Figure 8–8 is a DTI reconstruction of the AF, as well as two other association tracts, the inferior longitudinal fasciculus and uncinate fasciculus. The AF is the arched pathway (hence "arcuate") with one leg of the arch in the temporal lobe, from which fibers run slightly back and up into the parietal lobe before turning forward to end as the other leg of the arch in the posterior part of the frontal lobe. Four cortical areas are connected by the AF: Wernicke's area (temporal lobe), the angular and supramarginal gyri (parietal lobe), and Broca's area

(frontal lobe). This is a more or less standard way to describe the AF, as a fiber tract connecting the receptive language areas (Wernicke's area and possibly parts of the angular and supramarginal gyri) to the expressive area (Broca's area). In fact, the connections as well as the notion of "receptive" and "expressive" language areas of the brain are much more complicated than this simple but appealing picture (Bernal & Ardila, 2009; Catani & Mesulam, 2008).

The AF has a prominent role in theories of speech and language functions in healthy and diseased brains. The most influential of these theories is referred to as the Wernicke-Geschwind model (Geschwind, 1965), in which the comprehension area of the brain (Wernicke's area) is connected to the expressive region (Broca's area) by means of the AF. In this model, acoustic properties of spoken words are first analyzed in the primary auditory cortex and then sent to Wernicke's area to convert this "raw" analysis into meaning. The meaningful phonetic sequences thus identified—the words—can be transferred to Broca's area for production via the AF. In the Wernicke-Geschwind model, this sequence of processing centers (cortical cell bodies) and pathways (fiber tracts) is fully engaged when a person is asked to imitate a spoken word or series of words. Neurologi-

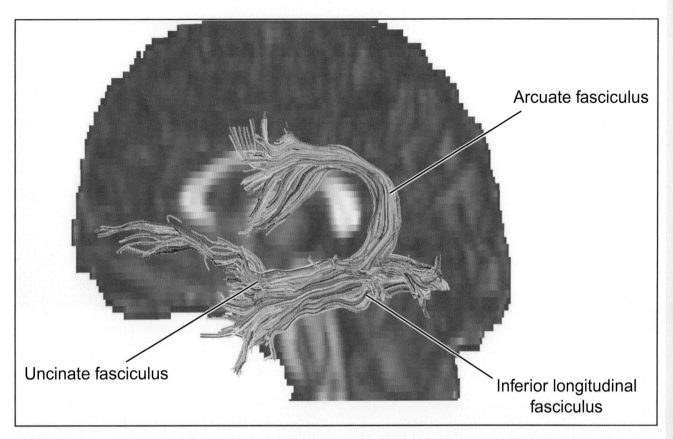

FIGURE 8–8. DTI image showing the arcuate fasciculus (the arched fiber tract contained within the superior longitudinal fasciculus), which runs from the temporal/parietal lobe to the frontal lobe), inferior longitudinal fasciculus (which runs from the occipital to the temporal lobe), and the uncinate fasciculus (which runs from the temporal to the frontal lobe).

cally intact individuals with a healthy primary auditory cortex and Wernicke's area have no problem with this task, because they can analyze phonetic (speech sound) properties, comprehend meaning, and transfer this information via the AF to the brain region specialized for speech production. When the AF is damaged by neurological disease, various aspects of speech/language performance may be impaired. If the damage is restricted to the tract, leaving Wernicke's and Broca's areas intact (healthy), the speech/language problem may be described as a "disconnection syndrome" because the main receptive area has been disconnected from the main expressive area of the brain. This disconnection impairs a patient's ability to imitate spoken words or sentences, even with healthy Wernicke's and Broca's areas.

The Wernicke-Geschwind model (Geschwind, 1965) has exerted a profound influence on scientific and clinical thinking on the role of brain structures for speech and language. A more contemporary view is that speech and language functions of the brain are far more complex than suggested by the Wernicke-Geschwind model (Tremblay & Dick, 2016).

Striatal Tracts

Deep within the cerebral hemispheres, there are several clusters of cell bodies, collectively referred to as *subcortical nuclei* (below the cortex). One group of these nuclei includes components of the *basal ganglia* (sometimes called *basal nuclei*). The *thalamus*, itself a collection of many nuclei, is another major subcortical nucleus. Beneath the cortical rind of gray matter, these nuclei appear as collections of gray matter within the extensive white matter of the cerebral hemispheres. *Striatal tracts* are fiber tracts connecting the cortical gray matter and the subcortical nuclei of the basal ganglia. It is useful to think of these fiber tracts as forming a connection loop between cortical and basal ganglia structures. This loop plays an important role in motor control and in speech motor control in particular (and possibly aspects of language production). Also, there are striatal fiber tracts that connect individual nuclei of the basal ganglia, as well as nuclei of the basal ganglia and the thalamus.

Commissural Tracts

Commissural tracts connect a specific region of one hemisphere with its similar topographical region in the other hemisphere. The wording of this description is purposely careful, because of the notion of *lateralization of function*. Brain regions having the same locations in the two hemispheres most likely do not have the same function. For example, Broca's area has a sister region in the right hemisphere, but it is not called Broca's area. Nevertheless, these two frontal lobe regions are connected across the hemispheres by fibers running in the corpus callosum. The same can be said for the other cortical regions described above; they are all connected across the hemispheres by the corpus callosum, but the connection does not imply connection for identical function.

The corpus callosum is a massive and complex bundle of fibers. A classic view of the corpus callosum is the one viewed in the midsagittal plane (see Figure 8–4, top right), where the front-to-back extent of the tract appears as a thick length of arched white matter, shaped somewhat like a flattened letter "C" turned on its right side. The frontmost and backmost parts of the corpus callosum are the *genu* and *splenium*, respectively. Between the genu and splenium is the central, main bulk of the corpus callosum, called the *body*. At the genu, the corpus callosum has a curl of fibers (one end of the "C") pointing slightly downward and toward the back of the cerebral hemispheres; this backward-directed curl is called the *rostrum*.

The front and back reaches of the corpus callosum, as seen in the midsagittal section of the cerebral hemispheres, do not extend to the front and back "poles" (end points) of the hemispheres. Nevertheless, fiber tracts extend from the corpus callosum forward and backward into the most anterior regions of the frontal lobe and most posterior regions of the occipital lobes, connecting these regions across the hemispheres. Finally, although in the midsagittal plane the body of the corpus callosum is beneath cortical tissue, the connecting fibers project upward to reach cortical layers at the top of the hemispheres. The extension of corpus callosum fibers into the front and back parts of the hemispheres, as well as to the top of the cortex, is shown in the sagittal plane, DTI image of Figure 8–9. The "flat" part of the tract, corresponding to the view in Figure 8–4 of the medial part of the corpus callosum, is seen toward the front of the brain in Figure 8–9, and

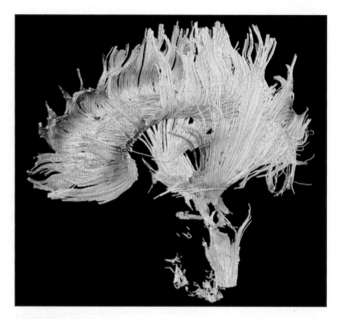

FIGURE 8–9. DTI image of the corpus callosum, showing the fibers extending up toward the dorsal surface of the hemispheres as well as into anterior and posterior parts of the hemispheres.

the upcurled fibers reaching to cortical layers are seen all along the length of the tract.

Descending Projection Tracts

Descending projection tracts include the corticobulbar and corticospinal tracts, as well as tracts running from cortical regions to the thalamus (corticothalamic tracts; see Table 8–1). Figure 8–10 shows in a schematic coronal view the descending corticobulbar and corticospinal fiber tracts. The corticobulbar tract (*bulbar* is a term used to indicate the brainstem), represented in Figure 8–10 by the solid pink and orange lines, includes fibers originating in cortical neuronal cell bodies that make a first synapse in one of the several brainstem motor nuclei. The corticospinal tract, represented in Figure 8–10 by the dashed blue lines, includes fibers originating in the cortex that make a first synapse in motor cells of the spinal cord. Many of these motor neurons in the brainstem and spinal cord issue axons that leave the CNS to innervate muscles of the body.

As the corticobulbar and corticospinal tracts descend from the cortex to lower regions of the CNS, their location within the brain is designated by use of different terms. For example, fibers of the corticobulbar and corticospinal tracts issue from cell bodies all over the cortex and form a fan-like pattern called the *corona radiata*. The fibers of the corona radiata make up the

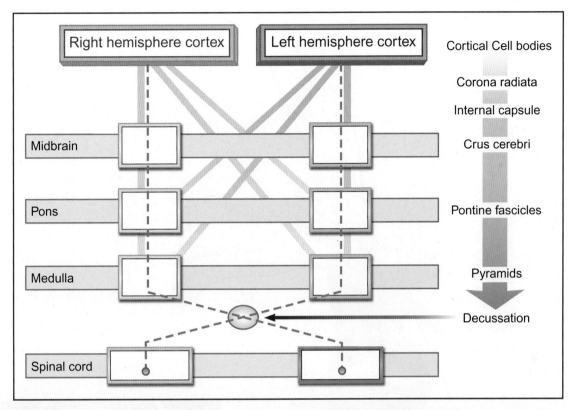

FIGURE 8–10. Schematic coronal view of the descending corticobulbar (*thick pink and orange lines*) and corticospinal (*dashed blue lines*) tracts. The corticobulbar tracts are both ipsilateral and contralateral, sending axons to brainstem nuclei on the same and opposite side as their cortical origin. The corticospinal tract is primarily contralateral, crossing at the decussation of the pyramids and sending axons to ventral horn nuclei in the spinal cord on the side opposite the cortical origin.

The Final Common Pathway

What is this? The last path we will all travel? No, it is a term used when referring to a certain part of the motor system, the part containing nuclei of cell bodies whose axons go directly to muscles. The term *motor neuron* is often reserved for the cells in these nuclei, which receive information primarily from descending fiber tracts coming from the cortex. They are the last stop before motor commands are sent via cranial and spinal nerves to muscles in the jaw, lips, rib cage wall, and other parts of the speech mechanism and

body. The idea of a final common pathway recognizes that a particular motor nucleus in the brainstem or spinal cord may receive input from several different sources. The output of these motor nuclei to muscles is subject to a "net effect" of all those different inputs. The idea of a final common pathway in motor systems was originally formulated by the famous neurophysiologist Charles Sherrington and described in his then-revolutionary, 1906 text, *The Integrative Action of the Nervous System.*

large majority of white matter immediately below the cortex. The corona radiata is represented schematically in the right column of Figure 8–10 and in the more anatomically correct image of Figure 8–11. As the fibers in the corona radiata descend, they gather into a relatively

tight bundle that passes between subcortical nuclei to reach the more inferior brainstem and spinal cord. The sagittal view in Figure 8–11 (top image) shows the corona radiata merging into this tight bundle. This part of the descending tracts, where the corticobulbar

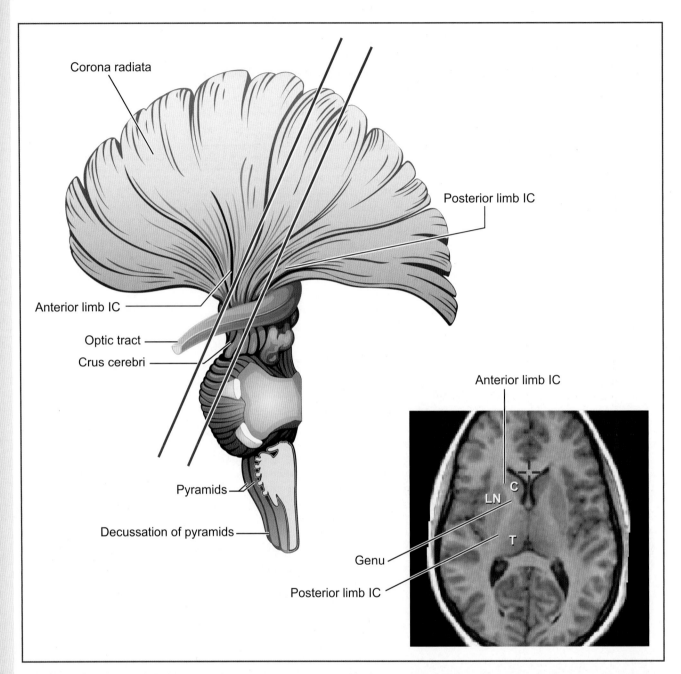

Corona radiata

Posterior limb IC

Anterior limb IC

Optic tract

Crus cerebri

Anterior limb IC

Pyramids

LN C

Decussation of pyramids

T

Genu

Posterior limb IC

FIGURE 8–11. *Upper left*, view of fibers of the corona radiata descending in the cerebral hemispheres and gathering into a narrow bundle called the internal capsule (IC) to pass between several subcortical nuclei, en route to the brainstem. *Lower right*, horizontal section of cerebral hemispheres (anterior is toward the top of the image) showing the boomerang shape of the internal capsule. The anterior and posterior limbs plus the genu of the internal capsule are labeled. C = caudate nucleus; LN = lenticular nucleus; T = thalamus.

and corticospinal tracts pass through a narrow channel whose medial borders are the thalamus and caudate nucleus, and whose lateral border is the lentiform (globus pallidus and putamen) nucleus, is called the *internal capsule*. Figure 8–10 shows the schematic location of the internal capsule along the descending tracts, and

Figure 8–11, right image, shows a horizontal section in which the internal capsule is viewed between the thalamus and putamen (medial border) and the lentiform nucleus (lateral border).

The coronal slices in previous figures show the internal capsule at a single location along the front-to-back extent of the cerebral hemispheres (e.g., top right of Figure 8–2, not labeled in the figure). A greater appreciation for the distribution of these fiber tracts is gained from careful examination of Figure 8–11 (upper left), where the front of the head is toward the left of the image. Here the cortical tissue has been stripped away to reveal the fibers of the corona radiata and internal capsule. Even though the internal capsule is the tightly gathered merger of the many fibers of the corona radiata, the internal capsule can be described as having an anterior, middle, and posterior part (IC, for internal capsule in Figure 8–11). The precise location of a coronal slice therefore determines which part of the internal capsule is displayed. Like so many other parts of the brain, the internal capsule is not a random jumble of fibers but rather is arranged systematically based on the cortical origin of the fibers. In a horizontal (axial) slice (inset, lower right of Figure 8–11), the internal capsule in each hemisphere has a boomerang shape with the angle of the boomerang most medial and the two arms extending away from this angle anterolaterally and posterolaterally. To provide a rough idea of the systematic arrangement of fibers within the internal capsule, most corticobulbar fibers associated with control of facial, jaw, tongue, velopharyngeal, and laryngeal muscles run through a compact bundle close to or within the angle (called the genu) of the internal capsule. In contrast, fibers descending to motor neurons in the spinal cord are mostly located in the posterior limb of the internal capsule.

Descending fibers leave the internal capsule and continue their downward path in the *cerebral peduncles*, a tract in the central part of the midbrain. The largest portion of these fibers runs in the *crus cerebri*, an anterior part of the cerebral peduncles. (The terms *cerebral peduncles* and *crus cerebri* are occasionally used interchangeably; see Figure 8–11.) The fibers then continue through the pons in small bundles, called fascicles, and are gathered back together in the medulla as the pyramids. Some descending fibers in the cerebral peduncles, pontine fascicles, and medulla leave the tract to make synapses with motor nuclei in the midbrain, pons, and medulla; these fibers belong to the corticobulbar tract, and the synapses they make within the brainstem define the termination of this tract. The fibers continuing into the spinal cord belong to the corticospinal tract; these make synapses in the ventral gray matter of the spinal cord, where spinal motor neurons are found.

The path of the corticospinal tract is shown for one side of the brain in Figure 8–12; the path on the other side of the brain is a mirror image of the one shown. Fibers in the corticospinal tract descend from the cortex until the majority (about 80%) cross to the other

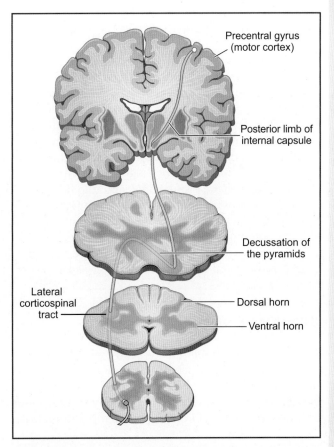

FIGURE 8–12. Pathway of corticospinal tract. The green pathway shows the tract originating in the cortex of one hemisphere and descending on the same side until it reaches the medulla where about 80% of the fibers cross over to the opposite side to descend in the lateral corticospinal tract. The pathway on the other side of the hemisphere is a mirror image of the one shown. Descending fibers leave the corticospinal tract at all segments of the spinal cord to make synapses with ventral horn cells (spinal motor neurons). The purple fiber shown leaving the spinal cord at the lowest level represents axons sent via peripheral nerves to muscles.

side at the decussation of the pyramids, a landmark on the ventral surface of the medulla created by the crossing fibers (see Figure 8–16, later in the chapter). The fact that so many fibers from one cerebral hemisphere eventually travel in the spinal cord on the side opposite to their cortical origin, and innervate motor neurons on that opposite side, accounts for the well-known fact that the left hemisphere controls limbs on the right side, and the right hemisphere controls limbs on the left side. In Figure 8–12, the descent of the corticospinal tract through the internal capsule to its cross-over point within the inferior medulla is represented by the green line.

Upper Versus Lower Motor Neuron Lesions

There are motor neurons in the cortex, the brainstem, and the spinal cord. Cortical motor neurons send long axons to cells in both the brainstem and the spinal cord, which in turn send axons into the peripheral nervous system, where they terminate on muscle fibers. Muscle control problems can result from damage anywhere along this path from cortex to muscle fiber. Neuroscientists and neurologists have professional jargon to refer to sites of lesions along these motor pathways. *Upper motor neuron* lesions are those occurring in the cortical motor neurons or in the axons they issue prior to making synapses with the motor neurons in the brainstem or spinal cord. *Lower motor neuron* lesions are those occurring in the nuclei of the brainstem or motor cells of the spinal cord, or in the axons they issue and the peripheral nerves in which those axons travel, or even at the location of the nerve–muscle fiber connection. *Upper* motor neuron lesions result in muscles with excessive muscle tone while at rest and hypersensitive reflexes. *Lower* motor neuron lesions generally result in loss of muscle mass (wasting or atrophy), small muscle twitches visible to the naked eye (called *fasciculations*), and in some cases low muscle tone at rest. In both upper and lower motor neuron lesions, the affected muscles tend to be weak.

Ascending Projection Tracts

Ascending fiber tracts are typically associated with sensory pathways, which can be thought of as projection tracts from points below to points above. Sensory events begin in an end organ in the body that responds to touch, pressure, vibration, pain, temperature, taste, odor, light, sound, and position and movement of a body structure (called proprioception, see sidetrack called Muscle Spindles).

The somatosensory pathways constitute a major portion of the ascending projection tracts. These tracts run in the opposite direction from the descending projection tracts. The "points below" are the end organs,

Muscle Spindles

Skeletal muscle is striated muscle; when viewed with a high-powered microscope, these muscles resemble a series of bands, or "striae." Voluntary muscles—those associated with conscious control, such as muscles of the fingers, arms, and legs—are composed of striated tissue. In contrast, smooth muscle such as that found in the gut is not striated and not under conscious control. Skeletal muscles contain small organs (about 5 mm long) called muscle spindles that are embedded in the muscle tissue. The sense of proprioception—the ability to detect the position and motion of a limb resulting from muscle contraction—is due to muscle spindle function (Macefield & Knellwolf, 2018). A simple example of muscle spindle function is its critical role in the stretch reflex. When a physician hammer-taps your patellar tendon, located immediately below the kneecap, the tendon is stretched and transmitted to muscle fibers in the quadriceps, which are attached to the upper part of the tendon. The spindles sense the stretch and send a signal to the spinal cord to issue a motor command to contract the quadriceps, to a degree that restores the length of the muscle before it was stretched by the tap. Muscle spindles code the degree and velocity of the stretch, which occurs naturally during movement—they don't need to be triggered by the tap of a reflex hammer. When the tens or hundreds of muscle spindles in a given muscle send signals on muscle stretch (and its opposite, shortening) back to the brainstem or spinal cord, fine adjustments are made in the degree and velocity of change in muscle length. Thus, it comes as no surprise that muscles that create very precise and fast movements, such as those that control eye movement, and fine finger movement, have a high density of muscles spindles. The masseter muscle (Chapter 5) also has a dense distribution of muscle spindles. Why? The force of masseter muscle contraction must be scaled precisely for bite force. When the jaw bites, different foods (or whatever is bitten) offer a wide range of hardness to forces applied by the jaw. Biting force can be adjusted precisely by muscle spindle signals when the masseter muscle is stretched a lot (by hard foods, such as nuts) or stretched minimally (by a piece of banana).

where stimuli are sensed, and the "points above" include several synapses along the ascending pathway with a final destination in the cortex.

There are two major somatosensory pathways for stimuli sensed below the neck (that is, in the torso or limbs). One of these, the posterior column-medial lemniscal tract (Blumenfeld, 2010), carries sensory information from one side of the body. This sensory information enters the spinal cord after making a first synapse in a dorsal root ganglion. The fibers ascend in the spinal cord until reaching the dorsal part of the medulla (the medulla is the lowest part of the brainstem, at the top of the spinal cord), where the fibers make a synapse and then cross to the opposite side to ascend through the brainstem and thalamus before terminating in the primary sensory cortex and surrounding areas. Sensation from one side of the body is therefore processed in the cortex on the opposite side of the brain. Note the parallel to the corticospinal tract, which carries motor commands to the opposite side of the body. The descending corticospinal tract crosses over on the ventral surface of the medulla, whereas the ascending posterior column-medial lemniscus tract crosses over in the dorsal (posterior) part of the medulla. This ascending tract carries information on fine touch, vibration, and joint position.

A second ascending pathway for sensory stimuli entering the spinal cord is called the anterolateral tract. This tract carries information on pain, temperature, and "crude" touch (Blumenfeld, 2010) and, like the posterior column-medial lemniscus tract, conveys this information to the cortex on the side opposite to the stimulation.

Both the posterior column-medial lemniscus and anterolateral tracts eventually send their information to the thalamus, where synapses are made and fibers sent to the cortex. Visual and auditory ascending fibers, carrying information from the retina (vision) and hair cells (audition), also make a final synapse in the thalamus before projecting to the visual and auditory cortical areas. All of the ascending fibers pass through the internal capsule and make synapses in the thalamus. The thalamus then sends this information, via the thalamocortical tract, to the cortex. The thalamocortical tract is a significant component of the white matter in the cerebral hemispheres.

SUBCORTICAL NUCLEI AND CEREBELLUM

The subcortical nuclei include the various structures of the basal ganglia (also referred to as the basal nuclei), the thalamus, the hypothalamus, and other nuclei of the limbic system (such as the amygdala). The cerebellum is also subcortical but is typically discussed separately from subcortical structures. In this section, the focus is on the basal ganglia, thalamus, and cerebellum.

Basal Ganglia

The basal ganglia include the caudate and putamen nuclei (which together constitute the striatum), the globus pallidus (which, paired with the putamen, is referred to as the lenticular or lentiform nucleus—see Figure 8–11), the subthalamic nucleus, and the substantia nigra. Technically, the substantia nigra is not a subcortical nucleus (that is, below the cortex but within the cerebral hemispheres) but rather is a brainstem nucleus, because it is located in the ventral midbrain. The substantia nigra is included here as a subcortical nucleus because of its close anatomical and functional connection with the striatum and subthalamic nucleus.

The gross anatomy of the basal ganglia can be better appreciated in a coronal slice of the cerebral hemispheres. Figure 8–13 (left) shows a "zoomed" artist's rendition of a coronal slice from the right side of the brain, roughly midway between the front and back of the brain. The image on the right shows the full slice from which this closeup is taken. The traditional shading difference between nuclei and tracts is shown, with nuclei and cortical cells appearing darker and fiber tracts lighter. The caudate, putamen, globus pallidus, substantia nigra, and subthalamic nucleus are labeled in the images, as is the thalamus. The thalamus is not considered a basal ganglia structure but is shown here for orientation purposes and because of its role in the processing of basal ganglia function (see below). Note the location of the putamen, deep to the insula; in this coronal slice, the putamen is the most lateral of the basal ganglia nuclei. Just medial to the putamen is the globus pallidus, and together these two structures form a curved, lens-like mass of cells, explaining why the combined nuclei are called the lentiform or lenticular nucleus. Superior and medial to the lentiform nucleus and just lateral to the lateral ventricle is the caudate nucleus, which appears in this slice as a small, pear-shaped mass. Recall that the caudate and putamen are together called the striatum. Inferior and medial to the lentiform nucleus is the aptly named subthalamic nucleus. (Note its position relative to the massive thalamus.) Inferior to the subthalamic nucleus, the relatively long, oblique strip of darkened tissue is the substantia nigra, located ventrally in the superior part of the midbrain.

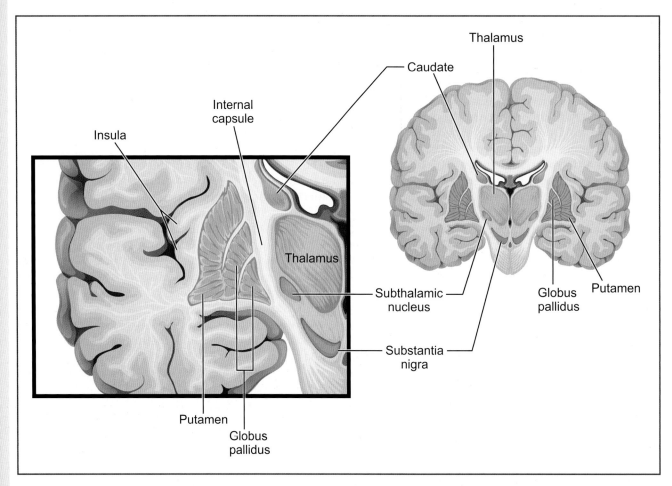

FIGURE 8–13. Structures of the basal ganglia shown in an artist's rendition, one closeup (*left*), the other the whole coronal slice (*right*) from which the zoomed view is taken.

Basal Ganglia or Basal Nuclei?

Language usage is *conventional*. If a sufficient number of people agree on the meaning of a word or phrase, its meaning is established for that language community, and technical analysis of language is, well, meaningless. Much of this textbook is about speech; in German, speech is *sprache*, in French *parle*, in Mandarin Chinese *yanyu*, in Korean *mal*, and in Russian *rech*. No one of these words captures the idea of "speech" more accurately than any other, and no one of the words is intrinsically "right." Technical analysis of which word may be "right" will not reveal an answer because there is none. The words mean *speech* because speakers of the languages agree on the meaning. So it is with the term *basal ganglia*, even if the term is technically a misnomer. Technically, a ganglion is a cluster of cell bodies just outside of the CNS, but the components of the basal ganglia (caudate, putamen, and so forth) are within the CNS. In a grave, lumbering statement issued in 1998, the International Federation of Associations of Anatomists (IFAA) declared that the term *basal nuclei* should be used for this collection of structures due to the error of referring to these cell groups as *ganglia* (Sarikcioglu, Altun, Suzen, & Oguz, 2008). Unfortunately for the IFAA, most scientists are not paying attention. In a PubMed search done by one of your authors on July 10, 2020, using the key words *basal ganglia* and restricting the search to articles published from July 2010 to the present (giving the scientific community plenty of time to respect the 1998 IFAA proclamation), 12,984 "hits" were obtained. In contrast, the key words *basal nuclei* produced only 126 "hits." In this text, we side with the majority, choosing convention over technical accuracy. We choose and use the term *basal ganglia*.

A pale white strip of tissue separates the lentiform nucleus from the more medial caudate, thalamus, subthalamic nucleus, and substantia nigra. This is the internal capsule.

The specific appearance of basal ganglia structures, and in some cases the presence of a structure in a particular coronal slice, depends substantially on the location of the slice along the anteroposterior axis of the cerebral hemispheres. A conceptual appreciation for this dependency can be gained by studying Figure 8–14, a sagittal-view drawing of the complex configuration of basal ganglia structures (in which the front of the brain is to the left). Cerebral cortex and cerebral white matter have been eliminated from the figure, leaving the structures of the basal ganglia "floating" free from their moorings within the cerebral hemispheres. Note the C-shaped form of the caudate nucleus, how the nucleus is massive toward the front of the hemispheres and narrows as it curls toward the back of the brain and turns around to point forward. The tail of the caudate nucleus points so far forward that it terminates ventral to the globus pallidus. The image also shows the caudate and putamen nuclei joined at the anterior end of the nuclei and splitting apart as the image is viewed from left to right (that is, from anterior to posterior within the cerebral hemispheres). The channel between the caudate and putamen, created as they separate, is the internal capsule. Note the strands of light pink tissue bridging the spaces between the caudate and putamen, running across the region where the descending and ascending fibers of the internal capsule are located. In fixed-brain slices, these strands appear as gray streaks across the white matter of the internal capsule, especially in coronal slices taken near the anterior edge of the basal ganglia. This streaked or striated appearance of the internal capsule gives the name striatum to the putamen and caudate nuclei.

Basal ganglia structures receive information from the cortex, process that information, and send it back to the cortex via the thalamus. This pathway is referred to as the cortico-striatal-cortical loop. The general function of this loop is to refine motor commands issued from the cortex via processing in basal ganglia structures.

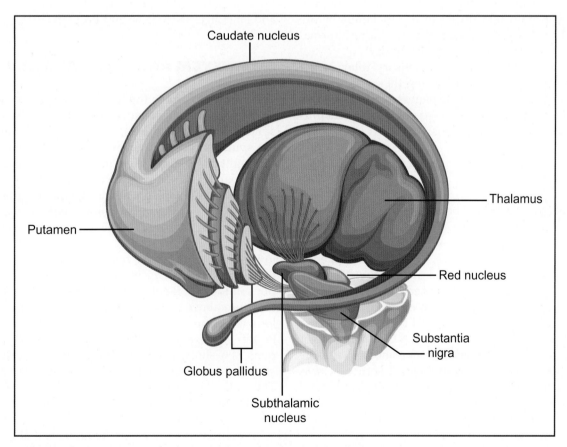

FIGURE 8–14. Sagittal-view drawing of the complex configuration of the basal ganglia and adjacent structures. Front is to the left. Green lines show fiber tracts running between the nuclei. The four light pink strands toward the front of the basal ganglia structures show cell body connections between the anterior caudate and putamen.

This refinement may involve aspects of both planning and execution of a motor act.

Thalamus

Figure 8–13 shows the thalamus as a massive group of nuclei on either side of the midline of the hemispheres; the two thalami surround the third ventricle. When viewed from the side (see Figure 8–14), the thalamus appears as an egg-shaped structure. The thalamus is a collection of specialized nuclei, many of which relay a specific type of sensory information from lower parts of the brain to specific cortical areas. For example, auditory and visual nuclei within the brainstem send information to specialized nuclei within the thalamus, which in turn relay this information to auditory and visual cortical areas. Similarly, sensory fibers carrying tactile information from the limbs and torso enter the spinal cord and ascend in the dorsal columns described above; fibers in this tract make synapses within dorsal column nuclei, which send tracts through specialized nuclei in the thalamus to the somatosensory regions of the cortex. Tactile information from the head and neck travels via brainstem nuclei to the thalamus before delivery to appropriate cortical areas. Taste information is also relayed through the thalamus.

The thalamus is the main sensory relay of the brain; all sensory roads connecting the outside world to the cortex go through the thalamus (except olfaction, the sense of smell). As discussed above, the thalamus also contributes to motor plans.

Cerebellum

The cerebellum is located below the occipital lobe and posterior to the brainstem. The cerebellum has two lobes and can be distinguished from other parts of the brain by its unique appearance, which has been likened to a cauliflower (Figure 8–15, lower image). The surface of the cerebellum is composed of a series of very slim tissue slabs, separated from each other by parallel, narrow fissures. In a prepared (fixed) brain, these tissue slabs—called *folia* (plural of *folium*, a thin layer or leaf)—can be separated from one another with the careful use of dissecting instruments. In principle, this is similar to separating adjacent gyri of the cerebral cortex to look into the sulci between them, but cerebellar folia are much more tightly packed and difficult to separate by hand.

Like the cerebral hemispheres, the cerebellar lobes have an outer cortex (gray matter), as well as white matter and nuclei deep within the cortical mantle. The structure and function of the cerebellum are exceedingly complex. Of interest here is its relevance to motor control, including speech motor control.

The cerebellum is connected via fiber tracts to the spinal cord, brainstem, and cortex. The cerebellar peduncles, massive bundles of axons seen on the ventral and lateral surfaces of the brainstem (see Figures 8–16 and 8–17, later in the chapter), are the connections between the cerebellum and the rest of the CNS. The cerebellum, like the basal ganglia, is connected to the cortex by means of a loop that runs from cortex to cerebellum and back to the cortex. This cortico-cerebello-cortical loop is thought to play a primary role in movement coordination. Patients with cerebellar damage typically have balance problems, produce jerky movements, and have difficulty producing and maintaining steady movement rhythms. The cerebellum plays an important role in the sequencing and timing of speech sounds, in coordination of chewing movements, and even in language production. Damage to the cerebellum can result in a motor speech disorder called *ataxic dysarthria* that is characterized by impaired coordination among articulatory movements. For a review of the cerebellum and its role in speech and language, see Mariën and Borgatti (2018).

BRAINSTEM AND CRANIAL NERVES

The brainstem can be thought of as a stalk of nervous system tissue, connected above to the cerebral hemispheres and its contents, and connected below to the spinal cord. Refer again to Figure 8–3, where the midsagittal MR image (right image) shows a dotted red line separating the top of the brainstem from the bulk of the cerebral hemispheres. In this midsagittal view, identification of the major components of the brainstem is made easy by the bulging, middle part of the brainstem called the *pons*. If a horizontal line is drawn lower and parallel to the red dotted line in Figure 8–3, through the nose of the imaged person, it intersects the pons in the middle of its bulge. The smaller, narrower structure above the pons, the midbrain (mesencephalon), is the most superior component of the brainstem; its top end extends to the dotted red line. Below the pons is a short, narrow column of tissue called the *medulla* (sometimes referred to as the *medulla oblongata*). The medulla is the most inferior component of the brainstem, and its inferior border is contiguous with the superior boundary of the spinal cord.

An artist's rendition of the brainstem and nearby structures in the sagittal plane is shown in the lower part of Figure 8–15. Note the location of the cerebellum, posterior to the pons and medulla and beneath the

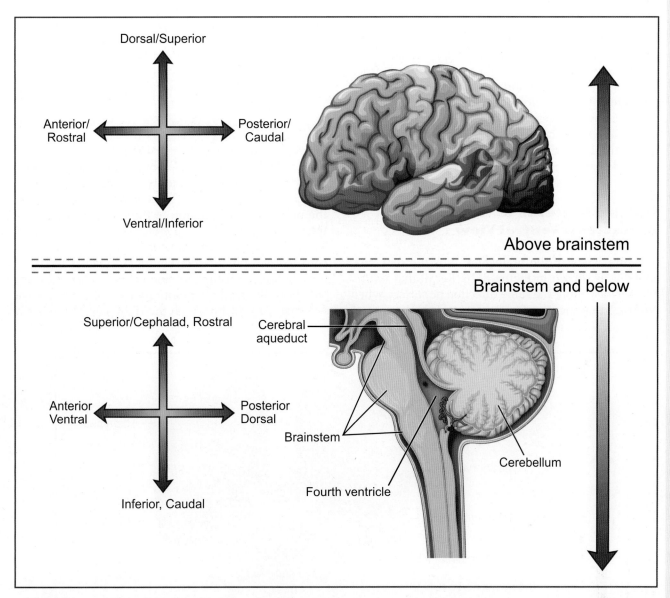

FIGURE 8–15. The cerebral hemispheres (*top*) and the brainstem, cerebellum, and upper part of spinal cord (*bottom*). Both images are shown in the sagittal plane.

occipital lobe of the cerebral hemispheres. At the top of the brainstem, a narrow, dark brown canal can be seen running through the midbrain, posterior to the superior part of the pons. This canal expands below into a larger cavity separating the cerebellum from the pons and medulla. The narrow canal is the *cerebral aqueduct*, and the cavity into which it expands is the *fourth ventricle*. These cavities are part of the ventricular system through which cerebrospinal fluid (CSF) flows.

The brainstem is small compared to the cerebral hemispheres but contains cells and tracts critical to a wide variety of sensorimotor behaviors, as well as to consciousness, mood, and basic vegetative functions.

A great deal of nervous system tissue with a broad range of functions is packed into the small volume of the brainstem, and it is precisely these close quarters that explain why blood deprivation to the brainstem—as in the case of brainstem strokes—can have such devastating consequences. Of special interest to the speech-language pathologist and audiologist are the nuclei and fiber tracts of the brainstem associated with a subset of the 12 paired cranial nerves. These brainstem structures and the nerves associated with them control muscles of the head and neck and sensation (including hearing) from the same structures. Speaking, swallowing, and hearing are very much dependent on the integrity of brainstem structures and the cranial nerves.

In this section, the cranial nerves are first described as surface features of the brainstem; other surface features of the ventral and dorsal brainstem are also presented. This is followed by consideration of 7 of the 12 cranial nerves and their associated brainstem nuclei. The seven cranial nerves described more fully below are those with relevance to speaking, swallowing, and hearing.

Surface Features of the Brainstem: Ventral View

A ventral view of the brainstem, plus the thalamus above it, is shown in Figure 8–16. Recall that *ventral* and *anterior* imply the same direction or surface when referring to structures from the top of the brainstem down through the spinal cord. The view in Figure 8–16 is therefore the one obtained if the midsagittal views of Figures 8–3 and 8–15 are rotated counterclockwise 90 degrees, resulting in the observer looking at the front, or ventral/anterior surface, of the brainstem.

Ventral Surface of Midbrain

Prominent surface features of the ventral midbrain include the *cerebral peduncles* (often called the *crus cerebri*, although this term is not technically equivalent to the cerebral peduncles). The cerebral peduncles are the midbrain continuation of the massive, long fiber tract running from cortical motor cells to motor nuclei in both the brainstem (corticobulbar tract) and spinal cord (corticospinal tract). Figure 8–16 labels the cerebral peduncle on the left side of the midbrain (right side from the reader's point of view); of course, there is a matching peduncle on the right side of the brain

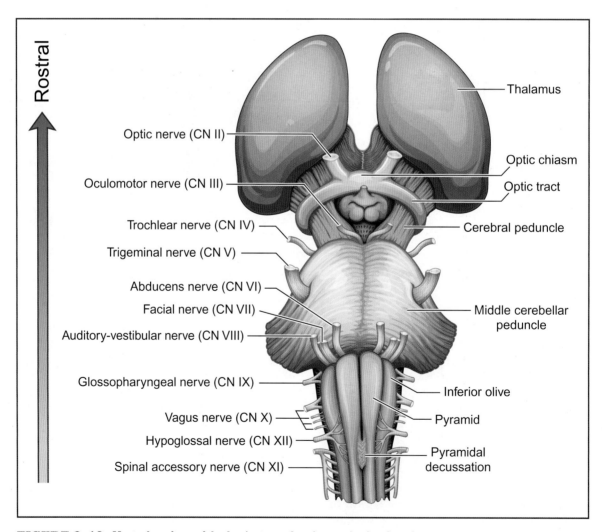

FIGURE 8–16. Ventral surface of the brainstem, showing major landmarks.

because both hemispheres issue a descending tract to motor nuclei in the brainstem and spinal cord. As shown in Figure 8–16, the cerebral peduncles enter the pons and continue through the middle part of the brainstem below the ventral surface.

The *optic chiasm* is located at the midline of the ventral surface of the midbrain. The optic chiasm is the location where the two optic nerves (paired cranial nerve II) meet before continuing into the cerebral hemispheres as the optic tracts. In Figure 8–16, the optic nerves have been cut because this view of the brainstem is drawn with more anterior structures—principally the face and neck—removed. The optic nerves originate at the retinas, and the destination of the optic tracts (which originate at the optic chiasm) is the occipital lobes of the cerebral hemispheres. Figure 8–16 shows the optic nerves entering the chiasm, where about half the fibers from each eye continue to the hemisphere on the same side as the eye, and the other half cross over to the opposite hemisphere. Each optic tract, therefore, carries fibers from both eyes, and a visual "field" from each eye is represented in both hemispheres.

Two additional features on the ventral surface of the midbrain are cranial nerves III (oculomotor nerve) and IV (trochlear nerve). The oculomotor nerve emerges from the midbrain at its junction with the pons, and the trochlear nerve exits the brainstem on its dorsal surface and circles around to be visible on the ventrolateral aspect of the brainstem, as shown in Figure 8–16. These cranial nerves are critical to the control of eye movements.

Ventral Surface of Pons

The anatomical structures that define the ventral surface of the pons are the thick bands of fibers running more or less horizontally across this surface (see Figure 8–16). These fiber tracts create the bulge of the pons and consist of three separate tracts called the *superior*, *middle*, and *inferior cerebellar peduncles*. The middle cerebellar peduncle (labeled in Figure 8–16) is the largest of these tracts and forms the bulk of the ventral surface of the pons. Collectively, the three cerebellar peduncles connect the cerebellum to the spinal cord, brainstem, and thalamus. The *pons*, a word meaning *bridge*, is well named because it serves as a bridge from the cerebellum to each major part of the CNS.

The other major landmarks on the ventral surface of the pons include the roots of four cranial nerves. Figure 8–16 shows these four nerves cut shortly after they emerge from the brainstem; they include cranial nerves V (trigeminal), VI (abducens), VII (facial), and VIII (auditory-vestibular). Cranial nerve V emerges as a large root from the middle of the pons, on its ventro-lateral aspect. Cranial nerves VI, VII, and VIII emerge between the lower edge of the pons and upper edge of the medulla, in a medial-to-lateral order, with VI being most medial and VIII most lateral. The roots of these three cranial nerves are included as surface features of the ventral pons because the nuclei from which they arise are completely (VI, VII) or partially (VIII) within the pons (see below, Figure 8–18).

Ventral Surface of Medulla

The ventral surface of the medulla shows two pairs of prominent columns. The two most medial columns are called the *pyramids*. The pyramids are the continuation into the medulla of the corticobulbar and corticospinal tracts. As noted above, these tracts descend in the midbrain as the crus cerebri and in the pons as pontine fascicles, below the ventral surface. The pyramids are the corticobulbar and corticospinal fibers emerging from inside the pons and organized in the medulla as the relatively long, medial columns on its ventral surface.

Toward the inferior border of the medulla, Figure 8–16 shows a landmark labeled "Pyramidal decussation." This is where the large majority of corticospinal fibers (roughly 80%) from one pyramid cross over to the other pyramid before their descent into the spinal cord. Fibers originating in the left cerebral hemisphere descend on the left side until crossing to the other side via the pyramidal decussation. Fibers from the right hemisphere descend on the right side before crossing to the left side via the decussation. The fibers from both hemispheres form an X-like pattern as they cross at the bottom of the medulla; in fact, the word *decussate* means the crossing of two "paths" that form an "X." The boundary between the medulla and the spinal cord is at the inferior edge of the pyramidal decussation.

Four cranial nerves are attached to the medulla and are landmarks on its ventral and ventrolateral surface. The most superior of these is cranial nerve IX (glossopharyngeal), shown exiting the right side of the lateral medulla just lateral to the inferior olive, a nucleus within the medulla that creates a columnar bulge on the surface. The column that forms the inferior olive, as shown of the right side of Figure 8–16, is just lateral to the column formed by the pyramid.

Just inferior to the exit point of cranial nerve IX is cranial nerve X (vagus), attached to the medulla as a group of rootlets just lateral to the inferior olive. Cranial nerve XII (hypoglossal) is below the exit point of cranial nerve X but more medial, exiting the medulla in the first fissure lateral to the midline. Finally, the most inferior of the nerves exiting the ventral surface of the medulla is cranial nerve XI (spinal accessory nerve, sometimes called the accessory nerve), which like cranial nerves IX and X emerges from the fissure just lateral to the inferior olive.

Surface Features of the Brainstem: Dorsal View

A dorsal view of the brainstem, plus the thalamus above it, is shown in Figure 8–17. Recall that *dorsal* and *posterior* imply the same direction or surface when referring to structures from the top of the brainstem down through the spinal cord. The view in Figure 8–17 is obtained when the midsagittal views of Figures 8–3 and 8–15 are rotated clockwise 90 degrees, so that the

back—the dorsal/posterior surface—of the brainstem is facing the observer. The cerebellum has been removed from this figure, as it would block a clear view of the dorsal surface of the brainstem. Cranial nerves attached to the medulla can be seen in this dorsal view, because they extend outward from their point of attachment on the ventral surface, as described above.

Dorsal Surface of Midbrain

Prominent surface features of the dorsal midbrain include the *superior* and *inferior colliculi* and the root of cranial nerve IV (trochlear), as shown in Figure 8–17. The superior and inferior colliculi are paired bumps forming the roof of the midbrain, jointly referred to as

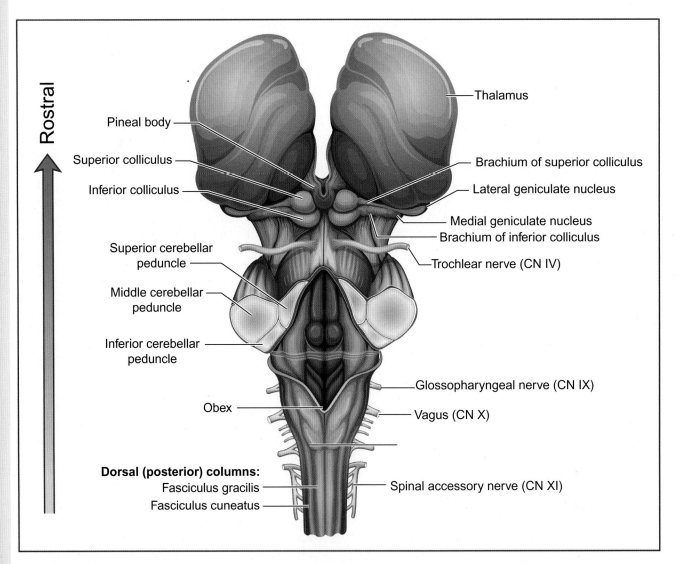

FIGURE 8–17. Dorsal surface of the brainstem, showing major landmarks. The cerebellum has been removed for this view and the cerebellar peduncles are shown with cuts prior to their entry point to the cerebellum.

the *corpora quadrigemina*. If the midsagittal MR image (see Figure 8–3, right) and artist's rendition (see Figure 8–4, lower left) are reexamined, these bumps can be seen on the small island of tissue that is separated from, and dorsal to, the bulk of the midbrain. The narrow channel separating the bulk of the midbrain from these dorsal bumps is the cerebral aqueduct, one of the series of cavities in the brain through which CSF is circulated.

The superior and inferior colliculi are nuclei along the visual and auditory pathways of the brain, respectively. These nuclei relay visual (superior colliculus) and auditory (inferior colliculus) information from more inferior nuclei in the brainstem to nuclei in the thalamus.

The root of cranial nerve IV (trochlear) emerges from the inferior border of the dorsal midbrain, close to the midline. Figure 8–17 shows the paired nerves running laterally from their roots; as noted above, the nerves wrap around the brainstem and can be seen in the ventral view as well (see Figure 8–16).

Dorsal Surface of Pons

Recall that the ventral surface of the pons is formed by fibers of the three cerebellar peduncles, which connect regions of the cerebral hemispheres, the brainstem, and the spinal cord to the cerebellum. These fiber tracts wrap around the brainstem on their way to the cerebellum. The dorsal view of the brainstem in Figure 8–17 shows these peduncles cut, because the cerebellum has been removed. Note the diamond-shaped cavity surrounded superiorly and laterally by the cerebellar peduncles and laterally and inferiorly by the medulla. This cavity is the *fourth ventricle*, which is part of the ventricular system that circulates CSF through the CNS. The fourth ventricle can also be seen in the midsagittal images of Figures 8–3 and 8–4.

Dorsal Surface of Medulla

Several bumps and bands of tissue can be seen in the floor of the fourth ventricle (colored dark brown in Figure 8–17), especially below the cut level of the inferior cerebellar peduncle. The floor of the fourth ventricle is its ventral wall, as seen in Figure 8–17; the roof of the fourth ventricle is its dorsal wall, formed largely by the cerebellum, especially along or close to the midline.

Cranial Nerves and Associated Brainstem Nuclei

Table 8–2 lists the 12 cranial nerves, their associated nuclei (which are primarily in the brainstem), and their major function(s). Figure 8–18 is a dorsal view of the brainstem showing the mediolateral locations and superior-inferior extents of the cranial nerve nuclei. The drawing does not indicate the position of the nuclei along the ventral-to-dorsal (anterior-to-posterior) dimension of the brainstem, as would be seen in a transverse section.

Some of the cranial nerves have purely sensory function, some purely motor function, and some both sensory and motor functions. In Table 8–2, those cranial nerves with purely sensory function (CN I, II, and VIII) are listed in normal font and those with purely motor function (CN III, IV, VI, XI, and XII) in bold font. Those having both motor and sensory function are called mixed nerves and are listed in italicized font.

Two of the cranial nerves (I and II) are not directly associated with nuclei in the brainstem. Cranial nerves I (olfactory) and II (optic) are both sensory and have their cell bodies in ganglia outside the brainstem, close to their specialized receptors. One cranial nerve with purely motor function, cranial nerve XI (accessory), has its nuclei in the upper part of the cervical spinal cord. The remaining cranial nerves have motor nuclei within the brainstem or, in the case of sensory components, ganglia whose projections are to nuclei within the brainstem.

The remainder of this section focuses on just seven of the cranial nerves (V, VII, VIII, IX, X, XI, and XII). These are singled out because of their relevance to speaking, swallowing, and hearing.

Cranial Nerve V (Trigeminal)

Cranial nerve V is a mixed nerve (both sensory and motor function) with three major divisions—ophthalmic, maxillary, and mandibular. The trigeminal nerve emerges from the ventrolateral surface of the pons as a large root (see Figure 8–16) containing sensory and motor fibers. A short distance away from the brainstem, the root separates into three major branches. The ophthalmic and maxillary divisions are purely sensory, carrying information on touch, pressure, and pain from the mid and upper face (including the forehead, front part of the scalp, and eyeball), maxillary teeth, sinuses, and meninges (coverings of the CNS; see below). The mandibular division contains both sensory and motor fibers. The sensory fibers of the mandibular division carry information on touch, pressure, and pain from the lower teeth, the skin of the lower face, the anterior two thirds of the tongue, the external auditory meatus, and parts of the pinna. The sensory division also carries information from specialized sensory organs (muscle spindles) in the jaw-closing muscles to a sensory

TABLE 8–2. Cranial Nerves, Their Associated Brainstem Nuclei, and General Function(s).

Nerve (Name)	Nuclei	Function(s)
I (Olfactory)	Olfactory Bulb[a]	Olfaction
II (Optic)	Midbrain[b]	Vision
III (Oculomotor)	**Oculomotor; Edinger-Westphal**	**Eye movement, pupil size and accommodation**
IV (Trochlear)	**Trochlear**	**Eye movement (one muscle)**
V (Trigeminal)	*Motor n. of V*	*Control of jaw muscles (closers and opener), mylohyoid m., tensor veli palatine m., tensor tympani m.*
	Sensory n. of V	*Sensation from entire face, teeth, palate, gums, anterior two-thirds of tongue*
VI (Abducens)	**Abducens**	**Eye movement (single muscle)**
VII (Facial)	*Facial motor n.*	*Control of muscles of facial expression and stapedius m.*
	Sup. Salivatory n.	*Control of salivary glands*
	Sensory n. of V	*Possible sensation from parts of external ear and parts of tonsils*
	N. solitarius	*Taste from anterior two-thirds of tongue*
VIII (Auditory-vestibular)	Cochlear n.	Audition
	Vestibular n.	Balance
IX (Glossopharyngeal)	*N. ambiguus*	*Control of stylopharyngeus m.*
	Sensory n. of V	*Sensation from parts of external ear, medial surface of eardrum, upper pharynx, posterior one-third of tongue*
	Salivatory n.	*Control of salivatory glands*
	N. solitarius	*Detection of chemical and pressure changes in blood; taste to posterior one-third of tongue*
X (Vagus)	*N. ambiguus*	*Control of velopharyngeal, pharyngeal, and laryngeal muscles*
	Sensory n. of V	*Sensation from meninges, parts of external ear and ear canal, external surface of eardrum, pharynx, and larynx*
	Dorsal motor n.	*Control of smooth muscle and glands of pharynx, larynx, heart, and digestive system*
	N. solitarius	*Sensation from heart, digestive system, esophagus, and trachea*
XI (Accessory)	**Accessory spinal n. (upper cervical cord)**	**Control of sternocleidomastoid and trapezius m.**
XII (Hypoglossal)	**Hypoglossal n.**	**Control of three of the four muscles of the tongue and all intrinsic muscles**

Note. Nerves that are purely sensory are in regular font, nerves that are purely motor are in bold font, and mixed nerves (with both sensory and motor function) are in italicized font.

[a] The olfactory nerve has sensory receptors embedded within the cribriform plate of the ethmoid bone, and the "nuclei" are in the olfactory bulbs (Figure 8–4, lower left image), which are located on the base of the frontal lobe, external to the brainstem. The olfactory "nerve" is therefore really the olfactory "tract" but is typically called a "nerve."

[b] The optic nerve does not make connections with brainstem nuclei in the sense of cranial nerves III–XII but rather sends fibers from the retina (the sensory receptors) to the lateral geniculate nucleus of the thalamus, which "forwards" this information to the visual cortex. Some optic nerve fibers go to the midbrain, where information is used by cranial nerves III, IV, and VI to control eye movements.

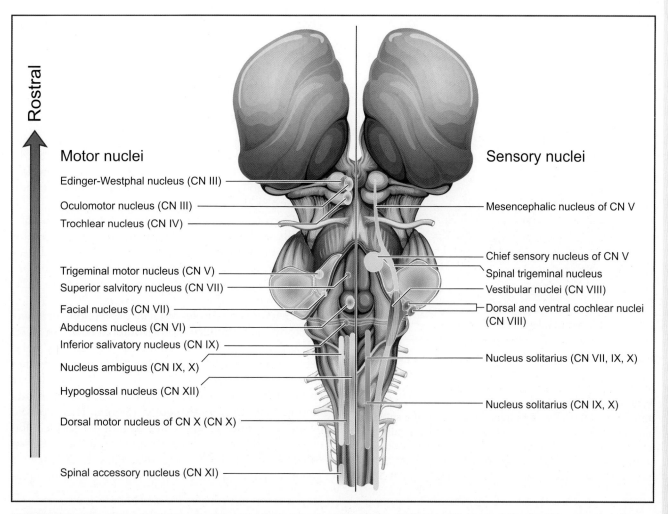

FIGURE 8–18. Dorsal view of brainstem showing locations of nuclei associated with cranial nerves. Motor nuclei are shown on the left side of the brainstem and sensory nuclei on the right side. This view allows an estimate of the location of nuclei along the medial-to-lateral plane of the brainstem, as well as the length of nuclei along the inferior-superior dimension of the brainstem but does not provide information on nuclei location along the anteroposterior (that is, ventral-dorsal) dimension.

nucleus in the brainstem, the mesencephalic nucleus of V (Figure 8–19). These specialized organs are an important component of an orofacial reflex called the jaw-jerk reflex. The motor part of the mandibular division innervates the jaw closing muscles and the single jaw-opener for speech (anterior belly of the *digastric* muscle), the *palatal tensor* muscle, the *tensor tympani* muscle, and the *mylohyoid* muscle (see Chapters 3, 4, and 5).

The motor fibers of cranial nerve V are derived from the trigeminal motor nucleus (also called the motor nucleus of V), located in the pons roughly midway between its superior and inferior borders (see Figure 8–18, left side). In a transverse section of the pons, the trigeminal motor nuclei are found ventral to the floor of the fourth ventricle and somewhat lateral to the midline; this can be seen in Figure 8–20. The motor

fibers run laterally from the two nuclei, exit the pons on the same side as the nuclei (e.g., the left motor nucleus generates a motor tract on the left side of the pons), and innervate muscles on the same side of the head (that is, ipsilaterally).

As shown in light green on the right side of Figure 8–18, the sensory nucleus of V runs the entire length of the brainstem, from midbrain to medulla. The sensory nucleus of V is separated into three main parts, including the mesencephalic nucleus of V in the midbrain, the chief (or principal) sensory nucleus in the pons, and the spinal trigeminal nucleus in the lower pons and length of the medulla.

Here is a simple account of the functions of the three parts of the sensory nucleus of V. The chief (principal) sensory nucleus in the pons receives information on touch and pressure from the face, tongue, teeth, and other facial structures whose sensory function is served by the trigeminal nerve. The spinal trigeminal nucleus receives information on pain and temperature from these same areas, as well as touch and pressure information from small regions of the head and neck. The mesencephalic (midbrain) nucleus of V is specialized for receiving fibers originating in the muscle spindles of the jaw-closing muscles.

Cranial Nerve VII (Facial)

The facial nerve is a mixed nerve. The fibers of the facial nerve originate in the facial motor nucleus, located in the mid-pons. This nucleus is slightly ventral and lateral to the abducens nucleus, as labeled on the left side of Figure 8–21.

The tract issued from the facial motor nucleus runs dorsally in the brainstem before exiting on the ventral surface between the pons and medulla. The dorsal course wraps around the abducens nucleus before heading ventrally toward the exit point (Figure 8–21, tract shown in yellow).

Virtually all muscles of facial expression are innervated by the voluntary motor component of the facial nerve, issued from the facial motor nucleus. The facial nerve also innervates the stapedius muscle, which attaches to the neck of the stapes in the middle ear and pulls on it reflexively in response to acoustic events having extremely high sound energy. The acoustic (stapedius) reflex protects hair cells in the cochlea, the end organ of hearing, from extremely loud sounds (see sidetrack titled (Re)Flexing Your Ears in Chapter 6). The innervation of the stapedius muscle from the same

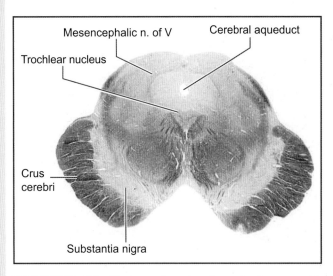

FIGURE 8–19. Horizontal section through a human midbrain, roughly halfway between its superior and inferior boundaries. The slice is prepared with a process that stains fiber tracts dark (note the crus cerebri at the anterior [ventral] edge of the slice) and nuclei light (note the substantia nigra, just posterior to the crus cerebri). The small hole in the center and somewhat posterior part of the section is the cerebral aqueduct, the passageway through which CSF flows from the third to fourth ventricles (see also Figure 8–32).

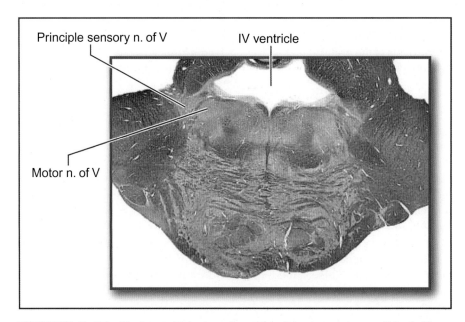

FIGURE 8–20. Horizontal section through a human pons, roughly halfway between its superior and inferior boundaries. This section was made to intersect the motor nucleus of V (see relative inferior-superior location of motor nucleus of V in Figure 8–18).

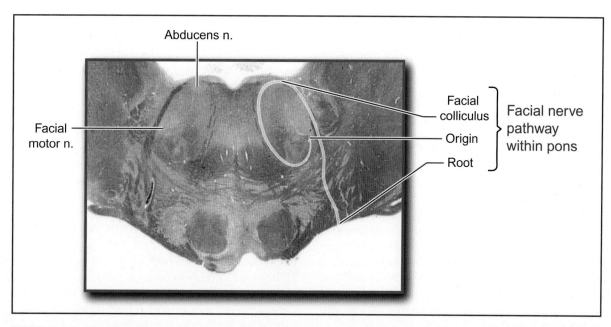

FIGURE 8–21. Horizontal section through a human pons, inferior to the cut shown in Figure 8–20. The section was made to intersect the facial motor nuclei and the abducens nuclei (see relative inferior-superior location of these two motor nuclei in Figure 8–18). The pathway shown in yellow (on the right side) is the tract leading from the facial motor nucleus to the exit of cranial nerve VII on the ventral surface of the brainstem, at the junction between the medulla and pons. Note the looping of the pathway around the abducens nucleus, in the floor of the fourth ventricle, before the tract turns anteriorly toward its exit point from the brainstem.

pool of fibers that supply muscles of facial expression is useful anatomical knowledge when a clinical profile includes both facial paralysis and absence of the acoustic reflex.

Cranial nerve VII also carries autonomic motor fibers to glands that secrete tears and saliva. The term *autonomic* is reserved for nervous system function that is not voluntary. The motor cells for this part of cranial nerve VII are found in the superior salivatory nucleus (see Figure 8–18, left side, small nucleus colored brown in pons, superior to the abducens nucleus). The salivatory axons exit the brainstem with the rest of the facial nerve fibers. Examples of involuntary motor functions controlled by fibers of cranial nerves include production of saliva (cranial nerve IX), regulation of blood pressure (cranial nerves IX and X), and activation of sweat glands (cranial nerve X).

The sensory component of cranial nerve VII includes general touch and pressure, as well as taste. Sensory innervation for touch and pressure is limited to small regions of the external ear, including the ear canal and the external surface of the eardrum. Sensory fibers from these regions make an initial synapse in a ganglion outside the brainstem, within the skull, and enter the brainstem through the root of cranial nerve VII. These fibers terminate in the chief sensory nucleus of V (see Figure 8–18, right side). Taste fibers innervate the ante-

rior two-thirds of the tongue, have an initial synapse in the same ganglion as other sensory fibers, and enter the brainstem with other sensory fibers through the root of cranial nerve VII, terminating in the nucleus solitarius.

Knowledge of the voluntary motor function of cranial nerve VII is important to speech-language pathologists. As one example, the motor component of cranial nerve VII controls the *orbicularis oris* muscles and the associated muscle complex (including muscles such as the *mentalis, levator anguli oris*, etc.; see Chapter 5) that are critical to the production of vowel contrasts that depend on labial configuration, as well as labial motions and configurations for consonants such as /p/, /b/, /f/, and /v/. These muscles, as well as muscles of the cheeks, also have an important role in swallowing.

Cranial Nerve VIII (Auditory-Vestibular)

The auditory-vestibular nerve is sensory. This cranial nerve has a double name because it carries information to the brainstem from the hearing, head position, and balance parts of the inner ear. Specifically, cranial nerve VIII carries nerve fibers from both the cochlea and semicircular canals to ganglia and subsequently to the brainstem (see Chapter 6, Figure 6–2).

The two nerve bundles of cranial nerve VIII approach and enter the dorsolateral aspect of the brainstem close to the junction of the medulla and pons (the pontomedullary junction). Figure 8–22 shows a transverse section of the brainstem, slightly inferior to the pontomedullary junction and therefore technically in the medulla. Note the entry point of the auditory portion of cranial nerve VIII and the close proximity of the cerebellum to the inferior, dorsolateral surfaces of the pons. The narrow space between the pons and cerebellum is referred to as the *cerebellopontine angle*.

Fibers of the cochlear (auditory) division of cranial nerve VIII synapse on cells in the cochlear nuclei (two on each side), located just below the dorsolateral surface of the pontomedullary junction (see Figure 8–22). Fibers from the vestibular division of the nerve synapse on cells of the vestibular nuclei (four on each side), located dorsally, more or less facing the ventral surface of the cerebellum. In the inferior-superior dimension shown on the right side of Figure 8–18, the vestibular nuclei (in purple) extend well above and below the pontomedullary junction.

The *central auditory pathways* consist of fiber tracts and several intervening nuclei connecting the cochlear nuclei to auditory cortical regions. A signal moves along the auditory pathway from the cochlea to the auditory nerve, from the auditory nerve to the cochlear nuclei, and from the cochlear nuclei to several other nuclei in the brainstem, the last of which are the inferior colliculi in the midbrain. The inferior colliculi send their information to the medial geniculate bodies of the thalamus, which sends information to the primary auditory cortex. Signals are processed from the auditory nerve through the brainstem quickly, with about a 5- to 6-ms lag between the firing of auditory nerve fibers and firing of cells in the inferior colliculus. An audiometric test called the auditory brainstem response (ABR), in which electrical signals generated by nervous system structures are measured with scalp electrodes and amplifiers, takes advantage of these very rapid but measurable transit times along the auditory nerve and brainstem pathways.

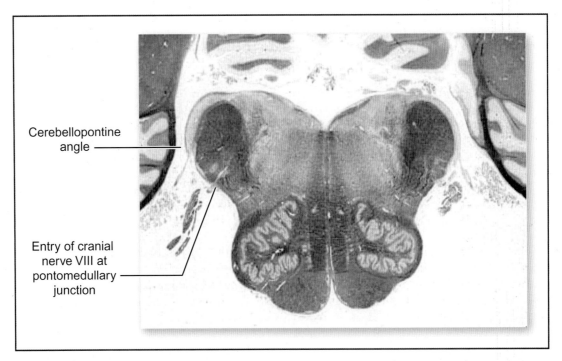

Cerebellopontine angle

Entry of cranial nerve VIII at pontomedullary junction

FIGURE 8–22. Horizontal section through a human brainstem, in the upper medulla just below its junction with the pons. This section shows the brainstem tissue surrounded by cerebellar tissue—note the small white space at the midline, between the posterior edge of the brainstem tissue and the more posterior cerebellar tissue (that is, a ventral surface of the cerebellum), which is part of the fourth ventricle. The section also shows the entry point of cranial nerve VIII to the brainstem, as well as the small, lateral space between the lower pons and the surrounding cerebellar tissue; this space is the cerebellopontine angle. The coiled nuclei in the ventrolateral part of the brainstem section are the inferior olivary nuclei whose most lateral "bend" forms the inferior olive landmark on the ventral surface of the brainstem (see Figure 8–16).

Cranial Nerve IX (Glossopharyngeal)

The glossopharyngeal is a mixed nerve. It is attached to the upper medulla in a groove on the lateral, ventral surface of the brainstem (see Figure 8–16). Voluntary motor fibers of cranial nerve IX originate in the superior portion of the nucleus ambiguus, a long column of motor neuron cells located in a cross-sectional view about midway between the ventral and dorsal surfaces of the medulla. Figure 8–18, left side, shows the nucleus ambiguus extending throughout the entire vertical length of the medulla. The motor component of cranial nerve IX innervates a single pharyngeal muscle, the *stylopharyngeus*. As described in Chapter 4, contraction of the paired *stylopharyngeus* muscles may lift and widen the pharyngeal tube. The specific role of this muscle in speech production is unknown, but it almost certainly plays a role in swallowing by shortening the pharyngeal tube (Meng, Murakami, Suzuki, & Miyamoto, 2008).

The glossopharyngeal nerve also has an autonomic motor component. The inferior salivatory nucleus in the upper medulla and close to the midline gives off fibers that exit the brainstem along with the voluntary motor fibers derived from the nucleus ambiguus. The autonomic fibers separate from the fibers en route to the *stylopharyngeus* muscle, the former innervating cells in the parotid gland. The parotid is the largest salivary gland of the head and neck and is located at —actually wrapped around—the ramus of the mandible (see Chapter 7, Figure 7–5). When stimulated by the autonomic fibers of cranial nerve IX, the gland secretes saliva into the oral and pharyngeal cavities.

The sensory component of the glossopharyngeal nerve transmits information on touch, temperature, and pressure from the posterior one-third of the tongue, parts of the pharynx, and the external ear and surface of the eardrum facing the middle ear cavity. The various sensory fibers serving these regions make first synapses in a pair of related ganglia, then enter the brainstem together at the root of cranial nerve IX (see Figure 8–16) and terminate in the brainstem, within the spinal part of the sensory trigeminal nucleus (see Figure 8–18). Cranial nerve IX also has an autonomic sensory component, part of which carries taste information from the posterior one-third of the tongue to cells at the top of the solitary nucleus. The other autonomic sensory component of cranial nerve IX conveys information on blood gases and blood pressure from receptors near the split of the common carotid artery into the internal and external carotid arteries (see Chapter 2, and below). Fibers from these receptors go to cells at the bottom of the solitary nucleus.

Cranial Nerve X (Vagus)

Cranial nerve X is a mixed nerve. It is attached to the brainstem as a series of roots in the same lateral groove as cranial nerve IX, immediately inferior to the latter nerve (see Figure 8–16). Also like cranial nerve IX, the voluntary motor fibers of the vagus nerve originate in cells of the nucleus ambiguus (see Figure 8–18). These cells and the fibers they give rise to innervate the *pharyngeal constrictor* muscles, the *palatal levator*, the *salpingopharyngeus*, the *palatopharyngeus* and *palatoglossus* muscles, and the intrinsic muscles of the larynx (*cricothyroid*, *thryoarytenoid*, *posterior cricoarytenoid*, *lateral cricoarytenoid*, and *arytenoid*) (see Chapters 3 through 5). The voluntary muscle component of cranial nerve X clearly plays an important role in speaking and swallowing, given its control of muscles that adjust the dimensions of the velopharyngeal port and the pharyngeal lumen, control tongue motion, and alter the tension and configuration of the vocal folds.

Cranial nerve X also has an autonomic motor component. Most of these fibers arise from the dorsal motor nucleus of X, which like the nucleus ambiguus forms a column throughout the medulla. The dorsal motor nucleus of X is medial to the nucleus ambiguus, more dorsal (hence its name), and close to the floor of the fourth ventricle. Fibers arising from cells in the dorsal motor nucleus of X (and possibly from a small region of the nucleus ambiguus as well) stimulate mucous glands within the pharynx and larynx, as well as glands within the gut and other organs. Autonomic motor function, with fibers derived from the dorsal motor nucleus of X, is also supplied by cranial nerve X for control of the smooth (nonvoluntary) muscle of the heart and gut.

Information on touch, pressure, and temperature is carried by sensory fibers from the pharynx, larynx, parts of the external ear and eardrum, and the meninges from the posterior part of the cerebral hemispheres. Like touch, pressure, and temperature information traveling in any cranial nerve (see information above on cranial nerves V, VII, and IX), these sensory fibers make initial synapses in ganglia outside the brainstem, enter the brainstem via the nerve roots for cranial nerve X, and travel to the lower part of the sensory nucleus of V.

Cranial nerve X includes an autonomic sensory component that carries sensation from the gut. These sensations are not conscious, as in the case of touch or pressure, but may result in a sense of "feeling good" or "feeling bad" (Wilson-Pauwels, Akesson, Stewart, & Spacey, 2002). Autonomic fibers also arise from chemoreceptors, baroreceptors (receptors sensitive to pressures), and the mucosal surfaces of the larynx. This information makes a first synapse in a pair of ganglia, which sends fibers into the brainstem at the point of attachment of the vagus roots and subsequently to the nucleus solitarius (see Figure 8–18, right side, dark green column).

Cranial Nerve XI (Spinal Accessory Nerve)

Cranial nerve XI, which is purely motor, is called the spinal accessory nerve because its motor neurons are located in the ventral horn of upper segments of the cervical spinal cord, rather than in the brainstem. Figure 8–18 shows the approximate location of this column of spinal cells, called the spinal accessory nucleus, extending four or five cervical segments down from the junction of the medulla and spinal cord. Note how the spinal accessory nucleus is in line with the columnar nucleus ambiguus in the medulla.

Why is a nerve with cells of origin in the spinal cord considered a cranial nerve? First, the nerve supplies motor innervation to two muscles of the head and neck, the *sternocleidomastoid* muscle and the *trapezius* muscle. The former muscle turns the head and lifts the chin toward the side opposite the contraction (when the right *sternocleidomastoid* contracts with its sternum end fixed, the head is turned and lifted toward the left side, and vice versa), and the latter muscle produces rotation of the scapula and raises the arm above the shoulder. Second, many authors regard the accessory nucleus as a continuation of the nucleus ambiguous, which innervates so many of the important muscles of speaking and swallowing. Third, the fibers issued from the accessory nucleus emerge from the spinal cord and ascend into the skull to travel with fibers of cranial nerves IX and X. Note in Figure 8–16 how the several rootlets of the accessory nerve emerge from the same groove as the rootlets of cranial nerves IX and X and travel superiorly along the edge of the spinal cord. Cranial nerves IX, X, and XI exit (or, in the case of the sensory components of IX and X, enter) the skull, as a group, through the same opening.

Cranial Nerve XII (Hypoglossal)

Cranial nerve XII is a motor nerve, innervating all the intrinsic muscles and all but one of the extrinsic muscles of the tongue (the exception being the *palatoglossus* muscle, innervated by cranial nerve X). The fibers of cranial nerve XII originate in the hypoglossal nucleus, a column of motor cells near the midline of the medulla (see Figure 8–18). Axons from these cells run ventrally and laterally to emerge as cranial nerve

XII on the ventral surface of the medulla, in the sulcus immediately lateral to the midline (see Figure 8–16).

The control of both intrinsic and extrinsic tongue muscles by cranial nerve XII means that virtually any lingual behavior relevant to speech production or swallowing is ultimately vested in the integrity of this nerve and its brainstem nuclei. This includes both fine adjustments to create the precise configurations required for the grooved tongue of fricatives such as /s/ and /sh/, larger-scale adjustments of tongue position associated with distinctions between (for example) front and back vowels, and the complex activity of the tongue during the initial phase of swallowing.

CORTICAL INNERVATION PATTERNS

This section describes the innervation of brainstem motor nuclei by cortical cells, specifically of the motor nuclei associated with speech- and swallowing-related muscles of the head and neck. As described above, these nuclei include the motor nucleus of V (trigeminal), the facial motor nucleus, the nucleus ambiguus, the spinal accessory nucleus, and the hypoglossal nucleus. The cortical innervation of the oculomotor nuclei (oculomotor, trochlear, and abducens nuclei) is not discussed here, nor is the innervation of nuclei associated with outflow of the autonomic system (salivatory nuclei, dorsal motor nucleus of X).

Table 8–3 summarizes the innervation patterns for the five paired brainstem motor nuclei that control speech and swallowing musculature of the head and neck. When both members of a specific motor nucleus pair receive input from the left and right motor cortices (from the primary motor cells in both the left and right hemispheres), the nuclei are bilaterally innervated. Table 8–3 classifies the motor nucleus of V, part of the facial motor nucleus, the nucleus ambiguus, and the accessory nucleus as receiving bilateral innervation. For example, both motor nuclei of V—on the left and right sides of the pons—receive corticobulbar projections from both the left and right hemispheres. Stated in another way, the left motor nucleus of V receives an ipsilateral projection from the left cerebral cortex and a contralateral projection from the right cerebral cortex. Similarly, the right motor nucleus of V receives an ipsilateral projection from the hemisphere and a contralateral projection from the left hemisphere.

Table 8–3 shows the innervation of the facial motor nucleus to be both contralateral and bilateral. The facial motor nucleus contains cells specific to muscles of the upper face and cells specific to muscles of the lower face. Cells for control of the lower facial muscles

TABLE 8–3. Cortical Innervation Patterns of the Brainstem Motor Nuclei for Speech Musculature

Motor Nucleus	Innervation
Motor nucleus of V (V)	Bilateral
Facial motor nucleus (VII)	Bilateral (upper face)
	Contralateral (lower face)
Nucleus ambiguus (IX, X, XI)	Bilateral
Accessory nucleus (XI)	Bilateral (*sternocleidomastoid* muscle)
	Contralateral (*trapezius* muscle)
Hypoglossal nucleus (XII)	Contralateral

Note. The cranial nerves associated with these motor nuclei are indicated in parenthesis.

receive only contralateral innervation from the cortex, whereas cells for control of the upper facial muscles receive bilateral innervation from the motor cortex. Raising your eyebrows in surprise, for example, is the result of commands from both sides of the motor cortex to both facial motor nuclei. In contrast, movement of the corner of your right lower lip is produced by commands only from the left motor cortex to the right facial motor nucleus.

Like the facial motor nucleus, the accessory nucleus has both contralateral and bilateral innervation from the motor cortex. There is some dispute about the pathways from the motor cortex to the upper regions of the cervical spinal cord, where the accessory nucleus is located, but the most conservative view seems to be that the *sternocleidomastoid* muscle is innervated bilaterally and the *trapezius* muscle contralaterally (DeToledo & David, 2001; see Wilson-Pauwels et al., 2002, for a different interpretation).

The hypoglossal nucleus, which controls muscles of the tongue, is the only motor nucleus of the brainstem with strictly contralateral innervation from the motor cortex. Tongue cells in the left motor cortex innervate cells in the right hypoglossal nucleus, and vice versa (see sidetracks called Why Innervation Patterns Matter: Part I and Part II).

Why Innervation Patterns Matter: Part I

Innervation patterns have significance for clinical signs of neurological disease. Because the brainstem motor nuclei innervate the speech muscles ipsilaterally—that is, motor nuclei on the left side of the brainstem innervate muscles on the left side of the head and neck, and motor nuclei on the right side of the brainstem innervate muscles on the right side of the head and neck—knowledge of the innervation of the brainstem nuclei by cortical structures can lead to important clues concerning where a lesion is located in neurological disease. These clues include the appearance of head and neck structures at rest and their performance during voluntary maneuvers. For example, a unilateral, cortical lesion of cells that control muscles of the face should not result in a deficit of upper face control but may result in a loss of lower face control on the side opposite the lesion. The unilateral cortical lesion will cause loss of input to the facial motor nucleus on the same side (ipsilateral to the lesion) and to the facial motor nucleus on the opposite side (contralateral to the lesion), but these facial motor nuclei still receive healthy input from the undamaged motor cortex on the other side of the brain, allowing for more or less normal appearance and functional muscle contraction for muscles of the upper face. The unilateral cortical damage does, however, result in a deficit in appearance and control of the lower face contralateral to the lesion. This is because the cells in the facial motor nucleus that control lower face muscles receive cortical input only from the contralateral hemisphere.

Why Innervation Patterns Matter: Part II

Unlike the case of bilateral innervation reviewed in the preceding sidetrack, a unilateral lesion of tongue cells in the motor cortex should result in an observable deficit. The contralateral-only innervation of the hypoglossal nuclei suggests this expectation. For example, a unilateral lesion among tongue motor neurons in the right motor cortex affects the strength of muscles on the left side of the muscular complex of the tongue. A simple test of the integrity of tongue motion is to request an individual to protrude her tongue, in a straight line. In the neurologically healthy individual, the tongue is centered as it is protruded, balanced by the roughly equivalent strength of the paired musculature (primarily the *genioglossus* muscle)

producing the protrusion. In a person with a unilateral cortical lesion in tongue cells, the tongue muscles on the side opposite the lesion are weak; therefore, when the tongue is protruded from the mouth, the healthy side pushes the tongue "away from the lesion." For example, a lesion in the left motor cortex results in weakness of the *genioglossus* muscle on the right side of the tongue, which causes the tongue to deviate rightward when protruded from the mouth, away from the left-side cortical lesion. The tongue deviates toward the weak side during a protrusion gesture because the "strong" genioglossus on the left side of the tongue is not balanced by an equally strong genioglossus on the right side of the tongue.

SPINAL CORD AND SPINAL NERVES

Spinal Cord

The spinal cord includes gray and white matter and extends as a long column of tissue from the first cervical vertebrae (C1) to the first or second lumbar vertebrae (L1, L2). The superior edge of the spinal cord is continuous with the inferior edge of the medulla. Although the inferior edge of the spinal cord terminates at L1 or L2, the protective coverings of the brain and spinal cord, including the dura and arachnoid mater—labeled in Figure 8–23 and discussed below in the section Meninges, Ventricles, Blood Supply—continue nearly to the bottom of the sacral vertebrae. The space enclosed within the meningeal coverings below the inferior termination of the spinal cord is filled with CSF.

A vertical segment of spinal cord tissue, plus its protective coverings and nerves exiting and entering the cord, is shown in Figure 8–23. The view is from the front and slightly above and to the right of a horizontal (transverse) slice across the cord. The roughly H-shaped, darker part seen in this transverse slice is composed of clusters of neuron cell bodies (gray matter), and the whitish area surrounding these cells (white matter) are axons ascending and descending in the spinal cord and entering and leaving the spinal cord. The specific form of the H-shaped cluster of cell bodies varies by the level of the spinal cord at which a horizontal slice is made. The slice shown in Figure 8–23 is at the lower end of the cervical cord; the gross ana-

tomical facts described in the next paragraph apply to any level of the cord.

The anterior (ventral) midline of the spinal cord is defined by the *anterior median fissure*; the corresponding midline groove on the posterior (dorsal) aspect of the spinal cord is the *posterior median septum*. At any level of the spinal cord, the H-shaped cluster of cell bodies is more or less symmetrical with respect to these anterior and posterior median landmarks.

The spinal cord gray matter in Figure 8–23 appears as paired posterior horns and paired anterior horns. The "horns" are the clusters of cell bodies in the ventral (anterior) or dorsal (posterior) halves of the transverse section. Dorsal horn cells are typically sensory, receiving input from axons traveling from peripheral body structures to the spinal cord, and ventral horn cells issue axons that exit the spinal cord to provide motor innervation to muscles.

The white matter of the spinal cord is a dense composition of axons running in many different directions. In any transverse section, spinal cord white matter includes axons entering and leaving the cord, ascending and descending in the cord, and even traveling between cell bodies within the cord. The details of each of these fiber tracts are outside the scope of this text, but as in the cerebral hemispheres, the fibers are arranged systematically and can be described by a general "geography" within any section of the cord. For example, the corticospinal tract, which originates in the primary motor cortex and other parts of the frontal lobe and continues through the internal capsule until most of the fibers decussate in the medulla, descends

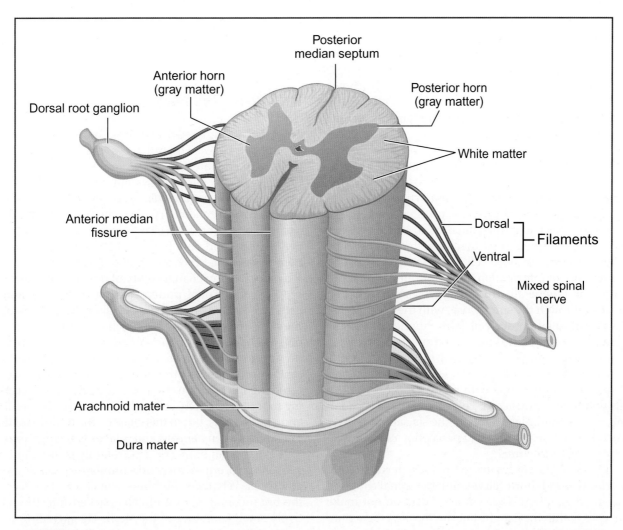

FIGURE 8–23. View of a section of the spinal cord from the front and slightly above a horizontal cut through the lower cervical cord. The horizontal cut shows the central gray matter in an H-shaped pattern and the white matter surrounding it. The dorsal and ventral root filaments entering and leaving the spinal cord, respectively, are shown, as are the meningeal coverings.

as a fairly tight bundle in the lateral part of the spinal cord. At each level of the spinal cord, this *lateral corticospinal tract* issues axons to the anterior horn cells on the same side. Recall that a small proportion (about 20%) of motor fibers originating in the motor cortex do not decussate in the medulla but rather continue into the spinal cord on the same side as their origination. These fibers form the *anterior corticospinal tract*, which runs in the anterior (ventral) part of the spinal cord white matter, just lateral to the anterior median fissure. Other motor tracts in the spinal cord are not discussed here.

Sensory fibers that ascend from posterior (dorsal) horn cells in the spinal cord run primarily in the posterior (dorsal) white matter columns lateral to the posterior median septum. These fibers synapse in the brainstem, followed by a synapse in the thalamus before projecting to cortical sensory cells. The fibers carry information on touch, pain, and temperature that originates from peripheral body structures.

Spinal Nerves

As shown in Figure 8–23, spinal nerves are attached to each segment of the spinal cord and have the following general organizational scheme. Dorsal root filaments (filaments are small bundles of nerve fibers) that carry sensory information enter the spinal cord close to the most posterior (dorsal) tip of the spinal gray matter. Ventral root filaments, which carry motor information, exit the spinal cord lateral to the anterior median fissure, close to the most anterior border of the anterior (ventral) horns. At each segment of the spinal cord, several of these nerve filaments are gathered into a single nerve bundle just outside the cord. Figure 8–23 shows the sensory (dorsal) filaments as red fibers entering the spinal cord, and the motor (ventral) filaments as blue fibers exiting the spinal cord.

At a short distance from the entrance or exit of these nerves into or from the spinal cord, there is a ganglion for each spinal nerve. Those entering the dorsal root ganglia contain the first synapses for sensory fibers from peripheral structures en route to the nerve root that enters the spinal cord. When sensory fibers enter the spinal cord, therefore, the synapse they make in a posterior horn cell is the *second* synapse in the sequence of information transfer from periphery to cortex. This is generally true for all sensory information in transit through the spinal cord, with the exception of sensory information derived from muscle spindles in voluntary muscle of the limbs and trunk. Sensory fibers from muscle spindles embedded in limb and trunk muscles bypass a synapse in dorsal root ganglia and make direct connections with posterior (dorsal) horn cells within the spinal cord. This increases the speed of limb reflexes and plays a role in the sensation of body structure position in space and perception of the movement of body structures.

Figure 8–23 shows motor nerves derived from anterior (ventral) horn cells exiting the spinal cord and entering a ganglion. These motor fibers do not make synapses within the ganglia but run through them bundled together with sensory fibers. Beyond the ganglia, toward the periphery, motor and sensory fibers associated with the spinal cord always run together; spinal nerves are therefore mixed (both sensory and motor) nerves. For example, the spinal nerves associated with the *internal intercostal* and *external intercostal* muscles are derived from the 1st (T1) through 11th (T11) thoracic segments (Chapter 2, Table 2–2). Sensory fibers from receptors in these muscles carry information back to the spinal cord concerning touch, pressure, and stretch (the latter via muscle spindles). Motor fibers in these nerves control the contraction properties of the muscles. In general, the level at which a spinal nerve exits the spinal cord is consistent with the body level of the structures innervated by the nerves. Thus, arm and hand muscles are innervated by spinal nerves from cervical segments of the cord, rib cage wall muscles by spinal nerves from thoracic segments, and abdominal wall muscles from lumbar segments. Two well-known exceptions to this general rule are the diaphragm, which corresponds in position to the lower level of the thoracic cord but is innervated from the third through

fifth cervical segments of the spinal cord, and the feet and legs, which are innervated from lumbar segments of the spinal cord.

NERVOUS SYSTEM CELLS

The CNS is composed of fluids, blood vessels, and several cell types. The cell types can be divided into the two major categories of *neurons* and *glial cells*. All the cells of the nervous system sit in a bath of fluids—called the *extracellular space*—with very precise, yet changeable, chemistry. This chemistry is regularly changed on a short-term basis—in fact, millions of times per second—and on a long-term basis as well. Interactions between neurons and glial cells contribute to both the precision and changeability of this chemical profile.

The traditional understanding of the difference between the two major types of cells is that neurons are the signaling cells in the brain, whereas glial cells function as support and nourishment for the neurons and do not transmit signals. Signaling cells are those that send information to other cells and are also capable of receiving information from one or many cells. According to recent research, some glial cells may also receive and send signals, but in this chapter, the traditional distinction between neurons and glial cells is emphasized.

The human brain contains roughly 80 to 95 billion neurons and either the same number or many more glial cells. Whatever numbers one chooses to accept, the brain contains a lot of cells packed into the relatively small container of the skull. The signaling cells send and receive a staggering amount of information per unit time and in doing so generate and expend a tremendous amount of energy.

There is practical value in understanding the structure and physiology of nervous system cells because many neurological diseases with consequences for speech, language, hearing, and swallowing behavior are explained partly or largely in terms of dysfunction of basic cellular anatomy and physiology. In addition, pharmacological and other treatments for these diseases often target aspects of basic cellular physiology. The following sections cover the structure and function of glial cells and neurons, the nature of neuronal potentials (resting and action), synaptic transmission and neurotransmitters, and the neuromuscular junction.

Glial Cells

Figure 8–24 shows a neuron and selected glial cells with which it shares brain space. The primary role of glial cells, according to present understanding, is to support the integrity of the signaling cells—the neurons—in a number of ways. Glial cells come in several forms, including *astrocytes*, *oligodendrocytes*, and others, as listed in Table 8–4.

The most numerous glial cells are *astrocytes*, shown in Figure 8–24 by a star-shaped cell with appendage-like projections from a central body. (Other subtypes of astrocyte may have different forms.) Astrocytes were at one time thought of as not much more than biological filler material between neurons, but recent research suggests a much more important role for these cells. This role includes a contribution to the control of the chemical makeup of the extracellular environment, including regulation of the molecules permitted to pass

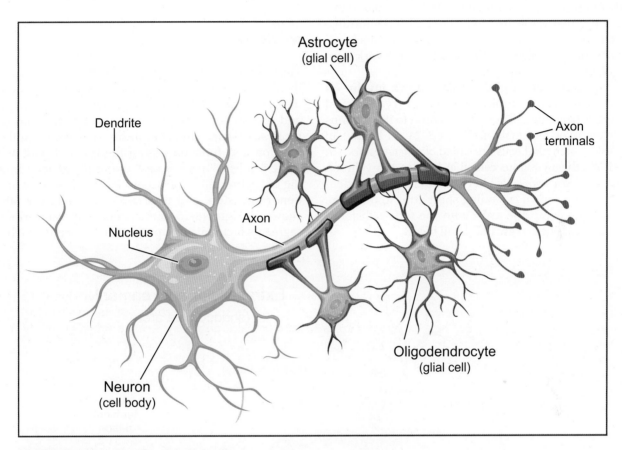

FIGURE 8–24. Neuron and glial cells.

TABLE 8–4. Types and General Functions of Glial Cells and Neurons

Type	Function
Glial Cells	Nonsignaling
Astrocytes	"Anchor" neurons to blood supply
	Regulate neuron extracellular environment
Oligodendrocytes (Schwann cells in PNS)	Myelin forming
Microglia	Remove dead material
Ependymal	Produce cerebrospinal fluid
Neurons	Signaling
Many types	

from the blood supply of the brain to the extracellular fluid. In addition, astrocytes form protective barriers around synapses (locations where information is transmitted from one neuron to another), apparently to ensure that neurotransmitters (chemicals used in neural communication) released at a particular synapse ("connections" between neurons) do not spread to other locations where they are not needed or where they might interfere with other transmissions. Astrocytes also play a role in removal of excess neurotransmitter after it has been released and provide "anchors" for neurons, as if they are the skeletal framework from which neurons are hung.

Another type of glial cell lays down myelin on axons, the narrow projections that carry electrical impulses from the cell body of a neuron to its terminus (labeled "axon terminals" in Figure 8–24, see below). In the CNS, such glial cells are called *oligodendrocytes*. (In the PNS, the analogous cells that lay down myelin on nerves are *Schwann* cells.) In Figure 8–24, the oligodendrocytes are shown extending short arms to the axon. These arms wrap the axon with the fatty substance myelin, described in greater detail below.

Other glial cells (not shown in the figure) include those responsible for removing dead material in the brain; these are called microglia. Finally, the fluid-filled ventricles of the brain contain ependymal cells along their walls. These cells generate the fluid (CSF) that flows through the ventricles. Technically, ependymal cells are not glia because their embryological origin is different from the origins of astrocytes and oligodendrocytes.

Neurons

The structure of the neuron is critical to understanding its normal physiology and how it may be affected by disease. Figure 8–25 is a schematic image of a neuron and several of its component structures. Neurons differ in size, shape, and complexity, depending on their location and function within the brain. This is why Table 8–4 lists "many types" under the general heading of "neurons." All neurons have a cell body (soma), dendrites, axon, and a terminal segment, the latter shown in Figure 8–25 within a shaded oval. Terminal segments include many projections, the ends of which

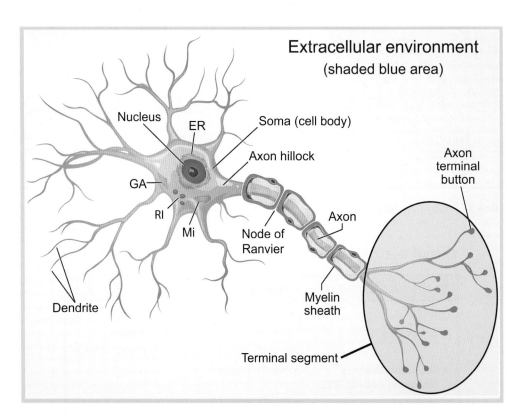

FIGURE 8–25. Neuron showing structures within the soma (ER = endoplasmic reticulum; Mi = mitochondria; GA = Golgi apparatus; RI = ribosomes) that manufacture proteins and neurotransmitters, as well as other components of the neuron. The myelin sheath is not continuous across the entire length of the axon; the small gaps between adjacent myelin wraps are called nodes of Ranvier. Note the many dendrites associated with the soma; also note the complex terminal segment of the neuron.

are called "terminal buttons." Throughout this chapter, "terminal segment" is used to describe this part of a neuron. The extracellular fluid in which neurons are contained is shaded blue in Figure 8–25.

Structures inside the neuron are its *intra*cellular components. The intracellular components of a neuron are separated from the extracellular environment by a membrane with special properties. The membrane is impermeable to a number of different types of molecules but can change its permeability to those molecules by the action of substances manufactured within the cell body.

Cell Body (Soma)

The cell body or *soma* is typically a relatively large, spherical structure. To call the cell body "relatively large" is to describe the size of a tiny structure in a brain-world of other tiny structures. A typical soma is about 20 μm in diameter (0.000020 meters, perhaps 100 times smaller than the diameter of a poppyseed).

Inside the cell body is the nucleus, as well as a number of critical structures called *organelles*. Among the organelles shown in Figure 8–25 are mitochondria (Mi), endoplasmic reticula (ER: where reticulum is the singular), Golgi apparatus (GA), and ribosomes (RI). Collectively, the organelles serve the neuron's metabolic functions, generate proteins that affect the properties of cell membranes, and manufacture and transport neurotransmitters to the terminal segment of axons.

The membrane that separates the cell body and its contents from the extracellular environment is composed of lipids (fatty and/or oily substances that are insoluble in water). Embedded in the membrane are protein molecules. The membrane's permeability to various molecules can be changed very rapidly by the action of these proteins. Changes in cell membrane permeability are critical to understanding the neuron's basic function of conducting electrical impulses from the soma to terminal segment (see below, section on Action Potential). More advanced information on the function of organelles, the synthesis of neurotransmitters, and their transport from soma to terminal segment is presented in Bear et al. (2016) and Kandel et al. (2012).

The cell body gives off microtubules that extend like railroad tracks within the axon to the terminal segment. Proteins and other substances synthesized in the cell body are transported to the terminal segment by means of the microtubules.

Dendrites

As shown in Figure 8–25, many short projections from the cell body extend into the extracellular space. These are *dendrites*, and the entire set of them extending from the cell body is called the *dendritic tree*. The membranes of dendrites contain protein molecules that are called *receptors*. Receptors detect neurotransmitters and in many cases are "tuned" to specific neurotransmitters. The section on Synaptic Transmission and Neurotransmitters provides information on how the terminal segment of one neuron interacts with the dendritic tree of another nearby neuron.

Axon and Terminal Segment

Axons can be truly short (less than a millimeter) or exceptionally long (close to a meter). Axons emerge from the cell body as a narrow projection that ends just before the terminal segment. Proteins and other substances synthesized in the cell body are transported to the terminal segment via the microtubules. The axon is the means by which a neuron transmits an electrical impulse from the cell body to the terminal segment.

The proteins that are synthesized in the cell body and transported down the axon are stored in "packets" within the terminal segment. These packets are called synaptic vesicles. Synaptic vesicles are tiny, membrane-encased packets of neurotransmitter, critical to the transfer of information from one neuron to another.

Axons are typically wrapped in myelin, the fatty substance produced by oligodendrocytes (see Table 8–4). Figure 8–25 shows the myelin wrapping to be discontinuous along the axon, so that intervals of myelin-covered axon are interrupted by small breaks. These small breaks are called *nodes of Ranvier*. The myelin wrapping and nodes of Ranvier improve conduction speed of electrical impulses from cell body to terminal segments (explained in more detail below). Most axons in the CNS and PNS are myelinated, but certain functional systems (such as the pathways responsible for pain and temperature perception) have a fair number of unmyelinated axons.

Synapse

Figure 8–26 illustrates the essential features of a synapse. The typical synapse is composed of the terminal segment of one neuron, the dendritic tree of another, and the space between these structures.

The structure of a synapse has a *presynaptic membrane*, a *postsynaptic membrane*, and the small space between them, called the *synaptic cleft*. The presynaptic membrane encases the terminal segment and separates it from the synaptic cleft; the postsynaptic membrane covers the dendrites of another neuron and separates it from the synaptic cleft. The synaptic cleft is in the extracellular fluid (fluid outside of the neurons) and may also contain substances that join the presynaptic and postsynaptic membranes.

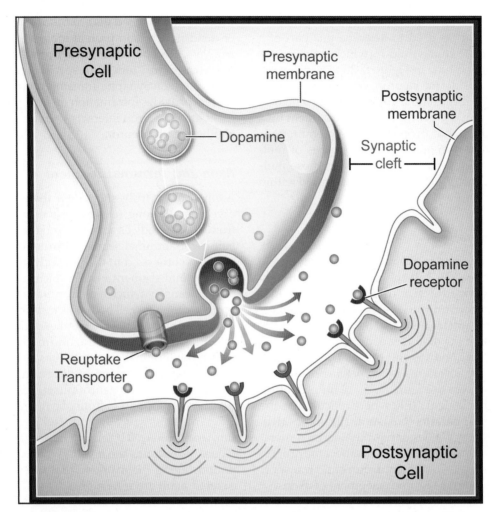

FIGURE 8–26. Essential features of a synapse. The drawing shows a terminal segment, whose covering is called the presynaptic membrane. Inside the segment are packets containing neurotransmitter molecules, illustrated in this drawing by dopamine molecules. The postsynaptic membrane, associated with a different neuron, is shown in light salmon and separated from the presynaptic membrane by a small gap filled with extracellular fluid called the synaptic cleft. Embedded within the postsynaptic membrane are receptors often specialized for a particular neurotransmitter, in this example dopamine. The dopamine released from the presynaptic membrane binds to the dopamine-tuned receptors on the postsynaptic membrane. Excess neurotransmitter that is released into the synaptic cleft is restored to the terminal segment by a reuptake transporter. Once inside the terminal segment, the recovered neurotransmitter is repackaged for later use.

Presynaptic Membrane

The presynaptic membrane is the cell wall at the end of the axon; it encases the synaptic vesicles within the terminal segments. In Figure 8–26, synaptic vesicles are shown as light brown spheres that contain dopamine neurotransmitter molecules. Embedded within the presynaptic membrane are special proteins that under the right conditions allow synaptic vesicles to attach to the membrane and "dump" their neurotransmitter contents into the synaptic cleft. A single terminal segment may contain synaptic vesicles storing different kinds of neurotransmitters; individual neurons are not limited to a single neurotransmitter. Structures in the presynaptic membrane, called reuptake transporters, take back neurotransmitter that is not used in synaptic transmission. The recovered neurotransmitter is repackaged in synaptic vesicles and used for future synaptic activity. The presynaptic membrane can be thought of as the component of a synapse from which neural signals are sent.

Postsynaptic Membrane

The postsynaptic membrane is the receiving part of a synapse, where signals sent from the presynaptic membrane of one neuron are picked up for processing by another neuron. Like the presynaptic membrane, the postsynaptic membrane is partly composed of protein molecules that serve the specialized purpose of receiving neurotransmitter signals. The molecules embedded in the postsynaptic membrane form receptors that in many cases are specialized for the detection of particular neurotransmitters. A postsynaptic membrane of a single neuron may contain receptors specialized for a variety of neurotransmitters.

Synaptic Cleft

The synaptic cleft is the intercellular "space" between the presynaptic and postsynaptic membranes. The scare quotes emphasize the miniature width of the synaptic cleft (between 20 and 50 millionths of a millimeter). The cleft includes a meshwork of proteins that not only serves as the medium through which a neurotransmitter is conveyed from the presynaptic to postsynaptic membranes but also attaches the two membranes. The presynaptic membrane, synaptic cleft, and postsynaptic membranes are bound together as an anatomical unit.

Resting Potential, Action Potential, and Neurotransmitters

Information is transmitted in the nervous system by the conversion of electrical energy into neurochemical energy, which is subsequentially transformed back into electrical energy. It is the changeable characteristics of cell membranes that hold the key to understanding how neurons send electrical signals from the soma to the terminal segment. The following paragraphs present a simple overview of this signaling process.

Resting Potential

Figure 8–27 shows a schematic neuron with a focus on the chemical, ionic environment of the soma when the neuron is at rest (not stimulated). Some ions have a positive electrical charge, whereas others have a negative electrical charge. The two most important of the positively charged ions in the extracellular fluid are potassium ($K+$) and sodium ($Na+$). Within the cell body, in the intracellular fluid, a group of unspecified negatively charged ions is shown. Note that the ionic environment depicted in Figure 8–27 is relative; that

is, because $K+$ and $Na+$ ions are shown to be restricted to outside the soma does not actually mean that these ions are not also within the cell body. Rather, after ionic equilibrium is established, it means that the positive ions ($K+$ and $Na+$) are more highly concentrated in the extracellular fluid than in the intracellular fluid.

At rest, the membrane of a neuron cell body is relatively permeable (allowing easy passage) to $K+$ molecules. On the other hand, the membrane is not permeable to $Na+$ molecules or the negatively charged ions concentrated inside the soma. The selective membrane permeability to $K+$ is the result of openings, like tiny pores, within the membrane that are specifically available for the passage of $K+$ molecules. These special openings are a relatively constant characteristic of the cell membrane.

The presence of $K+$ openings helps explain how "ionic equilibrium," the equal and opposite electrical forces across the cell membrane that define the resting state of the cell, is achieved. Before ionic equilibrium is established, $K+$ molecules are concentrated *inside* the soma; their numbers inside the soma are much greater than in the extracellular fluids. Ions with unequal concentrations in two locations always seek to establish equilibrium of concentration between the locations. Because of the unequal concentration of $K+$ inside and outside the soma, the permanent openings to $K+$ within the cell membrane result in more $K+$ traffic outward to the extracellular fluid, as compared with traffic inward to the intracellular fluid. When more $K+$ molecules pass out of the soma than move into it, the result is a more negative charge within the soma relative to outside the soma. A critical phase in this process of net $K+$ movement to the extracellular fluid is when the tendency of the positively charged ions to leave the soma is exactly balanced by the negative electrical charge inside the soma. When this occurs, equilibrium is reached and the movement of $K+$ ions ceases. This can be likened to two forces pulling with identical magnitudes in opposite directions. One force is exerted by $K+$ molecules as they "run down" their concentration gradient from inside to outside the soma. The other force is exerted by the increasing concentration of negative ions in the soma, which creates a force to pull back the positively charged ions $K+$ ions leaving the soma.

The balance of these two oppositely directed forces establishes the resting potential of the undisturbed (resting) neuron. Potentials refer to voltage differences between two points, and the absolute difference in electrical potential between the inside and outside of the cell body is roughly 70 millivolts (mV) (0.070 volts). Because the voltage inside the soma is lower relative to outside the soma, the resting potential of a neuron is expressed with a negative sign, roughly −70 mV. Under

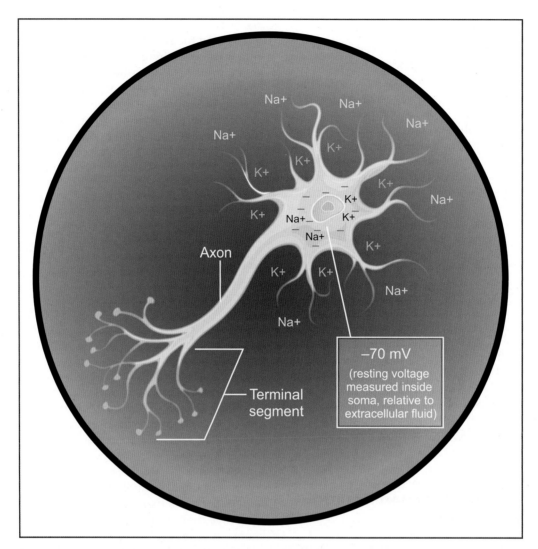

FIGURE 8–27. A neuron showing the relative distribution of negative and positive ions inside the soma versus the extracellular fluid. K+ = potassium; Na+ = sodium.

these conditions, the neuron does not fire impulses down its axon and its membrane is said to be *polarized*.

Action Potential

The description of the action potential presented below is schematic; for greater detail on the molecular basis of the action potential, Kandel et al. (2012) is an excellent source. An action potential is the change of the negative resting potential to a positive value and the subsequent return of the potential to a negative resting value. Changes in membrane potential occur in response to stimulation of a sensory organ as a result of touch, sound, or light, to give a few examples, or as a result of exposure of the neuron's membrane to neurotransmitters released by another, nearby neuron. The action potential occurs very rapidly (on the order

of 1/1,000th of a second, that is, 1 ms) and propagates down the length of the axon to its terminal segment. The arrival of the action potential at the terminal segment causes packets of neurotransmitter to be released into the synaptic cleft.

Figure 8–28 shows a diagram of an action potential. The x-axis is time (units = ms) and the y-axis is voltage (units = mV). The red trace shows the voltage measured, as a function of time, inside the soma relative to the voltage in the surrounding extracellular fluid as a function of time. The narrow, blue-shaded rectangle extending across the time axis between roughly −60 mV and −80 mV shows a range of resting membrane potentials, with a center potential of −70 mV (resting potentials are not always exactly −70 mv). In this drawing, the action potential trace begins within this narrow range of resting potentials. Less than half a mil-

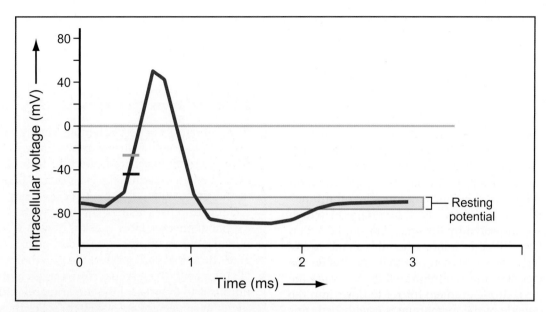

FIGURE 8–28. Diagram of an action potential, showing intracellular voltage (in mV) on the *y*-axis and time (in ms) on the *x*-axis. The range of resting potential values is shown by the blue rectangle centered on an intracellular voltage around −70 mV. The short, dark purple horizontal line shows the voltage change that must be reached to produce the "all-or-none" action potential, and the short green horizontal line shows the cell potential at which the K+ channels are opened to begin the process of reestablishing the resting potential, as described in the text. Both events are examples of voltage-gated membrane permeabilities to specific ion flows.

lisecond after the beginning of the trace, the potential moves in the positive direction, toward zero, as a result of stimulation of the neuron. The membrane potential begins to change in the positive direction because the stimulation causes the membrane to become permeable to Na+ ions, which previously have been unable to pass through the membrane to enter the soma. The new permeability of the membrane to Na+ allows the positive ions to flow into the soma, to establish equilibrium of positive ions on the inside and outside of the soma membrane. These initial openings are limited, however, allowing only a modest flow on Na+ ions down its concentration gradient, toward the inside of the soma. This is why the membrane potential begins to change in a positive direction.

The real action in the action potential begins, however, when the changing membrane potential reaches a value of roughly −45 mV. At this voltage level, a threshold effect occurs and a huge number of Na+ channels in the membrane are instantly opened, allowing a rush of Na+ into the soma. The sudden rush of Na+ into the soma when the voltage threshold is reached guarantees depolarization of the neuron, and the "firing" of the action potential down the axon to the terminal segment. This is called the "all or none" principle: Changes in the membrane potential below the threshold do not guarantee an action potential, but when

threshold is reached, the action potential *must* happen. This threshold is indicated in Figure 8–28 by the short, horizontal, dark purple bar that crosses the rising action potential trace.

The term *voltage-gated sodium channel* refers to a special membrane pore that is switched on when the membrane voltage threshold is reached. Considering the thousands and thousands of voltage-gated channels on each neuron membrane, their simultaneous opening at the threshold voltage allows a great deal of Na+ to rush into the soma. As seen in Figure 8–28, this causes the potential to shoot up past zero, perhaps as high as +40 mV, *depolarizing* the membrane in less than 1 ms. A depolarized membrane is one in which the normal (resting) negative potential is "flipped" into the positive region for a very brief interval. A depolarized membrane—the action potential—initiates the conduction of electrical impulses down the axon, to the terminal segment.

As shown in Figure 8–28, the action potential is not only defined by the rapid increase from a negative to positive membrane potential but also by the reversal of this process and a return to a negative potential within the resting range. The return to a negative potential may, for a brief time, reach a value that is slightly *more negative* than the average resting potential of −70 mV. Why does this happen? First, when the action potential approaches its peak positive value, the Na+ channels are closed as suddenly as they were opened at the threshold value. This is another voltage-gated channel effect. The cessation of Na+ ions rushing into the soma initiates the process of repolarizing the cell membrane. But another mechanism is equally if not more important in repolarizing the membrane potential, and this is related to the large number of voltage-gated K+ channels in the cell membrane. Very shortly after the threshold voltage has been reached and the Na+ channels have been instantly opened, the depolarization triggers a relatively slow opening (on a "neuron-time" scale, that is) of K+ channels; the voltage at which this occurs is indicated by the green bar on the action potential trace. Keep in mind, when the membrane is strongly depolarized—when positive ions inside the membrane are far more concentrated than outside the membrane—a strong gradient for K+ to flow from the inside to outside of the membrane is established; this is the reverse of the gradient direction during the resting potential. When the voltage-gated K+ channels are turned on shortly after depolarization, by the time the action potential has reached its maximum value, the K+ channels are wide open and ready to allow these positive ions to rush out of the soma into the extracellular fluid. This drives the membrane potential into the negative range, often below the resting potential value of around −70 mV. This hyperpolarized state is seen in Figure 8–28 between roughly 1 and 2 ms along the time scale. During this brief time, the neuron is said to be *refractory*, or relatively unresponsive to stimulation, because the electrical potential is more negative than it is at rest.

When the cell membrane is depolarized, propagation of the action potential from soma to terminal segment is not continuous but appears to make its way down the myelinated portion of the axon in a series of "jumps." The jumps are due to the anatomy of a myelinated neuron, as shown in Figure 8–25. Recall that most axons are wrapped in myelin, which functions as an electrical insulator to the flow of current down the axon resulting from the voltage changes that define the action potential. Myelin is wrapped around axons in sections, with tiny interruptions (the nodes of Ranvier) at regular intervals. When measured by sensitive electrodes and voltage monitors, the action potential appears to jump down the axon from one node of Ranvier to the next. This is referred to as *saltatory transmission* (the word *saltatory* having a Latin origin meaning leaping or dancing). The net effect of the myelin and the jumping action potential is to make transmission of electrical impulses from soma to terminal segment very, very fast. Healthy myelin wrapping is critical to an efficiently and effectively functioning nervous system; demyelinating diseases such as multiple sclerosis slow neural transmission and may cause a range of sensory and motor problems.

Faster Than the Speed of . . .

Nerves conduct action potentials very, very quickly. A general rule is that myelinated axon fibers conduct impulses faster than unmyelinated fibers, and within the class of myelinated axons, those with larger axonal diameters conduct impulses faster than those with smaller axonal diameters. How quick is quick? The ulnar nerve, a mixed (motor and sensory) nerve that exits the spinal cord around the first thoracic (T1) segment of the spinal cord, carries motor impulses to muscles of the forearm and pinky finger at a speed of at least 60 m/s. For those of you who do not like metric, that's about 134 miles per hour. Closer to home, the facial nerve conducts motor impulses at a speed of roughly 50 m/s; the motor part of the trigeminal nerve (to jaw muscles) conducts at a rate of about 55 m/s. Some nerve fibers conduct at slower speeds, such as those that lack a myelin wrapping or have just a thin myelin sheath; these are primarily fibers that carry the sensations of pain and temperature, and their conduction speeds may be no more than 20 m/s. Everyone has had the experience of touching something hot and realizing it only after what seems to be a long time. This is because thinly or unmyelinated temperature pathways conduct impulses relatively slowly, so the time between stimulation of the temperature receptors and recognition of the heat seems relatively long.

Synaptic Transmission and Neurotransmitters

The following discussion focuses on action potentials in the CNS, in which the properties of neuron membranes and their ability to change polarity (electrical charge) are largely dictated by the chemicals to which they are exposed. Signaling in the nervous system—sending messages from one area of the nervous system to another—is a recurring process of energy conversion.

When the action potential (electrical energy) reaches the terminal segment of an axon, it initiates processes that cause neurotransmitter (chemical energy) to be released into the synaptic cleft. In the synaptic cleft, these chemicals bathe the membrane of an adjacent neuron's dendrites and, in so doing, affect the membrane properties. The effect on the membrane properties is to open or close ion channels, which may result in a change in the membrane's potential for creating (depolarization) or inhibiting (hyperpolarization) electrical energy. The constant and widespread demand for energy conversion and consumption in the brain explains why in humans, the metabolic requirements of brain function are disproportionately large. An often used example that makes this point is that the typical weight of a human brain (~3.2 pounds) is about 2% of total body weight, but its activity consumes about 20% of the energy required for functioning of the *entire* body.

When an action potential propagates down an axon and reaches the terminal segment, a series of chemical reactions (not described here) cause some of the packets to breach the presynaptic membrane and dump their neurotransmitter contents into the synaptic cleft. This is represented in Figure 8–26 as the pale blue medium between the terminal segment and the postsynaptic membrane (curved, purplish surface) of a dendrite. The dendritic membrane is studded with special organs, shown in Figure 8–26 as small spikes with semicircular receptacles reaching into the synaptic cleft. These special organs are neurotransmitter receptors, typically "tuned" for specific neurotransmitter types. Some of the neurotransmitter molecules in the synaptic cleft bind to the dendritic receptors that are tuned to their chemical properties. The binding of neurotransmitter molecules to these receptor sites is shown by the blue dots sitting within the semicircular receptacles.

The effect of neurotransmitters on the dendritic membrane is to modify the permeability of the membrane. Some neurotransmitters make the membrane more permeable to positive ions, which result in an action potential. The neurochemical gating of ion channels is directly analogous to the voltage-dependent gating described above; the difference is in what causes the channels to open. A neurotransmitter that binds to receptors on the postsynaptic membrane and "flips" the negative resting potential to a positive one—that induces an action potential—is referred to as an *excitatory* effect, because it causes the postsynaptic neuron to fire. Other neurotransmitters close membrane channels that, under other circumstances, permit positive ions to flow into the cell body. This makes the membrane potential more negative (hyperpolarized), which inhibits the production of an action potential. The neurotransmitters that hyperpolarize membrane potentials are called *inhibitory*.

The energy conversion that produces excitatory and inhibitory signaling in the nervous system is much more complicated than the simple model shown in Figure 8–26. In the real brain-world, each neuron in the CNS receives input from many neurons and delivers output to many neurons. Each neuron has many dendrites and many terminal segments. Neuronal activity is even more complex because many neurons are not specialized for a particular neurotransmitter. Rather, they have dendritic receptors for multiple neurotransmitters (even for subtypes of the same neurotransmitter) and may package more than one neurotransmitter in their terminal segments. The receptors on the dendrites may be tuned to both excitatory and inhibitory neurotransmitters, and the terminal segments may contain neurotransmitter packets of both types. How does this work?

Think of the many inputs converging on the dendrites of a single neuron as summing their effects on the dendritic membrane, with the net effect determining the dendritic membrane potential. The dendrites of a single neuron may receive thousands of excitatory inputs from multiple neurons and thousands of inhibitory inputs from other (or the same) neurons. When there are more excitatory inputs than inhibitory inputs, the net effect is excitatory and an action potential is generated in the neuron receiving the multiple inputs. The opposite net effect silences the neuron, maintaining or exaggerating the negative membrane potential. Summed over millions and millions of neurons, the state of brain activity at any given moment is a statistical process involving net inputs and outputs.

The complex, statistical nature of neuron excitation and inhibition allows the CNS to control actions and perceptions with spectacular precision and integration. It also allows the brain to adjust its excitation and inhibition patterns over time with new stimulation, such as occurs during speech and language development in children. The statistical activity of the 80-plus billion neurons in the CNS is well suited to learning. For the relevance of statistical brain activity in speech, hearing, and language, see Gervain and Geffen (2019) and Plante and Gomez (2018).

Neurochemically gated ion channels in neuron membranes are sensitive to a range of neurotransmitter types. Some well-known (and well-studied) neurotransmitters are listed in Table 8–5, together with their primary function (excitatory or inhibitory) and primary role in behavior. It is important to understand the use of the term *primary* function and role when consulting this table. A neurotransmitter such as acetylcholine may have a primary excitatory function but still be able to produce inhibitory effects when binding to specialized, inhibitory receptors. Similarly, a particular neurotransmitter may play a primary role in motor control (such as dopamine or acetylcholine), yet also have major roles in functions such as memory and attention.

TABLE 8–5. Well-Studied Neurotransmitters in the Human Brain, Their Primary Function, and the Behaviors Linked to Them

Neurotransmitter	Primary Function	Behaviors
Glutamate	Excitatory	Widespread (memory, learning)
GABA	Inhibitory	Widespread (muscle tone)
Dopamine	Excitatory	Motor, mood, reward
Norepinephrine	Excitatory	Mood, attention, sleep, pain
Epinephrine	Excitatory, inhibitory	Blood pressure, airway diameter
Serotonin	Excitatory, inhibitory	Mood, arousal
Acetylcholine	Excitatory	Muscle contraction (sk)
	Inhibitory	Muscle contraction (ht)

Note. GABA = gamma aminobutyric acid; sk = skeletal; ht = heart.

Neuromuscular Junction

The neuromuscular junction is a special type of synapse in the PNS. It is the location at which the terminal segments of motor axons make contact with specialized receptors on the surface of muscle tissue. A schematic drawing of a neuromuscular junction is shown in Figure 8–29, where contact is made between a terminal segment of a motor axon and muscle fibers. A specialized structure at this point of contact is called a motor endplate, which contains specialized receptors sensitive to the neurotransmitter acetylcholine. As shown in Figure 8–29, packets of acetylcholine are stored in the terminal segments of motor nerve axons. When an action potential travels down a motor nerve axon and reaches the terminal segment, acetylcholine is released into the synaptic cleft separating the terminal segment from the motor endplate. At a neuromuscular junction, therefore, the terminal segment is the presynaptic membrane and the motor endplate is the postsynaptic membrane, and these membranes are separated by a synaptic cleft. The release of acetylcholine into the synaptic cleft results in binding of the neurotransmitter to the specialized acetylcholine receptors embedded in the motor endplate. This binding opens positive-ion channels in the muscle tissue membrane, resulting in a postsynaptic action potential that causes the underlying muscle fibers to slide across each other. This is the micro view of what happens when a motor endplate is depolarized; the macro view is that the summed effect of the terminal segments of many motor axons releasing acetylcholine onto many motor endplate receptors makes a muscle contract and exert force.

MENINGES, VENTRICLES, AND BLOOD SUPPLY

This section presents information on the coverings of the brain; the cavities within the CNS that produce, contain, and transport CSF; and the brain's blood supply. These three major areas of brain anatomy and physiology are considered together because of their tightly interrelated functions.

Meninges

The cerebral hemispheres, the brainstem, and the spinal cord are masses of cells and fiber tracts encased by layers of nonneural tissue. These casings serve a protective function, as well as several other functions related to metabolic activities of neural tissue. The cerebral hemispheres, cerebellum, brainstem, and spinal cord float inside this protective housing. The layers of tissue providing this protective function are collectively called the meninges (the plural of the Greek word *meninx*, meaning *membrane*).

An artist's rendition of the anatomical relationship of the cortex and its underlying white matter to the meninges is shown in Figure 8–30 (bottom image). Imagine this rectangular slab of multilayered tissue to be extracted from the top part of the head, a centimeter or two posterior to the top of the forehead and viewed at an angle in the coronal and horizontal planes. This perspective shows white matter toward the inferior edge of the slab and the cortical layer of gray matter above it. The labels for white matter and cerebral cortex are shown on the left side of the slab.

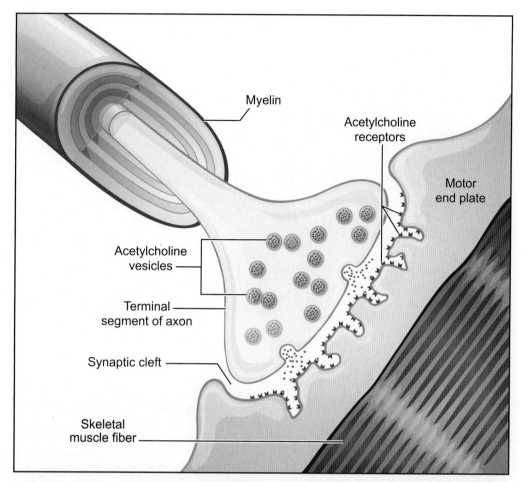

FIGURE 8–29. A neuromuscular junction, the specialized synapse at the junction between a peripheral motor nerve and muscle tissue. The terminal segment containing packets of the neurotransmitter acetylcholine is the presynaptic component of the synapse, and the motor endplate is the postsynaptic component. Embedded within the motor endplate are specialized receptors for acetylcholine. When acetylcholine released by the presynaptic membrane binds to receptors in the motor endplate, the muscle fibers are depolarized and slide across each other, resulting in muscle contraction.

Above the cortex and its underlying white matter are multiple layers of tissue, the top layer being the skin of the scalp and its protruding hairs, beneath which is a relatively thick, bony layer—the skull. Immediately beneath the skull is the most superficial layer of the meninges, the dura mater; deep to this layer is the arachnoid mater, followed by the pia mater, the deepest layer of the meninges. The dura, arachnoid, and pia mater layers form the meninges of the brain.

Dura Mater

The term *dura mater* means *tough mother*, an appropriate term that captures the leathery, hide-like texture of the tissue. Figure 8–30 (bottom image) shows the dura mater as tissue in two layers, the more superficial of which is called the periosteal layer, the deeper one the meningeal layer. The periosteal layer of the dura mater adheres to the underside of the bony skull, whereas the meningeal layer is in contact with the arachnoid mater.

The description of the dura mater as a two-layered meningeal structure is more than excessive anatomical detail. As shown on the coronal face of the slab (bottom image in Figure 8–30), the meningeal layer separates from the periosteal layer toward the midline of the slab, to form a barrier between the left and right hemispheres. Note how as the bilayered dura mater approaches the midline, the meningeal layers on either side dip inferiorly and form a nearly vertical separation

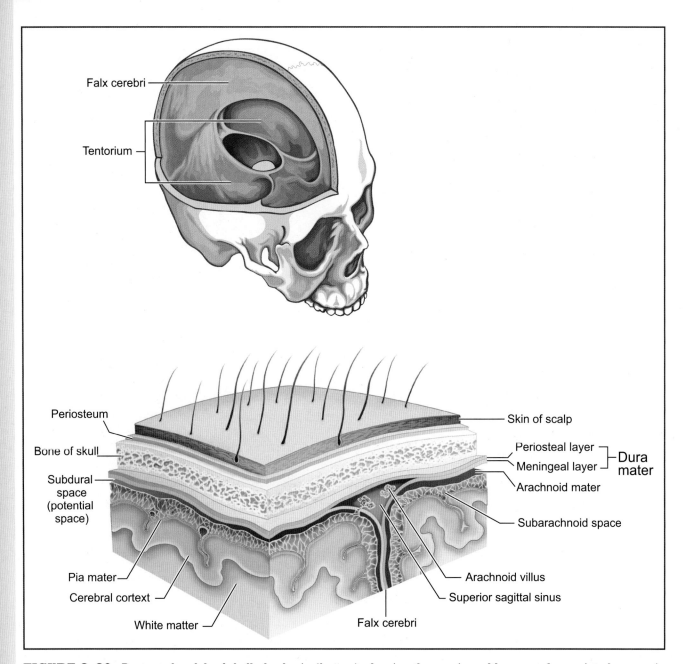

FIGURE 8–30. Rectangular slab of skull plus brain (*bottom*), showing the meningeal layers and associated spaces in relation to the underlying nervous system tissues. The various folds of the dura mater are shown (*top*) with all brain tissue removed; note the falx cerebri and the tent-like covering—the tentorium cerebelli—of the brainstem and cerebellum created by the infoldings of the dura mater.

between the tissues of the two hemispheres. This partition is called the *falx cerebri*. When viewed in the sagittal plane, the falx cerebri forms a sheet having the shape of the letter C rotated 90 degrees clockwise. The anterior-to-posterior extent of the falx cerebri is roughly the same as the anterior-to-posterior extent of the corpus callosum, which is located immediately ventral to the inferior edge of the falx. The falx cerebri is shown in a separate image at the top of Figure 8–30, an image drawn with all brain tissue removed from the contents of the skull cavity. In this image, the darker gray folds depict infoldings of the meningeal layer of the dura mater.

Another separation of the meningeal layer of the dura mater from the periosteal layer forms the *tentorium cerebelli*. This part of the dura mater is like a tent (hence, *tentorium*) draped over the brainstem, separating it from the cerebral hemispheres. The tentorium cerebelli also forms a boundary between the cerebellum and the ventral surface of the occipital lobes. Although the configuration of the tentorium cerebelli is difficult to appreciate in a two-dimensional drawing, Figure 8–30, top image, shows the tent-like structure with an opening in the middle, formed by the infoldings of the meningeal layers of the dura. The cerebral hemispheres are above this opening, the brainstem and cerebellum below it. The posterior edge of the opening is the midline of the dural covering separating the cerebellum from the ventral surfaces of the occipital lobes. When you hear the term *supratentorial*, reference is being made to a structure or disease process (such as a stroke or tumor) above the opening between the cerebral hemispheres and brainstem. *Infratentorial* refers to structures or disease processes below this opening, in the brainstem and/or cerebellum.

The dura mater serves a protective function for the neural tissue of the CNS. The dura encases the CSF in which the cerebral hemispheres and brainstem float. As discussed in the next section, CSF circulates throughout the CNS. One prominent region within which the fluid circulates is immediately below the second layer of the meninges, the arachnoid mater.

Arachnoid Mater

The arachnoid mater is a thin membrane attached to the underside of the dura matter; below this membrane is a small space in which CSF circulates. As shown in the bottom image of Figure 8–30, the subarachnoid space is a honeycombed chamber. The typical thickness of this space, extending from the arachnoid membrane to the pia mater below, is roughly 5 to 6 mm but varies quite a bit depending on where the measurement is taken. The honeycombed appearance results from delicate membranes extending from the arachnoid layer that is adhered to the underside of the dura, down to the pia mater. These membranes, together with the CSF circulating in the subarachnoid space, create a spongy cushion that protects the underlying neural tissue against damage.

Although not shown in Figure 8–30, arteries enter and veins exit brain tissue via the subarachnoid space. Arteries distribute blood to brain tissue via smaller vessels that penetrate the deepest layer of the meninges (the pia mater). Veins in the subarachnoid space carry blood away from the brain, into sinuses created by the separation of the two layers of the dura mater. The major venous return of blood to the heart is located in these sinuses; a cross section of one such sinus, the superior sagittal sinus, is shown in Figure 8–30.

Pia Mater

The pia mater, the deepest layer of the meninges, is a thin membrane that adheres closely to the surface of the cerebral hemispheres, following its curvatures and fissures. In a fixed brain prepared for dissection, in which the dura and arachnoid have been removed, the pia is often intact and appears as a filmy, milky-colored membrane that can be "pinched" away from the gyri and sulci. The pia mater is so closely adherent to the cortical surface that it is sometimes not immediately apparent on casual inspection by eye.

Meninges and Clinically Relevant Spaces

Clinically, the meninges are often referenced when there is bleeding in one of the spaces between the layers of these protective coverings. These are "potential spaces" in the sense of not having any measurable volume until something causes them to expand and create a "real" space. For example, the undersurface of the skull and the top surface of the dura are normally tightly bound to one another, but the potential space between them, called the epidural space, may be filled by blood when an artery bleeds. Similarly, the potential space between the dura and arachnoid membrane can be filled by blood when an artery or vein bleeds. The term *subdural hematoma* refers to pooled blood in the space between the dura and arachnoid membrane of the meninges. Any collection of blood within the meningeal spaces can exert pressure on the underlying brain tissue and cause impaired function, including speech, language, hearing, and/or swallowing deficits.

Ventricles

The meningeal layers, as described above, include the honeycombed subarachnoid space filled with CSF. CSF is produced, circulated, and delivered back to the venous system (the drainage of blood from brain to heart) within a system of interconnected ventricles located deep within the cerebral hemispheres and brainstem. CSF also flows through a central canal in the spinal cord.

The ventricular system and associated conduits are shown in Figure 8–31. This sagittal view of the hemispheres and brainstem has been made transparent for better appreciation of the location and configuration of the ventricular system. The lateral ventricle is the complexly shaped green structure, the third ventricle is shown in light blue, the cerebral aqueduct in purple, and the fourth ventricle in reddish orange. Below the fourth ventricle, in darker blue, is the *foramen*

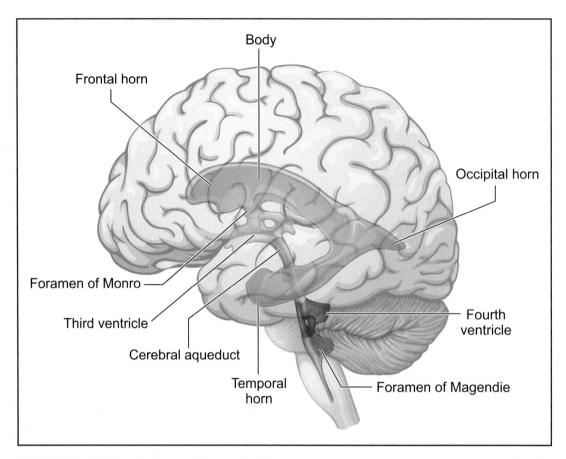

FIGURE 8–31. Sagittal view of the cerebral hemispheres, brainstem, and cerebellum showing the location and configuration of the ventricles. Lateral ventricles are in green, third ventricle in light blue, cerebral aqueduct in purple, and fourth ventricle in reddish orange. The dark blue part of the ventricular system, seen inferior to the fourth ventricle, includes the beginning of the central canal of the spinal cord as well as other conduits through which CSF flows back up to the subarachnoid spaces in the cerebral hemispheres.

of Magendie and a downward projection that becomes the central canal of the spinal cord. Figure 8–32 shows these structures in a coronal view, looking from the front of the cerebral hemispheres toward the occipital lobes, and color-coded in the same way as in Figure 8–31. This view shows the lateral ventricles (green) to be paired, symmetrical structures in the two hemispheres, and the third ventricle and cerebral aqueduct to be midline (axial) structures. The fourth ventricle is a chamber between the brainstem and cerebellum and is symmetrical with respect to both halves of the brainstem.

Lateral Ventricles

The sagittal view of Figure 8–31 shows the lateral ventricle to be a large, reversed C-shaped chamber occupying deep locations in all four lobes of the brain. The

frontal horn of the lateral ventricle is in the frontal lobe, the body is in both the frontal and parietal lobes, and an occipital horn extends into the occipital lobe. The lower part of the reversed-C shape is the temporal horn of the lateral ventricle, which extends anterolaterally into the temporal lobe from the junction of the body and occipital horn.

Some notable landmarks are associated with the complex shape of the lateral ventricle. For example, the corpus callosum, the massive fiber tract that connects cells in one hemisphere to cells in the other hemisphere, is located just superior to the upper edge of the frontal horn and body of the lateral ventricle (see Figure 8–4, upper right). The caudate nucleus, a component of the basal ganglia (see Figure 8–3), is the lateral boundary of the lateral ventricle and follows its inverted C shape (see Figure 8–14) from the frontal lobe to its curl into the temporal lobe.

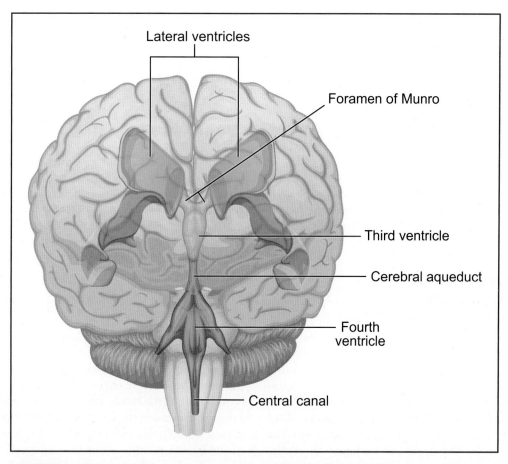

Lateral ventricles

Foramen of Munro

Third ventricle

Cerebral aqueduct

Fourth ventricle

Central canal

FIGURE 8–32. Coronal view of the cerebral hemispheres, brainstem, and cerebellum, looking from the front to the back of the hemispheres, and drawn to show the configuration of the ventricles. Color coding of the ventricles is the same as in Figure 8–31.

Third Ventricle

In the sagittal view of Figure 8–31, the third ventricle is shown in blue as a flattened, complexly shaped cavity. The coronal view of Figure 8–32 shows the lateral ventricles connected to the third ventricle by paired, narrow conduits, both called the *foramen of Munro*. The foramina (plural of foramen) join in the midline to form a single channel that drains CSF from the lateral ventricles into the third ventricle. In addition to its role in the transport of CSF throughout the CNS, the third ventricle is an important anatomical landmark because it is the medial boundary of the two thalami (see the coronal view of Figure 8–3, in which the lateral ventricles are the two wing-like cavities next to the caudate nuclei, and the third ventricle is the narrow slit between the thalami). There is often a connection between the left and right thalami *through* the third ventricle; this is shown in Figure 8–31 as the circular opening in the third ventricle depicted in the same

color as the brain tissue. This connection is called the interthalamic adhesion.

Cerebral Aqueduct, Fourth Ventricle, and Other Passageways for CSF

At the posterior, inferior end of the third ventricle, roughly at the top of the midbrain, the cavity narrows and forms the cerebral aqueduct, shown in purple in Figures 8–31 and 8–32. This narrow channel courses through the midbrain and opens up in the pons and medulla as a complexly shaped cavity called the fourth ventricle. The fourth ventricle is just posterior to much of the pons and medulla, and anterior to the cerebellum. Think of this fluid-filled cavity as a boundary between the cerebellum and the lower two divisions of the brainstem.

The fourth ventricle has several outlets that deliver CSF to the spinal cord and the subarachnoid space covering the cerebral hemispheres. In Figures 8–31 and

8–32, the thin blue passageway extending down from the fourth ventricle is the beginning of the central canal of the spinal cord. In horizontal cross sections of the spinal cord (such as Figure 8–23), this canal is seen as the small circle in the center of the section, surrounded by gray matter. CSF flows through the canal and collects toward the bottom of the vertebral column in a small cavity below the inferior termination of spinal cord tissue, which is a few segments higher than the termination of the vertebral column.

Two additional conduits projecting from the fourth ventricle in posterolateral directions can be seen in Figure 8–32. These are passageways from the fourth ventricle into the subarachnoid space around the cerebral hemispheres.

Production, Composition, and Circulation of CSF

CSF is primarily generated by the choroid plexus cells in the lateral ventricles. The choroid plexus cells are suspended from the roof of the lateral ventricles and generate roughly half a quart of CSF every 24 hours. CSF travels from the lateral ventricles via the foramen of Monro to the third ventricle and then via the cerebral aqueduct to the fourth ventricle. Some fluid from the fourth ventricle continues inferiorly into the central canal of the spinal cord, and some exits via the lateral passageways shown in Figure 8–32 to circulate in the subarachnoid space surrounding the cerebral hemispheres. CSF is constantly recirculated throughout the ventricular system. Because the subarachnoid space can hold only about one-third of the volume of CSF produced by the choroid plexus, a mechanism exists to drain CSF from the brain into the bloodstream. Figure 8–30 (bottom image) includes a small structure labeled *arachnoid villus* (plural, *villi*), also called *arachnoid granulations*. There are many arachnoid villi that extend from the subarachnoid space into the sinuses created by separation of the two layers of the dura mater. The arachnoid villi "dump" circulating CSF from the subarachnoid space into the venous system, effectively draining off excess CSF and maintaining a healthy pressure inside the ventricles and subarachnoid spaces. The draining of CSF into the venous system also serves the purpose of carrying neural waste products—brain "trash" generated as neural and glial cells perform their metabolic tasks—out of the brain to be dissolved harmlessly in blood returning to the heart.

CSF is a clear fluid containing many different kinds of molecules, including proteins, chemical elements such as magnesium, chloride, potassium, and sodium, and other substances such as glucose, urea, and carbon dioxide. Normal values are available for each of these substances and may be used as reference data when spinal tap fluid is analyzed as part of a diagnostic workup for diseases such as meningitis or certain cancers.

Blood Supply of Brain

A frequently used organizing principle for describing the blood supply to the brain is to divide it into anterior versus posterior circulation. The anterior circulation is supplied by the internal carotid artery and its branches, and the posterior circulation is supplied by the basilar artery and its branches. Both anterior and posterior circulations originate in major arteries emerging from the heart.

Anterior Circulation

The aorta, the largest artery in the body, emerges from the heart and ascends in the thorax before turning around and descending toward the abdomen. At the top of the aortic arch, two major arteries arise and move blood toward the head. These are the common carotid arteries, one being the left common carotid artery (supplying the left side of the face and the left hemisphere of the brain) and the other the right common carotid artery. For the sake of clarity, Figure 8–33 shows only the left common carotid artery and the left hemisphere; the anatomical facts on the right side are identical to the ones described in the next paragraph.

As the common carotid artery ascends in the neck, it bifurcates (splits into two branches) roughly at the level of the mandible. One branch is the external carotid artery, which provides blood to structures such as the pharynx, tongue, face, and eyes. The other branch appears in Figure 8–33 as a continuation of the common carotid artery; this is the internal carotid artery, a main source of blood supply to the brain. Note how the internal carotid artery makes several sharp turns when it reaches the ventral surface of the temporal lobe. One of these is shown in Figure 8–33 as a hard right turn, along the line of the sylvian fissure. This branch of the internal carotid artery is called the middle cerebral artery (MCA). The MCA supplies blood to the lateral surfaces of the temporal and parietal lobes, as well as part of the frontal lobe; this blood supply includes the cortical regions associated with speech, language, and hearing skills. Another branch of the internal carotid artery is the anterior cerebral artery (ACA), shown in Figure 8–33 as a slight leftward and then upward turn off the main path of the internal carotid artery. The ACA supplies blood to medial portions of the frontal

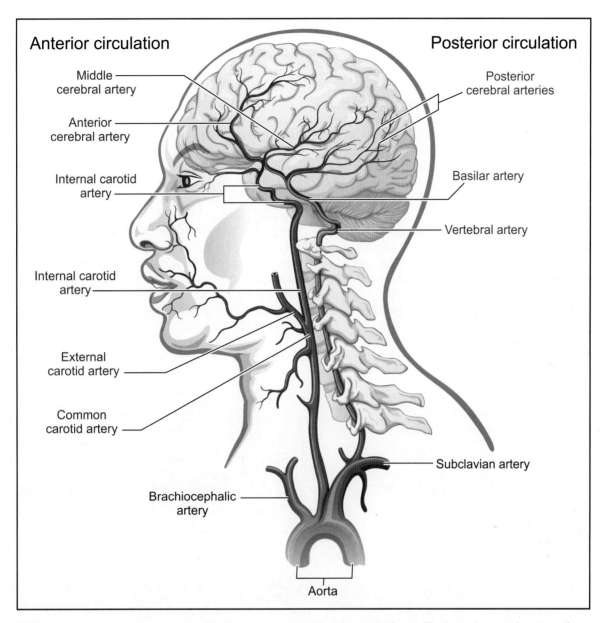

FIGURE 8–33. Arterial supply of the brain, shown originating at the heart. The anterior supply comes from the internal carotid artery, and the posterior supply from the basilar artery.

and parietal lobes, much of the corpus callosum, and portions of basal ganglia structures. The importance of the MCA in speech, language, and hearing function is discussed below.

Posterior Circulation

The posterior circulation is originally derived from the subclavian artery (Figure 8–33). The subclavian artery is a major branch of the aortic arch, supplying blood to the arm on the same side as the artery. The vertebral artery arises from the subclavian artery and ascends the neck through small openings in the ventral portions of the cervical vertebrae. When it reaches the base of the skull, the vertebral artery passes through the major opening on the base of the skull, called the *foramen magnum,* through which also pass the spinal cord and medulla. The vertebral artery continues to ascend on the ventral surface of the medulla until it joins with the vertebral artery from the other side, at the junction of the medulla and pons. The joining of the two vertebral arteries forms the basilar artery.

Before the vertebral arteries join at the junction of the medulla and pons, they deliver blood to one part of the cerebellum and the lateral part of the medulla via the posterior inferior cerebellar artery (PICA). The PICA is shown in Figure 8–34, which presents a view of the ventral surface of the cerebral hemispheres, the cerebellum, and the medulla and pons, as well as an illustration of the joining of the two vertebral arteries to form the basilar artery. As the basilar artery ascends the pons, it issues two more branches, the anterior inferior cerebellar artery (AICA) and the superior cerebellar artery (SCA). The AICA supplies blood to parts of the pons and the central part of the cerebellum, whereas the SCA serves the upper part of the cerebellum and some parts of the midbrain.

The basilar artery provides the posterior circulation for the cerebral hemispheres by issuing the posterior cerebral artery (PCA; see Figures 8–33 and 8–34). The PCA provides blood to the posterior parts of the cerebral hemispheres, including the occipital lobes, and parts of the thalamus and corpus callosum.

Circle of Willis

A view of the arterial anatomy on the base of the brain (see Figure 8–34) shows the ACA and MCA, both major branches of the internal carotid artery, and the PCA, the main branch of the basilar artery. These arteries, along with connecting arteries, form the circle of Willis, a continuous passageway for blood flow. The circle of Willis is illustrated in isolation in Figure 8–35.

Follow the basilar artery up the pons and note where the PCA branches off into the left and right hemispheres; both PCAs give off a branch called the posterior communicating artery (PComm), which links to the MCA. The MCA is labeled on the left side of Figure 8–35, and a comparison of the left and right sides makes it obvious that the MCA can be considered a continuation of the internal carotid artery. The ACAs connect from the MCA to the anterior part of the brain, and the two ACAs are connected via the anterior communicating artery (AComm).

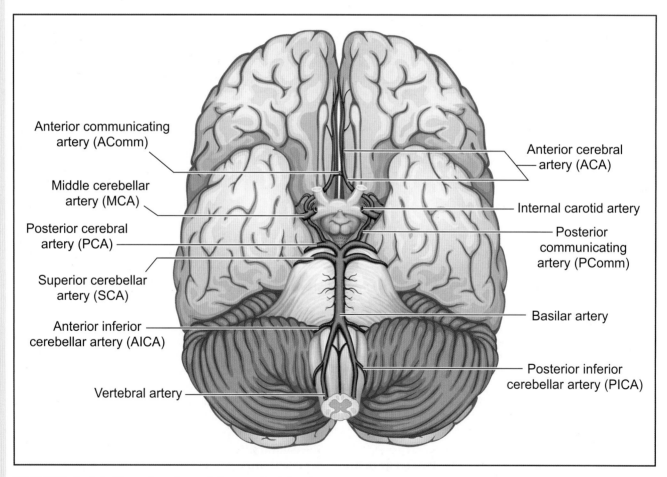

FIGURE 8–34. Ventral surface of the cerebral hemispheres, showing the paired vertebral arteries ascending the medulla, their junction at the base of the pons to form the basilar artery, and some of the important branches into the brainstem and cerebellum. The circle of Willis can also be seen in this drawing (see also Figure 8–35).

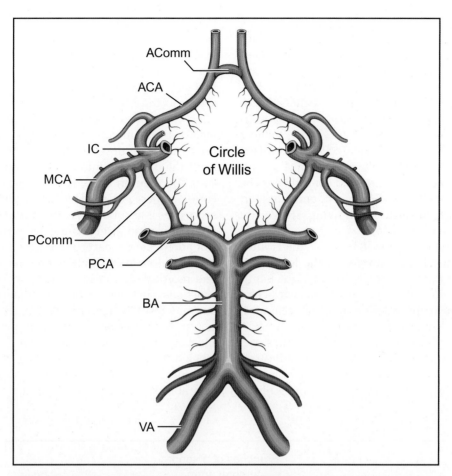

FIGURE 8–35. Isolated view of the circle of Willis showing its formation from the main blood supply sources to the brain: the basilar artery (posterior supply; BA) and internal carotid arteries (anterior supply; IC). The circle is completed by linking arteries (posterior cerebral artery, PCA; posterior communicating artery, PComm; middle cerebral arteries, MCA; anterior cerebral artery, ACA; and anterior communicating artery, AComm). The vertebral arteries (VA) supply blood to the basilar artery.

Blood at the base of the brain can flow in a circular pattern because the two main, paired branches of the carotid artery (ACA, MCA) and the one main, paired branch of the basilar artery (the PCA) are connected by communicating arteries. The circular blood flow in the circle of Willis has the capability of compensating for loss of blood flow from one of the main blood supplies to the brain. For example, blockage of the internal carotid on one side of the circle of Willis could, in theory, be compensated for by increased flow from the basilar artery, because both main arteries contribute to the circular blood flow pattern. This may be especially important in cases of temporary blockage. The classic description of circle of Willis anatomy must be taken with a grain of salt because there is a good deal of variation across individuals in the actual components and configuration of this circular arrangement. Some scientists believe this anatomical variation across individuals may help explain racial and ethnic differences in stroke risk (Eftekhar et al., 2006).

MCA and Blood Supply to the Dominant Hemisphere

The MCA is of particular interest to speech-language pathologists and audiologists because it supplies blood to much of the lateral surfaces of the cerebral hemispheres. More specifically, the MCA is the source of blood for the perisylvian speech, language, and hearing areas of the dominant hemisphere (the left hemisphere, in about 95% of the population). Blockage of the left MCA, or of one of its more local branches or associated small vessels deeper in the brain, has the potential to affect brain tissue critical to normal communication function. Many strokes associated with deficits in speech, swallowing, and language production and reception (comprehension) are the result of loss of blood flow in the left MCA or its branches. Motor speech disorders (dysarthria and apraxia of speech) resulting from stroke have been reviewed by Spencer and Brown (2018), Knollman-Porter (2008), and Ballard et al. (2016). The effects of stroke on language behaviors, such as language expression and comprehension, are reviewed by O'Sullivan, Brownsett, and Copland (2019). Swallowing disorders following stroke are described in Cohen et al. (2016).

Figure 8–36 shows how the MCA distributes branches across the lateral surface of the left hemisphere; the same pattern applies to the right hemisphere. Note how the MCA emerges on the surface of the hemisphere near the anterior tip of the temporal lobe and the lower surface of the frontal lobe. The MCA courses along the sylvian fissure, posteriorly and superiorly, giving off an upper branch and a lower branch. The upper branch supplies blood primarily to frontal lobe tissue, whereas the lower branch distributes blood to parietal lobe tissue. Note also the offshoots from the main trunk of the MCA to the temporal lobe.

In theory, a blockage to blood flow can occur at any point along the course of the MCA and its branches. Blockages at the sharp turn from the internal carotid artery to the MCA (a more or less right-angle bend) affect the entire distribution of blood to the lateral surface of the hemisphere. Blockages can also occur in the turn to the upper or lower branches of the MCA or in the offshoots into the temporal lobe. An overly simplified, but in many cases clinically useful, way to correlate these potential blockages with functional consequences is as follows. A blockage at the turn from the internal carotid artery to the MCA deprives the anterior and posterior parts of the left hemisphere of blood and therefore affects both expressive (anterior lesions) and receptive (posterior lesions) speech and language functions. Such a large area of damaged perisylvian tissue may result in a global aphasia, the massive disruption of both production and comprehension abilities. Blockage at the junction of the MCA and the offshoot labeled "MCA upper branch" (see Figure 8–36) may be expected to have a primary influence on production ability, whereas blockage at the junction of the

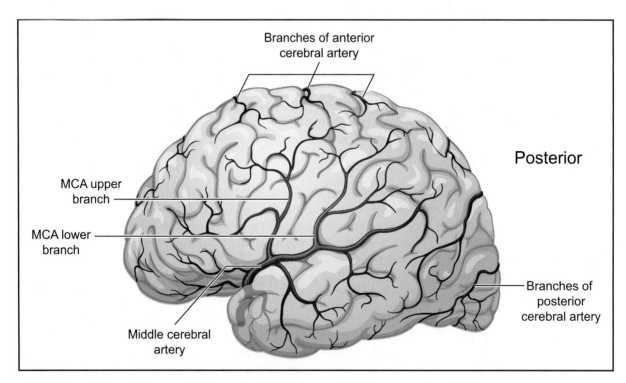

FIGURE 8–36. Distribution of middle cerebral artery (MCA) branches across the lateral surface of the left hemisphere. As the MCA emerges on the surface of the hemisphere between the anterior tip of the temporal lobe and lower, posterior lip of the frontal lobe, it gives off upper and lower branches as labeled in the figure. Branches of the anterior cerebral artery (ACA) and posterior cerebral artery (PCA) are also shown.

MCA and the offshoot labeled "MCA lower branch" might be associated with a primary receptive problem. This is consistent with the idea of anterior and posterior lesions in the dominant hemisphere producing primarily production and comprehension problems, respectively. Although overly simplified, this view is consistent with certain diagnostic categories of communication function following left hemisphere damage due to stroke.

The MCA also is a significant source of blood supply for structures deep within the cerebral hemispheres. A general view of the distribution of MCA blood supply to the contents of the cerebral hemispheres is given in Figure 8–37, which is a coronal section roughly midway between the front and back of the hemispheres. The left side of the section shows labeled brain structures, and the right side shows the source of blood supply to these structures from the main components of the circle of Willis (MCA, ACA, PCA). The purple shaded regions indicate the areas of the hemispheres supplied by the upper and lower branches of the MCA, including the cortical regions on the lateral surface of the hemisphere and the underlying white matter of the coronal radiata. Deep branches of the MCA (shown in light bluish gray) provide blood to the caudate, putamen, parts of the globus pallidus, and parts of the internal capsule. Speech and language problems plus limb deficits on the right side of the body, a frequently observed

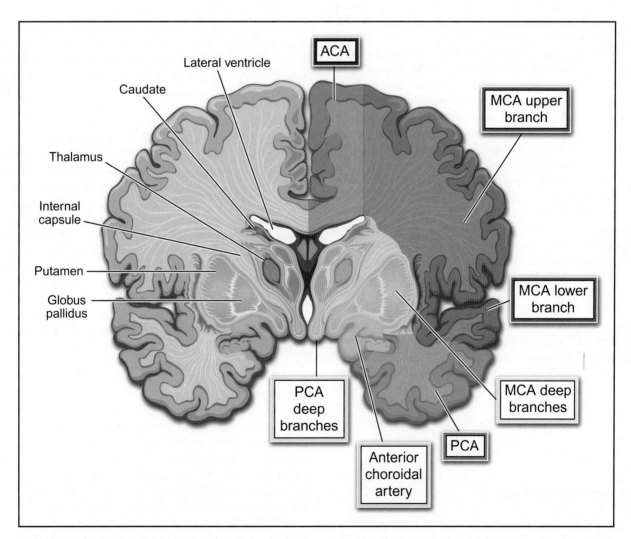

FIGURE 8–37. Distribution of cerebral artery supply to both surface and internal components of the cerebral hemispheres, shown in a coronal slice made roughly midway between the anterior and posterior ends of the hemispheres. The left side of the slice shows labels for subcortical structures; the right side of the slice identifies the arteries supplying different regions. MCA = middle cerebral artery; PCA = posterior cerebral artery; ACA = anterior cerebral artery.

combination in stroke clinics, are explained by interruptions of MCA blood flow, which affect the perisylvian areas (speech and language) and the internal capsule (limbs). Regions of the internal capsule, caudate, and globus pallidus are supplied by the anterior choroidal artery, an offshoot of the internal carotid artery close to the branching of the MCA at the base of the brain. The PCA supplies the ventral part of the temporal lobe, with deeper branches of the PCA supplying the thalamus and hypothalamus. The most dorsal and medial aspects of the cerebral hemispheres are supplied by the ACA.

Blood-Brain Barrier

In most parts of the body, substances flowing in the bloodstream can be transferred to tissue by passing through the walls of the vessels, directly into the tissue. However, the walls of vessels in the brain are different from walls of vessels in other parts of the body. Brain blood vessels have a structure that forms a protective barrier against chemicals or toxins that have the potential to destabilize the neurochemistry of the brain. This *blood-brain barrier* is especially relevant when certain drugs are administered to alleviate symptoms and signs of a CNS disease. For example, Parkinson's disease is to a large degree a result of reduction of the neurotransmitter dopamine in the brain. Dopamine is manufactured by cells in the substantia nigra and plays an important role in the normal functioning of basal ganglia structures. To address the reduction of dopamine in the brain, why not administer a drug, orally, with the molecular composition of dopamine? As it turns out, dopamine molecules are blocked by the blood-brain barrier. In the 1960s, scientists figured out that a precursor of dopamine—a chemical compound that is one of the steps in the neuronal synthesis of dopamine—was able to cross the blood-brain barrier. Patients were given this precursor, called L-DOPA, which crossed the blood-brain barrier. Once in the brain, L-DOPA was converted into dopamine. In this case, knowledge of the blood-brain barrier and the chemical transformations in the synthesis of dopamine permitted an effective treatment for some symptoms associated with Parkinson's disease.

CLINICAL NOTES

Decades of clinical experience and research have resulted in a good, if not perfect, understanding of the CNS basis of Parkinson's disease (PD). PD is the second most common degenerative diseases of the CNS—second only to Alzheimer's disease—with an overall rate per year 14 new cases per 100,000 people. Above the of age 65, the rate of newly diagnosed cases is nearly three times the overall rate (Ascherio & Schwarzchild, 2016). PD is classified as a degenerative disease because the damage in the brain and the associated signs and symptoms worsen over time.[2] A significant component of the degeneration in PD is a cumulative reduction of the neurotransmitter dopamine, which plays a critical role in movement (see Table 8–4). The reduction of dopamine is particularly relevant to effective function of the basal ganglia, the group of subcortical nuclei so critical to movement control (see section above on Basal Ganglia).

PD is almost always diagnosed based on a triad of signs that includes tremor (repetitive shaking), rigidity (stiff muscles), and bradykinesia (slowness of movement). Speech and swallowing are also affected in PD; speech becomes soft and "mumbly," both of which reduce speech intelligibility and have a profound impact on communication. Swallowing becomes less efficient in preventing food from entering the lungs, with a heightened risk of aspiration pneumonia.

Pharmacological (drug) treatment is by far the treatment of choice for PD, at least in the early stages of the disease. The preferred drug (generically, carbidopa-levodopa) increases the amount of dopamine in the CNS, with the goal of compensating for its loss due to the disease process. The drug is not a cure because it does not prevent the progression of the disease, but it does slow the progress of the signs and symptoms of PD. The drug is known to be effective in reducing the stiffness and slow movement in the limbs. On the other hand, there is controversy about the degree to which drug therapy improves speech and/or swallowing problems or even if there is any effect on the respiratory, laryngeal, and pharyngeal-oral functions required for speech and swallowing (Brabenec, Mekyska, Galaz, & Rektorova, 2017).

Another treatment that may be used for people with severe signs and symptoms—people who have difficulty making *any* movement—and for whom drug therapy has stopped working to relieve symptoms is called deep brain stimulation (DBS). DBS is a surgical treatment that highlights the clinical relevance of understanding brain anatomy and physiology.

DBS is implemented by inserting electrodes deep into the cerebral hemispheres, with a frequent implantation target of the subthalamic nucleus (STN), which

---

[2]In medical diagnosis and description, signs refer to observable and measurable events, such as tremor (e.g., observation of a tremor is a sign; measurement of a tremor is the rate of back-and-forth movement). Symptoms refer to behaviors experienced by a patient but not necessarily observable, such as fatigue or depression.

is part of the basal ganglia (see Figure 8–13). The electrodes are connected by a wire to a voltage generator that delivers electrical pulses to the STN, as illustrated in Figure 8–38. Once properly implanted, the electrodes are stimulated with a voltage source—under control by the patient via a handheld device—to reduce stiffness and slowness. Why does stimulation of the STN work in many people?

The answer lies in the knowledge that the several nuclei of the basal ganglia function as a *network* to control movement—the nuclei of the basal ganglia are interconnected, and the performance of one nucleus of the basal ganglia depends on performance of the others. Some of the nuclei exert inhibitory influence on other nuclei, and some exert excitatory influence. Now let us apply this knowledge to the use of DBS to treat signs and symptoms of PD. In a healthy brain, the STN sends excitatory

signals to a subgroup of cells in the globus pallidus, increasing the activity of the latter cells. Recall that the basal ganglia form a loop with the cortical areas that control movement: Cortical commands for movement control are delivered to the basal ganglia network, which processes and delivers them via the globus pallidus to the thalamus. Thus, the globus pallidus is the output of the loop. The thalamus sends the output, refined by processing in the basal ganglia, back to the cortical regions that initially issued the commands. The result of this processing is the kind of movement control we expect in healthy individuals—scaled correctly, precise, and with effective coordination.

Interestingly, in the cortico-striatal-cortico loop, the output of the globus pallidus is *inhibitory* to the thalamus. Thus, greater activity in the globus pallidus delivers more inhibited movement signals to the thalamus, which the thalamus passes on to the cortex. In the

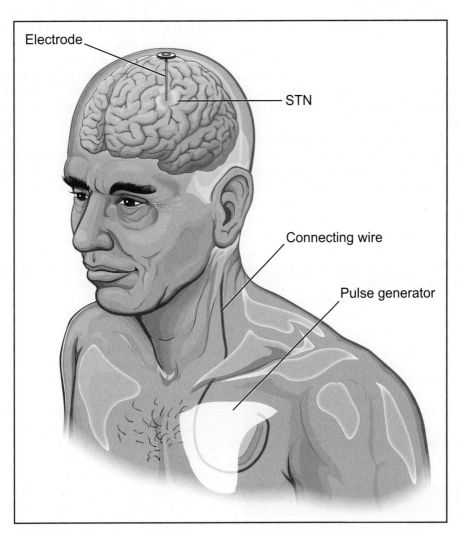

FIGURE 8–38. Implantation of electrode in STN, pulse generator, and connecting wire. The pulse generator and connecting wire are embedded under the skin.

healthy brain, this inhibition is presumably "scaled" for movements of proper size. Here is where the role of the STN in PD enters the picture. The STN is *excitatory* to the globus pallidus. The greater the activity of STN, the greater the inhibitory output of the globus pallidus to the thalamus. Another inhibitory effect in the basal ganglia network is that of the striatum (caudate and putamen) on the STN. The proper function of the striatum is impaired by the loss of dopamine. Hence, in PD, the activity of the STN is *disinhibited*, as a result of greater excitation to the STN from the striatum. The loss of normal inhibition of the STN excites the globus pallidus to abnormally high levels, which are reflected in a weak output to the thalamus, and this weak output is forwarded to the cortex. The motor commands in the brain of a person with PD are therefore more inhibited than the motor commands in a healthy brain, resulting in the small and slow movements that are among the hallmark features of the disease.

DBS targets the STN to reduce its activity, via stimulation delivered through the implanted electrodes. The electrical signals interfere with normal STN activity, thus decreasing its excitatory effect on the globus pallidus. In other words, the reduced STN activity makes the globus pallidus activity less inhibitory, which results in movements that are less underscaled than they are in the absence of DBS.

DBS is often effective in relieving profoundly serious movement problems in PD. Unfortunately, there is great controversy concerning its success in treating the speech and swallowing impairments associated with PD. There is even evidence that in some patients, DBS may worsen speech and/or swallowing function (see review and results of Aldridge, Theodoros, Angwin, & Vogel, 2016; di Biase & Fasano, 2016; Sidtis, Van Lancker Sidtis, Ramdhani, & Tagliati, 2020; Yu, Takahashi, Bloom, Quaynor, & Xie, 2020).

This discussion shows how knowledge of brain anatomy (in this case, the basal ganglia), the complex function of brain networks in producing movement (the cortico-striatal-cortico loop), the role of neurotransmitters in the brain (dopamine), and the concepts of excitation and inhibition are relevant to the expertise of a speech-language pathologist who engages in professional communication with other members of a heath care team. The knowledge also increases the skill of diagnosing and treating speech and swallowing disorders in PD.

REVIEW

The chapter begins with a summary of general concepts, including central and peripheral nervous system (CNS and PNS), anatomical planes and directions,

white and gray matter, tracts and nuclei, nerves and ganglia, afferent and efferent, and lateralization and specialization of function.

The cerebral hemispheres include cortical tissue (gray matter), fiber tracts (white matter), and subcortical nuclei (gray matter); the surface of the cerebral hemispheres is defined by gyri (hills) and sulci (valleys).

Each cerebral hemisphere has four lobes, including the frontal, parietal, temporal, and occipital lobes; regions within three of these lobes have been proposed as serving specialized roles in speech, language, and hearing.

Two other areas of cortical tissue—the insula and components of the limbic system—play important roles in speech, language, hearing, and swallowing.

Cerebral white matter is composed of many types of tracts (association, striatal, commissural, descending, and ascending) that connect different parts of the CNS.

The arcuate fasciculus, a massive association tract, connects temporal/parietal lobe cortical areas to regions in the frontal lobe and has a major role speech and language function.

Descending tracts from the cortex to the brainstem (corticobulbar tract) and spinal cord (corticospinal tract) innervate lower motor neurons that represent the final common pathway to muscles of the speech mechanism, as well as other structures in the head, neck, and trunk.

Ascending tracts are primarily associated with sensory pathways and carry information about touch, pain, light, sound, temperature, odor, taste, vibration, and proprioception.

The basal ganglia are subcortical nuclei (nuclei within the cerebral hemispheres and above the brainstem) that are connected to the cortex via loops and are important to aspects of speech sensorimotor control such as the refinement and programming of motor behavior.

The thalamus is the major relay for all sensory information (except smell) ascending in the CNS to the cortex and is also the primary output to the cortex for delivery of information processed in the basal ganglia and for sensory fibers ascending through the spinal cord and brainstem.

The cerebellum is connected to the spinal cord, brainstem, and subcortical nuclei by means of the cerebellar peduncles; output from the thalamus sends information to the cerebral cortex, and the cortex sends information to the cerebellum, creating a cortico-cerebellar-cortical loop that contributes to the coordination of complex motor behavior and balance, and it possibly plays a role in programming motor sequences such as successive articulatory gestures.

The brainstem, a stalk of tissue connecting the spinal cord to the cerebral hemispheres and cerebellum, has three levels, including (from superior to inferior) the midbrain (mesencephalon), pons, and medulla, each containing sensory and motor nuclei, as well as descending, ascending, and crossing fiber tracts.

Prominent features on the ventral and dorsal surfaces of the brainstem are entrance and exit locations of 10 of the 12 cranial nerves, including those associated with control of head and neck muscles that are part of the speech mechanism (cranial nerves V, VII, IX, X, XI, XII) and are associated with hearing and balance (cranial nerve VIII).

The 12 cranial nerves have numbers and names—olfactory (I), optic (II), oculomotor (III), trochlear (IV), trigeminal (V), abducens (VI), facial (VII), auditory-vestibular (VIII), glossopharyngeal (IX), vagus (X), spinal accessory (XI), and hypoglossal (XII)—and are composed of motor, sensory, or both motor and sensory fibers that transmit information between the CNS and the body.

Cranial nerves III to XII are associated with specific nuclei in the brainstem or, in one case (cranial nerve XI), with nuclei in the upper cervical spinal cord.

The spinal cord, which is continuous with the inferior border of the medulla and extends from the first cervical vertebrae to the upper lumbar vertebrae, contains central gray matter consisting of neuron cell bodies (sensory cells in the dorsal horn, motor cells in the ventral horn) and surrounding white matter consisting of axons that supply the muscles of the breathing apparatus as well as other voluntary musculature of the limbs and torso, as well as fibers associated with sensation.

Cells in the nervous system include signaling cells (neurons) and glial cells (astrocytes, oligodendrocytes, Schwann cells) that provide metabolic and protective support to the neurons and ependymal cells that secrete CSF.

Neurons, or signaling cells, are composed of a cell body (soma), dendrites, an axon, and a terminal segment and usually communicate with each other by conversion of electrical-to-neurochemical energy, which is then converted back to electrical energy.

An action potential is initiated at the dendrites, which depolarizes the soma, causing electrical energy to be propagated down the axon to the terminal segment (presynaptic membrane), where neurotransmitter is released into the cleft between the terminal segment and the dendrites of an adjacent neuron (postsynaptic membrane), with the presynaptic/synaptic cleft/postsynaptic structures and conversion of electrical-to-chemical-to-electrical energy called a synapse.

The neuromuscular junction is where a motor nerve makes contact with a motor endplate attached to muscle fiber and where acetylcholine is released by the terminal segment of the peripheral nerve to bind to special receptors embedded in the motor endplate, thereby causing an action potential to be generated in the muscle fiber, which causes it to shorten (contract).

The meninges, which include the dura mater, arachnoid mater, and pia mater, are protective coverings of the cerebral hemispheres, brainstem, and spinal cord.

CSF flows throughout the ventricular system, which includes the lateral ventricles, third ventricle, fourth ventricle, and central canal of the spinal cord.

The blood supply of the brain includes an anterior and posterior supply, with one of the most important anterior arteries for speech, language, and hearing function being the middle cerebral artery.

The posterior blood supply of the brain furnishes blood to the brainstem, cerebellum, and some posterior structures within the cerebral hemispheres.

Deep brain stimulation (DBS) is sometimes used to manage the signs and symptoms of Parkinson's disease; however, it is not clear that DBS improves speech and swallowing function.

REFERENCES

Ackermann, H., & Riecker, A. (2010). The contributions of the insula to speech production: A review of the clinical and functional imaging literature. *Brain Structure and Function, 214,* 419–433.

Aldridge, D., Theodoros, D., Angwin, A., & Vogel, A. P. (2016). Speech outcomes in Parkinson's disease after subthalamic nucleus deep brain stimulation: A systematic review. *Parkinsonism & Related Disorders, 33,* 3–11.

Ascherio, M., & Schwarzchild, M. A. (2016). The epidemiology of Parkinson's disease: Risk factors and prevention. *The Lancet Neurology, 15,* 1257–1272.

Ballard, K. A., Azizi, L., Duffy, J. R., McNeil, M. R., Halaki, M., O'Dwyer, N., . . . Robin, D. A. (2016). A predictive model for diagnosing stroke-related apraxia of speech. *Neuropsychologia, 81,* 129–139.

Bear, M. F., Connors, B. W., & Paradiso, M. A. (2016). *Neuroscience: Exploring the brain* (4th ed.). Riverwoods, IL: Wolters Kluwer.

Bernal, B., & Ardila, A. (2009). The role of the arcuate fasciculus in conduction aphasia. *Brain, 132,* 2309–2316.

Blumenfeld, H. (2010). *Neuroanatomy through clinical cases* (2nd ed.). Sunderland, MA: Sinauer Associates.

Brabenec, L., Mekyska, J., Galaz, Z., & Rektorova, I. (2017), Speech disorders in Parkinson's disease: Early diagnostics and effects of medication and brain stimulation. *Journal of Neural Transmission (Vienna), 124,* 303–334. https://doi.org/10.1007/s00702-017-1676-0

Catani, M., & Mesulam, M. (2008). The arcuate fasciculus and the disconnection theme in language and aphasia: History and current state. *Cortex, 44,* 953–961.

Cohen, D. L., Roffe, C., Beavan, J., Blackett, B., Fairfield, C. A., Hamdy, S., . . . Bath, P. M. (2016). Post-stroke dysphagia: A review and design considerations for future trials. *International Journal of Stroke, 11,* 399–411.

Conturo, T. E., Lori, N. F., Cull, T. S., Akbudak, E., Snyder, A., Z., Shimony, J. S., . . . Raichle, M. E. (2008). Tracking neuronal fiber pathways in the living human brain. *Proceedings of the National Academy of Sciences USA, 96,* 10422–10427.

Culham, J. C., & Valyear, K. F. (2006). Human parietal cortex in action. *Current Opinion in Neurobiology, 16,* 205–212.

Deacon, T. W. (1997). *The symbolic species: The co-evolution of language and the brain.* New York, NY: W. W. Norton.

DeToledo, J. C., & David, N. J. (2001). Innervation of the sternocleidomastoid and trapezius muscles by the accessory nucleus. *Journal of Neuro-Ophthalmology, 21,* 214–216.

di Biase, L., & Fasano, A. (2016). Low-frequency deep brain stimulation for Parkinson's disease: Great expectations or false hopes? *Movement Disorders, 31,* 962–967.

Eftekhar, B., Dadmehr, M., Ansari, S., Ghodsi, M., Nazparvar, B., & Ketabchi, E. (2006). Are the distributions of variations of circle of Willis different in different populations? Results of an anatomical study and review of literature. *BMC Neurology, 6,* 22. https://doi.org/10.1186/1471-2377-6-22

Gervain, J., & Geffen, M.N. (2019). Efficient neural coding in auditory and speech perception. *Trends in Neuroscience, 42,* 56-65.

Geschwind, N. (1965). Disconnection syndromes in animals and man. *Brain, 88,* 237–294.

Heimer, L., & Van Hoesen, G. W. (2006). The limbic lobe and its output channels: Implications for emotional functions and adaptive behavior. *Neuroscience and Biobehavioral Reviews, 30,* 126–147.

Hickok, G. (2009). The functional neuroanatomy of language. *Physics of Life Reviews, 6,* 121–143.

Kandel, E. R., Schwartz, J. H., Jessel, T. M., Siegelbaum, S. A., & Hudspeth, J. A. (2012). *Principles of neural science* (5th ed.). New York, NY: McGraw-Hill.

Knollman-Porter, K. (2008). Acquired apraxia of speech: A review. *Topics in Stroke Rehabilitation, 15,* 484–493.

Langers, D. R. M., Backe, W. H., & van Dijk, P. (2007). Representation of lateralization and tonotopicity in primary versus secondary human auditory cortex. *NeuroImage, 34,* 264–273.

Macefield, V. G., & Knellwolf, T.P. (2018). Functional properties of human muscle spindles. *Journal of Neurophysiology, 120,* 452–467.

Mariën, P., & Borgatti, R. (2018). Language and the cerebellum. *Handbook of Clinical Neurology, 154,* 181–202.

Meng, H., Murakami, G., Suzuki, D., & Miyamoto, S. (2008). Anatomical variations in stylopharyngeus muscle insertions suggest interindividual and left/right differences in pharyngeal clearance function of elderly patients: A cadaveric study. *Dysphagia, 23,* 251–257.

O'Sullivan, M., Brownsett, S., & Copland, D. (2019). Language and language disorders: Neuroscience to clinical practice. *Practical Neurology, 19,* 380–388.

Papanicolaou, A. C., Rezaie, R., & Simos, P. G. (2019). The auditory an association cortex and language evaluation methods. *Handbook of Clinical Neurology, 160,* 465–479.

Plante, E., & Gomez, R. L. (2018) Learning without trying: The clinical relevance of statistical learning. *Language, Speech, and Hearing Services in the Schools, 49,* 710–722.

Price, C. J. (2010). The anatomy of language: A review of 100 fMRI studies published in 2009. *Annals of the New York Academy of Sciences, 1191,* 62–88.

Rasmussen, T., & Milner, B. (1977). The role of early left-brain injury in determining lateralization of cerebral speech functions. *Annals of the New York Academy of Sciences, 299,* 355–369.

Ridderinkhof, K. R., Ullsperger, M., Crone, E. A., & Nieuwenhuis, S. (2004). The role of the medial frontal cortex in cognitive control. *Science, 306,* 443–447.

Sarikcioglu, L., Altun, U., Suzen, B., & Oguz, N. (2008). The evolution of the terminology of the basal ganglia, or are they nuclei? *Journal of the History of the Neurosciences: Basic and Clinical Perspectives, 17,* 226–229.

Saur, D., Kreher, B. W., Schnell, S., Kümmerer, D., Kellmeyer, P., Vry, M. S., . . . Weiller, C. (2008). Ventral and dorsal pathways for language. *Proceedings of the National Academy of Sciences of the United States, 18,* 18035–18040.

Schmahmann, J. D., Smith, E. E., Eichler, F. S., & Filley, C. M. (2008). Cerebral white matter: Neuroanatomy, clinical neurology, and neurobehavioral correlates. *Annals of the New York Academy of Sciences, 1142,* 266–309.

Sherrington, C. S. (1906). *The integrative action of the nervous system.* New Haven, CT: Yale University Press.

Sidtis, J. J., Van Lancker Sidtis, D., Ramdhani, R., & Tagliat, M. (2020). Speech intelligibility during clinical and low frequency. *Brain Sciences, 10,* 26.

Spencer, K. A., & Brown, K. A. (2018). Dysarthria following stroke. *Seminars in Speech and Language, 39,* 15–24.

Swanson, S. J., Sabsevitz, D. S., Hammeke, T. A., & Binder, J. R. (2007). Functional magnetic resonance imaging of language in epilepsy. *Neuropsychology Review, 17,* 491–504.

Takai, O., Brown, S., & Liotti, M. (2010). Representation of the speech effectors in the human motor cortex: Somatotopy or overlap? *Brain and Language, 113,* 39–44.

Tervaniemi, M., & Hugdahl, K. (2003). Lateralization of auditory-cortex functions. *Brain Research Reviews, 43,* 231–246.

Tremblay, P., & Dick, A. S. (2016). Broca and Wernicke are dead, or moving past the classic model of language neurobiology. *Brain and Language, 162,* 60–71.

Wilson-Pauwels, L., Akesson, E. J., Stewart, P. A., & Spacey, R. D. (2002). *Cranial nerves in health and disease.* Hamilton, Ontario: B. C. Decker.

Yu, H., Takahashi, K., Bloom, L., Quaynor, S. D., & Xie, T. (2020). Effect of deep brain stimulation on swallowing function: A systematic review. *Frontiers in Neurology, 11,* 1–13.

Zilles, K., Armstrong, E., Schleicher, A., & Kretschmann, H. J. (1988). The human pattern of gyrification in the cerebral cortex. *Anatomy and Embryology, 179,* 173–179.

Index

Note: Page numbers in **bold** reference non-text material